New Drug
Approval Process

DRUGS AND THE PHARMACEUTICAL SCIENCES

DRUGS AND THE PHARMACEUTICAL SCIENCES

A Series of Textbooks and Monographs

1. Pharmacokinetics, *Milo Gibaldi and Donald Perrier*
2. Good Manufacturing Practices for Pharmaceuticals: A Plan for Total Quality Control, *Sidney H. Willig, Murray M. Tuckerman, and William S. Hitchings IV*
3. Microencapsulation, *edited by J. R. Nixon*
4. Drug Metabolism: Chemical and Biochemical Aspects, *Bernard Testa and Peter Jenner*
5. New Drugs: Discovery and Development, *edited by Alan A. Rubin*
6. Sustained and Controlled Release Drug Delivery Systems, *edited by Joseph R. Robinson*
7. Modern Pharmaceutics, *edited by Gilbert S. Banker and Christopher T. Rhodes*
8. Prescription Drugs in Short Supply: Case Histories, *Michael A. Schwartz*
9. Activated Charcoal: Antidotal and Other Medical Uses, *David O. Cooney*
10. Concepts in Drug Metabolism (in two parts), *edited by Peter Jenner and Bernard Testa*
11. Pharmaceutical Analysis: Modern Methods (in two parts), *edited by James W. Munson*
12. Techniques of Solubilization of Drugs, *edited by Samuel H. Yalkowsky*
13. Orphan Drugs, *edited by Fred E. Karch*
14. Novel Drug Delivery Systems: Fundamentals, Developmental Concepts, Biomedical Assessments, *Yie W. Chien*
15. Pharmacokinetics: Second Edition, Revised and Expanded, *Milo Gibaldi and Donald Perrier*
16. Good Manufacturing Practices for Pharmaceuticals: A Plan for Total Quality Control, Second Edition, Revised and Expanded, *Sidney H. Willig, Murray M. Tuckerman, and William S. Hitchings IV*
17. Formulation of Veterinary Dosage Forms, *edited by Jack Blodinger*
18. Dermatological Formulations: Percutaneous Absorption, *Brian W. Barry*
19. The Clinical Research Process in the Pharmaceutical Industry, *edited by Gary M. Matoren*
20. Microencapsulation and Related Drug Processes, *Patrick B. Deasy*
21. Drugs and Nutrients: The Interactive Effects, *edited by Daphne A. Roe and T. Colin Campbell*
22. Biotechnology of Industrial Antibiotics, *Erick J. Vandamme*
23. Pharmaceutical Process Validation, *edited by Bernard T. Loftus and Robert A. Nash*
24. Anticancer and Interferon Agents: Synthesis and Properties, *edited by Raphael M. Ottenbrite and George B. Butler*
25. Pharmaceutical Statistics: Practical and Clinical Applications, *Sanford Bolton*

ADDITIONAL VOLUMES IN PREPARATION

New Drug Approval Process

Fourth Edition
Accelerating Global Registrations

edited by
Richard A. Guarino, M.D.
Oxford Pharmaceutical Resources, Inc.
Totowa, New Jersey, U.S.A.

MARCEL DEKKER, INC.   NEW YORK · BASEL

The third edition was published as *New Drug Approval Process: Third Edition, The Global Challenge.*

Although great care has been taken to provide accurate and current information, neither the author(s) nor the publisher, nor anyone else associated with this publication, shall be liable for any loss, damage, or liability directly or indirectly caused or alleged to be caused by this book. The material contained herein is not intended to provide specific advice or recommendations for any specific situation.

Trademark notice: Product or corporate names may be trademarks or registered trademarks and are used only for identification and explanation without intent to infringe.

Library of Congress Cataloging-in-Publication Data
A catalog record for this book is available from the Library of Congress.

ISBN: 0-8247-5041-1

This book is printed on acid-free paper.

Headquarters
Marcel Dekker, Inc., 270 Madison Avenue, New York, NY 10016, U.S.A.
tel: 212-696-9000; fax: 212-685-4540

Distribution and Customer Service
Marcel Dekker, Inc., Cimarron Road, Monticello, New York 12701, U.S.A.
tel: 800-228-1160; fax: 845-796-1772

Eastern Hemisphere Distribution
Marcel Dekker AG, Hutgasse 4, Postfach 812, CH-4001 Basel, Switzerland
tel: 41-61-260-6300; fax: 41-61-260-6333

World Wide Web
http://www.dekker.com

The publisher offers discounts on this book when ordered in bulk quantities. For more information, write to Special Sales/Professional Marketing at the headquarters address above.

Current printing (last digit):

10 9 8 7 6 5 4 3 2 1

PRINTED IN THE UNITED STATES OF AMERICA

To the victims of the tragic events of September 11, 2001, and to all our brave military who gave their lives and who proudly serve to protect our freedom and democracy. Let us never forget.

Preface

The impact of the global registration concept is still in the neonatal phase. The International Committee on Harmonization (ICH) and the subsequent implementation of its outcome will take time before the approvals of worldwide registrations for new pharmaceutical products can occur simultaneously. The interchange of information and the acceptance and adaptation of guidelines and regulations specific to drug, device, and biological product development need to be completely understood before the ideal common technical document can be readily accepted on an international scale.

This fourth edition of *New Drug Approval Process*, subtitled *Accelerating Global Registrations*, approaches each aspect of the processes required to obtain new product approval globally. Included is a comprehensive presentation of regulatory, clinical, and statistical mechanics involved in completing New Pharmaceutical Product Applications for prescription and generic drugs, devices, and biologics. Congruently, we address the way to expedite these processes and the strategic discipline necessary to achieve these difficult tasks.

We discuss the systems in which the dissemination of information to achieve a uniform way to educate the personnel involved in completing these duties. The authors selected to address the new drug approval process not only are knowledgeable in the academic writing of their specialties but also have the practical knowledge that can only come from years of successes and failures. They impart this knowledge so that readers can apply and use this information in their jobs with a clear understanding of their scientific and legal responsibilities.

The content, assembly, and strategic approach in filing U.S. and global submissions of Investigational and New Drug Applications (INDs/NDAs), Biologic License Applications (BLAs), Abbreviated New Drug Applications (ANDAs), and Supplemental New Drug Applications (SNDAs) are detailed in a step-by-step format. The essential aspects of the nonclinical, preclinical, and clinical development of products are carefully detailed and are integrated with the regulatory requirements for expediting new drug approvals. Within these submissions, Chemistry, Manufacturing, and Controls (CMC) become one of the most important issues. Therefore special attention is devoted to the CMC section for NDAs and ANDAs.

Good Clinical Practice (GCP) regulations in the United States and the ICH guidelines, which meet safety, ethical and efficacy requirements, are comprehensively covered in the clinical research development chapters. Investigator, sponsor, and monitor obligations are detailed and applied practically. Institutional Review Boards (IRBs), Independent Ethics Committees (IECs), and Informed Consent (IC) will be discussed fully along with the sponsors', investigators', and monitors' legal responsibilities in the approval, implementation, and retention of the legal documents required for these processes. The Health Insurance Portability and Accountability Act (HIPAA) has become an essential consideration in the recruitment, identification, pre-screening, and retention of subjects involved in clinical research. This edition addresses the impact HIPAA will have on the handling of patient data and on the use of existing databases.

The way we communicate electronically, coupled with new concepts and methodologies in global clinical development, will dramatically influence how pharmaceutical products are registered worldwide. Educating different societies on the techniques to meet international regulations will not be an easy task and will require immediate attention. The common technical document (CTD) and guidelines of the ICH are getting us closer to this goal, but there are still many differences to resolve. Educating the personnel involved in new product development and how this can be accomplished through technology change and e-learning is discussed in chapters on effective methodologies in expediting new product approvals.

New Drug Approval Process, *Fourth Edition*, addresses all the essentials, latest requirements, and techniques necessary to submit new pharmaceutical product applications globally. The text details the regulations, guidelines, and procedures that must be incorporated and adhered to in order to expedite and gain product approval. Moreover, it introduces a new approach of how to communicate effectively and integrate the world of pharmaceutical personnel on all aspects of new drug development. The future of international regulatory requirements and new product submissions is considered from every aspect by each contributing author. Readers will gain an education as well as an understanding of how to apply their research capabilities resourcefully now and in the future.

I sincerely thank the authors and contributors who have cooperated in the preparation of this fourth edition of *New Drug Approval Process*. In particular, a special thanks goes to Patricia Birkner and Barbara Connizzaro for their diligent efforts and insight in the preparation of this edition.

Richard A. Guarino, M.D.

Introduction

The global discovery and approval of new drugs, devices, and biologics will revolutionize the availability of health care products worldwide. The crucial areas of vaccines and blood safety, critical to our public health, coupled with such cutting-edge biologic scientific areas as gene therapy and tissue transplant will play a major part in these new product discoveries. These must be made available to the entire world population. The pharmaceutical industry's aggressiveness in marketing these products will also be a major factor in how fast these products become available internationally. Bureaucratic agencies regulating these products will also play a part in how fast they are approved for the global market.

The opportunity to accomplish this task has been greatly enhanced with the introduction of guidelines and recommendations formulated by the International Committee of Harmonization (ICH). This committee established safety, efficacy, and quality guidelines for new drug development in order to expedite international registrations. These guidelines give a basis for uniformity of data, developed for pharmaceutical products, that will be used as evidence for product approvals.

Notwithstanding these guidelines, which create the foundation necessary for new product approval internationally, each country's regulations for new product approval must be considered and incorporated within global submissions. For example, in the United States, the Food and Drug Administration expects that all U.S. and foreign data supporting safety and efficacy for new product submissions meet the regulatory standards required by this agency. Other countries might require that a percentage of clinical research be conducted in that country before approval of products is granted. In conjunction with these demands, regulatory and clinical personnel are continually confronted with the challenge of submitting data that will meet and support the requirements for global new product approvals. Each person who plays a role in the process of new product development is aware of what must be done to meet these regulatory requirements and puts forth a great deal of time, effort, and expense to achieve these goals. However, in many instances they are not entirely in agreement on *how to do it.*

Pharmaceutical companies and related industries are actively seeking new ways to decrease the time and costs for the development and approval of new products. The ability to submit applications for new products simultaneously in more than one country would greatly ease these goals. Bureaucratic agencies that approve these products are also cooperating by reviewing submissions more rapidly, with a new emphasis on accepting international data in order to avail new products to the world population. Personnel involved in new product development are working more closely with regulatory agencies to facilitate their needs and requests so that less time is involved in the approval process. Therefore a thorough understanding of all the regulations and guidelines and of how to effectively implement the intricate steps in new drug development is vital.

There are many components in the drug, device, and biologic approval process that must be defined, documented, and understood. The knowledge one may gain from reading a book or taking a course can only be considered a basis of what is needed in getting a new product approved. It is only from experience of trial and error and constant training and retraining that one is capable of expressing enough understanding to hope for a successful product submission and approval.

The personnel working in the pharmaceutical industries are of a particular breed. Above all, they *must love detail.* Detail, in this industry, is the underlying key to achieving many of these components. Every facet of new drug development must be examined and reexamined with the greatest care and understanding. Each regulatory aspect must be seriously applied in the overall product development. All clinical research must reflect the primary goal of human safety and investigator and sponsor integrity. The sponsors must assure the quality of all the data within the submissions. Lastly, the constant changes in the process of new product development must be rapidly distributed and applied.

These golden guidelines are detailed, defined, explained, resolved and practically applied in this new edition of *New Drug Approval Process.*

Richard A. Guarino, M.D.

Table of Contents

ix

Contributors

Patricia Blaine, R.R.T., M.Ed. Blaine Pharmaceutical Services, Inc., Matawan, New Jersey, U.S.A.

Mark Bradshaw, Ph.D. Covance, Inc., Princeton, New Jersey, U.S.A.

Brian J. Chadwick LookLeft Group, New York, New York, U.S.A.

Martha R. Charney, Ph.D. Piedmont Consulting Group, LLC, Menlo Park, California, U.S.A.

Robert P. Delamontagne, Ph.D. EduNeering, Inc., Princeton, New Jersey, U.S.A.

Kenneth A. Getz, M.S., M.B.A. CenterWatch, Inc., Boston, Massachusetts, U.S.A.

Albert A. Ghignone, M.S., M.B.A. AAG, Inc., Easton, Pennsylvania, U.S.A.

Rochelle L. Goodson R. L. Goodson Consulting, Inc., New York, U.S.A.

Richard A. Guarino, M.D., K.M. Oxford Pharmaceutical Resources, Inc., Totowa, New Jersey, U.S.A.

Kent Hill, Ph.D. Biopharma Consulting Ltd., Colwyn Bay, United Kingdom

Earl W. Hulihan, M.Ed.   Regulatory Consulting Services, META Solutions, Inc., Warren, New Jersey, U.S.A.

Duane B. Lakings, Ph.D.   Drug Safety Evaluation Consulting, Inc., Elgin, Texas, U.S.A.

Edith Lewis-Rogers   META Solutions, Inc., Warren, New Jersey, U.S.A.

Andrea G. Procaccino   Johnson & Johnson Pharmaceutical Research & Development, LLC, Titusville, New Jersey, U.S.A.

Max Sherman   Sherman Consulting Services, Warsaw, Indiana, U.S.A.

Evan B. Siegel, Ph.D.   Ground Zero Pharmaceuticals, Inc., Irvine, California, U.S.A.

William M. Troetel, Ph.D.   Regulatory Affairs Consultant, Mount Vernon, New York, U.S.A.

Timothy Urschel, M.B.A.   EpiGenesis Pharmaceuticals, Inc., Cranbury, New Jersey, U.S.A.

John T. Zenno   Regulatory Services, Inc., Yardley, Pennsylvania, U.S.A.

New Drug
Approval Process

1

Drug Development Teams

Duane B. Lakings
Drug Safety Evaluation Consulting, Inc., Elgin, Texas, U.S.A.

I. INTRODUCTION

The drug discovery and development process requires the close interaction of a large number of scientific disciplines for as many as 10 to 12 years. Most pharmaceutical and biotechnology firms employ teams to guide the processes involved in taking a discovery lead through the various preclinical and clinical drug development stages for making the drug candidate into a therapeutic product. The responsibilities of these project teams include, but are not limited to,

1. Reviewing research results from experiments conducted by any of the various scientific disciplines
2. Integrating new research results with previously generated data
3. Planning research studies to further characterize a drug candidate
4. Preparing a detailed drug development plan, including designation of key points or development milestones, generating a timeline for completion, and defining the critical path
5. Monitoring the status of research studies to ensure that they are being conducted according to the timeline and critical path in the development plan and, if appropriate, modifying the plan as new information becomes available
6. Comparing research results and development status and timelines with drug candidates under development by competitors
7. Conducting appropriate market surveys to ensure that the development of a drug candidate is economically justified and continues to meet a medical need

8. Reporting the status of the drug development program to manage-
    ment and making recommendations on the continued development
    of the drug candidate

This chapter discusses the various types of project teams that are involved in
the drug discovery and development process. Also included is a detailed
example of a drug development logic plan for what many developmental
pharmaceutical scientists consider to be the most difficult and time- and
resource-consuming drug candidate to develop into a therapeutic product.

II. DRUG DISCOVERY PROJECT TEAM

A company makes a decision to enter into a new disease area or to expand an
existing therapeutic area on the basis of new research findings, an unmet
medical need, or marketing surveys. The responsible department, commonly
a therapeutic disease group such as cardiovascular, CNS, cancer, infectious
diseases, or metabolic diseases, assigns researchers to the new project—
usually chemists to synthesize compounds and pharmacologists or biologists
to evaluate the leads in in vitro or in vivo models of the disease. This small
group of researchers is the first project team and is commonly called a discovery project team. Their primary responsibility is to identify lead compounds or classes of compounds worthy of continued research and that are
patentable, i.e., have unique, previously undisclosed chemical structures. The
initial effort may consist of screening existing compounds in the company's
archives or libraries of compounds, obtained by use of combinatorial
chemistry techniques, for activity. The primary end point used in this assessment is the biological activity or potency of the various compounds in the
disease model. The pharmacology results are shared with the chemists, who
then prepare analogues of the most active compounds to identify the
pharmacophore (i.e., the chemical moiety of the compounds responsible for
the biological activity) and to explore further the SAR.

Once a lead or class of leads has been identified, the discovery team
commonly grows to include other scientific disciplines to characterize more
fully the possibility of developing the leads of interest. The other disciplines
include, but are not limited to,

1. Analytical chemistry to define the physical and chemical properties
    of the leads and to provide preliminary information on the
    solubility and stability of the potential drug substances
2. Pharmacokinetics, which normally include bioanalytical chemis-
    try, to assess the absorption or delivery and disposition profiles of
    the leads in animal models using the route of administration

projected for clinical studies and drug metabolism using in vitro systems to assess the extent of metabolism by the various drug metabolism enzymes

3. Toxicology, possibly including safety pharmacology and genotoxicity, to evaluate the potential for the leads to cause adverse effects in in vitro or cell-based systems and in vivo or animal models and to determine that the dose levels that cause toxicity are substantially greater than the dose levels needed to elicit the desired pharmacological effect

4. Biopharmaceutics to study the formulation potential of the leads and to ensure that the compounds can be effectively delivered by the proposed clinical route of administration

The results from the preliminary or lead optimization studies conducted by these disciplines are integrated with the biological activity data from the pharmacologist. If stability, delivery, metabolism, or toxicity problems are encountered, the chemists use the previously generated SAR information to modify the structure of the lead without destroying the site(s) required for biological activity of the compound. The new compounds are evaluated for potency and to ensure that the undesirable structural attribute, which causes the developability problem, has been deleted or minimized. Then the other scientific disciplines check the new lead(s) to ensure that the structural change did not adversely affect desirable characteristics and did substantially alter the previously defined undesirable characteristics. This iterative process continues until a lead compound (or a small group of leads) is identified.

The discovery project team compiles the generated information and presents the results to management. At this stage, the drug discovery team normally recommends that a lead candidate be entered into formal preclinical development. However, that is not always the case. In the experience of this author, the results from the various scientific disciplines can be at odds with each other, with one group pushing for continued development while another thinks the potential for successful development is too low to justify the expenditure of additional resources. For example, the discovery and development of renin inhibitors as antihypertension agents were, and in some cases may still be being, evaluated by a number of pharmaceutical companies. The discovered leads, which were structurally modified small peptides, were very potent in inhibiting renin and thus interfering with the renin–angiotensin cascade, resulting in an antihypertension effect. However, biological activity correlated and increased with the lipophilicity of the modified peptides. The most potent leads had few, if any, polar groups to provide aqueous solubility, preventing the compounds from being delivered to the intestinal wall for absorption. When absorption enhancers were used to administer the leads to animal models of hypertension, the compounds had sufficient absorption to reduce blood pressure. The results from drug delivery and pharmacokinetic evaluations of these same leads showed very low bioavailability, usually less than 10%, which was also quite variable, at times more than 200% of the amount absorbed. This difference in the developability potential of renin inhibitors caused a number of pharmaceutical companies to stop research in this area, whereas other companies continued their efforts to find inhibitors with acceptable delivery characteristics and without unacceptable decreases in potency. This effort has been somewhat successful with a new generation of renin inhibitors now in development.

Once the discovery project team's recommendation for preclinical development of a lead candidate is accepted by management, this team is either disbanded or continues its efforts to discover other compounds with attributes that could identify a next-generation lead. Many of the discovery project team members become members of the more formal preclinical development project team.

III. PRECLINICAL DRUG DEVELOPMENT PROJECT TEAM

One of the first tasks after management's acceptance of a lead candidate as a drug candidate is the establishment of the preclinical drug development team. Commonly, the researchers from the various scientific disciplines involved on the discovery project team are assigned by their departments to the new team, but not always. Some companies have defined groups that support discovery research and others that conduct nonclinical and clinical developmental studies. In this case, the newly assigned project team member needs to be "brought up to speed" by the researcher who had been providing support to the discovery team. This approach allows departments to separate the non-definitive, or non-GLP-regulated, discovery research effort from the more definitive, or GLP-directed, drug development effort and to develop research-ers with expertise in one or the other area. However, complete transfer of knowledge and experience is not always possible, and "ownership" of and "champions" for a particular compound or disease area are lost. Having the same researcher or research group involved in all aspects of the drug discovery and development process provides continuity of effort but requires a possible dilution of scientific expertise. The best approach (each approach has its attributes and demerits) has been under discussion at pharmaceutical houses for years. This issue will probably continue to be a point of contention for researchers wanting to develop a specific expertise or to be involved in all aspects of the drug discovery and development processes. This problem is not as prevalent at biotechnology firms or small pharmaceutical companies, where researchers have to wear many hats and are commonly involved in many phases of the drug discovery and development process.

In addition to the scientific disciplines, e.g., pharmacology, chemistry, toxicology, drug metabolism, and pharmacokinetics, and biopharmaceutics, involved on the discovery team, the preclinical drug development team has a number of new players. These new players include, among others,

1. A management-assigned project team leader and coordinator who are responsible for the development of the drug candidate
2. Regulatory affairs and quality assurance experts to ensure that the developmental studies meet regulatory agency requirements and are conducted according to regulatory agency regulations and guidelines, including ICH guidelines
3. A clinical research scientist to provide input into study designs so that the generated results support the proposed clinical program and to initiate development of clinical safety and tolerance and efficacy protocols and the investigator's brochure
4. An analytical chemistry researcher to develop assays and characterize the drug substance and proposed drug product
5. Manufacturing scientists to scale up the synthesis of the drug candidate and provide sufficient GLP- or GMP-quality material for regulatory-driven research studies
6. A marketing person to determine that the drug candidate has a potential market niche in light of what other companies are developing or drugs that are already on the market for the disease indication

One of the first charges of the preclinical development project team is to prepare a drug development plan, which lists all the studies considered necessary for the successful development of a drug candidate. Based on the disease indication (life-threatening or non–life-threatening), the drug candidate type (small organic molecule or macromolecule), the length of therapy (acute or chronic), and the route of administration (oral, intravenous, dermal, pulmonary, etc.), each of the scientific disciplines prepares a list of proposed research studies, usually in the order to be conducted and with the predicted duration of time needed for completion. All of the studies are combined into a drug development logic plan (a sample is presented later in this chapter). The initial drug development plan is put together with key points or milestones in mind. These key points are commonly submission of an IND, completion of phase 2 clinical trial studies, and submission of an NDA. The first plan is very detailed for the preclinical development, with less definition for the clinical and nonclinical stages of development and for the manufacturing effort.

The individual department lists are combined with the studies ordered according to time required and dependence on the results from other studies. For example, before a subchronic toxicology study can be conducted, acute toxicology study results need to be available to define dose levels and frequency of dosing; sufficient GLP- or GMP-quality drug substance and drug product have to be available or will be available to dose the test species at the desired levels for the duration of the study; and acceptable analytical and bioanalytical chemistry methods should be in place to provide support for formulation assessment and toxicokinetics, which require preliminary pharmacokinetic information to determine the correct or optimal sampling times. Thus the subchronic toxicology study does not depend only on when the toxicologist and his/her group can conduct the study but also on when other disciplines have completed supportive research studies and are available to support the toxicology effort.

Once the development studies are listed and integrated into a logic plan, the next aspect is to develop a timeline. Based on the overall plan, each department determines when it can start a proposed study and when the results of the experiment can be expected. This information is added to the development plan and the time to completion, and to reach predefined milestones, such as filing an IND or completion of phase 2 clinical studies, are determined. The timeline identifies the critical path, that is, the research studies that are rate limiting, and the department or departments involved. Commonly, the departments on the critical path are manufacturing, then toxicology, and finally clinical. Other scientific disciplines that have a key component to the development process can also be on the critical path. Normally, management and project team leadership want the development time to be as short as possible, which is only logical and justifiable, as a single day of development time for a product with projected yearly sales of $365 million is worth $1 million in revenue. In addition, once a patent has been filed, each day of development time decreases the patent life by a day, reducing the overall sales revenue for a product. Thus departments attempt to be off the critical path unless absolutely necessary and will often modify their projected start or completion dates for studies in order to move off the critical path. The completed drug development plan, with defined milestones and critical path, is presented to, and accepted by, management.

The drug development plan has to be a living document and subject to change or modification as results from research studies become available. Unexpected or negative data will usually require additional studies to answer or explain more fully the observations. These additional studies may, and probably will, affect the development timeline and possibly the critical path. Typically, the status of a drug development project is formally presented to management on a semiannual or annual basis, provided no unexpected results or surprises are generated. Special meetings with management are held to

present and discuss problems that are encountered, to make recommendations on how to overcome the problems, and to request the additional resources that may be needed to solve or correct the problems.

One of the final responsibilities of the preclinical drug development
project team is to prepare an IND and to submit the appropriate documents
to the FDA or other regulatory agency. As the development of the drug
candidate moves into the clinic, the preclinical project team often becomes a
clinical project team.

IV. CLINICAL DRUG DEVELOPMENT PROJECT TEAM

After the IND is submitted, the project team is again expanded to include new
players. Some of the old players, such as chemistry and pharmacology, have
decreased roles but may continue to serve on the team to provide scientific
expertise when new problems arise. The roles of many project team members
substantially expand. The new players and expanded roles of members include

1. Physicians who will conduct phase 1, 2, and 3 clinical trial studies
   or serve as medical monitors if these studies are conducted by a
   CRO
2. Clinical research associates who coordinate and monitor the phase
   1, 2, and 3 studies and ensure that the appropriate documents,
   such as case report forms, are correctly prepared
3. Manufacturing scientists to coordinate the development of the drug
   substance and drug product production facilities and to ensure that
   all the necessary processes are in place and appropriately validated
4. Quality control researchers to ensure that the appropriate assays
   are developed, validated, and in place to support the manufacturing program
5. Statisticians to assist in designing clinical protocols and in evaluating generated results from both nonclinical and clinical studies
6. Clinical pharmacokinetic experts to support phase 1 studies and to
   design and conduct pharmacokinetic studies in special populations
7. Marketing personnel to continue evaluating the status of competitor's drug candidates and the potential of the developmental
   candidate to fill a medical need and to prepare for product launch

The drug development plan is updated, with emphasis now placed on the
clinical and manufacturing aspects, either of which could be on the critical
path. The nonclinical program continues but, with the exception of carcinogenicity studies, is rarely rate limiting. As the results from phase 1 and phase 2
clinical trials become available, special nonclinical or even clinical studies may
be needed to evaluate clinical observations. These may include unexpected

adverse experiences (AEs) or reactions (ARs) in volunteers or patients; pharmacokinetic differences between human and animal models; or correcting unforeseen problems, such as unacceptable or highly variable delivery in humans or the inability to scale up the manufacturing process using the proposed methods. For example, this author was a project team member for the development of a CNS drug candidate for anxiety. Phase 1 single-dose, dose-escalating studies in human volunteers produced no safety or tolerance issues. Thus phase 1 multiple-dose studies were initiated and planning for phase 2 efficacy studies started. Bioanalytical chemistry analyses of clinical specimens for the parent drug and a known metabolite showed the presence of an unidentified drug metabolite. Pharmacokinetic evaluation of the new metabolite suggested that the compound had an estimated apparent terminal disposition half-life of more than 7 days and thus would accumulate after multiple-dose administration, possibly leading to adverse experiences. Analogues of the parent drug candidate were prepared and the metabolite was identified. Pharmacology testing showed the metabolite to be almost as biologically active as the drug candidate and, because of the accumulation aspect, was efficacious at lower doses. Toxicology evaluation demonstrated that the metabolite had a safety profile similar to the parent compound and thus had a better therapeutic ratio when combined with the lower dose required for pharmacologic activity. Biopharmaceutic and pharmacokinetic studies showed that the metabolite had acceptable bioavailability. These results suggested that the metabolite might be a better drug candidate than the parent. A preclinical program was initiated on the metabolite and after a delay of only a few months, the metabolite entered the clinic as a drug candidate with a better chance of success than the original compound.

The final responsibility of the clinical project team is to ensure that all the research studies are appropriately documented in technical reports or scientific publications and to compile this information, along with the necessary nonclinical and clinical summaries, into an NDA submission that is formatted in compliance with the ICH guideline on common technical documents. After submission, the project team, usually through the regulatory affairs department of the company, interacts with the regulatory agency and provides answers to any questions. If requested, the project team designs and conducts the necessary research studies to support the submission. Once the NDA has been approved, the final responsibility of the clinical development team is to coordinate the launch of the new therapeutic agent.

V. DRUG DEVELOPMENT LOGIC PLAN

One of the primary functions of the project team is to coordinate the various studies necessary for the successful development of a drug candidate and to ensure that the timeline for development is on schedule, both for time and budget. As mentioned above, this coordination is usually accomplished by preparing a detailed drug development logic plan and monitoring the research process. The required studies and the extent of the development plan depend on at least four criteria of the proposed drug candidate, which are

1. Drug candidate type (macromolecule such as a protein, polypeptide, or oligonucleotide or small organic molecule commonly referred to as an NCE)
2. Disease indication (life-threatening, such as AIDS, some cancers, some cardiovascular and CNS indications, or non-life-threatening, such as hypertension, diabetes, anti-inflammatory agents, antibacterial agents)
3. Therapy duration (acute, with one or a few doses being sufficient for treatment, or chronic, with prolonged administration necessary to mediate the disease process)
4. Route of administration (intravenous such as a bolus injection or an infusion, or nonintravenous, such as oral, pulmonary, subcutaneous, intramuscular, dermal, etc.)

These four criteria form a matrix of 16 possible drug candidate types. A generic drug development plan for what most drug development scientists consider to be the most difficult drug candidate to develop successfully is shown in the appendix. The timelines for the various studies and their integration into a formal drug development plan are compound specific and dependent on the availability of resources within the various departments at the company or at CROs if some of the research effort is to be outsourced. Similarly, the designation of key milestone events and the critical path are compound and company specific. However, the information provided in the sample logic plan can be used as a template to generate a logic plan for the other 15 drug candidate types. Depending on the drug candidate type, some of the listed studies, such as absolute bioavailability for a candidate to be administered intravenously or carcinogenicity studies for a candidate to be administered acutely for a life-threatening disease, may not be necessary. Other studies, such as biological potency, immunogenicity, and immunotoxicity evaluations for a macromolecule, may be required.

VI. CONCLUSION

This chapter has described the various project teams and their responsibilities, including the generation, implementation, and monitoring of a drug development plan, in the drug discovery and development processes. The large number of scientific disciplines required for the successful development of a drug candidate into a therapeutic product makes the use of project teams a common practice within the pharmaceutical and biotechnology industry. The abilities of the members to communicate the results from their research efforts and to integrate the results from other disciplines into their study designs are important aspects of the project team environment.

APPENDIX: DRUG DISCOVERY AND DEVELOPMENT LOGIC PLAN EXAMPLE

Logic Plan Drug Candidate Characteristics

A. Candidate: New chemical entity (small organic molecule)
B. Indication: Non-life-threatening disease
C. Therapy: Chronic administration
D. Dosing Route: Nonintravenous

I. Drug Discovery Stage

A. Chemistry or Synthesis

1. Generate drug discovery lead(s) using rational approaches, such as random screening, nonrandom screening, drug metabolism, or clinical observations, or using combinatorial chemistry libraries.

2. Modify lead(s) by identification of pharmacophore and synthesis of analogues; functional group changes; SAR of lead candidate analogues; structure modification, such as homologation, chain branching, ring-chain transformation, and bioisosterism to increase potency and therapeutic ratio; and QSAR.

3. Determine drug–receptor interactions using techniques like molecular modeling and x-ray crystallography.

B. Pharmacology or In Vitro and Animal Model Efficacy

1. Using in vitro techniques, evaluate requirements for activation and dependency on dosing schedule and route of administration; calculate inhibitory concentrations, e.g., IC_{50} and IC_{90}, for each system evaluated; assess potential for resistance to lead candidate(s); determine synergistic, additive, or antagonistic drug–drug interactions during combination therapy, if appropriate; evaluate possible cytostatic or cytotoxic concentrations of lead candidate(s) on various cell types (bone marrow, stem cells, and immune system cells).

2. Define and characterize an animal model(s) that mimics the human disease to be evaluated and determine appropriate end points for assessment of biological activity.

3. Evaluate in vivo dose–response range, including dose–response comparison of lead candidates; determine pharmacologically active doses, e.g., ED_{50} or ED_{10} ; and therapeutic ratio when combined with no-observable-toxic-effect or minimum-toxic-effect dose level.

4. Conduct other in vivo evaluations including, but not limited to, dosing regimen dependency; route of administration and formulation dependency; and spectrum of activity, disease status, cross-resistance profile, combination therapy for synergy or antagonism, and special models.

II. Drug Developability Stage

A. Preliminary formulation evaluation (may not be started until preclinical development is initiated).

1. From pharmacology results and proposed clinical program, select route of administration (oral, pulmonary, intramuscular, subcutaneous, transdermal, ocular, vaginal, buccal, sublingual, etc.) and formulation type to be dosed (solution, suspension, tablet, capsule, granulation powder, microspheres, microemulsion, depot drug, etc.).

2. Evaluate excipients, including concentration and potential for interaction.

3. Select and evaluate formulation process(es), such as tableting, granulation, lyophilization, or microencapsulation.

4. Prepare prototype formulation.

5. Confirm formulation composition, including, but not limited to, drug substance content, drug substance stability, excipient levels, water, and residual solvents, using appropriately characterized methods.

6. Measure formulation physical properties, such as hardness, size, size distribution, morphology.

7. Measure formulation function, such as release or disintegration profile and nonrelease properties like taste-masking.

8. Develop and characterize stability-indicating analytical chemistry method.

9. Define and implement preliminary solubility and stability studies on drug substance and proposed drug product.

B. Preliminary Bioanalytical Chemistry Method Development

1. Select bioanalytical chemistry technique (LC/MS/MS, HPLC, GC, ELISA, etc.).

2. Select physiological matrix (plasma, serum, whole blood, urine).

3. Characterize bioanalytical chemistry method, including sample preparation procedure, for linearity, sensitivity, specificity, precision, and accuracy.

4. Conduct preliminary stability study of drug candidate in selected physiological matrix(ces).

C. Preliminary Pharmacokinetic and Bioavailability Assessments

1. Evaluate distribution and disposition in pharmacology animal model species after intravenous and proposed clinical route of administration.

2. Evaluate pharmacokinetics and bioavailability (drug delivery) in toxicology rodent and nonrodent animal species after intravenous and proposed clinical route of administration.

D. Toxicology

1. Evaluate single-dose or dose-escalation acute toxicity in rodent species.

2. Evaluate single-dose or dose-escalation acute toxicity in nonrodent species.

3. Conduct safety pharmacology studies, if appropriate.

4. Conduct genotoxicity evaluations, if necessary.

E. Drug Metabolism

1. Evaluate potential for drug metabolism by CYP450 isozymes and other enzyme systems.

2. Study potential for conjugation, e.g., glucuronidation, sulfation, acetylation, etc.

3. Determine extent of protein binding.

III. Preclinical Drug Development Stage

(Note: If developability assessment studies listed above have not been conducted, these studies should be included in the preclinical drug development stage.)

A. Drug Candidate Characterization

1. Validate stability-indicating analytical chemistry method and other assays.

2. Generate impurity profile and identify impurities in drug substance and proposed drug product.

3. Study stress stability for drug substance and proposed drug product.

B. Formulation Development

1. Review preliminary pharmacokinetics and histology (local reaction) results and modify formulation, if necessary, using GLP- or GMP-quality drug substance.

2. Characterize and optimize modified formulation for excipients, pH, processing, etc.

C. Bioanalytical Chemistry Method Validation

1. Validate developed method for specificity, sensitivity, range of reliable results, precision, and accuracy for each physiological matrix type and for each species.
2. Evaluate protein binding in blood/plasma obtained from animal species and humans.
3. Determine drug candidate stability in selected physiological matrices from time of collection to time of assay.

D. IND-Directed Toxicology Studies

1. Determine safety pharmacology profile in CNS, cardiovascular, respiratory, renal, and gastrointestinal systems.
2. Evaluate genetic toxicology.
3. Conduct local irritation studies.
4. Determine occupational toxicology (dermal, eye irritation, skin sensitization).
5. Perform subchronic (2– or 4–week) study in a rodent species using proposed clinical route of administration. Study should have a toxicokinetic component.
6. Perform subchronic (2– or 4–week) study in a nonrodent species using proposed clinical route of administration. Study should have a toxicokinetic component.
7. Perform subchronic (13–week) study in a rodent species using proposed clinical route of administration. If appropriate, include a toxicokinetic component.
8. Perform subchronic (13–week) study in a nonrodent species using proposed clinical route of administration. If appropriate, include a toxicokinetic component.
9. Design and conduct additional confirmatory or specialized studies, as warranted.

E. Pharmacokinetics and Drug Metabolism

1. Evaluate absolute bioavailability, distribution and disposition, and linearity of kinetics over toxicology dose range, i.e., dose proportionality, in pharmacology and toxicology animal species.
2. Synthesize and characterize radiolabeled drug candidate.
3. Using radiolabeled drug candidate, determine mass balance, including metabolite profiling and route(s) of elimination, in toxicology animal species.

 4. Isolate and identify major metabolites and if appropriate, evaluate pharmacologic and toxicologic activity of metabolites.
 5. Correlate in vitro metabolism using liver and other appropriate enzyme systems from animal models and humans.
 6. Provide toxicokinetic support to toxicology studies.

F. Mechanism of Action Studies

 1. Study effect on cell cycle or replication cycle.
 2. Determine intra- or extracellular site of action.
 3. Evaluate requirements for enzyme activation or inhibition for desired pharmacologic response.
 4. Perform enzyme–substrate kinetic studies, if appropriate.
 5. Assess intracellular site of action using compartmentalization experiments.

G. Manufacturing Program

 1. Obtain COAs on raw materials.
 2. Define, evaluate, and scale up manufacturing process for drug substance.
 3. Validate formulation process procedures such as mixing, sterilization, lyophilization, closure, resolubilization.
 4. Prepare various CMC sections for IND.
 5. Make phase 1 clinical supplies using GLP or GMP process.
 6. Test clinical supplies for composition, required characteristics, and function.
 7. Release phase 1 clinical supplies to clinic.

H. Quality Control Processes

 1. Validate analytical chemistry method(s) for drug substance, including identity tests and impurity profile.
 2. Validate analytical chemistry method(s) for drug product, including impurity profile.
 3. If appropriate, validate analytical chemistry method(s) for key intermediates in drug substance manufacturing process.
 4. Develop and validated analytical chemistry methods for excipients.

I. Clinical

 1. Prepare phase 1 clinical protocol and outlines of phase 2 and 3 clinical programs.
 2. Prepare investigator's brochure.
 3. Prepare and submit IND to regulatory agency.

IV. Nonclinical Drug Development Stage (Conducted Concurrently with Clinical Development)

A. Chronic and Reproductive Toxicology

    1. Conduct chronic (9–month) nonrodent toxicology study.

    2. Conduct chronic (6–month) rodent toxicology study or combined rat chronic toxicity/carcinogenicity (2–year) study.

    3. Perform mouse carcinogenicity study, if necessary.

    4. Evaluate reproductive/development toxicity in rats or other appropriate rodent species (Segments I, II, and III).

    5. Evaluate reproductive/development toxicity in rabbits or other appropriate nonrodent species (Segment II).

    6. Design and conduct additional confirmatory or specialized studies, as warranted.

B. Pharmacokinetics and Drug Metabolism

    1. Using radiolabeled drug candidate, perform tissue distribution, with whole body autoradiography, in rodents after single-dose and multiple-dose (if appropriate) administration.

    2. Provide toxicokinetic support as necessary, including, but not limited to, feto-placenta transfer and lacteal secretion studies to support reproductive toxicology.

    3. Isolate and identify metabolite(s), if appropriate, in toxicology animal species and humans.

    4. Evaluate pharmacokinetics of metabolite(s) to support pharmacologic and toxicologic evaluation of metabolites, if appropriate.

    5. Conduct in vitro and in vivo enzyme-induction and enzyme-inhibition studies in animal models, if appropriate.

C. Mechanism of Action

    1. Conduct additional mechanism of pharmacologic action studies, if necessary.

    2. Conduct additional mechanism of toxicologic action studies, if necessary.

V. Clinical Drug Development Stage (Conducted Concurrently with Nonclinical Development)

A. Phase 1 Safety and Tolerance Study

    1. Obtain IRB approval for phase 1 study.

    2. Prepare and release clinical supplies.

3. Develop and validate bioanalytical chemistry method for drug candidate and known metabolites in human physiologic fluid specimens.

4. Conduct single-dose and multiple-dose escalation evaluation of drug candidate in normal human volunteers.

5. Study pharmacokinetics of drug candidate and known metabolites in humans after single-dose and multiple-dose administration.

6. Develop and validate surrogate and biochemical marker method(s), if appropriate.

7. Design and conduct mass balance study in human volunteers using an appropriately labeled drug candidate.

B. Phase 2 Efficacy Studies

1. Prepare phase 2 efficacy study protocols and obtain IRB approval.

2. Conduct multiple-dose evaluation of drug candidate efficacy in patients with disease indication.

3. Determine surrogate and biochemical marker levels in human physiologic fluid specimens.

4. Design and conduct relative bioavailability studies if drug product used in early phase 2 is changed for later phase 2 and 3 clinical trials.

C. Phase 3 Definitive Safety and Efficacy Studies

1. Prepare phase 3 clinical protocols and obtain IRB and regulatory agency approvals.

2. Conduct randomized, double-blind, placebo-controlled studies in patients with disease indication using at least two dose levels of proposed drug product.

3. Perform pharmacokinetic studies in special population (geriatric or pediatric age groups, renal or hepatic impaired patients, various ethnic groups, and drug–drug interaction studies) groups, if appropriate.

4. Determine surrogate or biochemical marker levels in human physiologic fluid specimens.

5. Collate all information and prepare NDA for submission to regulatory agency.

D. Phase 4 Studies

1. Design phase 4 protocols for product extensions for new indications or improved/modified delivery profile/route and obtain appropriate approvals.

2. Conduct randomized, double-blind, placebo-controlled studies in patients with new disease indication.

3. Conduct bioequivalence or bioavailability comparison studies for novel formulation assessment.

VI. Manufacturing (Conducted Concurrently with Nonclinical and Clinical Development)

A. Raw Materials

    1. Identify critical components, intermediates, and suppliers.
    2. Negotiate supply and certify vendors.
    3. Conduct site audit for selected vendors.
    4. Determine shelf life of raw materials.

B. Scale-Up and Engineering

    1. Identify synthesis and formulation methods, including definition of equipment, processes, scale.
    2. Define processes and validate for fill, finish, and packaging.
    3. Determine procedure for waste disposal, including appropriate environmental assessments.
    4. Determine number of batches required to support development program and product launch.

C. Documentation

    1. Generate table of contents for manufacture and control documents.
    2. Generate appropriate standard operating procedures.
    3. Develop validation protocols.
    4. Prepare regulatory documents, such as IND, yearly updates, and NDA.
    5. Conduct validation efforts, including preparation of progress reports.

D. Drug Substance

    1. Define production timeline for drug substance supplies for formulation development, stability, toxicology, and clinical studies.
    2. Determine characterization (content, purity, identify) and specification (acceptance and rejection) requirements.

E. Stability

    1. Evaluate drug substance stability, including protocol preparation, approval, and study conduct.
    2. Evaluate drug product stability, including protocol preparation, approval, and study conduct.

F. Sterilization (if appropriate)

    1. Select and evaluate sterilization methods.
    2. Select dose levels and location for sterilization.

    3. Prepare sterilization protocol and obtain necessary approvals.

    4. Develop and validate quality control methods for sterilization.

G. Packaging and Labeling

    1. Identify each component in drug product.

    2. Define process for assemble and fill method.

    3. Generate labeling and package insert requirements.

2

Nonclinical Drug Development: Pharmacology, Drug Metabolism, and Toxicology

Duane B. Lakings
Drug Safety Evaluation Consulting, Inc., Elgin, Texas, U.S.A.

I. INTRODUCTION

The discovery and development of a novel therapeutic agent, whether a small organic molecule or a macromolecule such as a protein and oligonucleotide, require scientific expertise from a number of different disciplines and an enormous amount of time and money. While humans may be the ultimate test species to ascertain the safety and efficacy of a potential new therapeutic agent, research studies in animal models are necessary to determine whether a drug candidate has a pharmacological property that might mediate a human disease process and that the test article does not have a toxicity profile that could cause adverse experiences in humans at pharmacological doses. Present estimates suggest that about 10 to 12 years and more than $800 million (with this cost including the amount expended on drug candidates that "died" during development) are needed to discover and develop a novel therapeutic agent. Figure 1 presents the relationship between the dollars spent and the time of development. As shown, the drug discovery and preclinical, or animal, phases are relatively inexpensive compared to the clinical and nonclinical phases of development.

Historically, for every 100 compounds screened for biological activity in animal models, only one has the necessary pharmacology and safety profiles for evaluation in humans. Of those compounds tested in humans, only about 1 in 10 is successfully brought to the marketplace. This poor rate of success

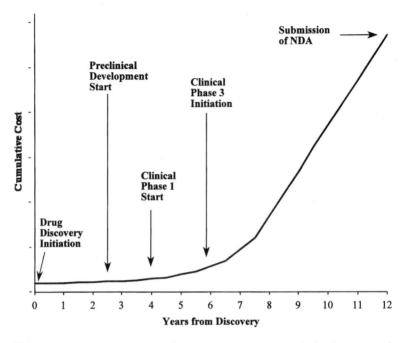

Figure 1 Time and cost profile for the discovery and development of a drug candidate.

has been attributed to a number of factors, a primary one being that animals are not truly predictive of biological activity and/or safety in humans. The problem, however, may be that insufficient time and resources are put into characterizing a discovery lead or drug candidate in pharmacology, drug metabolism, and toxicology animal models to select the compound with the desired druglike attributes for successful development and then to evaluate critically the results from preclinical animal studies to ensure that a compound with developability problems does not enter into clinical studies until those demerits are resolved. Instead of a rush from the first sign of biological activity in an in vitro pharmacology test to clinical trial evaluation, careful design, conduct, and interpretation of preclinical pharmacology, pharmacokinetic, and toxicology animal studies will detect "loser" candidates much earlier. This will allow precious time and resources to be devoted to finding development candidates with a better chance than 1 in 10 of successfully completing clinical studies and becoming a marketed therapeutic agent. Being able to identify the 999 losers of the 1,000 discovery leads that have a potentially desirable biological activity as early as possible in the development process will save substantial time and resources.

This chapter describes the biological aspects of the nonclinical research programs of the drug development process. The chapter has been organized along the timeline for the nonclinical drug discovery and development process, with the major subsections being pharmacology or drug discovery, developability assessment, preclinical or pre-IND development, and nonclinical or post-IND development. The information presented should help drug development researchers to design experiments to evaluate discovery leads and drug candidates as they progress from drug discovery through the nonclinical research studies required for successful drug development and to determine which nonclinical research studies need to be conducted in order to support regulatory agency submissions.

II. OVERVIEW OF DRUG DISCOVERY AND DEVELOPMENT

Normally, the biological aspects of the drug discovery and development processes can be subdivided into four distinct stages. The first is drug discovery, in which the pharmacology or biological activity of a discovery lead is explored in in vitro models or more appropriately in defined and characterized animal models, showing that the compound, or class of compounds, mediates a disease process and thus has potential human therapeutic benefit. This stage should also include preliminary studies to characterize the developability, which may include studies on delivery, metabolism, acute toxicity, preliminary pharmacokinetics, and initial formulation development of a lead candidate or to select the optimal lead from a group of compounds with similar pharmacological properties [1,2]. The second stage consists of preclinical development, in which the safety (including subchronic toxicology, pharmacokinetics, drug metabolism, and deliverability) of a drug candidate is studied in animal models. Additional pharmacology studies may also be conducted during this stage to optimize the route and frequency of administration, determine the pharmacological mechanism of action, and further explore the candidate's pharmacology profile for other possible disease indications. During the early (phase 1 and 2) clinical studies, the third stage of the process includes the initial human experiments to define the drug candidate's safety, tolerance, and pharmacokinetics in normal volunteers and the candidate's efficacy in patients. In addition, the nonclinical research program is continued to extend the scientific database on the toxicity, metabolism, and delivery of the drug candidate. The final, fourth stage involves definitive safety and efficacy (phase 3) clinical studies in humans; carcinogenicity and reproductive toxicology studies in animals with supportive toxicokinetic experiments; and,

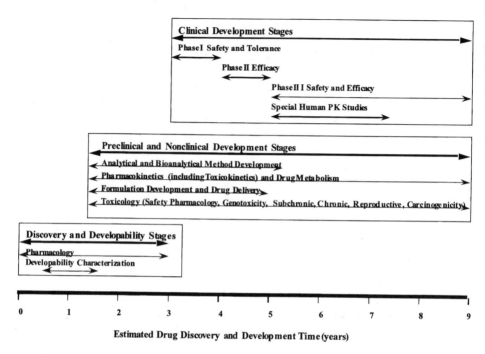

Figure 2 Interaction and timing of the various stages in the biological aspects of the drug discovery and development process.

where appropriate, human pharmacokinetic studies to evaluate potential changes in the extent and duration of delivery and disposition profiles caused by age, gender, race, interaction with other drugs, disease state, and hepatic and renal dysfunction. Figure 2 shows the interactions among these various biological stages. Each of these areas may also include a number of special experiments designed to confirm and extend results on a drug candidate's pharmacology, pharmacokinetic, and safety profiles.

III. PHARMACOLOGY

The drug discovery process has undergone enormous changes during the past few years. After years of first synthesizing individual compounds, then purifying and obtaining physical and chemical characterization of the new chemicals, and finally testing the NCEs in in vitro and in vivo pharmacological models of a particular human disease, the pharmaceutical and biotechnology industry has embraced rationally designed combinatorial chemistry as a way to generate large numbers of organic compounds for evaluation. Combinatorial chemistry techniques include

1. Having a large number of similar reactions taking place simultaneously in multiple-well reaction vessels, where the mixing of reagents and postreaction workup can be automated

2. Combining a mixture of reactants in the same reaction vessel to produce a library of products in a single vial and testing overlapping libraries to find those mixtures that contain active components

3. Using solid-phase chemistry, with the reactant attached to a support, and multistep syntheses, in which appropriate reagents are passed over the reactant on the support to prepare single or multiple products that are cleaved from the support and split and mixed so that subsequent steps have multiple starting materials

With these techniques, libraries have been created of many classes of NCEs, some of which include, but are not limited to, peptides, peptoids, prostaglandins, imidazoles, alkaloids, heparins, oxazoles, benzodiazepines, and β-lactams.

The combinatorial chemistry–generated library is then screened for biological activity, usually in an in vitro system, in which a known biochemical process, which is thought to mimic a human disease or disorder, is agonized or antagonized. The increased number of compounds or mixtures of compounds to be tested has required pharmacologists to devise novel techniques to screen rapidly for biological activity. Because the amount of material available from combinatorial chemistry syntheses is small (i.e., usually microgram quantities), miniaturization of the biological test system is a necessary first requirement. The large number of compounds makes automation of the tests the second requirement. The use of first 96-well, then 384-well, and now 1536-well or larger titer plates and robotics to add the appropriate small amounts of combinatorial chemistry libraries and reagents, including the material that generates the signal for a positive result, provides such a system for rapid assessment of biological activity for a large number of compounds. Those library vessels that elicit a positive or negative response, depending on the biological test being conducted, are identified and the compound(s) of interest is isolated and identified.

After a sufficient quantity of the active compounds discovered during the screening process have been synthesized, purified, identified, and characterized, additional studies are conducted to evaluate more fully the pharmacology of the lead. This more classic approach to evaluating the biological potency of a lead is referred to as SAR assessment. An important requirement in SAR determination is having or developing an animal model that correlates to, or mimics, a disease or disorder in humans. Developing these animal models can be time consuming and expensive and is often complicated by the fact that the model may not simulate the disease as manifested in humans. Many important human diseases, including psychoses, depression, Alzheimer's disease, AIDS, and many cancers, do not yet have predictive animal models. After the animal model has been characterized, various dose levels of the lead(s), identified from screens of combinatorial chemistry libraries or other sources, are administered to the test species, and a dose–response curve is generated. The most commonly used end point is the dose that provides a 50% response (the ED_{50}). Structural analogues of the lead(s) are frequently synthesized and tested in the same model to generate a family of curves with varying biological potencies or ED_{50}s. The lead with the greatest biological activity is frequently selected for further development. However, at this point, many unanswered questions exist. Some of these concerns are

1. Does the animal model reflect, in most or all aspects, the disease in humans?

2. Is the delivery or extent of exposure of all the leads similar, so that the generated dose–response curves accurately predict the compound with the greatest in vivo potency?

3. Are the route and frequency of administration and the formulation used to dose the test species similar to those proposed for human evaluation?

4. Do the leads have similar pharmacokinetic and drug metabolism profiles, so that the durations of exposure to the pharmacologically active compounds are similar?

5. Do any of the leads produce unacceptable toxicity in organs of physiological systems not involved in the desired pharmacology of the compounds?

Before the more formal and definitive preclinical development begins, attempts should be made to answer as many of these questions as possible. The following section discusses the drug developability experiments that can be conducted relatively quickly and cheaply to ascertain whether the lead(s) has the necessary biopharmaceutical, or druglike, characteristics needed for further development.

IV. DRUG DEVELOPABILITY ASSESSMENT

Completed drug discovery research studies indicate that a compound, or class of compounds, mediates a disease process and has potential as human therapeutic agent. Is this lead compound now ready to be transferred from the discovery area to a preclinical development group? Should additional, nondefinitive experiments be conducted to characterize more fully the properties of the lead candidate? If more studies are considered necessary, what experiments should be done?

This section describes some of the biological research experiments that could, and in most cases should, be conducted to evaluate the potential of a lead compound to become a developmental candidate or to select the optimal compound from a group of discovery leads. Figure 3 shows where these developability experiments fit into the drug discovery and development process. These nondefinitive developability studies may also uncover problems that have to be resolved before the definitive preclinical development studies required to support an IND submission are started and before the clinical protocols to evaluate the safety and efficacy of the drug candidate in humans are designed.

Before the preclinical drug development program is begun and because each discovery program is company and compound specific, a number of questions should be asked and answered so that the research studies, both

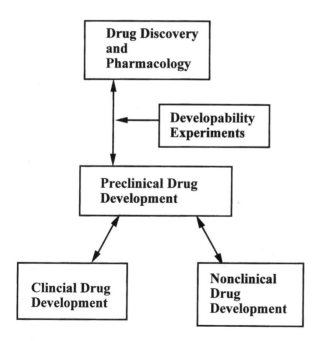

Figure 3 How drug developability experiments fit into the drug discovery and development process.

types and designs, may be planned effectively and the timelines for their completion can be determined. These questions include

1. What is the human disease indication for the candidate?
2. What is the proposed route and frequency of dosing for the candidate in human clinical studies?
3. What is the estimated pharmacological active substance concentration in physiological fluids and how long should that concentration be maintained so that the desired biological response can be obtained?
4. What, if any, are the biological markers to monitor toxicity or therapeutic effectiveness in nonclinical and clinical studies?
5. What definitive preclinical studies need to be completed before a human clinical program can be initiated?
6. What is the projected timeline for the completion of the preclinical studies and for submission of the IND?

Additional questions need to be considered, including whether the drug candidate can be synthesized and purified in sufficient quantity to support a development program, how to document and validate these processes, how to characterize and document the identity of and impurities present in the drug substance and the proposed drug product, and how to determine the stability of the drug substance and the proposed drug product. However, these questions are outside the scope of this discussion.

At least six scientific disciplines are involved in the developability characterization of a discovery lead or group of leads. As shown in Fig. 4,

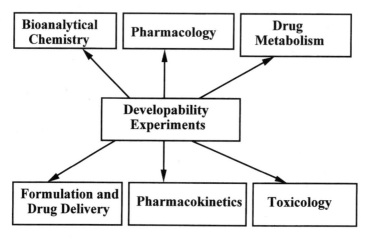

Figure 4 Scientific disciplines necessary for drug developability assessment.

these disciplines are in vivo pharmacology, bioanalytical chemistry method development, nonclinical formulation assessment and delivery, animal pharmacokinetics, drug metabolism, and toxicology. The following sections discuss each of these scientific disciplines in more detail. The discussion is for a single discovery lead; if more than one lead is being evaluated to select the lead with the most druglike properties, depending on a variety of factors such as disease indication, route and frequency of dosing, etc., for further development, similar experiments should be conducted on each lead.

A. Pharmacology

Preliminary pharmacology evaluations in in vitro or animal models will have shown that a lead interacts with a biological process suggestive of human therapeutic benefit. Depending on the design and extent of these early studies, additional pharmacology studies may be needed to characterize further the dose, or physiological fluid concentration, response curve using the proposed clinical route and frequency of administration. If possible, these pharmacology studies should be conducted in at least two species to show that the biological response is not species dependent. The ED_{50} dose should be determined and that value, divided into the no-observable-toxic-effect dose in the same animal species, described in the section on toxicology, estimates a therapeutic ratio or index. If the therapeutic ratio is one or less, a lead will most likely elicit adverse effects in addition to the beneficial response. Unless the lead is for the treatment of a life-threatening disease, such as AIDS, some cancers, or certain CNS indications, a low therapeutic ratio is a warning sign that the lead may not have the necessary properties for further development. A therapeutic ratio of five, preferably ten, or more indicates that a lead will most likely produce a pharmacological response before causing dose-limiting toxicities.

If possible, these developability pharmacology studies should be conducted with dosing to steady state unless the frequency of dosing to be used in clinical trials is as a single-dose therapeutic. The number of doses required to reach steady state depends on the lead's pharmacokinetic profile in the same animal model. These multiple-dose studies provide information on the frequency of dosing necessary to maximize the biological response. This is particularly important for compounds that inhibit an enzymatic system or are effective only during certain phases of the cell cycle.

These pharmacology evaluations assist in the selection of dose levels and route and frequency of administration for preliminary and definitive toxicology studies and for initial phase 1 safety and tolerance human trials. If the effective pharmacological dose is unknown, underdosing and achieving no-therapeutic-response or overdosing and being unable to define a no-observable-toxic-effect dose are undesirable possibilities. In such cases, the development of a potential beneficial therapeutic agent could be inappropriately discontinued.

B. Bioanalytical Chemistry Method Development

If not already available, a bioanalytical chemistry method needs to be defined and characterized for the quantification of the lead in physiological fluids. This assay can then support experiments in some of the other scientific disciplines involved in assessing the developability of the lead and, after appropriate validation, the preclinical, nonclinical, and clinical development of a selected drug candidate. For preliminary studies, a bioanalytical chemistry method should be characterized to demonstrate the range of reliable results, the lower and upper limits of quantification, specificity, accuracy, and precision. In addition, evaluations on the matrix to be used (blood, plasma, serum) should be conducted and the stability of the lead in each matrix should be determined.

The first step in characterizing a bioanalytical chemistry method is to select the analytical technique. For a compound with a molecular weight of less than 2000, instrumental methods such as LC/MS/MS (a very sensitive and specific technique and the most common method employed by the pharmaceutical industry), or HPLC and GC with a variety of detectors, including ultraviolet, fluorescence, flame ionization, and electron capture, may be used. A macromolecule (large peptide, protein, or oligonucleotide) may require an ELISA or RIA method. Samples in assay diluent and in a physiological fluid and over a large concentration range should be analyzed to show that the technique produces an appropriate signal to detect the analyte and to determine the potential interference caused by the matrix, i.e., assay specificity. The ability to quantify a lead in a physiological fluid may depend on the matrix. For example, serum is a poor choice when the analyte interacts with clotting factors. The matrix that gives the best recovery and has the least interference when the compound is added to whole blood should be selected.

The specificity of an assay evaluates the potential interferences from matrix components and from the different animal species to be used in pharmacology and toxicology experiments. Samples from each species to be studied are analyzed neat (with no added compound) and fortified with known amounts of the lead, and the results are calculated using a standard curve prepared in assay diluent. The responses obtained from the neat samples indicate the level of interference from each matrix, and the calculated amounts in the fortified samples show the difference in absolute recovery from the matrix compared with the candidate in buffer. If the absolute recovery is low, i.e., less than 50%, and/or highly variable, i.e., greater than 25%, the assay may not have the desired characteristics to quantify the lead in collected specimens. Additional development should be expended on such a method so that the assay will provide reliable results that can be used to evaluate the pharmacokinetic profile of the lead.

Acceptable results from the above experiments suggest whether a bioanalytical chemistry method should be able to quantify a lead in a physiological matrix. The range and reliability of quantification are assessed through the preparation and analysis of standard curves, prepared in either diluted or undiluted matrix, and multiple samples fortified at two or more concentrations. The standard curve responses that can be described by a mathematical equation (linear, quadratic, sigmoidal) define the range of reliable results. The lower limit of quantification is the lowest signal that can be accurately measured above background and should not be confused with the limit of detection, which is the lowest level that can be detected. The upper limit of quantification is the highest signal that can be defined by the response curve. The fortified samples provide information on precision, defined as the ability to obtain similar calculated concentrations from samples containing the same amounts of analyte, and accuracy, which is the ability to predict the actual concentration of the analyte in a sample.

The ability to measure a lead in a physiological fluid is not useful if the compound is unstable during collection, processing, storage, or sample preparation. Thus a nondefinitive stability study should be conducted to ensure that the compound does not degrade in blood during processing to obtain plasma or serum, during the time (hours, days, and weeks) and under the conditions (room temperature, refrigerated, frozen at −20 °C or −80 °C) that specimens may be stored until analyzed, and during sample preparation. The design of stability experiments is usually compound specific. The results ensure that measured concentrations in unknown specimens reflect the amount of lead present at the time of collection. Successful completion of the above experiments will characterize methods for use in evaluating a lead in animal models. If a lead is selected for further development, the method will need to be validated [3,4] for each matrix and for each species before being used to support definitive toxicology, drug metabolism, or pharmacokinetic studies.

C. Early Nonclinical Formulation Development and Delivery

Nonclinical formulation definition and the drug delivery characteristics of a lead are not usually studied in detail during the transition from discovery to development. The experiments necessary to define an acceptable formulation depend on the proposed clinical route of administration and usually require substantial quantities, i.e., milligram or gram amounts, of the lead. For a compound to be administered by intravenous injection or infusion, the formulation needs to be compatible with blood so that the compound does not precipitate when administered and has minimal local toxicity. Leads that are highly lipophilic or have limited aqueous solubility are the most likely compounds to have these types of problems. A low extent of, or a high variability in, absorption can cause problems for leads administered by other routes, such as oral, subcutaneous, and dermal. For compounds that are poorly absorbed, the amount reaching the site of action may be insufficient to elicit or to maintain a desired pharmacological response. If the absorption is variable and the therapeutic ratio is low, a toxic response may be observed in some animals. Experiments conducted by the author have shown that when the extent of absorption is 50% or more and the variability of absorption is less than 50% of the amount absorbed, which gives a 25% to 75% range of absorption, the lead should have acceptable bioavailability for further development. For leads with an extent of absorption less than 25% of the administered dose or a variability of absorption of more than 100% of the amount absorbed, other formulations with absorption enhancers or solubilizers might be evaluated to improve the drug delivery profile. If improvement in the drug delivery profile is not possible, the chances that a lead with low, variable absorption will become a therapeutic product are greatly reduced. The candidacy of such a compound should be carefully considered.

An analytical chemistry method should be developed and validated for the quantification of a lead in nonclinical formulations and should predict whether the compound degrades from the time of preparation to the time of dosing. A method with this ability is a stability-indicating assay. The physical and chemical properties of the lead usually suggest a technique (heat, light, pH) that can degrade the compound. Samples stored under nondegrading and degrading conditions are assayed by the stability-indicating assay and, if possible, by another technique that can also determine if the original compound is present in the sample. If the lead is not stable, formulation excipients possibly can be added to prevent the degradation, or the formulations can be maintained under conditions that provide sufficient stability for testing in animal models. However, when a lead has limited stability in nonclinical formulations, the development of a clinical formulation with a sufficient shelf-life for marketing is problematic. Again the candidacy of such a compound should be carefully considered.

For proteins and other large molecules, degradation may include changes in the secondary or tertiary structure, provided that rearrangement back to the original, biologically active structure does not occur. Stability-indicating assays for macromolecules should assess structural changes that cause reductions in biological activity. However, a protein may have a number of amino acids removed from one or both ends of the molecule and still retain some, and possibly all, biological activity relative to the intact protein. This chemically modified peptide may have a different drug delivery profile or be more toxic than the parent protein. Structural modifications may not be apparent if biological activity alone is used to determine the amount of the macromolecule in a formulation. Thus experiments to demonstrate that an assay method is stability-indicating need to be carefully designed and conducted. For macromolecules, a specific chemical assay, such as HPLC or ELISA, and a biological potency assay may be necessary to determine the concentration and stability of a compound in a formulation.

The stability-indicating assay should be used to determine the amount of the lead in nonclinical formulations used for dosing animals in preliminary pharmacokinetic, drug metabolism, and toxicology studies. For single-dose studies, samples from each formulation at each dose level can be collected before dosing and after the completion of dosing. For multiple-dose studies, samples from each formulation used can be collected before the first dose and after the last dose or at selected other times. Results from these analyses ensure that the formulations contain the desired amount of the lead, that the concentrations do not change during the dosing period, and that the animals are receiving the appropriate dose levels. Without an acceptable nonclinical formulation, the extent and variability of delivery may make interpretation of results from developability studies meaningless and prevent the continued development of a potentially useful therapeutic agent.

The best formulation is of little use if the lead is not effectively delivered to the site of biological action. One of the primary reasons that discovery leads are not successful drug candidates is limited or insufficient transport across various membranes from the site of dosing to the site of activity. Only compounds administered intravenously to mediate a disease indication expressed in the cardiovascular system do not have to cross at least one membrane in order to reach the site of action. Thus assessments of a lead's ability to cross membranes should be conducted as early as possible. Many pharmaceutical companies use delivery potential as a key indicator for whether or not a discovery lead should move into preclinical development. A number of in vitro models are available to evaluate the delivery potential of a lead. For a lead to be administered orally, the Caco-2 model is most commonly employed. The Caco-2 cells mimic the cell wall of the GI tract and can be used to estimate the rate and extent of diffusion across membranes. Recently, a lipophilic membrane technique has been defined and shown to be equally predictive of transport across membranes. Other in vitro systems are available to evaluate transport across other membrane types, including the blood–brain barrier, the lung, and the skin.

Since most membranes are lipophilic in nature, a lead has to have some lipophilic characteristics in order to diffuse effectively into and across the membrane. However, in order to reach the membrane, the lead has to be dissolved in the surrounding medium, which is aqueous. Thus the lead also needs some hydrophilic properties in order to have sufficient aqueous solubility to be transported to the membrane. An estimate of a lead's ability to have both the lipophilic and hydrophilic characteristics necessary for effective delivery, primarily from the GI tract, can be determined from the chemical structure of the compound and using what is commonly called Lipinski's Rules of Five, which are four rules with cutoff numbers that are 5 or multiples of 5. These rules are

1. A molecular weight of less than 500 Dalton
2. A log P (octanol–water coefficient) of less than 5
3. Hydrogen-bond donors (sum of hydroxyl and amine groups) less than 5
4. Hydrogen-bond receptors (sum of nitrogen and oxygen atoms) less than 10

While these rules may be somewhat predictive of a lead's ability to cross membranes, not all compounds having the desired characteristics are orally absorbed or effectively transported across membranes, and laboratory experiments are required to determine if a lead will effectively be delivered to the site of biological action.

D. Preliminary Animal Pharmacokinetics

The first animal pharmacokinetic study confirms that the bioanalytical chemistry method is useful in characterizing the absorption and disposition profiles of the lead. The animal species for this study is usually the same as that used in pharmacology evaluations, most likely a rodent. A study design for a lead that has pharmacological activity when administered orally to rats may consist of dosing at least two rats with intravenous bolus injections at a dose level between 25% and 50% of the pharmacologically active dose and dosing at least two rats orally at the pharmacologically active dose. Serial blood samples, collected from each rat and processed to obtain the desired physiological fluid, are analyzed by the bioanalytical chemistry method. The plasma concentration versus time profiles after intravenous dosing provide preliminary information on the distribution and disposition kinetics of the lead. These intravenous results certify that the assay method is useful for quantifying the lead in specimens obtained from animals, predict the concentration range that can be expected in animal specimens, and assist in determining the sampling times to be used in more definitive animal pharmacokinetic experiments. The plasma concentration versus time profiles after oral dosing provide preliminary information on the absorption kinetics and the absolute bioavailability of the lead. The design of additional animal pharmacokinetic studies depends on the results of the preliminary animal pharmacokinetic study, the theoretical kinetic profile needed to produce the desired pharmacology response, and the results from preliminary toxicology experiments.

For most drug development programs, toxicology studies in two or more species are necessary. In this case, preliminary animal pharmacokinetic studies should be conducted in each species projected for use in animal safety studies. If differences in delivery or disposition exist between species and result in an enhanced or decreased toxicology profile, the pharmacokinetics may explain, in part, the different toxicology profiles. If possible, physiological fluid specimens should be obtained from animals in the preliminary toxicology studies to determine the extent and uniformity of exposure, which is termed toxicokinetics. Normally, three or four specimens from each animal are sufficient for toxicokinetic evaluations, but this level of sampling may not be possible for all studies. A single specimen at one collection time can be obtained from one or two animals in a dose group and the other animals in that dose group can be sampled at other times. Analyses of these specimens provide data on the extent of exposure but not on the uniformity of exposure within a dose group. For multiple-dose studies, specimens are usually obtained after the first dose and after the last, or next to last, dose. The results provide information on possible changes in exposure and on the accumulation potential of the lead or drug candidate and can be used to design multiple-dose animal pharmacokinetic and tissue distribution studies. If the change in disposition or accumulation is substantial, modification of the dosing regimen may be necessary to obtain the desired concentration profile after dosing to steady state.

E. Preliminary Drug Metabolism

The number and design of drug metabolism studies needed to characterize the fate of a lead or drug candidate in the body depend on the results from preliminary animal pharmacokinetic and toxicology studies. Commonly, the results from these in vivo experiments are not available during earlier developability assessments, and in vitro drug metabolism evaluations are utilized to determine the metabolic stability and the extent of metabolism of a lead and to compare the extent of metabolism among various species, including humans. These in vitro experiments can be conducted in a variety of systems, including CYP450 isozymes (the enzymes responsible for most oxidative metabolism of drugs), microsomes, hepatocytes, or liver slices. Since hepatocytes contain both phase 1 (oxidative, hydrolysis, and reduction) and phase 2 (conjugation) metabolism systems and can be relatively easily obtained from pharmacology and toxicology animal species and from humans, many researchers select this model for the first assessment of metabolism. If the results from hepatocytes show extensive metabolism, additional in vitro experiments are usually conducted first in microsomes to ascertain if oxidative metabolism is present and then in isolated CYP450 isozymes to determine which enzyme or enzymes are responsible. Extensive metabolism is not necessarily a death knell for a lead. If rapid clearance from the body is a desired attribute for effectively treating a disease indication, metabolism to inactive metabolites may be advantageous. However, for most disease indications, extensive metabolism may prevent delivery of a pharmacologically active substance to the site of biological action in sufficient concentration to produce the desired response. Thus a lead that is extensively metabolized may not be successful as a drug candidate.

Another reason for conducting in vitro metabolism studies early is to determine if species differences are present. Evaluating metabolism in the pharmacological and proposed toxicological animal species and in humans assists in selecting the species that are similar, at least in metabolism, to humans for definitive toxicology studies. If an animal species has limited metabolism while humans may have extensive metabolism, pharmacological and/or toxicological metabolites may be responsible for some or all of the biological activity or adverse effects in humans, and these responses would not be observed in the animal model. Conversely, if an animal species has extensive or different metabolism compared to humans, the safety profile in that species would probably not be predictive of safety in humans.

If desired, which is sometimes the case when metabolism is extensive, the metabolites generated from in vitro systems can be isolated and identified. After preparation of sufficient quantities for additional testing, these metabolites can be evaluated for pharmacological and/or toxicological potential. This author, like many drug development researchers, has found metabolites with equal or greater biological activity when compared to the parent compound. At times, these pharmacological activity metabolites have more druglike attributes than the parent and can be developed either as a replacement of the parent or as a second-generation drug candidate.

F. Acute Toxicology Studies

Toxicology studies are conducted to define the safety profile of a candidate and include definition of the no-observable-toxic-effect dose, maximum tolerated dose or MTD, potential organs of toxicity, and potential biochemical markers to detect and track toxic events. Most developmental compounds that do not become therapeutic products have unacceptable toxicity in animals and/or humans. Before the definitive toxicology studies needed to support an IND submission are initiated, a number of in vitro and animal experiments can be conducted to characterize the potential toxicity of the candidate. These early toxicology evaluations are usually conducted in the same species as used in pharmacology evaluations. As mentioned earlier, the lowest dose that has no toxicity, or an acceptable level of toxicity, is compared with the dose that gives the desired pharmacological response in the same animal species to obtain a therapeutic ratio or index for that species.

A toxicology program to obtain toxicological characterization of a discovery lead should be accomplished through close interaction with the efforts of other scientists conducting developability experiments. Before drug safety studies are conducted, a sufficient quantity of the lead should be available and characterized so that testing is conducted with a known compound. If the lead requires formulation before dosing, the formulation should be the same for each study. If a change in the synthesis, purification, or formulation is necessary to improve the biopharmaceutical properties of the lead or the drug delivery profile, then some of the early toxicology studies should be repeated with the new formulation to determine whether the safety profile has been altered. These early safety studies do not need to be, but in many cases are, conducted according to GLP requirements. However, these experiments should be designed and conducted as close as possible to the processes used for definitive GLP toxicology studies. Then the results will be scientifically defensible and useful in predicting the toxicity expected from the GLP studies. Examples of the early toxicology studies needed to characterize a lead include the following.

1. In Vitro Toxicology Assessments

When a number of discovery leads has been identified and need to be further evaluated to select the optimal lead for further evaluations, the potential for toxic effects may be determined using in vitro techniques, such as cell-based systems or microarrays. By incubating various concentrations of the leads with cells, such as the pharmacological target cell, hepatocytes, etc., and measuring an adverse effect, such as cell death or change in cell function, the compounds can be stratified as to toxicological potential. Similarly, microarrays that have systems considered predictive of toxic events can be used to determine which leads "turn on" these systems. While most, if not all, toxicologists think these in vitro systems cannot be used to predict toxicology in animal models or humans, the results may be useful in evaluating a group of discovery leads to determine which lead may have a more acceptable profile compared to the others.

2. Acute Single-Dose Tolerability Studies

To evaluate the qualitative and quantitative single-dose toxicity of a lead, a single dose at a number of dose levels is administered by the proposed clinical route and the animals are observed for 14 days after dosing. The acute study is not an LD_{50} study, which is not needed for overall risk assessment according to an ICH guideline [5]. This ICH guideline suggests that the drug candidate dose levels include at least one that produces pharmacological activity and one that causes overt evidence of major or life-threatening toxicity and that a vehicle control group is included. The acute toxicity study should evaluate both the intravenous route and the intended clinical route of administration, unless the clinical route is intravenous. The studies should be conducted in two relevant mammalian species, rodent and nonrodent, and unless scientifically unjustifiable, they should use equal numbers of males and females for each species evaluated. The test species is observed for 14 days after dosing and, as with all toxicology studies, all signs of toxicity with time of onset, duration of symptoms, and reversibility are recorded. Also, the time to first observations of lethality is recorded. Gross necropsies are performed on all animals sacrificed moribund, found dead, or terminated after 14 days of observation and the results are presented by group. An evaluation of results should include all observations made and a discussion of the toxicological findings and their implications to humans, taking into account the pharmacology of the lead, the proposed human therapeutic use and dose, and experience with related drugs. The highest no-toxic-effect dose and the highest nonlethal dose are noted.

3. Dose-Range-Finding Studies

The doses for definitive toxicology studies are defined in dose-range-finding studies. These experiments usually include four dose levels, with the highest level being the dose that did not cause acute toxicity, and a vehicle control group, and they are conducted in each species proposed for use in definitive toxicology studies. For rodents, dose groups usually have 6 to 10 animals, 3 to 5 animals per sex. For nonrodent species, normally beagle dogs or nonhuman primates, the number of animals in each dose group is commonly four, 2 animals per sex. Endpoints for dose-range-finding studies may include, but are not limited to, weight loss, activity changes, clinical chemistry changes, and histology and pathology evaluations at necropsy. The primary goal of these studies is to determine an MTD. The route of administration and the frequency and duration of dosing are determined from the expected clinical use of the compound.

4. Pilot 14-Day Studies

A dose level that causes toxic changes, such as morbidity or salivation, and one that produces the no-toxic-effect are determined during 14-day studies. For a lead or drug candidate to be used for a non-life-threatening clinical indication, at least two animal species are tested, one rodent and one nonrodent. The information gained by these studies is used to model the definitive

GLP toxicology studies so that these experiments are conducted with a cost-efficient design and are data productive. These early toxicology studies can also evaluate the potential for antibody production, if the lead might be antigenic, and clinical chemistry changes in physiological parameters (electrolyte or biochemical imbalances, changes in liver enzymes). These data may identify potential biological markers that can be used in definitive toxicology and clinical studies to evaluate and possibly predict adverse effects.

Organs that are the targets of toxicity may be identified during the above toxicology studies by a full histology workup of animals in each dose group and from the results obtained from the analyses of clinical chemistry samples (discussed in more detail in the preclinical toxicology section). The level of the lead in the identified target organs of toxicity can be determined by the drug metabolism group in an attempt to correlate the observed toxicity with high or accumulated concentrations of the compound, providing a potential toxicodynamic correlation. If possible, investigations into the biochemical mechanism of identified toxicity should be initiated. Results from these experiments can provide insight into potential toxicities in definitive toxicology studies, identify biological markers that predict a toxic event, and suggest conditions in human patients where administration of the lead or drug candidate is contraindicated. If results from the early toxicology studies show that a lead has an unacceptable level of toxicity, the development candidacy of such a compound should be carefully considered.

5. Safety Pharmacology and Genotoxicity

If desired, the safety of a lead can be further assessed by conducting safety pharmacology and/or genotoxicity studies, which are described in more detail in the section on preclinical development. These studies, which are to be completed prior to the initiation of human clinical testing, are more commonly conducted after selection of a drug candidate. However, if some discovery leads are considered "equal" after other developability assessments have been completed, the results from safety pharmacology or genotoxicity studies may be able to identify the optimal lead or determine that some leads do not have the desired profile and should not be selected as the drug candidate.

G. Drug Development Candidate Selection

Many discovery leads are transferred to the preclinical development process with insufficient characterization to assess their development potential. This lack of knowledge usually results in poorly designed experiments that are not data productive and that, in many cases, have to be repeated when the drug candidate shows unexpected toxicity, low and variable delivery, instability or solubility problems, or unacceptable pharmacokinetic and drug metabolism profiles. In all too many cases, the recognition of these problem areas results in termination of development for a potentially useful therapeutic agent. At best, the problems encountered cause a delay, at times substantial, in the development of a candidate while additional studies are conducted to elucidate the causes of the problems and minimize their effects. Then the definitive development experiments have to be repeated.

The developability experiments in the six scientific disciplines shown in Fig. 4 can more fully characterize a discovery lead before the compound enters the definitive preclinical, and then the nonclinical and clinical, drug development processes. The experimental designs could also be used, with minor modifications, to evaluate a group of compounds and thus to select the lead with the best characteristics, i.e., the most druglike attributes and the fewest demerits, for further development. With appropriate planning and commitment of resources, these studies can usually be completed in 3 to 6 months if major problems are not encountered in one or more of the scientific areas.

If these developability experiments are completed as part of the transition from discovery to development, compounds that do not have the characteristics necessary to become therapeutic agents can be identified early and prevented from entering the development process. Analogues of a compound with unacceptable characteristics can be evaluated to find a development candidate that has better properties. In addition, the results from the developability studies will allow the preclinical development studies to be designed and conducted in a timely, cost-efficient manner and thus most likely allow the candidate to have an earlier entry into the clinic.

V. PRECLINICAL DRUG DEVELOPMENT

Before entering into a clinical evaluation program, a drug candidate is subjected to a number of preclinical studies to further define and characterize its safety profile. The results from the pharmacology, developability, and preclinical studies are documented in technical reports or scientific publications and used to prepare a regulatory agency submission for the initiation of human clinical trials. All of the preclinical studies, described in the sections below, and nonclinical studies, discussed in the following section, need to be conducted according to GLP regulations.

If the experiments described in the developability assessment section have not been completed, many of these studies should be conducted after the drug candidate has been selected. The results from these early studies are needed to design effectively the more definitive preclinical studies, particularly the toxicology and drug metabolism evaluations needed to support an IND submission.

A. Good Laboratory Practice

Research studies intended for submission to a regulatory agency are to be conducted according to GLP regulations, as published by regulatory authorities in all the leading pharmaceutical markets, such as the United States (the FDA regulations applicable to GLPs are provided in Title 21 Code of Federal Regulations, Part 58), the European Community, and Japan. Good Laboratory Practice regulations are very similar worldwide; however, researchers are cautioned to review the regulations for the marketing area to ensure that the completed studies are in compliance.

GLP regulations concern standard methods, facilities, and controls used in conducting preclinical and nonclinical laboratory studies and are used to assure the quality and integrity of generated data. The standards relate to both the design and the conduct of the research studies and the qualifications of the personnel and facilities involved with all aspects of the experiments. The GLPs necessitate that

1. SOPs are written for all routine or standard practices in the laboratory.
2. All personnel involved with the studies are sufficiently trained and experienced to perform their assigned functions.
3. An adequate number of personnel are available to conduct the study.
4. The facilities are appropriately designed and maintained.
5. A group, commonly called quality assurance or QA, monitors and checks the results from the studies to ensure that the experiments are conducted in compliance with the regulations.

B. Bioanalytical Chemistry

The bioanalytical method, defined and characterized during developability assessment, can be used to support definitive pharmacokinetic and toxicology studies after the assay has been appropriately validated for each physiological matrix and each species to be evaluated. The validation experiments need to address and define acceptance and rejection criteria for the range of reliable results, the lower limit (and if appropriate as for an ELISA or RIA method, the upper limit) of quantification, accuracy, precision, specificity, and recovery and should include appropriate stability studies. These stability studies will ensure that the analyte is stable in the physiological matrix from the time of collection to the time of analysis. Guidelines for validation of a bioanalytical method have been published [3,4]. ICH guidelines [6,7] have been issued for validation of analytical procedures and can be used for guidance for validation of bioanalytical chemistry methods. The validated method should be documented in a test assay procedure and supported by appropriate SOPs. Also, the results from the validation experiments should be documented in a technical report and included in the IND submission.

C. Pharmacokinetic and Bioavailability Experiments

Pharmacokinetic and bioavailability (absolute and relative) experiments are usually designed and conducted to evaluate dose proportionality over the dose range used, or expected to be used, in toxicology studies and possible species-to-species differences in pharmacokinetic profiles. With the incorporation of one or two intravenous dose levels into the study protocol, the drug candidate's absolute bioavailability can also be determined, and information on the linearity of absorption, distribution, and disposition kinetics can be obtained. If more than one drug formulation is to be used in toxicology studies (e.g., an oral solution for rodent studies and tablets or drug in capsules for dosing the larger nonrodent species), relative bioavailability experiments comparing the formulations can determine if the extent of delivery is similar or different and thus can make extrapolation of pharmacology and toxicity results between animal species meaningful and useful in designing the later nonclinical studies and phase 1 safety and tolerance studies in humans.

D. Drug Metabolism

Drug metabolism or ADME evaluations determine absorption (how a compound gets into the body), distribution (where the compound goes), disposition (how long the compound stays), metabolism (whether the compound is changed and to what), and elimination (how the compound is removed or cleared): the fate of a compound in the body.

Drug metabolism experiments in animal species used or to be used in toxicology studies are conducted using an appropriately labeled compound, usually a radioactive isotope such as carbon-14. At times, drug metabolism studies are conducted with a less than desirable radiolabel, such as ^{125}I on a protein or ^3H at a potentially exchangeable site on an NCE. However, the results obtained from these studies can be misleading, reflecting the distribution and disposition of the label and not the drug candidate or metabolites. For more reliable results, the radiolabeled compound should be radiochemically pure and stable and have a specific activity high enough to be measurable after dosing. Also, the label needs to be in a position where it does not affect the physical, chemical, or pharmacological properties of the candidate and is not lost during phase 1 (oxidation, reduction, cleavage) or phase 2 (conjugation) metabolism. Before animals are dosed, the radiochemical purity needs to be evaluated and the stability in physiological matrices should be studied. If the radiolabel is nonmetabolically removed from the compound, the results from the drug metabolism experiments, or other studies using the labeled compound, will have little, if any, meaning or usefulness in the determination of the metabolic fate of the drug candidate.

If the candidate has a slow disposition phase, suggesting distribution into some extravascular tissues, or if the early toxicology experiments identify potential organs of toxicity, a preliminary mass balance combined with tissue distribution study can be designed to evaluate the radioactivity level versus time profile in selected tissues, such as liver, kidney, fat (for a lipophilic candidate), muscle, skin, heart, and brain and to determine the primary route(s) and rate(s) of elimination. The results from this preliminary metabolism study can also be used to more effectively design (i.e., selection of time points and matrices for evaluation) the definitive mass balance and tissue distribution studies needed for supporting regulatory agency submissions.

The total radioactivity minus the parent compound concentration (determined by the bioanalytical chemistry method) in a specimen (plasma, serum, urine, bile) estimates the amount of metabolites present. If the difference is minimal and does not change over time, the extent of metabolism is low. For plasma or serum specimens, a small difference indicates that metabolites are not present in systemic circulation. For bile or urine specimens, high levels of radioactivity suggest a primary route of elimination for the parent and metabolites. For a drug candidate cleared primarily by metabolism, a preliminary metabolite profile in urine and bile can determine the amount of each potential metabolite. When the level of a metabolite in a matrix is high, i.e., greater than 5% of the parent, attempts to isolate and identify the metabolite should be undertaken and the results compared with in vitro drug metabolism studies, if conducted. After sufficient quantities of the metabolites are available, the metabolite's pharmacological and toxicological activity potential can be evaluated, providing possible additional information on the pharmacological and toxicological mechanism of action for the drug candidate.

One of the first metabolism studies conducted should be protein binding in animal and human physiological fluid. The pharmacological and toxicological activity of a drug candidate is usually attributed to the free or unbound fraction in systemic circulation and not to the total drug content, which includes both free and bound drug. The unbound drug is the species that passes through the cell walls of blood vessels and is distributed to various organs, including the pharmacological and toxicological sites of actions. The free and bound fractions of a drug candidate are in equilibrium, so that as the free drug is removed from systemic circulation, the bound drug disassociates to maintain the free-to-bound ratio. A drug candidate that is highly and tightly bound, e.g., more than 95%, to blood proteins may not have sufficient distribution to attain the necessary concentration at the site of action to elicit a pharmacological effect. If this is the case, a bioanalytical chemistry method that quantifies unbound drug may be needed so that the pharmacokinetic profile of the free fraction can be evaluated. For a drug with a protein binding of less than 95%, the amount of free drug and the equilibrium process generally provide a good correlation between total drug concentration in systemic circulation and pharmacological or toxicological responses.

The two most common drug metabolism studies are mass balance and tissue distribution. Mass balance studies are usually conducted in both the rodent and the nonrodent species used for toxicology evaluations, whereas tissue distribution is performed only in the rodent. For mass balance, a radio-labeled compound is administered to the test species and urine, feces, and, if necessary, expired air are collected at intervals and counted for total radio-activity. Commonly used intervals are 0–4, 4–8, 8–12, 12–24, and then daily, up to 168 hours or until more than 95% of the administered dose has been excreted. Depending on the pharmacokinetic profile of the candidate, other collection intervals can be selected to give a better picture of the excretion profile. For tissue distribution, a radiolabeled compound is administered to the test species, and after predefined times, usually 2, 4, 8, 24, and 48 hours, the test species is sacrificed, and tissues are collected, processed, and counted for total radioactivity. The tissues commonly evaluated are similar to those collected during necropsy in toxicology studies (listed in Table 1) plus the carcass. A routine aspect of most tissue distribution studies, in fact a technique that is being used by some pharmaceutical companies to replace tissue distribution studies, is quantitative whole body autoradiography (QWBA). Recent advances in QWBA allow this technique to quantify low levels of radioactivity in tissues. Some researchers think that QWBA should com-pletely replace the classic tissue distribution study to profile the organs and systems that are exposed and may accumulate the drug candidate and its metabolites.

These preclinical drug metabolism studies may also include metabolite profiling in plasma, selected tissues, urine, and bile to assess the distribution and disposition of potentially important metabolites, such as those having a level 5% or greater relative to the parent compound. Metabolite profiling requires a technique to separate the parent compound from metabolites and other endogenous compounds. For small organic molecules, HPLC is usually the method of choice. For macromolecules, gel or capillary electrophoresis techniques can be defined with sufficient resolution capability to separate the

Table 1 Tissues Collected at Necropsy and Prepared for Histopathological Evaluation

Tissue	Tissue
Adrenal glands	Pancreas
Aorta	Pituitary gland
Bone marrow (sternum)	Prostate gland (males)
Brain (usually at least three levels)	Rectum
Cervix/vagina (females)	Salivary gland (manidibular)
Epididymides (males)	Sciatic nerve
Esophagus	Skeletal muscle
Eyes with optic nerve	Skin from the abdomen
Femur with articular surface	Spinal cord (usually at least three levels)
Gallbladder	Spleen
Heart	Thymus
Large intestine	Thyroid and parathyroid
(including cecum and colon)	(when in same section)
Testes (males)	Tongue
Small intestine (including duodenum,	Stomach (including cardia, fundus, and
jejunum, and ileum)	pylorus)
Kidneys	Trachea
Liver	Uterus (females)
Lungs with bronchi	Urinary bladder
Lymph nodes	Gross lesions
Lacrimal gland	Seminal vessels (males)
Mammary gland (females)	Vertebra
Ovaries (females)	Injection site (if appropriate)

compounds. Those metabolites representing more than 5% of the parent compound are usually identified with such techniques as mass spectrometry and nuclear magnetic spectroscopy. After identification, those metabolites that might elicit a pharmacological or toxicological response can be synthesized and tested in appropriate animal models. Many novel drugs have been discovered during metabolite characterization of drug candidates. These new compounds may have attributes, such as better extent of delivery, longer or shorter disposition kinetics, less potential for accumulation, or better clearance properties, that make them better drug candidates than the parent compounds.

E. Toxicology

Before human clinical trials can be initiated, a number of toxicology studies need to be completed and documented in the IND submission. In addition to the studies listed above for toxicology developability assessment, preclinical toxicology studies include local tolerance, genotoxicity, safety pharmacology, and subchronic tests.

One of the most troublesome aspects in the interpretation of toxicology results is determining whether these data are predictive of safety in humans. Often, animal toxicology may not correlate with human safety because the observed adverse effects are species specific. For example, HMG-CoA reductase inhibitors induce cataracts, potentially a drug-candidate-killing effect, in beagle dogs but not in rats or monkeys. Human clinical use of these therapeutic agents also has not shown this adverse experience, suggesting that the beagle is susceptible to this problem but other species are not. Species specificity is sometimes discovered early in the development of a drug candidate, such as the drug developability phase discussed earlier, and can be used to design the early human trials to ascertain if humans also manifest the observed toxicity.

1. Local Tolerance

An ICH guideline [8] indicates that local tolerance evaluations are to be conducted in animals using the route of administration proposed for human clinical testing and that these evaluations are to be performed before human exposure. The assessment of local tolerance may be part of other toxicity studies.

2. Genotoxicity

Registration for marketing of pharmaceuticals requires an assessment of the drug candidate's genotoxic potential. Two ICH guidelines [9,10] have been issued for genotoxic testing, which includes in vitro and in vivo studies that are designed to determine if a compound induces genetic damage either directly or indirectly and by any of a number of mechanisms. Positive genotoxic compounds have the potential of being human carcinogens or mutagens, that is, these drug candidates may induce cancer or heritable defects. Three tests are recommended to evaluate the genotoxicity potential of a drug candidate: (1) a test for gene mutation in bacteria (the Ames test), (2) an in vitro cytogenetic evaluation of chromosomal damage by use of mammalian cells such as human lymphoblastoid TK6, CHO, V79, and AS52 cells or an in vitro mouse lymphoma L5178Y cell line tk assay, and (3) an in vivo study for chromosomal damage in rodent hematopoietic cells. Drug candidates that give negative results in these three tests are usually considered to have demonstrated an absence of genotoxic activity. Depending on the proposed therapeutic use, positive compounds may need to be and, probably should be, tested more extensively.

3. Safety Pharmacology

Safety pharmacology involves assessing the effects of a drug candidate for pharmacological activity on the functions of various organ systems other than the target system. Normally the organ systems that are evaluated are the cardiovascular, central nervous, and respiratory systems. Depending on the physical and chemical characteristics of the candidate and the route of administration, other systems to be evaluated include the renal/urinary, autonomic nervous, and gastrointestinal systems. Safety pharmacology studies need to be conducted [11] before human exposure and may be additions to other toxicology studies or separate studies.

4. Subchronic Toxicology

The FDA and most other regulatory agencies require subchronic toxicity studies in two species, one of which is a nonrodent, before human clinical trials are initiated. The recommended duration of the subchronic toxicity studies is related to duration of the proposed clinical trials. An ICH guideline [8] suggests the minimum duration of toxicity studies, shown in Table 2, needed to support phase 1, 2, and 3 clinical trials, in which humans are to be exposed to the drug candidate for varying durations.

The two most common species used in subchronic toxicology studies are the rat and the dog. The most common strain of rat used within the pharmaceutical and biotechnology industries is the Charles River CD rat, which is Sprague–Dawley derived and an outbred strain. Some companies use

Table 2 Duration of Multiple Dose Toxicology Studies Needed to Support Phase 1, 2, and 3 Clinical Trials

	Minimum duration of toxicity study	
Duration of clinical trial	Rodents	Nonrodents
Single Dose	2–4 weeks[a]	2 weeks
Up to 2 weeks	2–4 weeks[a]	2 weeks
Up to 1 month	1 month	1 month
Up to 3 months	3 months	3 months
Up to 6 months	6 months	6 months
Greater than 6 months	6 months	Chronic

[a] In Europe and the United States, 2 week studies are the minimum duration. In Japan, 2-week nonrodent and 4-week rodent studies are needed.
Note: Support for phase 3 clinical trails in Europe and for marketing in all regions required longer minimum duration toxicology studies than listed in the table.

the Fisher 244 albino rat, which is an inbred strain, because this strain does not grow as large as the Charles River CD rat. Other rodent species sometimes used for subchronic toxicity include the mouse and the hamster. The beagle dog, purebred and specifically bred for research, is the most common non-rodent species used in toxicology assessments. Cynomolgus and rhesus monkeys are also used as the nonrodent toxicology species, primarily by the biotechnology industry developing macromolecule therapeutics but also more and more frequently by pharmaceutical firms evaluating NCEs. The rabbit, which is commonly one of the species used in reproduction toxicology evaluations, has also been used as the nonrodent species for subchronic testing. During the past few years, significant advances have been made for effective dosing regimens of animals in toxicology studies. The most common route of administration for human therapy is oral, usually as tablets or capsules. Other routes include intravenous, pulmonary, dermal, subcutaneous, intramuscular, rectal, nasal, and buccal. Whatever the proposed route of administration for humans, the preclinical animal toxicology studies should use the same route of delivery. For rodents, oral dosing of tablets or capsules is not possible, but daily, or more frequent, oral gavage is a now standard technique. For larger species, the tablets or capsules can be placed in soft gelatin capsules and dosed. Present-day technology allows continuous infusion of both rodent and nonrodent species for evaluation of drug candidates to be administered as intravenous infusions. For other routes of administration, special techniques may be necessary to ensure that the test species is appropriately exposed to the test article.

Whenever possible, the proposed clinical formulation should be used in preclinical toxicology evaluations, because formulation excipients can be important in the extent and duration of delivery and in local tolerance. For oral dosing to rodents, the solid clinical formulation can be ground and the appropriate amount dissolved or suspended in water prior to gavaging. The most common dosing volume for rodents is 10 ml/kg, but other volumes can be used. The volume administered should be uniform for all dose groups, including the vehicle control group.

For rodent subchronic studies, 10 to 25 animals/sex/group are used, with the smaller groups used for shorter (2–4 week) studies and the larger groups for longer-term (more than 13 weeks) studies. If an interim sacrifice or a reversibility phase, which is a drug-free recovery phase, is incorporated into the study design, an extra 10 animals/sex are commonly added to each dose group, including the vehicle control group. For nonrodent subchronic studies, the number of animals/sex/group is usually three to six, depending on the length of the study and the expected toxicology profile.

Dose selection for subchronic and chronic toxicology studies should be based on the results from acute toxicity studies and pharmacokinetic evaluations. The three typical dose levels are (1) a no-toxic-effect level, which should be at least equivalent to, and hopefully a multiple of, the proposed human dose, (2) a dose level that produces a toxic effect in clinical observations, clinical pathology, or histopathological changes, and (3) a dose level between these two.

5. Formulation Analyses

Analyses of formulations for a drug candidate content are conducted to ensure that doses administered to animals in toxicology, pharmacokinetic, and drug metabolism studies have the proper amount of the drug candidate. Before these analyses are performed, a stability-indicating analytical method that can quantify the drug candidate in the formulation needs to be defined and validated [6,7] for sensitivity, linearity, precision, accuracy, and robustness. If the dosing formulation is changed between studies, revalidation of the analytical method for application to the new formulation is necessary.

For acute toxicity, single-dose pharmacokinetic, and single-dose drug metabolism studies, formulations for each dose level, including the vehicle control, are commonly analyzed before and after administration. If no apparent change in the drug candidate content is detected, the animals are assured to have been dosed with the appropriate amount of the compound. For subchronic and chronic studies, including carcinogenicity studies, and for multiple-dose pharmacokinetic and drug metabolism experiments, formulations for each dose level are analyzed for drug candidate content before the first dose, at predefined times during the course of the study, and after the last dose. If the length of study requires that the formulations be prepared periodically, content analyses need to be performed on some of the new formulations to ensure that the method of preparation provides a uniform drug candidate content. If the drug content in a formulation drops below or is above a predefined acceptance criterion (usually a range of 95% to 105% is considered acceptable), that formulation should not be used for dosing animals.

6. Toxicokinetics

For many years, the dose levels of a drug candidate administered to the test species in the various dose groups of a toxicology study were used to correlate the observed toxic effects with the drug candidate and to show that the effects increased with increasing dose. The administered dose levels were assumed to predict, and be proportional to, the amount of drug candidate that was in the body. However, for drug candidates that are poorly absorbed, have variable absorption, or show saturable absorption as the dose level increases, the administered dose has been shown not to be a uniform predictor of toxicity. Ensuring that test species have an increased exposure to the drug candidate as the dose levels increase has become a critical, and now standard, aspect of toxicology studies. Equally important is that the extent and duration of exposure are not changed after multiple-dose administration. An ICH guideline [12] has been issued on the generation of toxicokinetic data to support the development of a drug candidate. The objectives of toxicokinetics include

1. Describing the systemic exposure in each of the test species used in toxicology studies and showing how exposure relates to dose level and the time course of the study
2. Correlating the extent of exposure with toxicological findings and contributing to the assessment of these findings to clinical safety
3. Supporting the choice of test species and treatment regimen for nonclinical toxicology studies
4. Along with toxicity results, providing information on the appropriate design for subsequent nonclinical toxicity studies and human clinical trials

Toxicokinetic data, considered an integral part of a nonclinical program, can be obtained from the test species in a toxicology study or in specially designed supportive studies. The primary focus of toxicokinetic data is to assist in the interpretation of toxicity results and not on characterizing the basic pharmacokinetic parameters of the drug candidate being studied. Not all toxicology studies need to include a toxicokinetic component. If the extent and duration of exposure of a drug candidate in a particular formulation for a given test species has been generated for the dose level range to be used in a toxicity study, additional toxicokinetic evaluations are not generally necessary. Toxicology studies, which are usefully supported by toxicokinetics, include single-dose studies for which results from preliminary pharmacokinetic studies may be applicable; multiple-dose studies in which toxicokinetic data may predict whether multiple-dose pharmacokinetic studies are necessary; reproductive studies, which may use different test species that have an altered absorption and disposition profile due to pregnancy; and carcinogenicity studies, in which the test species may be dosed differently compared to other toxicology studies and changes in exposure can occur because of age.

7. Hematology, Clinical Chemistry, and Histopathology

Three important aspects for detecting and understanding the adverse effects observed during a toxicology study are hematology and clinical chemistry assays and histopathology evaluation of tissues collected at necropsy. Hematology parameters commonly evaluated include those listed in Table 3. These parameters should be determined periodically during the toxicity study, with the number of evaluations depending on the length of the study. Clinical chemistries routinely determined include those listed in Table 4. Urinalysis

Table 3 Hematology Parameters Evaluated During Toxicology Studies

Parameter	Abbreviation
White blood cell count	WBC
Red blood cell count	RBC
Hemoglobin concentration	HGB
Hematocrit	HCT
Mean corpuscular volume	MCV
Mean corpuscular hemoglobin	MCH
Mean corpuscular hemoglobin concentration	MCHC
Platelet count	PLT
Prothrombin time	PT
Activated partial thromboplastin time	APTT

Table 4 Clinical Chemistry Parameters Evaluated During Toxicology Studies

Parameter	Abbreviation
Total protein	TP
Triglycerides	TRI
Albumin	A
Globulin	G
Albumin/globulin ratio	A/G
Glucose	GLU
Cholesterol	CHOL
Total bilirubin	TBILI
Urea nitrogen	BUN
Creatinine	CREAT
Creatine phosphokinase	CPK
Alanine aminotransferase	ALT
Aspartate aminotransferase	AST
Alanine phosphatase	ALK
Gamma-glutamyltransferase	CGT
Lactate dehydrogenase	LDH
Calcium	Ca
Phosphorus	Phos
Sodium	Na
Potassium	K
Chloride	Cl

also may be performed but is usually limited to nonrodents and should include microscopical examination of sediment. Pretreatment clinical chemistry analyses and the number of determinations per group should be the same as for hematology. Depending on the pharmacology and toxicology profile of a drug candidate, other biological marker analyses can be included in addition to hematology and clinical chemistry evaluations. Results from these additional tests can provide information on physiological parameter changes caused by the drug candidate in animal models and may be used to evaluate pharmacological and toxicological effects during human clinical studies.

Tissues collected at necropsy and prepared for histopathological evaluation include those listed in Table 1. Routine sectioning and examination are recommended for all tissues from rodent and nonrodent animals used in subchronic and chronic studies. Requirements for special histopathology examination depend on adverse effects that are indicated by in-life clinical pathology changes and are usually on a case-by-case basis. Electron microscopy (EM) is a useful extension of light microscopic evaluation in determining morphological alteration of cellular structures not otherwise clearly visualized. Selected specimens can be processed for EM examination when use of this technique is justified. The application of EM to all tissues is considered impractical and unnecessary.

8. Immunogenicity

Many proteins, polypeptides, oligonucleotides, and other large molecules are immunogenic in the animal models used in pharmacology and toxicology evaluations. According to an ICH guideline [13], the potential for antibody formation should be determined during the conduct of subchronic toxicology studies to aid in the interpretation of results from these and later studies. Antibodies that are formed are characterized as to titer, number of responding animals, neutralizing or nonneutralizing, change in pharmacological or toxicological response, complement activation, and immune complex formation and deposition. If the observed immune response neutralizes the pharmacological or toxicological effects of the drug candidate, modification of the study design may be warranted. Because the induction of antibody formation in animal models is not predictive of a similar response in humans, no special significance to animal antibody formation should be ascribed unless the interpretation of results from pharmacology or safety studies is compromised. However, if antibodies are formed during animal studies, the potential for antibody formation in humans should be assessed during early clinical development to ensure that antibodies will not adversely affect the pharmacological profile and do not increase the potential toxicity of the drug candidate in humans.

VI. NONCLINICAL DRUG DEVELOPMENT

After a drug candidate enters into human clinical testing, information on the pharmacokinetics and toxicology of the compound in the relevant species finally becomes available. The results from pharmacology, developability, and preclinical drug development experiments should be reevaluated in light of this new information to ascertain if the animal models were predictive of the efficacy, safety, and pharmacokinetics in humans. If the animal results are extrapolative to humans, the remaining nonclinical animal studies are fairly straightforward and are conducted to provide supportive information on the safety of the drug candidate. However, if the early animal data do not extrapolate to the human situation, additional animal experiments should be designed and conducted to understand better and more fully the observed pharmacology and toxicology in humans. Considering the expense in both time and money to conduct nonclinical drug development studies, most pharmaceutical and biotechnology companies meet with the appropriate regulatory agencies to discuss the study designs and protocols and how dose levels were selected to avoid nonacceptance of regulatory agency submissions later on.

A. Pharmacokinetics

Unless justified from pharmacokinetic results from humans, additional animal pharmacokinetic studies are not usually conducted during nonclinical development. Types of animal pharmacokinetics that might be performed include

1. Multiple-dose pharmacokinetics to assess accumulation or changes in clearance caused by enzyme induction or inhibition
2. Bioavailability comparison when the formulation used in early toxicology or human studies is changed to alter the delivery profile of the drug candidate
3. Drug candidate metabolite distribution and disposition evaluations
4. Effect of food and time of feeding on the extent and duration of absorption
5. Drug–drug interaction if the animal model is considered predictive of humans

B. Drug Metabolism

After initiation of human clinical studies, drug metabolism studies are continued to build the database to show that the results from the animal models used to demonstrate the pharmacology and toxicology of the drug candidate can be extrapolated to the human situation. The most common drug metabolism studies conducted during nonclinical drug development are multiple-dose tissue distribution, additional characterization and evaluation of metabolites, and studies such as fetal-placental transfer and lacteal secretion, which are designed to support reproductive and developmental toxicology evaluations. Although most regulatory agencies agree that a single-dose tissue distribution study in rodents is needed to support the development of a drug candidate, and that this study often provides sufficient data on the distribution of the compound, a multiple-dose tissue distribution study may yield additional information [14]. This study, for which no consistent requirement currently exists, may be appropriate

1. When the apparent half-life of the drug candidate or a metabolite in organs or tissues significantly exceeds the apparent terminal disposition half-life in plasma and is more than twice the dosing interval in toxicity studies

2. When the steady-state concentrations of the drug candidate or a metabolite in systemic circulation, usually first detected from toxicokinetic results from multiple-dose toxicology studies, are substantially higher than predicted from single-dose pharmacokinetic studies

3. When the drug candidate is being developed for site-specific targeted delivery

4. When histopathology changes that were not predicted from shorter-term toxicology studies, single-dose tissue distribution studies, or pharmacology studies are observed

The study design for multiple-dose tissue distribution studies is usually compound and result specific and thus is determined on a case-by-case basis.

Reproductive and developmental toxicology studies are conducted to reveal the effect of the drug candidate on mammalian reproduction and whether potential reproductive risks may exist for humans. These reproductive studies commonly use pregnant rats and rabbits as the test species. To ensure that the dams and the fetuses are appropriately exposed to the drug candidate and metabolites [12], the dams can be dosed with radiolabeled compound, and the amount of radioactivity that crosses the placenta and into the fetuses at various times after dosing determined. If little or no radioactivity is detected in the fetuses, then the ability of animal reproductive studies to predict risks in humans has to be questioned, inasmuch as humans may have a different delivery profile from the animal models. Similarly, the exposure of the drug candidate to nursing pups can be ascertained after the dam is dosed with radiolabeled compound and the amount of radioactivity excreted in the milk is determined. If little or no radioactivity is detected in the dam's milk, then potential risk to nursing humans cannot be ascertained. When reproductive toxicology studies show no apparent effect, fetal-placenta transfer and lacteal secretion studies can be used to certify these findings and demonstrate that the animals were appropriately exposed to the drug candidate.

C. Toxicology

1. Chronic Studies

Regulatory agencies require chronic toxicity studies in two species, a rodent and a nonrodent, for drug candidates that are to be administered to humans for more than 3 months [8]. The two basic reasons for conducting chronic studies are to produce a toxic effect and to define a safety factor. The study should provide a dose–response relationship to effects resulting from prolonged exposure to the drug candidate and should reveal adverse effects that require a long exposure to be expressed or that are cumulative. Chronic studies often can be conducted in species whose metabolism is most similar to humans, because early human evaluations most likely have been completed before these chronic studies are initiated. The rat is the most common rodent species used in chronic studies, whereas the beagle dog and nonhuman primates are the usual nonrodent species. The dog, a carnivore, often metabolizes compounds differently from humans and should be used with caution. However, nonhuman primates have not been shown to have metabolic systems any closer to humans than most other laboratory animals. Monkeys are the preferred species for macromolecules, because they are similar to humans in anatomy and physiology.

The duration for chronic toxicology studies depends on the projected duration of administration to humans (Table 2). The present consensus according to the FDA [5] is that 6–month rodent and 9–month nonrodent studies are sufficient for drug candidates intended for long-term human use, provided the candidate is studied in rats, or other appropriate species, to evaluate the potential for tumor production, i.e., a carcinogenicity study.

Dose selection for chronic studies is very important, because regulatory agencies want one dose to be a no-toxic-effect dose level and another to show frank toxicity. Several approaches are available to select doses, as described in the section on carcinogenicity studies. However, the most common approach historically has been to use the MTD as the high-dose level for chronic toxicology studies. The MTD has been defined as the dose that, at a minimum, suppresses body weight gain by approximately 10%. The mid- and low-dose levels are based on the MTD and have usually been one quarter of the MTD for the mid-dose and one eighth of the MTD for the low dose. Using this approach, the low dose may be substantially above, but could even be below, the expected human therapeutic dose.

2. Reproductive and Developmental Toxicology

Reproductive and developmental toxicology studies are designed and conducted to reveal any effect of a drug candidate or a metabolite on mammalian reproduction and to ascertain the potential risks to humans. These studies evaluate male and female fertility, embryo and fetal death, parturition and the newborn, the lactation process, care of the young, and the potential teratogenicity of the drug candidate. Historically, these reproductive parameters have been evaluated in three types of studies, generally referred to as segment I, segment II, and segment III. Segment I evaluates fertility and general reproductive performance in rats. Segment II, commonly conducted in rats and rabbits, determines the embryo toxicity or teratogenic effects of the drug candidate. Segment III, designated the perinatal and postnatal study and normally conducted only in rats, assesses the effects of the drug candidate on late fetal development, labor and delivery, lactation, neonatal viability, and growth of the newborn. Other rodents and nonrodent species, such as mice, guinea pigs, mini pigs, ferrets, hamsters, dogs, and nonhuman primates, have been used to evaluate the reproductive toxicity of drug candidates.

According to an ICH guideline [15], the combination of studies selected needs to allow exposure of mature adults and all stages of development from conception to sexual maturity to conception in the following generation. This integrated sequence has been subdivided into various stages, which are designated (A) premating to conception, (B) conception to implantation, (C) implantation to closure of the hard palate, (D) closure of the hard palate to the end of pregnancy, (E) birth to weaning, and (F) weaning to sexual maturity. Using these designations, segment I evaluates stages A and B of the reproductive process, segment II studies stages C and D, and segment III detects adverse effects during stages C to F. A common practice is to combine segments I and III into a single study and conduct separate segment II studies in rats and rabbits. Segment I studies, designed to evaluate fertility and general reproductive performance (stages A and B), uses sexually mature male and female rats. Male fertility is determined by premating dosing of at least 4 weeks and with dosing continuing throughout the mating period. Histopathology of the testes and sperm analysis are used to detect effects on spermatogenesis [16]. Female fertility is determined by premating dosing of at least 14 days with dosing continuing during the mating period. A mating ratio of 1 to 1 is recommended, and documentation should allow identification of both parents of a litter. Copulation is evaluated daily by vaginal smears or by observation of the copulatory plug. Day 0 of gestation is when proof of copulation is discovered. Half of the females are sacrificed at a point after midpregnancy, usually day 13 of gestation, and are examined for the number and distribution of embryos in each uterine horn, embryos undergoing resorption, and the presence of empty implantation sites. Males are sacrificed at any time after mating and assurance of successful induction of pregnancy. The other half of the females are allowed to deliver normally and the litter size, number per litter alive or dead, and any abnormal observations during gross examination are noted.

Segment II, or teratology studies, are designed to ascertain if a drug candidate has potential for embryotoicity or teratogenic effects (stages C and D) and are conducted in a rodent and nonrodent species. The drug candidate is administered during the period of organogenesis, which is usually considered gestation day 6 to 15 for mice and rats and gestation day 6 to 18 for rabbits. Fetuses are delivered by Cesarean section a day or two before anticipated parturition. For rats, half of the fetuses are examined for visceral alterations and the other half are evaluated for skeletal abnormalities. For rabbits, microdissection techniques for soft tissue alterations allow all of the fetuses to be examined for both soft tissue and skeletal abnormalities.

Segment III studies are usually conducted only in rats and are designed to evaluate effects on perinatal and postnatal development of pups and on maternal function (stages C to F). The drug candidate is administered to the dams from implantation to the end of lactation (stages C to E). At the time of weaning, normally one male and one female offspring per litter are selected for rearing to adulthood and mating to assess reproductive competence. These offspring can also be evaluated by use of behavioral and other functional tests for the study of physical development, sensory functions and reflexes, and behavior. The dams and other pups are sacrificed at the time of weaning and evaluated histopathologically.

As with most toxicology studies, three dose levels and a vehicle control group are recommended for reproductive studies. Commonly, a dose-range-finding study, which can incorporate toxicokinetic evaluation, is conducted in pregnant animals, which may be more susceptible to toxic effects, to define the dose levels, one of which should produce frank signs of toxicity and another that should be a no-toxic-effect dose. As noted earlier, drug metabolism studies are sometimes conducted to demonstrate that the dams and the fetuses have been appropriately exposed to the drug candidate and metabolites.

3. Carcinogenicity

Carcinogenicity studies encompass most of the test species' life span and are designed to measure tumor induction in animals and to assess the relevant risk in humans [17]. These studies are normally conducted concurrently with phase 3 human clinical trials and are required by regulatory agencies when human exposure to a drug candidate is anticipated to be more than 6 months. For drug candidates being developed to treat certain life-threatening diseases, carcinogenicity studies may be concluded after marketing approval but should be started during human clinical testing. Carcinogenicity studies should be initiated earlier in the drug development process when

1. The drug candidate or a known metabolite is structurally related to a known carcinogen.
2. A special aspect of the drug candidate's biological action (e.g., members of the therapeutic class have shown a positive carcinogenic response) causes concern.
3. The drug candidate produces toxicities in early studies that are indicative of preneoplastic changes.
4. The drug candidate or a metabolite shows evidence of accumulation in organ systems.
5. Mutagenicity tests suggest that the drug candidate may be a potential carcinogen.

Some companies combine chronic toxicity and carcinogenicity studies in the rat by appropriately increasing the sizes of each dose group.

Mice and rats, with life spans of approximately 18 and 24 months, respectively, are normally used in carcinogenicity studies because of the economy of these species, their susceptibility to tumor induction, and the large database available on their physiology and pathology. If other nonclinical or clinical results suggest that the rodent is an inappropriate model, carcinogenicity studies in other species, such as the dog for the development of birth control drugs, can be conducted. An ICH guideline [18] suggests that one rodent (usually the rat) carcinogenicity study plus one other study, usually a subchronic or chronic in vivo rodent study, may be sufficient to ascertain the carcinogenicity potential of a drug candidate.

When feasible, the route of exposure in the test species should be the same as the clinical route of administration. An alternative route may be used if this route gives similar metabolism and systemic exposure, particularly to relevant organs, such as the lung for inhalation agents, as the clinical route. Supportive drug metabolism and toxicokinetic data are generally required for the selection of an alternative route of administration.

Standard carcinogenicity studies are generally inappropriate for biotechnology-derived pharmaceuticals [13]. Macromolecules, unless they are endogenous substances used as replacement therapy, may need to be evaluated for carcinogenic potential if indicated by treatment duration, clinical indication, and patient population. A variety of approaches, such as the ability to support or induce proliferation of transformed cells or to simulate growth of normal or malignant cells expressing a receptor for the drug candidate, can be used to assess risk and are usually compound specific. The study designs and protocols to evaluate the carcinogenicity potential of macromolecules should be discussed with the appropriate regulatory agencies before the evaluations are initiated.

Dose selection for carcinogenicity studies has been a topic of discussion for many years. According to an ICH guideline [19], the selected doses (1) should provide a test species exposure to the drug candidate that allows an adequate margin of safety over the human therapeutic exposure, (2) are tolerated without significant chronic physiological function impairment and are compatible with good survival, (3) are guided by a comprehensive set of animal and human data that focus on the properties of the drug candidate and the suitability of the test species, and (4) permit data interpretation in the context of proposed clinical use. In all cases, appropriate dose-ranging studies, usually of 90-day duration, need to be conducted.

The approaches that may be appropriate and are acceptable for dose selection include toxicity-based endpoints such as the MTD, pharmacokinetic endpoints, saturation of absorption, pharmacodynamic endpoints, maximum feasible dose, and additional scientifically defensible endpoints. For toxicity-based endpoints, general study design characteristics to establish the MTD include that

1. The rodent species/strains with metabolic profiles as similar as possible to that of humans should be used.
2. Dose-ranging studies should be conducted for both males and females for all strains and species to be tested in the carcinogenicity bioassay.
3. Dose selection is generally determined from 90–day studies with the route and method of administration that will be used in the bioassay.
4. Selection of an appropriate dosing schedule and regimen should be based on clinical use and exposure patterns, pharmacokinetics, and practical considerations.
5. Both the toxicity profile and any dose-limiting toxicity should be characterized, with consideration given to the occurrence of preneoplastic lesions or tissue-specific proliferative effects and disturbances in endocrine homeostasis.
6. Changes in metabolite profile or alterations in metabolizing enzyme activities (induction or inhibition) over time should be understood to allow for appropriate interpretation of results from the studies.

Systemic exposure of the drug candidate in the test species that represents a large multiple of human exposure, based on the plasma concentration versus time curve (AUC), at the maximum proposed human daily dose may be used for carcinogenicity study dose selection. The AUC is the most comprehensive pharmacokinetic endpoint, because this value includes both the plasma concentrations of the drug candidate and the residence time in vivo. For pharmacokinetic endpoints to be used for dose selection, the information needed to establish the recommended 25-fold ratio of rodent to human normalized (using mg/m^2 dose levels) AUC include that

1. Rodent pharmacokinetic data are derived with the use of the test species strains, the route of administration, and dose ranges planned for the carcinogenicity study.
2. Bioanalytical chemistry methods, which have been appropriately validated, are used to determine plasma concentrations of the drug candidate in both rodents and humans.
3. Pharmacokinetic data are derived from studies of sufficient duration to take into account potential time-dependent changes in pharmacokinetic parameters, which may be detected from toxicokinetic results obtained during the dose-ranging studies.
4. Documentation is available on the similarity of metabolism between the test species and humans.
5. In the assessment of exposure, scientific judgment is used to determine whether the AUC comparison is based on data for the parent, parent and metabolite(s), or metabolite(s), and justification for the decision is provided.
6. Interspecies differences in protein binding are taken into consideration when relative exposure is estimated.
7. Human pharmacokinetic data are obtained from studies encompassing the maximum recommended human daily dose.

For saturation of absorption to be used for dose selection, information that the absorption process has been saturated using the intended route of administration is necessary. These data can usually be obtained during well-designed pharmacokinetic studies that evaluate linearity of absorption and dose proportionality using the route and frequency of dosing projected for human clinical studies.

The use of pharmacodynamic end points for high-dose selection is considered to be highly compound specific and is considered for individual study designs on the basis of scientific merit. The high dose should produce a pharmacodynamic response in the test species that precludes further dose escalation but does not produce disturbances of physiology or homeostasis that would compromise the validity of the carcinogenicity study. Examples of such pharmacodynamic endpoints include hypotension and inhibition of blood clotting.

The use of maximum feasible dose for dose selection is usually applicable only to studies using dietary administration of the drug candidate. When routes other than dietary administration are used, the high dose may be limited because of practicality and local tolerance. The use of pharmacokinetic endpoints for dose selection should significantly decrease the need to select the high dose for carcinogenicity studies based on feasibility criteria.

The mid and low doses for a carcinogenicity study are to provide information for assessing the relevance of the study findings to humans. The low dose should be equal to, or a multiple of, the maximum dose proposed for human testing. The rationale for the selection of the low and mid dose needs to be provided on the basis of pharmacokinetic linearity and saturation of metabolic pathways, human exposure and therapeutic dose, pharmacodynamic response in the test species, alteration in the normal physiology of the test species, mechanistic information and the potential for threshold effects, and the unpredictability of toxicity progression observed in other toxicology studies.

VII. CONCLUSION

This chapter has provided information on the nonclinical aspects of the drug development process. As described, the biological stages of nonclinical development normally proceed linearly (1) from drug discovery, when the pharmacology of a lead candidate is evaluated in in vitro systems and/or animal models to show that the compound has the potential to mediate a human disease, (2) to developability assessment, which provides preliminary data on the pharmacokinetics, drug delivery, and toxicology of the discovery lead to ascertain if the compound has the necessary attributes and without substantial demerits to enter the drug development process, (3) to preclinical evaluations, when the necessary drug safety studies are conducted to support the submission of an IND, and (4) finally to nonclinical studies, which extend information on the metabolism and toxicity of the drug candidate and show that the earlier animal studies are predictive of human pharmacological and toxicological responses. Careful design, conduct, and interpretation of the results from these nonclinical research experiments normally determine which discovery leads have the necessary attributes to become marketed human therapeutic products. These experiments can be used to weed out those candidates that have unacceptable pharmacology or toxicology profiles before, or shortly after, the initiation of human clinical testing, but definitely before the start of phase 3 clinical studies, which are the most expensive aspect of drug development in terms of both time and dollars (Fig. 1). If most, or at least many, of the estimated 999 out of 1,000 "loser" candidates can be detected earlier in the drug development process and dropped from further evaluation, the precious time and resources needed to support clinical and nonclinical drug development studies can be devoted to drug candidates that have a greater potential of successfully completing the studies necessary for the submission of an NDA.

REFERENCES

1. Lakings DB. Making a successful transition from drug discovery to drug development. Part 1. Biopharm 1995; 87:20–24.
2. Lakings DB. Making a successful transition from drug discovery to drug development. Part 2. Biopharm 1995; 88:48–51.
3. Karnes HT, Shiu G, Shah VP. Validation of bioanalytical methods. Pharm Res 1991; 84:421–426.
4. Shah VP. Analytical methods validation: bioavailability, bioequivalence and pharmacokinetic studies. Pharm Res 1992; 94:588–592.
5. U.S. FDA's proposed implementation of ICH safety working group consensus regarding new drug applications. Federal Register. Vol. 57. No. 73. 15 April 1992; 13105–13106.
6. ICH Harmonised Tripartite Guideline (Q2A). Text on validation of analytical procedures. 27 October 1994.
7. ICH Harmonised Tripartite Guideline (Q2B). Validation of analytical procedures: methodology. 6 November 1996.
8. ICH Harmonised Tripartite Guideline (M3). Nonclinical safety studies for the conduct of human clinical trials for pharmaceuticals. 16 July 1997.
9. ICH Harmonised Tripartite Guideline (S2A). Guidance on specific aspects of regulatory genotoxicity tests for pharmaceuticals. 19 July 1995.
10. ICH Harmonised Tripartite Guideline (S2B). Genotoxicity: a standard battery for genotoxicity testing of pharmaceuticals. 16 July 1997.
11. ICH Harmonised Tripartite Guideline (S7). Safety pharmacology studies for human pharmaceuticals. 13 July 2001.
12. ICH Harmonised Tripartite Guideline (S3A). Note for guidance on toxicokinetics: the assessment of systemic exposure in toxicity studies. 27 October 1994.
13. ICH Harmonised Tripartite Guideline (S6). Preclinical safety evaluation of biotechnology-derived pharmaceuticals. 16 July 1997.
14. ICH Harmonised Tripartite Guideline (S3B). Pharmacokinetics: guidance for repeated dose tissue distribution studies. 27 October 1994.
15. ICH Harmonised Tripartite Guideline (S5A). Detection of toxicity to reproduction for medicinal products. 24 June 1993.

16. ICH Harmonised Tripartite Guideline (S5B). Toxicity to male fertility: an addendum to the ICH Tripartite Guideline on detection of toxicity to reproduction for medicinal products. 29 November 1995.

17. ICH Harmonised Tripartite Guideline (S1A). Guidelines on the need for carcinogenicity studies of pharmaceuticals. 29 November 1995.

18. ICH Harmonised Tripartite Guideline (S1B). Testing for carcinogenicity of pharmaceuticals. 16 July 1997.

19. ICH Harmonised Tripartite Guideline (S1C). Dose selection for carcinogenicity studies of pharmaceuticals. 27 October 1994.

3

The Investigational New Drug Application and the Investigator's Brochure

William M. Troetel
Regulatory Affairs Consultant, Mount Vernon, New York, U.S.A.

I. OVERVIEW

The Federal Food, Drug and Cosmetic Act prohibits the shipment of a new drug into interstate commerce unless there exists for that drug an approved NDA or an effective IND application. Unlike certain European countries, such as Germany and the United Kingdom, the existence of an IND is required regardless of the proposed phase of clinical trial. Thus even phase 1 trials to be conducted in the United States on volunteer subjects require the prior submission of an IND before that trial may be undertaken.

The requirements for the format and content of the IND application, as well as the requirements governing the use of the IND, are provided in Title 21 of the Code of Federal Regulations (21 CFR), Section 312. Unlike an NDA, the FDA does not formally "approve" an IND submission. If the FDA reviewers believe that the proposed clinical trial(s) submitted in the IND are acceptable from a safety and risk versus benefit viewpoint, the IND is "in effect," and the compound that is the subject of that IND may be shipped in interstate commerce for the purpose of conducting specific clinical trials. Drugs shipped under an IND have specific labeling requirements, and false or misleading statements, as well as any claims regarding safety and efficacy, are prohibited.

This chapter will provide information that is necessary to achieve a successful IND submission to the FDA. It will focus on the differences between the requirements for an IND submitted to permit a phase 1 trial as contrasted to IND submissions intended to support phase 2 or 3 clinical research. Finally, it will also detail the requirements for the investigator's brochure, the document that summarizes the known safety and efficacy information about the drug that will be submitted to potential investigators and to IRBs and as part of the IND document itself.

II. THE INVESTIGATIONAL NEW DRUG APPLICATION

A. Introduction

An IND may be submitted to the FDA by a commercial organization (the "sponsor") or by a clinical investigator (the "investigator"). The sponsor or investigator may not commercially distribute or test market an investigational new drug, nor may an investigation be unduly prolonged after the finding that the results of the investigation appear to establish sufficient data to support a marketing application. Under certain defined circumstances described in 21 CFR Part 312.7, a sponsor may charge the patient for an investigational drug, but this is atypical and can be done only after written approval from the FDA.

B. General Information Regarding INDs

1. Exemptions

The clinical investigation of a drug product that is lawfully marketed in the United States is exempt from the requirements of an IND providing all of the following apply: (1) the investigation is neither intended to be reported to the FDA as a well-controlled study in support of a new indication for use nor to be used to support any other significant change in the labeling for the drug, (2) if the drug that is undergoing investigation is lawfully marketed as a prescription drug product, the investigation is not intended to support a significant change in the advertising for the product, (3) the investigation does not involve a route of administration nor dosage level or use in a patient population or other factor that significantly increases the risks (or decreases the acceptability of the risks) associated with the use of the drug product, and (4) the investigation is conducted in compliance with the requirements for institutional review approval and the requirements for informed consent as discussed elsewhere in this book.

2. Labeling Requirements for an Investigational New Drug

Labeling for a drug covered by an IND will be discussed under the Chemistry, Manufacturing, and Control requirements for part 7 of the IND; however, independent of the use or indication for the drug and independent of the dosage form, all immediate packages of drug product supplied to a patient involved in an investigational trial require the following statement: "Caution: New Drug—Limited by Federal (or United States) law to investigational use." Additionally, the label or labeling (including the investigator's brochure) shall not bear any statement that is false or misleading possibly to represent the investigational new drug as being safe or effective for the purposes for which it is being investigated.

3. Waivers

In rare instances, the FDA may grant a waiver to the requirements for an IND on the basis of a justified request from the sponsor. Acceptable justification may include an explanation of why the sponsor's compliance is unnecessary or cannot be achieved or a description of an alternative means of satisfying the requirement. The FDA may grant such a request for a waiver if it determines that the sponsor's noncompliance would not pose a significant or unreasonable risk to the human test subjects.

4. Preconsultation Program

At this time, only one division within the Center for Drug Evaluation and Research, the Division of Antiviral Drug Products (DAVDP), has established a pre-IND consultation program. This program, established in 1988, is a proactive strategy designed to facilitate informal early communications between DAVDP and the potential sponsor of new therapeutics for the treatment of AIDS and life-threatening opportunistic infections, other viral infections, and soft tissue transplantations. Pre-IND advice may be requested for issues related to drug development plans, data needed to support the rationale for testing a drug in humans, the design of nonclinical pharmacology, toxicology, and drug activity studies, data requirements for IND applications, and regulatory requirements for demonstrating safety and efficacy. Details on requesting information about this program or on how to participate in this preconsultation program may be found on the internet.

For INDs to be submitted to other divisions, on the sponsor's request, the FDA will provide advice on specific matters relating to an IND. Examples may include advice on the adequacy of technical data to support an investigational plan, on the design of a clinical trial, and on whether proposed investigations are likely to produce the data and information needed to meet requirements for a marketing application. It should be noted, however, that unless the communication is accompanied by a clinical hold, FDA communications with a sponsor regarding pre-IND information is solely advisory and does not require any modification in the planned or ongoing clinical investigations or response to the agency.

5. Binders for IND Submissions

The FDA has specific requirements for the type and color of binders in which an IND may be submitted. All INDs and IND amendments are submitted to FDA in triplicate. The original IND submission (copy 1) is to be submitted in a red binder, and copies 2 and 3 are submitted in green and orange binders, respectively. Effective April 1, 1998, sponsors may contact the U.S. Government Printing Office (GPO) to order FDA IND, NDA, ANDA, and Drug Master File binders. The red binder is Form No. 2675, and the green and orange binders are Forms No. 2675a and 2675b, respectively. The GPO may be contacted by telephone at (202) 512-1800 or by mail at U.S. Government Printing Office, Washington, DC 20404-0001. In either instance, reference should be made to Program #B511-S. Details on the required specifications for the FDA's binders may also be obtained from the internet at http://www. fda.gov/cder/ddms/binders.htm.

6. Address for IND Submissions

An initial IND submission is to be sent in triplicate to the Central Document Room, Center for Drug Evaluation and Research, Food and Drug Administration, Park Building, Room 214, 12420 Parklawn Drive, Rockville, Maryland 20852. Upon receipt of the IND, the FDA will inform the sponsor which one of the divisions in the Center for Drug Evaluation and Research or the Center for Biologics Evaluation and Research is responsible for the IND.

Once the IND is in effect, amendments, reports, and other correspondence relating to matters covered by the IND should be directed to the appropriate division. The outside wrapper or cover letter of each submission should state what is contained in the submission, for example "IND Application," "Protocol Amendment," etc.

Specific address information relating to submission of applications for products subject to the licensing provisions of the Public Health Service Act of July 1, 1944, urokinase products, plasma volume expanders, coupled antibodies, and biological products that are also radioactive drugs are described in 21 CFR Part 312.140.

7. Availability for Public Disclosure of IND Data

The manner in which the FDA handles requests for disclosure of information to the public under the Freedom of Information Act is described in 21 CFR Part 312.130. The existence of an IND will not be disclosed by the FDA unless it has previously been publicly disclosed or acknowledged by the sponsor. However, upon request, the FDA will disclose to an individual to whom an investigational new drug has been given a copy of any IND safety report relating to the use in the individual.

C. Phases of Clinical Investigations

As noted previously, the FDA has clarified the requirements for an IND intended for phase 1 clinical trials compared with trials that are designed for phase 2 or 3 clinical programs. Table 1 provides information regarding the differences between the phases of investigation with respect to the size and scope of the particular phase. A more detailed description of the phases of investigation may be found in 21 CFR Part 312.21.

Phase 1 includes the initial introduction of an investigational new drug into humans. These studies are typically closely monitored and may be conducted in patients or in normal volunteer subjects. They are designed to determine the metabolism and pharmacological actions of the drug in humans and the side effects associated with increasing doses and sometimes to gain early evidence on effectiveness. The results of the phase 1 program concerning the drug's pharmacokinetic and pharmacological effects will be obtained to permit the design of well-controlled and scientifically valid phase 2 trials.

Phase 2 includes the controlled clinical studies conducted to evaluate the appropriate dose range and effectiveness of the drug for a particular indication in patients with the disease or condition under study and to determine the common short-term side effects and risks associated with the drug. Phase 2 studies are typically well controlled, closely monitored, and conducted in a relatively small number of patients, usually involving no more than several hundred subjects.

Table 1 Phases of Clinical Investigation

Phase	Number of patients	Length	Purpose	Percent of drugs successfully tested[*]
1	20–200	Several months	Mainly safety	70%
2	Up to several hundred	Several months to 2 years	Some short-term safety, dosage and effectiveness	33%
3	Several hundred to several thousand	1 to 4 years	Safety, dosage and effectiveness	25–30%

[*]For example, of 100 drugs for which IND applications are submitted to the FDA, about 70 will successfully complete phase 1 trials and go on to phase 2; about 33 of the original 100 will complete phase 2 and go to phase 3; and 25 to 30 percent of the original 100 will clear phase 3 (and, on average, about 20 of the original 100 will ultimately be approved for marketing).

Expanded controlled and uncontrolled trials comprise the phase 3 program. They are performed after preliminary evidence suggesting a knowledge of the proper dosage and effectiveness of the drug has been obtained and are intended to gather the additional information about effectiveness and safety needed to evaluate the overall benefit–risk relationship of the drug and to provide an adequate basis for physician labeling.

1. Phase 1

INDs for Phase 1 Studies. The FDA has assessed means to increase the efficiency of the drug development process without sacrificing the long-standing safety and efficacy standards expected by the public for their drug products to meet.

In November 1995, CDER and CBER issued a Guidance for Industry entitled Content and Format of Investigational New Drug Applications for Phase 1 Studies of Drugs, Including Well-Characterized, Therapeutic, Biotechnology-Derived Products. This guidance clarified the requirements for data and data presentation related to the initial entry into human studies in the United States of an investigational drug, including well-characterized therapeutic bio-technology-derived products. The FDA emphasized that the IND regulations allowed a great deal of flexibility in the amount and depth of various data to be submitted in an IND, depending in large part on the phase of investigation and the specific human testing being proposed. In some cases, the extent of that flexibility had not been appreciated by industry. Thus the guidance was developed to clarify many of the phase 1 IND requirements to help expedite the entry of new drugs into clinical testing by increasing transparency and by reducing ambiguity, inconsistencies, and the amount of information submitted, while providing the FDA with the data it needs to assess the safety of the proposed phase 1 study. According to the guidance, if the suggestions specified in the document are followed, typical IND submissions for phase 1 studies usually should not be larger than two to three 3-inch binders.

The most significant clarifications in the guidance document are (1) the explicit willingness of the FDA to accept an integrated summary report of toxicology findings based on the unaudited draft toxicologic reports of completed animal studies as initial support for human studies, and (2) specific manufacturing data appropriate for a phase 1 investigation. Because of the manufacturing and toxicological differences between well-characterized therapeutic biotechnology-derived products and other biological products, the FDA emphasized that the guidance applies only to drugs and well-characterized therapeutic biotechnology-derived products. For products not covered by this phase 1 guidance, it is recommended that the center responsible for the product be contacted for specific information.

Requirements for Protocols. The regulation requires submission of a copy of the protocol for the conduct of each proposed clinical trial. However, the regulations were changed in 1987 specifically to allow phase 1 study protocols to be less detailed and more flexible than protocols for phase 2 or 3 studies. This change recognized that these protocols are part of an early learning process and should be adaptable as information is obtained, and that the principal concern at this stage of development is that the study be conducted safely. The regulations state that phase 1 protocols should be directed primarily at providing an outline of the investigation: an estimate of the number of subjects to be included; a description of safety exclusions; and a description of the dosing plan, including duration, dose, or method to be used in determining dose. In addition, such protocols should specify in detail only those elements of the study that are critical to subject safety, such as (1) necessary monitoring of vital signs and blood chemistries, and (2) toxicity-based stopping or dose adjustment rules. The regulations also state that modifications of the experimental design of phase 1 studies that do not affect critical safety assessments are required to be reported to FDA only in the IND Annual Report.

Requirements for CMC Information. The IND regulations emphasize the graded nature of manufacturing and control information that is required to be submitted. Although in each phase of the investigation, sufficient information should be submitted to assure the proper identification, quality, purity, and strength of the investigational drug, the amount of information needed to make that assurance will vary with the phase of the investigation, the proposed duration of the investigation, the dosage form, and the amount of information otherwise available. For example, although stability data are required in all phases of the IND to demonstrate that the new drug substance and drug product are within acceptable chemical and physical limits for the planned duration of the proposed clinical investigation, if very short-term tests are proposed, the supporting stability data also can be very limited.

It is recognized that modifications to the method of preparation of the new drug substance and dosage form, and even changes in the dosage form itself, are likely as the investigation progresses. Emphasis in an initial phase 1 CMC submission should generally be placed on providing information that will allow evaluation of the safety of subjects in the proposed study. The identification of a safety concern or insufficient data to make an evaluation of safety is the only basis for a clinical hold based on the CMC section.

Reasons for concern may include (1) a product made with unknown or impure components, (2) a product possessing chemical structures of known or highly likely toxicity, (3) a product that cannot remain chemically stable throughout the testing program proposed, (4) a product with an impurity

profile indicative of a potential health hazard or an impurity profile insufficiently defined to assess a potential health hazard, or (5) a poorly characterized master or working cell bank. In addition, for preclinical studies to be
useful in assuring the safety of human studies, sponsors should be able to
relate the drug product being proposed for use in a clinical study to the drug
product used in the animal toxicology studies that support the safety of the
proposed human study. The following information will usually suffice for a
meaningful review of the manufacturing procedures for drug products used in
phase 1 clinical studies. As will be discussed later in this chapter, additional
information should ordinarily be submitted for review of the larger scale
manufacturing procedures used to produce drug products for phase 2 or 3
clinical trials or as part of the manufacturing section of an NDA.

The CMC Section Introduction. At the beginning of this section, the
sponsor should state whether it believes (1) the chemistry of either the drug
substance or the drug product, or (2) the manufacturing of either the drug
substance or the drug product, presents any signals of potential human risk. If
so, these signals of potential risks should be discussed. The steps proposed to
monitor for such risk(s) should be described or the reason(s) why the signal(s)
should be dismissed should be discussed. In addition, sponsors should
describe any chemistry and manufacturing differences between the drug product proposed for clinical use and the drug product used in the animal
toxicology trials that formed the basis for the sponsor's conclusion that it
was safe to proceed with the proposed clinical study. How these differences
might affect the safety profile of the drug product should be discussed. If there
are no differences in the products, that should be stated.

The Drug Substance. It should be noted that references to the current
edition of the USP-NF may be used to satisfy some of the requirements of this
section, when applicable. Information on the drug substance should be submitted in a summary report containing the following items:

1. Description: A brief description of the drug substance and some
evidence to support its proposed chemical structure should be submitted. It is
understood that the amount of structure information will be limited in the
early stage of drug development.
2. The name and address of its manufacturer: The full street address of
the manufacturer of the clinical trial drug substance should be submitted.
3. Method of preparation: A brief description of the manufacturing
process, including a list of the reagents, solvents, and catalysts used, should be
submitted. A detailed flow diagram is suggested as the usual most effective
presentation of this information. However, more information may be needed
to assess the safety of biotechnology-derived drugs or drugs extracted from
human or animal sources.

4. Tests and analytical methods: A brief description of the test methods used should be submitted. Proposed acceptable limits supported by simple analytical data (e.g., IR spectrum to prove the identity and HPLC chromatograms to support the purity level and impurities profile) of the clinical trials material should be provided. Submission of a copy of the certificate of analysis is also suggested. The specific methods will depend on the source and type of drug substance (e.g., animal source, plant extract, radiopharmaceutical,other biotechnology-derived products). Validation data and established specifications ordinarily need not be submitted at the initial stage of drug development. However, for some well-characterized therapeutic biotechnology-derived products, preliminary specifications and additional validation data may be needed in certain circumstances to ensure safety in phase 1.

5. Stability data: A brief description of the stability study and the test methods used to monitor the stability of the drug substance should be submitted. Preliminary tabular data based on representative material may be submitted. Neither detailed stability data nor the stability protocol should be submitted.

The Drug Product. It should be noted that references to the current edition of the USP-NF may be used to satisfy some of the requirements of this section, when applicable. Information on the drug product should be submitted in a summary report containing the following items:

1. A list of all components: A list of usually no more than one or two pages of written information should be submitted. The quality (e.g., NF, ACS) of the inactive ingredients should be cited. For novel excipients, additional manufacturing information may be necessary.

2. Quantitative composition: A brief summary of the composition of the investigational new drug product should be submitted. In most cases, information on component ranges is not necessary.

3. The name and address of the manufacturer: The full street address(es) of the manufacturer(s) and packager of the clinical trial drug product should be submitted.

4. Method of manufacturing and packaging: A diagrammatic presentation and a brief written description of the manufacturing process should be submitted, including the sterilization process for sterile products. Flow diagrams are suggested as the usual most effective presentations of this information.

5. Acceptable limits and analytical methods: A brief description of the proposed acceptable limits and the test methods used should be submitted. Tests that should be submitted will vary according to the dosage form. For example, for sterile products, sterility and nonpyrogenicity tests should be submitted. Submission of a copy of the certificate of analysis of the clinical

batch is also suggested. Validation data and established specifications need not be submitted at the initial stage of drug development. For well-characterized therapeutic biotechnology-derived products, adequate assessment of bioactivity and preliminary specifications should be available.

6. Stability testing: A brief description of the stability study and the test methods used to monitor the stability of the drug product packaged in the proposed container/closure system and storage conditions should be submitted. Preliminary tabular data based on representative material may be submitted. Neither detailed stability data nor the stability protocol need to be submitted.

7. Placebo: If any placebo dosage form is to be used in the phase 1 trial, diagrammatic, tabular, and brief written information should be submitted.

8. Labeling: A mock-up or printed representation of the proposed labeling that will be provided to investigators in the proposed clinical trial should be submitted. Investigational labels must carry a "caution" statement as stated earlier. The required statement reads "Caution: New Drug— Limited by Federal (or United States) law to investigational use."

9. Environmental assessment: The FDA believes that the great majority of products will qualify for a categorical exclusion. Sponsors who believe that their investigational product meets the exclusion categories under 21 CFR 25.24 should submit a statement certifying that their product meets the exclusion requirements and request a categorical exclusion on that basis. (For INDs submitted to CDER, it is recommended to review the FDA guidance entitled Guidance for Industry for the Submission of Environmental Assessments for Human Drug Applications and Supplements, November, 1995.)

Pharmacology and Toxicology Information. Pharmacology and drug distribution: This section of the phase 1 IND should contain, if known, (a) a description of the pharmacological effects and mechanism of action of the drug in animals, and (b) information on the absorption, distribution, metabolism, and excretion of the drug. The regulations do not describe the presentation of these data. A summary report, without individual animal records or individual study results, usually suffices. In most circumstances, five pages or less should be adequate for this summary. To the extent that such studies may be important to address safety issues or to assist in evaluation of toxicology data, they may be necessary; however, lack of this potential effectiveness information generally should not be a reason for a phase 1 IND to be placed on clinical hold.

Toxicology—integrated summary: The IND regulations require an integrated summary of the toxicological effects of the drug in animals and in vitro. The particular studies needed depend on the nature of the drug and the phase of human investigation. The regulations are not specific as to the nature of the report of toxicology data needed in an IND submission and the nature of the study reports upon which the report submitted to the IND is based. Also, the IND regulations are silent on whether the submitted material should be based on (1) "final, fully quality-assured" individual study reports, or (2) earlier, unaudited draft toxicological reports of the completed studies. In the past, most sponsors have concluded that a submission based on final fully quality-assured individual study reports is required, and a substantial delay in submission of an IND for several months is often encountered to complete such final fully quality-assured individual reports from the time the unaudited draft toxicological reports of the completed studies are prepared.

Moreover, although the regulation does not specifically require individual toxicology study reports to be submitted, referring only to an integrated summary of the toxicological findings, the requirement for a full tabulation of data from each study suitable for detailed review has led most sponsors to provide detailed reports of each study.

Although the GLP and quality assurance processes and principles are critical for the maintenance of a toxicology study system that is valid and credible, it is unusual for findings in the unaudited draft toxicologic report of the completed studies to change during the production of the "final" quality-assured individual study reports in ways important to determining whether use in humans is safe. Therefore, for a phase 1 IND, if final fully quality-assured individual study reports are not available at the time of IND submission, an integrated summary report of toxicological findings based on the unaudited draft toxicological reports of the completed animal studies may be submitted. This integrated summary report should represent the sponsor's evaluation of the animal studies that formed the basis for the sponsor's decision that the proposed human studies are safe. It is expected that the unaudited draft reports that formed the basis of this decision might undergo minor modifications during final review and quality assurance auditing. Full toxicology reports and individual study reports should be available to the FDA, upon request, as final fully quality-assured documents within 120 days of the start of the human study for which the animal study formed part of the safety conclusion basis. These final reports should contain in the introduction any changes from those reported in the integrated summary. If there are no changes, that should be clearly stated at the beginning of the final fully quality-assured report.

If the integrated summary is based upon unaudited draft reports, sponsors should submit an update to their integrated summary by 120 days after the start of the human studies identifying any differences found in the preparation of the final fully quality-assured study reports and the information submitted in the initial integrated summary. If no differences were found, that should be stated in the integrated summary update. In addition, any new finding discovered during the preparation of the final fully quality-assured individual study reports that could affect subject safety must be reported to the FDA as an IND safety report.

Usually, 10 to 15 pages of text with additional tables as needed should suffice for the integrated summary. It should represent a perspective on the completed animal studies at the time the sponsor decided that human trials were appropriate. Use of visual data displays (e.g., box plots, histograms, or distributions of laboratory results over time) will facilitate description of the findings of these trials. The summary document should be accurate contemporaneously with the IND submission (i.e., it should be updated so that if new information or findings from the completed animal studies have become known since the sponsor's decision that the proposed human study is safe, such new information should also be included in the submitted summary).

The integrated summary of the toxicological findings of the completed animal studies to support the safety of the proposed phase 1 human investigation should ordinarily contain the following information:

1.   A brief description of the design of the trials, dates of performance, and any deviations from the design in the conduct of the trials. Reference to the study protocol and protocol amendments may be adequate for some of this information.

2.   A systematic presentation of the findings from the animal toxicology and toxicokinetic studies. Those findings that an experienced expert would reasonably consider as possible signals of human risk should be highlighted. The format of this part of the summary may be approached from a "systems review" perspective (e.g., CNS, cardiovascular, pulmonary, gastrointestinal, renal, hepatic, genitourinary, hematopoietic, immunologic, and dermal). If a product's effects on a particular body system have not been assessed, that should be noted. If any well-documented toxicologic "signal" is not considered evidence of human risk, the reason should be given. In addition, the sponsor should note whether these findings are discussed in the Investigator's Brochure.

3.   Identification and qualifications of the individual(s) who evaluated the animal safety data and concluded that it is reasonably safe to begin the proposed human study. This person(s) should sign the summary attesting that it accurately reflects the animal toxicology data from the completed studies.

4.   A statement of where the animal studies were conducted and where the records of the studies are available for inspection, should an inspection occur.

5.   A declaration that each study subject to GLP regulations was performed in full compliance with GLPs or, if the study was not conducted in compliance with those regulations, a brief statement of the reason for the

noncompliance and the sponsor's view on how such noncompliance might affect the interpretation of the findings.

It should be noted that the information described in the last three points may be supplied as part of the integrated summary or as part of the full data tabulations described in the next section.

Toxicology—full data tabulation: The sponsor should submit, for each animal toxicology study that is intended to support the safety of the proposed clinical investigation, a full tabulation of data suitable for detailed review. This should consist of line listings of the individual data points, including laboratory data points, for each animal in these trials along with summary tabulations of these data points. To allow interpretation of the line listings, accompanying the line listings should be either (1) a brief (usually a few pages) description (i.e., a technical report or abstract including a methods description section) of the study, or (2) a copy of the study protocol and amendments.

In conclusion, this section has been included to assist sponsors who are preparing an IND submission for a phase 1 trial in the United States. Emphasis was provided on the requirements for submission of chemistry and manufacturing data for the drug substance and the drug product, and for information to be submitted regarding the pharmacological and toxicological assessments of the new drug candidate. If a sponsor has conducted phase 1 trials outside of the United States and believes that there are adequate human safety studies already available, it may not be necessary to conduct any phase 1 trials in the United States. In such a case, the sponsor would prepare an IND and include in the initial IND submission a clinical protocol for phase 2 or 3. This IND, because it will involve exposure of more patients to the drug for the purposes of safety testing as well as efficacy evaluations, will require a greater level and depth of manufacturing and nonclinical data. The next section will describe the requirements for such an advanced-stage IND.

2. Phase 2 or Phase 3

As noted in the previous section, the FDA's review of phase 1 submissions focuses on assessing the safety of those investigations. The review by the FDA for submissions of phase 2 and 3 trials will also include an assessment of the scientific quality of the clinical investigations and the likelihood that the investigations will yield data capable of meeting statutory standards for marketing approval.

The central focus of the initial IND submission will be on the general investigational plan and the protocols for specific human studies. Subsequent amendments to the IND that contain new or revised protocols should build logically on previous submissions and should be supported by additional information, including the results of animal toxicology studies or other human studies as appropriate. Annual reports to the IND will serve as the focus for reporting the status of studies being conducted under the IND and should update the general investigational plan for the coming year.

An IND goes into effect 30 days after the FDA receives the IND, unless the FDA notifies the sponsor that the investigations described in the IND are subject to a clinical hold. It is possible, but not usual, that there may be earlier notification by the FDA that the clinical investigations in the IND may begin. When the initial IND is filed, the FDA will notify the sponsor in writing of the date it receives the IND.

A sponsor may ship an investigational new drug to investigators named in the IND (1) 30 days after the FDA receives the IND, or (2) on earlier FDA authorization to ship the drug. Of course, an investigator may not administer an investigational new drug to human subjects until the IND goes into effect and there is compliance with the applicable requirements for the protection of human subjects, as described by the IRB and IC regulations.

Form FDA 1571. The initial IND and each amendment to the IND is to be submitted in triplicate and to include a completed copy of the 2-page form FDA 1571. A copy of this form is shown in Fig. 1. This form and many other FDA forms may be downloaded from the internet at http://forms.psc.dhhs.gov/fdaforms.htm.

The form contains 20 subitems, each of which must be completed. Items 1, 2, 3, 4, 7, 8, 14, 15, 18, 19, and 20 are self evident and need no further elaboration. Comments on the remaining items are justified.

Item 5 requires the name of the drug. It is cautioned that all names and codes that appear in the IND documentation be added to this space. It is not uncommon that, in the very early stages of preclinical development, a code name is used. As the drug advances in the preclinical stage, a generic name or modified code name may be used. If the early pharmacology or toxicology reports refer to the drug by the earlier code name, this too should be included in item 5.

Item 6, the IND number, will not be inserted at the time of the submission of the initial IND filing. Once the IND is filed, the FDA will assign an IND number, and the sponsor will be notified in writing of this number. From that point forward, every communication between the sponsor and the FDA should include this IND number.

A list of numbers of all referenced applications is needed in item 9. This list will include any referenced drug master files or references to other existing INDs or NDAs on file with the FDA. If the CMC section of the IND refers to the DMF of a container manufacturer for a particular container–closure system, the DMF number and, if possible, the specific pages within that DMF

DEPARTMENT OF HEALTH AND HUMAN SERVICES PUBLIC HEALTH SERVICE FOOD AND DRUG ADMINISTRATION **INVESTIGATIONAL NEW DRUG APPLICATION (IND)** *(TITLE 21, CODE OF FEDERAL REGULATIONS (CFR) PART 312)*	*Form Approved:* OMB No. 0910-0014. *Expiration Date: January 31, 2006* *See OMB Statement on Reverse.* **NOTE:** No drug may be shipped or clinical investigation begun until an IND for that investigation is in effect (21 CFR 312.40).

1. NAME OF SPONSER	2. DATE OF SUBMISSION
3. ADDRESS *(Number, Street, City, State and Zip Code)*	4. TELEPHONE NUMBER *(Include Area Code)*
5. NAME(S) OF DRUG *(Include all available names: Trade, Generic, Chemical, Code)*	6. IND NUMBER *(If previously assigned)*

7. INDICATION(S) *(Covered by this submission)*

8. PHASE(S) OF CLINICAL INVESTIGATION TO BE CONDUCTED:
☐ PHASE 1   ☐ PHASE 2   ☐ PHASE 3   ☐ OTHER _____
(Specify)

9. LIST NUMBERS OF ALL INVESTIGATIONAL NEW DRUG APPLICATIONS *(21 CFR Part 312)*, NEW DRUG OR ANTIBIOTIC APPLICATIONS *(21 CFR Part 314)*, DRUG MASTER FILES *(21 CFR Part 314.420)*, AND PRODUCT LICENSE APPLICATIONS *(21 CFR Part 601)* REFERRED TO IN THIS APPLICATION.

10. *IND submission should be consecutively numbered. The initial IND should be numbered "Serial number: 0000." The next submission (e.g., amendment, report, or correspondence) should be numbered "Serial Number: 0001." Subsequent submissions should be numbered consecutively in the order in which they are submitted.*	SERIAL NUMBER ___ ___ ___ ___

11. THIS SUBMISSION CONTAINS THE FOLLOWING: *(Check all that apply)*

☐ INITIAL INVESTIGATIONAL NEW DRUG APPLICATION (IND)   ☐ RESPONSE TO CLINICAL HOLD

PROTOCOL AMENDMENT(S):	INFORMATION AMENDMENT(S):	IND SAFETY REPORT(S):
☐ NEW PROTOCOL	☐ CHEMISTRY/MICROBIOLOGY	☐ INITIAL WRITTEN REPORT
☐ CHANGE IN PROTOCOL	☐ PHARMACOLOGY/TOXICOLOGY	☐ FOLLOW-UP TO A WRITTEN REPORT
☐ NEW INVESTIGATOR	☐ CLINICAL	

☐ RESPONSE TO FDA REQUEST FOR INFORMATION   ☐ ANNUAL REPORT   ☐ GENERAL CORRESPONDENCE

☐ REQUEST FOR REINSTATEMENT OF IND THAT IS WITHDRAWN, INACTIVATED, TERMINATED OR DISCONTINUED   ☐ OTHER _____
(Specify)

CHECK ONLY IF APPLICABLE

JUSTIFICATION STATEMENT MUST BE SUBMITTED WITH APPLICATION FOR ANY CHECKED BELOW. REFER TO THE CITED CFR SECTION FOR FURTHER INFORMATION.

☐ TREATMENT IND 21 CFR 312.35(b)   ☐ TREATMENT PROTOCOL 21 CFR 312.35(a)   ☐ CHARGE REQUEST/NOTIFICATION 21 CFR312.7(d)

FOR FDA USE ONLY

CDR/DBIND/DGD RECEIPT STAMP	DDR RECEIPT STAMP	DIVISION ASSIGNMENT:
		IND NUMBER ASSIGNED:

FORM FDA 1571 (1/03)   PREVIOUS EDITION IS OBSOLETE.   PAGE 1 OF 1

Figure 1 FDA Form 1571.

12. **CONTENTS OF APPLICATION**
This application contains the following items: *(Check all that apply)*

☐ 1. Form FDA 1571 *[21 CFR 312.23(a)(1)]*

☐ 2. Table of Contents *[21 CFR 312.23(a)(2)]*

☐ 3. Introductory statement *[21 CFR 312.23(a)(3)]*

☐ 4. General Investigational plan *[21 CFR 312.23(a)(3)]*

☐ 5. Investigator's brochure *[21 CFR 312.23(a)(5)]*

☐ 6. Protocol(s) *[21 CFR 312.23(a)(6)]*

    ☐ a. Study protocol(s) *[21 CFR 312.23(a)(6)]*

    ☐ b. Investigator data *[21 CFR 312.23(a)(6)(iii)(b)]* or completed Form(s) FDA 1572

    ☐ c. Facilities data *[21 CFR 312.23(a)(6)(iii)(b)]* or completed Form(s) FDA 1572

    ☐ d. Institutional Review Board data *[21 CFR 312.23(a)(6)(iii)(b)]* or completed Form(s) FDA 1572

☐ 7. Chemistry, manufacturing, and control data *[21 CFR 312.23(a)(7)]*

    ☐ Environmental assessment or claim for exclusion *[21 CFR 312.23(a)(7)(iv)(e)]*

☐ 8. Pharmacology and toxicology data *[21 CFR 312.23(a)(8)]*

☐ 9. Previous human experience *[21 CFR 312.23(a)(9)]*

☐ 10. Additional information *[21 CFR 312.23(a)(10)]*

13. IS ANY PART OF THE CLINICAL STUDY TO BE CONDUCTED BY A CONTRACT RESEARCH ORGANIZATION? ☐ YES ☐ NO

IF YES, WILL ANY SPONSOR OBLIGATIONS BE TRANSFERRED TO THE CONTRACT RESEARCH ORGANIZATION? ☐ YES ☐ NO

IF YES, ATTACH A STATEMENT CONTAINING THE NAME AND ADDRESS OF THE CONTRACT RESEARCH ORGANIZATION, IDENTIFICATION OF THE CLINICAL STUDY, AND A LISTING OF THE OBLIGATIONS TRANSFERRED.

14. NAME AND TITLE OF THE PERSON RESPONSIBLE FOR MONITORING THE CONDUCT AND PROGRESS OF THE CLINICAL INVESTIGATIONS

15. NAME(S) AND TITLE(S) OF THE PERSON(S) RESPONSIBLE FOR REVIEW AND EVALUATION OF INFORMATION RELEVANT TO THE SAFETY OF THE DRUG

I agree not to begin clinical investigations until 30 days after FDA's receipt of the IND unless I receive earlier notification by FDA that the studies may begin. I also agree not to begin or continue clinical investigations covered by the IND if those studies are placed on clinical hold. I agree that an Institutional Review Board (IRB) that complies with the requirements set fourth in 21 CFR Part 56 will be responsible for initial and continuing review and approval of each of the studies in the proposed clinical investigation. I agree to conduct the investigation in accordance with all other applicable regulatory requirements.

16. NAME OF SPONSOR OR SPONSOR'S AUTHORIZED REPRESENTATIVE	17. SIGNATURE OF SPONSOR OR SPONSOR'S AUTHORIZED REPRESENTATIVE	
18. ADDRESS *(Number, Street, City, State and Zip Code)*	19. TELEPHONE NUMBER *(Include Area Code)*	20. DATE

(WARNING: A willfully false statement is a criminal offense. U.S.C. Title 18, Sec. 1001.)

Public reporting burden for this collection of information is estimated to average 100 hours per response, including the time for reviewing instructions, searching existing data sources, gathering and maintaining the data needed, and completing reviewing the collection of information. Send comments regarding this burden estimate or any other aspect of this collection of information, including suggestions for reducing this burden to:

Food and Drug Administration	Food and Drug Administration	"An agency may not conduct or sponsor, and a
CBER (HFM-99)	CDER (HFD-94)	person is not required to respond to, a
1401 Rockville Pike	12229 Wilkins Avenue	collection of information unless it displays a
Rockville, MD 20852-1448	Rockville, MD 20852	currently valid OMB control number."

Please **DO NOT RETURN** this application to this address.

Figure 1 Continued.

containing information on the container–closure system being used, should be referenced. Similarly, if a previously filed IND or NDA contains pharmacological or toxicological data that support the safety of the present IND submission, reference by IND or NDA number, date, volume, and page numbers should be provided in this item.

Each IND submission is serially numbered. It should be noted that the initial filing of the IND is considered the "000" filing. Once the IND is filed, each amendment to the IND is given a progressively increasing serial submission number from 001 upward. When writing to the FDA about previous filings, the serial submission number may be used to reference the communication.

The appropriate box(es) briefly describing the submission should be checked in item 11. It is possible that one IND amendment may contain protocol amendments and information amendments. In such a case, the applicable boxes are marked. If the filing is for the initial IND, a response to a clinical hold, an initial or follow-up IND safety report, a response to an FDA request for information, an annual report, or general correspondence, the appropriate box should be checked. Finally, there is a box if the sponsor is requesting reinstatement of an IND that has been withdrawn, inactivated, terminated, or discontinued.

The second page of the form FDA 1571 contains items 12–20. Item 12 is a checklist table of contents. Any of the 10 items constituting this table of contents and contained in the specific IND submission for which the form is being prepared should be checked. An initial IND will most likely have all or a majority of the boxes checked. A protocol amendment will have items 1 and all or some of the items 6a–6d checked.

The transfer of obligations of GCP from a sponsor to a CRO is described in detail in 21CFR Part 312.52. A sponsor may transfer responsibility for any or all parts of the GCP obligations to a CRO. Any such transfer is to be described in writing. Conversely, any CRO that assumes any obligation of a sponsor for the requirements of GCP shall comply with the regulations and be subject to the same regulatory action as a sponsor for failure to comply with their assumed obligations. Thus the purpose of item 13 of the form FDA 1571 is to inform the FDA of whether any part of the clinical study is to be performed by a CRO and to identify whether the sponsor has transferred the obligations of compliance with GCP to that CRO. Finally, if the response is affirmative, the name and address of the CRO must be provided as part of the IND submission.

Items 16, 18, and 19 are to be completed only if the sponsor of the IND does not have a physical presence in the United States. It is not uncommon for a foreign-based company to sponsor an IND. However, when this occurs, the FDA must have the name, address, and telephone number of a contact person within the United States, as the FDA usually will not contact an overseas company directly. The contact person named by the sponsor may be either a representative within a United States affiliate office or a consultant working on behalf of the foreign sponsor.

IND Content and Format. As shown in Fig. 1, item 12 of the form FDA 1571 outlines the 10 parts of the IND. This section will detail the requirements for each of those parts and provide illustrations and examples of the items to be presented in the IND. It must be emphasized again that the information to be provided in the following sections represents more complete IND data to support a clinical program in phase 2 or 3. The lesser requirements for phase 1 trials have been discussed previously.

Table of Contents. Once the IND has been formatted and assembled, a detailed table of contents should be prepared. Depending on the size of the initial IND filing, this table of contents may be contained only in volume 1 or preferably included as the first pages of each of the IND volumes. The table of contents should be sufficiently detailed that an FDA reviewer can easily access any specific topic or report contained in the IND. It is also preferable to number sequentially the IND for each volume, rather than to number sequentially the entire IND. Thus, in reference to a specific report or in cross-referencing, it is necessary to provide the volume number and the page number.

The table of contents may have the following headings:

IND Part   Title of Information Provided   Volume   Page

Part 3: Introductory Statement and General Investigational Plan. On the form FDA 1571, the introductory statement appears as part 3 and the general investigational plan appears as part 4 in item 12 of the contents of application (see Fig. 1). This is inconsistent with the requirements as detailed in 21 CFR Part 312.23, inasmuch as the introductory statement and general investigation plan are listed only as part 3. Part 4 in the CFR is listed as "Reserved." Thus the option exists to combine these parts or to present them as separate entities. It is not important which way it is handled. The important thing is to have a clear and concise section, because, as the introduction to the IND, this section is likely to be read not only by the IND reviewers but also by the division director and others within the division.

The introductory statement and general investigational plan will contain the following:

1. A brief introductory statement giving the name of the drug and all active ingredients, the drug's pharmacological class, the structural formula of the drug (if known), the formulation of the dosage form(s) to be used, the route of administration, and the broad objectives and planned duration of the proposed clinical investigation(s).

2. A brief summary of previous human experience with the drug, with reference to other INDs if pertinent, and to investigational or marketing experience in other countries that may be relevant to the safety of the proposed clinical investigation(s).

3. If the drug has been withdrawn from investigation or marketing in any country for any reason related to safety or effectiveness, identification of the country(ies) where the drug was withdrawn and the reasons for the withdrawal.

4. A brief description of the overall plan for investigating the drug product for the following year. The plan should include the following: (1) the rationale for the drug or the research study, (2) the indication(s) to be studied, (3) the general approach to be followed in evaluating the drug, (4) the kinds of clinical trials to be conducted in the first year after the submission (if plans are not developed for the entire year, the sponsor should so indicate), (5) the estimated number of patients to be given the drug in those studies, and (6) any risks of particular severity or seriousness anticipated on the basis of the toxicological data in animals or prior studies in humans with the drug or related drugs.

Part 5: The Investigator's Brochure. This will be covered as a separate topic in this chapter.

Part 6: Protocols and Other Clinical Trial Information. It is necessary to provide at least one protocol in the initial IND submission. If more than one study is planned, a protocol for each planned study should be submitted. Protocols for studies not submitted initially in the IND should be submitted as a protocol amendment in a future IND serial submission. As noted in the discussion of phase 1 INDs, these protocols may be less detailed and more flexible than protocols for phase 2 and 3 studies. In phases 2 and 3, detailed protocols describing all aspects of the study should be submitted. A protocol for a phase 2 or 3 investigation should be designed in such a way that if the sponsor anticipates that some deviation from the study design may become necessary as the investigation progresses, alternatives or contingencies to provide for such a deviation are built into the protocols at the outset. For example, a protocol for a controlled short-term study might include a plan for an early crossover of nonresponders to an alternative therapy.

The requirements for a clinical protocol are described in detail in Chap. 10 of this book; however, a brief overview of the protocol content is provided here. A protocol is required to contain the following, with the specific elements and detail of the protocol reflecting the above distinctions depending on the phase of study.

1. A statement of the objectives and purpose of the study.

2. The name and address and a statement of the qualifications (curriculum vitae or other statement of qualifications) of each investigator, and

the name of each subinvestigator (e.g., research fellow, resident) working under the supervision of the investigator; the name and address of the research facilities to be used; and the name and address of each reviewing IRB. This information is neatly captured on FDA form 1572 provided in Fig. 2.

3.   The criteria for patient selection and for exclusion of patients and an estimate of the number of patients to be studied.

4.   A description of the design of the study, including the kind of control group to be used, if any, and a description of methods to be used to minimize bias on the part of subjects, investigators, and analysts.

5.   The method for determining the dose(s) to be administered, the planned maximum dosage, and the duration of individual patient exposure to the drug.

6.   A description of the observations and measurements to be made to fulfill the objectives of the study.

7.   A description of clinical procedures, laboratory tests, or other measures to be taken to monitor the effects of the drug in human subjects and to minimize risk.

This section can be best assembled by preparing various subparts. Part 6(a) will be the completed and signed clinical protocol written in compliance with the above suggestions. Part 6(b) can be the completed and signed form FDA 1572—Statement of Investigator. A copy of this form is provided in Fig. 2. This subpart can also contain the curriculum vitae of the principal investigator. It is up to the discretion of the sponsor as to whether it wishes to file the curricula vitae of all subinvestigators. However, for the sake of minimizing the size of the IND, the FDA is generally in agreement with a statement that all of the curricula vitae of subinvestigators are on file and any or all of the vitae are available upon request. Part 6(c) is a good place to provide the curricula vitae of the individuals named in items 14 and 15 of the Form FDA 1571, that is, the individual(s) responsible for monitoring the conduct and progress of the clinical investigations and the individual(s) responsible for review and evaluation of information relevant to the safety of the drug.

It should be emphasized that there is no requirement to provide the FDA at the time of the IND submission with copies of a specimen case report form or a specimen informed consent document. However, these are occasionally requested by the agency and should be immediately provided upon request.

Finally, on the introduction page to this section or in the cover letter, it is always a good idea to emphasize that the clinical trial supplies will not be shipped by the sponsor until there is documentation in hand to demonstrate

DEPARTMENT OF HEALTH AND HUMAN SERVICES PUBLIC HEALTH SERVICE FOOD AND DRUG ADMINISTRATION **STATEMENT OF INVESTIGATOR** *(TITLE 21, CODE OF FEDERAL REGULATIONS (CFR) PART 312)* (See instructions on reverse side.)	Form Approved: OMB No. 0910-0014. Expiration Date: January 31, 2006. *See OMB Statement on Reverse.*
	NOTE: No investigator may participate in an investigation until he/she provides the sponsor with a completed, signed Statement of Investigator, Form FDA 1572 (21 CFR 312.53(c)).

1. NAME AND ADDRESS OF INVESTIGATOR

2. EDUCATION, TRAINING, AND EXPERIENCE THAT QUALIFIES THE INVESTIGATOR AS AN EXPERT IN THE CLINICAL INVESTIGATION OF THE DRUG FOR THE USE UNDER INVESTIGATION. ONE OF THE FOLLOWING IS ATTACHED.

☐ CURRICULUM VITAE   ☐ OTHER STATEMENT OF QUALIFICATIONS

3. NAME AND ADDRESS OF ANY MEDICAL SCHOOL, HOSPITAL OR OTHER RESEARCH FACILITY WHERE THE CLINICAL INVESTIGATION(S) WILL BE CONDUCTED.

4. NAME AND ADDRESS OF ANY CLINICAL LABORATORY FACILITIES TO BE USED IN THE STUDY.

5. NAME AND ADDRESS OF THE INSTITUTIONAL REVIEW BOARD (IRB) THAT IS RESPONSIBLE FOR REVIEW AND APPROVAL OF THE STUDY(IES).

6. NAMES OF THE SUBINVESTIGATORS *(e.g., research fellows, residents, associates)* WHO WILL BE ASSISTING THE INVESTIGATOR IN THE CONDUCT OF THE INVESTIGATION(S).

7. NAME AND CODE NUMBER, IF ANY, OF THE PROTOCOL(S) IN THE IND FOR THE STUDY(IES) TO BE CONDUCTED BY THE INVESTIGATOR.

FORM FDA 1572 (1/03)   PREVIOUS EDITION IS OBSOLETE.   PAGE 1 OF 2

Figure 2 FDA Form 1572.

8. ATTACH THE FOLLOWING CLINICAL PROTOCOL INFORMATION:

☐ FOR PHASE 1 INVESTIGATIONS, A GENERAL OUTLINE OF THE PLANNED INVESTIGATION INCLUDING THE ESTIMATED DURATION OF THE STUDY AND THE MAXIMUM NUMBER OF SUBJECTS THAT WILL BE INVOLVED.

☐ FOR PHASE 2 OR 3 INVESTIGATIONS, AN OUTLINE OF THE STUDY PROTOCOL INCLUDING AN APPROXIMATION OF THE NUMBER OF SUBJECTS TO BE TREATED WITH THE DRUG AND THE NUMBER TO BE EMPLOYED AS CONTROLS, IF ANY; THE CLINICAL USES TO BE INVESTIGATED; CHARACTERISTICS OF SUBJECTS BY AGE, SEX, AND CONDITION; THE KIND OF CLINICAL OBSERVATIONS AND LABORATORY TESTS TO BE CONDUCTED; THE ESTIMATED DURATION OF THE STUDY; AND COPIES OR A DESCRIPTION OF CASE REPORT FORMS TO BE USED.

9. COMMITMENTS:

I agree to conduct the study(ies) in accordance with the relevant, current protocol(s) and will only make changes in a protocol after notifying the sponsor, except when necessary to protect the safety, rights, or welfare of subjects.

I agree to personally conduct or supervise the described investigation(s).

I agree to inform any patients, or any persons used as controls, that the drugs are being used for investigational purposes and I will ensure that the requirements relating to obtaining informed consent in 21 CFR Part 50 and institutional review board (IRB) review and approval in 21 CFR Part 56 are met.

I agree to report to the sponsor adverse experiences that occur in the course of the investigation(s) in accordance with 21 CFR 312.64.

I have read and understand the information in the investigator's brochure, including the potential risks and side effects of the drug.

I agree to ensure that all associates, colleagues, and employees assisting in the conduct of the study(ies) are informed about their obligations in meeting the above commitments.

I agree to maintain adequate and accurate records in accordance with 21 CFR 312.62 and to make those records available for inspection in accordance with 21 CFR 312.68.

I will ensure that an IRB that complies with the requirements of 21 CFR Part 56 will be responsible for the initial and continuing review and approval of the clinical investigation. I also agree to promptly report to the IRB all changes in the research activity and all unanticipated problems involving risks to human subjects or others. Additionally, I will not make any changes in the research without IRB approval, except where necessary to eliminate apparent immediate hazards to human subjects.

I agree to comply with all other requirements regarding the obligations of clinical investigators and all other pertinent requirements in 21 CFR Part 312.

**INSTRUCTIONS FOR COMPLETING FORM FDA 1572
STATEMENT OF INVESTIGATOR:**

1. Complete all sections. Attach a separate page if additional space is needed.

2. Attach curriculum vitae or other statement of qualifications as described in Section 2.

3. Attach protocol outline as described in Section 8.

4. Sign and date below.

5. FORWARD THE COMPLETED FORM AND ATTACHMENTS TO THE SPONSOR. The sponsor will incorporate this information along with other technical data into an Investigational New Drug Application (IND).

10. SIGNATURE OF INVESTIGATOR | 11. DATE

(WARNING: A willfully false statement is a criminal offense. U.S.C. Title 18, Sec. 1001.)

Public reporting burden for this collection of information is estimated to average 100 hours per response, including the time for reviewing instructions, searching existing data sources, gathering and maintaining the data needed, and completing reviewing the collection of information. Send comments regarding this burden estimate or any other aspect of this collection of information, including suggestions for reducing this burden to:

Food and Drug Administration
CBER (HFM-99)
1401 Rockville Pike
Rockville, MD 20852-1448

Food and Drug Administration
CDER (HFD-94)
12229 Wilkins Avenue
Rockville, MD 20852

"An agency may not conduct or sponsor, and a person is not required to respond to, a collection of information unless it displays a currently valid OMB control number."

Please **DO NOT RETURN** this application to this address.

FORM FDA 1572 (1/03)   PREVIOUS EDITION IS OBSOLETE.   PAGE 2 OF 2

Figure 2 Continued.

IRB approval, and that the drug will not be shipped to the clinical trial site until after the 30-day review period of the initial IND filing.

Part 7: Chemistry, Manufacturing, and Control Data. This section is also easier to review and better formatted with the use of subparts. Any number of approaches are acceptable; however, one logical formatting technique is to provide the CMC data for the drug substance as subpart (a), data for the drug product as subpart (b), information relating to any placebo formulations as subpart (c), labeling as subpart (d), and finally all environmental assessment information as subpart (e).

The emphasis of this part of the IND is to assure the proper identification, quality, purity, and strength of the investigational drug. As noted earlier in the section on the phase 1 IND, the amount of information needed to make that assurance will vary with the phase of the investigation, the proposed duration of the investigation, the dosage form, and the amount of information otherwise available. The FDA recognizes that modifications to the method of preparation of the new drug substance and dosage form and changes in the dosage form itself are likely as the investigation progresses. Therefore, as noted, the emphasis in an initial phase 1 submission should generally be placed on the identification and control of the raw materials and the new drug substance. Final specifications for the drug substance and drug product are not expected until near the end of the investigational process. Having said this, as drug development proceeds and as the scale or production is changed from the pilot-scale production appropriate for the limited initial clinical investigations to the larger scale production needed for expanded clinical trials, the sponsor should submit information amendments to update the initial information submitted on the chemistry, manufacturing, and control processes with information appropriate to the expanded scope of the investigation.

In May 2003, FDA issued a new and totally revised IND CMC guidance document entitled INDs for Phase 2 and Phase 3 Studies—Chemistry, Manufacturing and Controls Information. The goals of the guidance are to (1) ensure that sufficient data will be submitted to the FDA to permit assessment of the safety, as well as the quality, of the proposed clinical studies from the CMC perspective, (2) expedite the entry of new drugs into the marketplace by clarifying the type, extent and reporting of CMC information for phase 2 and 3 studies, and (3) facilitate drug discovery and development.

In addition to providing guidance on what CMC safety information should be submitted in IND information amendments, the guidance also provides details on the types of corroborating information that is more appropriately submitted to the IND Annual Report.

The recommendations in this guidance are intended to provide regulatory relief for IND sponsors by providing greater flexibility in the collecting and reporting of data and by avoiding redundant submissions. Four areas of regulatory relief are as follows:

- Certain information that traditionally has been submitted in information amendments would be identified as corroborating information and can be submitted in an annual report.
- The limited phase 2 corroborating information recommended in the guidance need not be submitted before initiation of phase 2 studies and can be generated during phase 2 drug development.
- The phase 3 corroborating information recommended in the guidance need not be submitted before the initiation of phase 3 studies and can be generated during phase 3 drug development.
- The corroborating information and a summary of CMC safety information submitted during a subject-reporting period would be included in the annual report. Therefore, there should be no need for general CMC updates at the end of phase 1 or phase 2.

Subpart (a)—Drug Substance: This section will contain a description of the drug substance, including its physical, chemical, or biological characteristics; the name and address of its manufacturer; the general method of preparation of the drug substance; the acceptable limits and analytical methods used to assure the identity, strength, quality, and purity of the drug substance; and information sufficient to support stability of the drug substance during the toxicological studies and the planned clinical studies. Reference to the current edition of the USP-NF may satisfy relevant requirements in this section.

By the time the clinical program has entered phase 3, the sponsor should provide a full description of the physical, chemical, and biological characteristics of the drug substance. For example, most of the following should be evaluated and submitted: solubility and partition coefficient, pKa, hygroscopicity, crystal properties/morphology, thermal evaluation, x-ray diffraction, particle size, melting point, and specific rotation stereochemical consideration. Proof of structure should include information on elemental analysis, conformational analysis, molecular weight determination and spectra for IR, NMR (1H and 13C), UV, MS, optical activity, and single crystal data (if available). For peptides and proteins, amino acid sequence, peptide map, and secondary and tertiary structure information should be available.

For the description of the synthesis or preparation of the drug substance, a detailed flow diagram containing chemical structures (including relevant stereochemical configurations), intermediates (either in situ or isolated), and significant side products, solvents, catalysts, and reagents should be submitted. For biotech or natural products, fermenters, columns, and other equipment/reagents should be identified. By late phase 2 or early phase

3, the synthetic process should be almost completely characterized, and the IND should therefore be able to contain a step-by-step description of the synthesis or manufacturing process, including the final recrystalization of the drug substance. The description should indicate the batch size (range) and descriptions of the types of equipment in which reactions will be carried out. Relative ratios of the reactants, catalysts, and reagents, as well as general operating conditions (time, temperature, pressures), are to be provided. Identification of steps at which all in-process controls are performed (with a complete description of the analytical methods and tentative acceptance criteria to be provided in the Process Control section) is also necessary.

Subparts (b) and (c)—Drug Product and Placebo: These sections require the submission of a list of all components. This may include reasonable alternatives for inactive compounds used in the manufacture of the investigational drug product and placebo, including those components intended to appear in the drug product and those that may not appear but are used in the manufacturing process and, where applicable, the quantitative composition of the investigational drug product, including any reasonable variations that may be expected during the investigational stage; the name and address of the drug product manufacturer and packager; a brief general description of the manufacturing and packaging procedure for the product; the acceptable limits and analytical methods used to ensure the identity, strength, quality, and purity of the drug product; and information sufficient to ensure the product's stability during the planned clinical studies. Reference to the current edition of the USP-NF may satisfy certain requirements in this subpart. There also should be a brief general description of the composition, manufacture, and control of any placebo used in a controlled clinical trial.

By the time the drug product is in phase 3, studies should be included to demonstrate the inherent stability of the drug product, and the ability to detect potential degradation products should be available. The analytical method should use a validated stability-indicating assay.

Subpart (d)—Labeling: A copy of all labels and labeling to be provided to each investigator should be submitted in the IND. This would include a mockup or printed representation of the proposed labeling and labels that will be provided to investigators to be used on the drug container. The investigational labels must also carry the standard "caution statement" as previously discussed.

Subpart (e)—Environmental Analysis Requirements: A claim for categorical exclusion under 21 CFR Section 25.30 or 25.31 or an environmental assessment under 21 CFR Section 25.40 should be provided.

Part 8: Pharmacology and Toxicology Information. This section of the IND must contain adequate information about pharmacological and toxicological studies of the drug involving laboratory animals or any studies conducted in vitro, on the basis of which the sponsor has concluded that it is reasonably safe to conduct the proposed clinical investigations. The kind, duration, and scope of animal and other tests required vary with the duration and nature of the proposed clinical investigations. Guidelines are available from the FDA that describe ways in which these requirements may be met. Such information must include the identification and qualifications of the individuals who evaluated the results of such studies and concluded that it is reasonably safe to begin the proposed investigations and a statement of where the investigations were conducted and where the records are available for inspection. As drug development proceeds, the sponsor is required to submit informational amendments, as appropriate, with additional information pertinent to safety.

With regard to formatting, this part of the IND may be divided into the following sections: Subpart (a): Pharmacology and Drug Disposition; Subpart (b)(i): Toxicology—Integrated Summary; Subpart (b)(ii): Full Toxicological Reports; and Subpart (c): Good Laboratory Practices Statement.

Subpart (a)—Pharmacology and Drug Disposition: This section should describe the pharmacological effects and mechanism(s) of action of the drug in animals and information on the absorption, distribution, metabolism, and excretion of the drug, if known.

Subpart (b)(i)—Toxicology: Integrated Summary: An integrated summary of the toxicological effects of the drug in animals and in vitro should be written. Depending on the nature of the drug and the phase of the investigation, the description is to include the results of acute, subacute, and chronic toxicity tests; tests of the drug's effects on reproduction and the developing fetus; any special toxicity test related to the drug's particular mode of administration or conditions of use (e.g., inhalation, dermal, or ocular toxicology); and any in vitro studies intended to evaluate drug toxicity. If the drug is to be studied in females of child-bearing potential in phase 2, complete investigations of the effect of the drug on fertility and reproductive performance should be a part of the IND submission.

Subpart (b)(ii)—Full Toxicological Reports: For each toxicology study that is intended primarily to support the safety of the proposed clinical investigation, a full tabulation of data suitable for detailed review should be submitted. The full reports must be quality assured by the QA unit of the laboratory that conducted the testing.

Subpart (c)—GLP Statement: For each nonclinical laboratory study subject to the GLP regulations under 21 CFR Part 58, a statement that the study was conducted in compliance with the good laboratory practice regulations, or, if the study was not conducted in compliance with those regulations, a brief statement of the reason for the noncompliance.

Part 9: Previous Human Experience. All previous human experience with the drug must be summarized. The information must include the following:

Subpart (a): If the investigational drug has been investigated or marketed previously, either in the United States or in other countries, detailed information about such experience relevant to the safety of the proposed investigation or to the investigation's rationale should be provided. If the drug has been the subject of controlled trials, detailed information on such trials that is relevant to an assessment of the drug's safety and effectiveness for the proposed investigational use should also be provided. Any published material that is relevant to the safety of the proposed investigation or to an assessment of the drug's effectiveness for its proposed investigational use should be provided in full. Published material that is less directly relevant may be supplied by a bibliography.

Subpart (b): If the drug is a combination of drugs previously investigated or marketed, the information required in the above section should be provided for each active drug component. However, if any component in such a combination is subject to an approved marketing application or is otherwise lawfully marketed in the United States, the sponsor is not required to submit published material concerning that active drug component unless such material relates directly to the proposed investigational use (including publications relevant to component–component interaction).

Subpart (c): If the drug has been marketed outside the United States, a list of the countries in which the drug has been marketed and a list of the countries in which the drug has been withdrawn from marketing for reasons potentially related to safety or effectiveness must be included.

Part 10: Additional Information. This section is necessary in only a small percentage of INDs to provide information on special topics, as listed below.

Drug Dependence and Abuse Potential: If the drug is a psychotropic substance or otherwise has abuse potential, a section describing relevant clinical studies and experience and studies in test animals is to be submitted.

Radioactive Drugs: If the drug is a radioactive drug, sufficient data from animal or human studies to allow a reasonable calculation of radiation-absorbed dose to the whole body and critical organs upon administration to a human subject are to be submitted. Phase 1 studies of radioactive drugs must include studies that will obtain sufficient data for dosimetry calculations.

Other Information: A brief statement of any other information that would aid evaluation of the proposed clinical investigations with respect to their safety or their design and potential as controlled clinical trials to support marketing of the drug.

Protocol and Information Amendments. As noted previously, the sponsor is required to wait 30 days after the submission of the initial IND before clinical investigations with the new drug may be instituted. Once the IND is in effect, all additional data and information submitted to that IND will be provided in the form of Protocol and Information Amendments, provided as sequentially numbered serial submissions.

Protocol Amendments. It is the obligation of the sponsor to amend the IND to ensure that the clinical investigations are conducted according to protocols included in the IND application. This section will describe the provisions under which new protocols may be submitted and the changes in previously submitted protocols that may be made.

New Protocol: Whenever a sponsor intends to conduct a study that is not covered by a protocol already contained in the IND, the sponsor shall submit to the FDA a protocol amendment containing the protocol for the study. Such a study may begin without delay provided two conditions are met: (1) the sponsor has submitted the protocol to FDA for its review, and (2) the protocol has been approved by the IRB with responsibility for review and approval of the study.

Changes in a Protocol: A sponsor shall submit a protocol amendment describing any change in a phase 1 protocol that significantly affects the safety of the subjects or any change in a phase 2 or 3 protocol that significantly affects the safety of the subjects, the scope of the investigation, or the scientific quality of the study. Examples of changes requiring an amendment under this paragraph include

1.   Any increase in drug dosage or duration of exposure of individual subjects to the drug beyond that in the current protocol or any significant increase in the number of subjects under study.

2.   Any significant change in the design of a protocol (such as the addition or deletion of a control group).

3.   The addition of a new test or procedure that is intended to improve monitoring for, or reduce the risk of, a side effect or an adverse event or the deletion of a test intended to monitor safety.

New Investigator: A sponsor shall submit a protocol amendment when a new investigator is added to carry out a previously submitted protocol. Once the investigator is added to the study, the investigational drug may be shipped to the investigator, and the investigator may begin participating in the study. The sponsor shall notify the FDA of the new investigator within 30 days of the investigator's being added.

It is important to note the distinction in timing of submissions to the IND for a protocol amendment and the addition of a new investigator. A sponsor must submit a protocol amendment for a new protocol or a change in protocol *before* its implementation. Protocol amendments to add a new investigator or to provide additional information about investigators may be grouped and submitted at 30-day intervals. When several submissions of new protocols or protocol changes are anticipated during a short period, the sponsor is encouraged, to the extent feasible, to include these all in a single submission.

Information Amendments. A sponsor shall report in an information amendment essential information on the IND that is not within the scope of a protocol amendment, IND safety reports, or annual report. Examples of information or data requiring an information amendment include new toxicology, chemistry, or other technical information or a report regarding the discontinuance of a clinical investigation. Information amendments to the IND should be submitted as necessary but, to the extent feasible, not more than every 30 days.

IND Safety Reports. Effective April 6, 1998, the FDA changed definitions associated with adverse experience reporting and the time frame for when IND safety reports must be provided to the FDA in relation to their occurrence.

At present, the following definitions of terms apply to this section:

Associated with the use of the drug means that there is a reasonable possibility that the experience may have been caused by the drug.

Disability is a substantial disruption of a person's ability to conduct normal life functions.

Life-threatening adverse drug experience means any adverse drug experience that places the patient or subject, in the view of the investigator, at immediate risk of death from the reaction as it occurred, i.e., it does not include a reaction that, had it occurred in a more severe form, might have caused death.

Serious adverse drug experience means any adverse drug experience occurring at any dose that results in any of the following outcomes: death, a life-threatening adverse drug experience, in-patient hospitalization or prolongation of existing hospitalization, a persistent or significant disability/incapacity, or a congenital anomaly/birth defect. Important medical events that may not result in death, be life-threatening, or require hospitalization may be considered serious adverse drug experiences when, based upon appropriate medical judgment, they may jeopardize the patient or subject and may require medical or surgical intervention to prevent one of the outcomes listed in this definition. An example would be blood dyscrasias or convulsions that do not result in in-patient hospitalization.

Unexpected adverse drug experience means any adverse drug experience, the specificity or severity of which is not consistent with the current investigator brochure; or, if an investigator brochure is not required or available, the specificity or severity of which is not consistent with the risk information described in the general investigational plan or elsewhere. For example, under this definition, hepatic necrosis would be unexpected (by virtue of greater severity) if the investigator brochure only referred to elevated hepatic enzymes or hepatitis. "Unexpected," as used in this definition, refers to an adverse drug experience that has not been previously observed (e.g., included in the investigator brochure) rather than from the perspective of such experience not being anticipated from the pharmacological properties of the product.

Review of safety information. An IND sponsor must review all information relevant to the safety of the drug obtained from any source, foreign or domestic, including information derived from any clinical or epidemiological investigations, animal investigations, commercial marketing experience, reports in the scientific literature, and unpublished scientific papers, as well as reports from foreign regulatory authorities that have not already been previously reported to the FDA by the sponsor.

There are two types of IND safety reports, written and telephone/facsimile reports. A written IND safety report is required for any adverse experience associated with the use of the drug that is both serious and unexpected; or for any finding from tests in laboratory animals that suggests a significant risk for human subjects including reports of mutagenicity, teratogenicity, or carcinogenicity. A telephone/facsimile report is required for any unexpected fatal or life-threatening experience associated with the use of the drug. The written report should be made as soon as possible but in no event later than 15 calendar days after the sponsor's initial receipt of the information. The report must clearly indicate the contents as an "IND Safety Report." A telephone/facsimile report must occur not more than 7 calendar days after receipt of the initial information. Any follow-up information obtained after initial notification must be submitted as soon as the relevant information is available. In the written IND safety report, the sponsor shall identify all safety reports previously filed with the IND concerning a similar adverse experience and provide an analysis of the significance of the adverse experience in light of the previous similar reports.

The FDA offers the opportunity for the sponsor to make a disclaimer to each IND safety report. The letter of transmittal of the initial and any follow-up reports should state that the information submitted does not necessarily reflect a conclusion by the sponsor or the FDA that the report or information constitutes an admission that the drug caused or contributed to an adverse experience. A sponsor need not admit, and may deny, that the report or information submitted by the sponsor constitutes an admission that the drug caused or contributed to an adverse experience.

Annual Reports.   In order to keep the FDA up to date with the progress of the IND, all sponsors are required to provide an annual report to the IND review division. This must be done within 2 months of the anniversary date that the IND went into effect. The annual report should be brief but summarize the progress of the investigations with the new drug.

This section will describe the information required for an annual report.

For each individual study, it is necessary to provide a brief summary of the status of each investigation in progress and each study completed during the previous year. The summary is required to include the following information for each study:

1. The title and protocol number of the study, its purpose, a brief statement identifying the patient population, and a statement as to whether the study is completed.

2. The total number of subjects initially planned for inclusion in the study; the number entered into the study to date, *tabulated by age group, sex, and race*; the number whose participation in the study was completed as planned; and the number who dropped out of the study for any reason. The requirement for tabulation by age group, sex, and race is a new annual report requirement effective February 1998.

3. If the study has been completed or if interim results are known, a brief description of any available study results.

The annual report will also contain summary information obtained during the previous year's clinical and nonclinical investigations including

1. A narrative or tabular summary showing the most frequent and most serious adverse experiences by body system

2. A summary of all IND safety reports submitted during the past year

3. A list of subjects who died during participation in the investigation, with the cause of death for each subject

4. A list of subjects who dropped out during the course of the investigation in association with any adverse experience, whether or not thought to be drug related

5. A brief description of what, if anything, was obtained that is pertinent to an understanding of the drug's actions, including, for example, information about dose response, controlled trials, and bioavailability

6. A list of the preclinical studies (including animal studies) completed or in progress during the past year and a summary of the major preclinical findings

7. A summary of any significant manufacturing or microbiological changes made during the past year

A description of the general investigational plan for the coming year to replace that submitted 1 year earlier should be submitted, as well as any revised Investigator's Brochure. If the drug is in phase 1, a description of any significant phase 1 protocol modifications made during the previous year and not previously reported to the IND in a protocol amendment should be identified. If applicable, a brief summary of significant foreign marketing developments with the drug during the past year, such as approval of marketing in any country or withdrawal or suspension from marketing in any country, is to be submitted. Finally, if desired by the sponsor, a log of any outstanding business with respect to the IND for which the sponsor requests or expects a reply, comment, or meeting may be included.

Clinical Holds and Withdrawal of an IND. The last thing a regulatory professional wants to receive from the FDA is the notification that, for one or more reasons, the IND has been placed on "clinical hold." When this occurs, a sponsor is not allowed to initiate or continue the clinical trial until the FDA has responded in writing that the clinical hold has been removed and the research program may begin. Thus a clinical hold is an order issued by the FDA to the sponsor to delay a proposed clinical investigation or to suspend an ongoing investigation. The clinical hold order may apply to one or more of the investigations covered by an IND. When a proposed study is placed on clinical hold, subjects may not be given the investigational drug. When an ongoing study is placed on clinical hold, no new subjects may be recruited to the study and placed on the investigational drug; patients already in the study should be taken off therapy involving the investigational drug unless specifically permitted by the FDA in the interest of patient safety.

Typically, a clinical hold is imposed prior to a phase 1 investigation if the FDA believes that human subjects are or would be exposed to an unreasonable and significant risk of illness or injury; if the clinical investigators named in the IND are not qualified by reason of their scientific training and experience to conduct the investigation described in the IND; if the Investigator's Brochure is misleading, erroneous, or materially incomplete; or if the IND does not contain sufficient information to assess the risks to subjects of the proposed studies. A clinical hold may occur during phases 2 or 3 for any of these reasons or if the FDA believes the plan or protocol for the investigation is clearly deficient in design to meet its stated objectives.

Details on the FDA's policy for the IND process and review procedures, including the handling of clinical holds, is presented in the FDA Manual of Policies and Procedures MAPP No. 6030.1, dated May 1, 1998. This document provides the general review principles for investigational new drugs, policies, and procedures for issuing and overseeing clinical holds of INDs and policies and procedures for processing and responding to sponsors' complete responses to clinical holds. With regard to withdrawal of an IND, this may be done at any time by a sponsor without prejudice. If a decision is taken to withdraw an IND, the FDA shall be notified in writing of this decision, all clinical investigations conducted under the IND shall be ended, all current investigators notified, and all stocks of the drug returned to the sponsor or otherwise disposed of at the request of the sponsor. If an IND is withdrawn for safety reasons, the sponsor shall promptly inform the FDA, all participating investigators, and all reviewing IRBs of the reasons for such withdrawal.

III. THE INVESTIGATOR'S BROCHURE

A. Introduction

The Investigator's Brochure (IB) is an important document, not only required as a part of the IND but also prepared for presentation to potential clinical investigators and ultimately for presentation to the investigator's IRB. The IB is a compilation of the clinical and nonclinical data on the investigational product that is relevant to the study of the product in human subjects. Its purpose is to provide the investigators and others involved in the trial with information to facilitate their understanding of the rationale for, and their compliance with, many key features of the protocol, such as the dose, dose frequency/interval, methods of administration, and safety monitoring procedures. The IB also provides insight to support the clinical management of the study subjects during the course of the clinical trial. The information should be presented in a concise, simple, objective, balanced, and nonpromotional form that enables a clinician or potential investigator to understand it and make his or her own unbiased risk–benefit assessment of the appropriateness of the proposed trial. For this reason, a medically qualified person should generally participate in the editing of an IB, but the contents of the IB should be approved by the disciplines that generated the described data.

The Efficacy Committee of the International Conference on Harmonization has prepared a final guidance (E6) entitled *Good Clinical Practice: Consolidated Guideline*. This document was issued by the FDA in April 1996, by both the Center for Drug Evaluation and Research and the Center for Biologics Evaluation and Research. This document should be consulted prior to completion of the final IB.

It is expected that the type and extent of information available will vary with the stage of development of the investigational product. If the investigational product is marketed and its pharmacology is widely understood by medical practitioners, an extensive IB may not be necessary. In this situation, a basic product information brochure, package insert, or labeling may be an appropriate alternative, provided that it includes current, comprehensive, and detailed information on all aspects of the investigational product that might be of importance to the investigator. If a marketed product is being studied for a new indication, an IB specific to that new use should be prepared.

The IB should be reviewed at least annually and revised as necessary in compliance with a sponsor's written procedures. The revised version should be included in the IND annual report. More frequent revision may be appropriate depending on the stage of development and the generation of relevant new information. However, in accordance with GCP, relevant new information may be so important that it should be communicated to the investigators, and possibly to the IRBs and the FDA, before it is included in a revised IB.

Generally, the sponsor is responsible for ensuring that an up-to-date IB is made available to the investigator(s), and the investigators are responsible for providing the up-to-date IB to the responsible IRBs.

The following provides the information that should be included in the IB.

1. Title Page

This should provide the sponsor's name, the identity of each investigational product (i.e., research number, chemical or approved generic name, and trade name(s) where legally permissible and desired by the sponsor), and the release date. It is also suggested that an edition number and a reference to the number and date of the edition it supersedes be provided.

TITLE PAGE OF INVESTIGATOR'S BROCHURE (Example)

Sponsor's Name: Product: Research Number: Name(s): Chemical, Generic (if approved)

Trade Name(s) (if legally permissible and desired by the sponsor) Edition Number:
Release Date:
Replaces Previous Edition Number:
Date:

2. Confidentiality Statement

The sponsor may wish to include a statement instructing the investigator/recipients to treat the IB as a confidential document for the sole information and use of the investigator's team and the IRB/IEC.

3. Contents of the Investigator's Brochure

The IB should contain the following sections, each with literature references where appropriate:

Table of Contents. An example of the Table of Contents is

TABLE OF CONTENTS OF INVESTIGATOR'S BROCHURE (Example)

Confidentiality Statement (optional) Signature Page (optional)

1. Table of Contents
2. Summary
3. Introduction
4. Physical, Chemical, and Pharmaceutical Properties and Formulation

5. Nonclinical Studies

    5.1. Nonclinical Pharmacology
    5.2. Pharmacokinetics and Product Metabolism in Animals
    5.3. Toxicology

6. Effects in Humans

    6.1. Pharmacokinetics and Product Metabolism in Humans
    6.2. Safety and Efficacy
    6.3. Marketing Experience

7. Summary of Data and Guidance for the Investigator NB: References on

    1. Publications
    2. Reports (these references should be found at the end of each chapter.) Appendices (if any)

Summary. A brief summary (preferably not more than two pages) should be given, highlighting the significant physical, chemical, pharmaceutical, pharmacological, toxicological, pharmacokinetic, metabolic, and clinical information available that is relevant to the stage of clinical development of the investigational product.

Introduction. A brief introductory statement should be provided that contains the chemical name (and generic and trade name(s) when approved) of the investigational product(s), all active ingredients, the investigational product(s) pharmacological class and its expected position within this class (e.g., advantages), the rationale for performing research with the investigational product(s), and the anticipated prophylactic, therapeutic, or diagnostic indication(s). Finally, the introductory statement should provide the general approach to be followed in evaluating the investigational product.

Physical, Chemical, and Pharmaceutical Properties and Formulation. A description should be provided of the investigational product substance(s) including the chemical and structural formula(e), and a brief summary should be given of the relevant physical, chemical, and pharmaceutical properties.

To permit appropriate safety measures to be taken in the course of the trial, a description of the formulation(s) to be used, including excipients, should be provided and justified if clinically relevant. Instructions for the storage and handling of the dosage form(s) also should be given. Any structural similarities to other known compounds should be mentioned.

Nonclinical Studies. The results of all relevant nonclinical pharmacology, toxicology, pharmacokinetic, and investigational product metabolism studies should be provided in summary form. This summary should address the methodology used, the results, and a discussion of the relevance of the findings to the investigated therapeutic and the possible unfavorable and unintended effects in humans.

The information provided may include the following, as appropriate, if known or available:

Species tested number and sex of animals in each group unit dose (e.g., milligram/kilogram [mg/kg]) Dose interval
Route of administration
Duration of dosing
Information on systemic distribution Duration of postexposure follow-up Results, including the following aspects:

Nature and frequency of pharmacological or toxic effects
Severity or intensity of pharmacological or toxic effects
Time to onset of effects
Reversibility of effects
Duration of effects
Dose response

Tabular format/listings should be used whenever possible to enhance the clarity of the presentation. The following sections should discuss the most important findings from the studies, including the dose response of observed effects, the relevance to humans, and any aspects to be studied in humans. If applicable, the effective and nontoxic dose findings in the same animal species should be compared (i.e., the therapeutic index should be discussed). The relevance of this information to the proposed human dosing should be addressed. Whenever possible, comparisons should be made in terms of blood/tissue levels rather than on a mg/kg basis.

Nonclinical Pharmacology. A summary of the pharmacological aspects of the investigational product and, where appropriate, its significant metabolites studied in animals should be included. Such a summary should incorporate studies that assess potential therapeutic activity (e.g., efficacy models, receptor binding, and specificity), as well as those that assess safety (such as special studies to assess pharmacological actions other than the intended therapeutic effect(s)).

Pharmacokinetics and Product Metabolism in Animals. A summary of the pharmacokinetics and biological transformation and disposition of the investigational product in all species studied should be given. The discussion of the findings should address the absorption and the local and systemic bioavailability of the investigational product and its metabolites, and their relationship to the pharmacological and toxicological findings in animal species.

Toxicology. A summary of the toxicologic effects found in relevant studies conducted in different animal species should be described under the following headings where appropriate:

Single dose Repeated dose Carcinogenicity Special studies (such as irritancy and sensitization) Reproductive toxicity Genotoxicity (mutagenicity)

Effects in Humans. A thorough discussion of the known effects of the investigational product(s) in humans should be provided, including information on pharmacokinetics, metabolism, pharmacodynamics, dose response, safety, efficacy, and other pharmacological activities. Where possible, a summary of each completed clinical trial should be provided. Information should also be provided regarding results from any use of the investigational product(s) other than in clinical trials, such as from experience during marketing.

Pharmacokinetics and Product Metabolism in Humans. A summary of information on the pharmacokinetics of the investigational product(s) should be presented, including the following, if available.

1. Pharmacokinetics (including metabolism, as appropriate, and absorption, plasma protein binding, distribution, and elimination)
2. Bioavailability of the investigational product (absolute, where possible, or relative) using a reference dosage form
3. Population subgroups (e.g., sex, age, and impaired organ function)
4. Interactions (such as product–product interactions and effects of food)
5. Other pharmacokinetic data (e.g., results of population studies performed within clinical trial[s]).

Safety and Efficacy. A summary of information should be provided about the investigational product's safety (including metabolites, where appropriate), pharmacodynamics, efficacy, and dose–response that were obtained from preceding trials in humans (healthy volunteers or patients). The implications of this information should be discussed. In cases where a number of clinical trials have been completed, the use of summaries of safety and efficacy across multiple trials by indications in subgroups may provide a clear presentation of the data. Tabular summaries of adverse drug reactions for all the clinical trials (including those for all the studied indications) would be useful. Important differences in adverse drug reaction patterns/incidences across indications or subgroups should be discussed.

The IB should provide a description of the possible risks and adverse drug reactions to be anticipated on the basis of prior experiences with the product under investigation and with related products. A description should also be provided of the precautions or special monitoring to be done as part of the investigational use of the product.

Marketing Experience. The IB should identify countries where the investigational product has been marketed or approved. Any significant information arising from the marketed use should be summarized (such as formulations, dosages, routes of administration, and adverse product reactions). The IB should also identify all the countries where the investigational product did not receive approval/registration for marketing or was withdrawn from marketing/registration.

Summary of Data and Guidance for the Investigator. This section should provide an overall discussion of the nonclinical and clinical data and should summarize the information from various sources on different aspects of the investigational product, wherever possible. In this way, the investigator can be given the most informative interpretation of the available data, with an assessment of the implications of the information for future clinical trials.

Where appropriate, the published reports on related products should be discussed. This could help the investigator to anticipate adverse drug reactions or other problems in clinical trials.

The overall aim of this section is to provide the investigator with a clear understanding of the possible risks and adverse reactions, and of the specific tests, observations, and precautions that may be needed for a clinical trial. This understanding should be based on the available physical, chemical, pharmaceutical, pharmacological, toxicological, and clinical information on the investigational product. Guidance should also be given to the clinical investigator on the recognition and treatment of possible overdose and adverse drug reactions, based on previous human experience and on the pharmacology of the investigational product.

CONCLUSIONS

This chapter has been prepared to describe in some detail the requirements of an IND application. Emphasis has been placed on the different requirements for the study of a drug in a phase 1 situation compared with a more advanced stage of drug research, that is, phases 2 and 3. Information relating to the submission of IND protocol and information amendments and IND annual reports has also been included. Finally, the newest guidance relating to the writing and content for an IB based on the International Conference on Harmonization has also been provided in detail.

4

General Considerations of the New Drug Application

Martha R. Charney
Piedmont Consulting Group, LLC, Menlo Park, California, U.S.A.

I. INTRODUCTION

An NDA is an application submitted to the United States FDA for permission to market a new drug product in the United States. The content of an NDA is designed to answer several questions: Does the new product provide a proven medical benefit? Are the associated risks acceptable compared to the benefits? Can the product be manufactured reproducibly and reliably? Are the data in the NDA reliable?

Since 1963, new drug products introduced into commerce in the United States have been the subjects of NDAs approved by the FDA, with some exceptions. For the approval of vaccines, traditional biological products (such as blood fractions), and genetically engineered biotechnical products, Biologics License Applications are used. They answer the same questions as NDAs about medical benefit, acceptable risks, and reliability of manufacturing and data. Generic drug products, which are designed to be equivalent to products already on the market, are subjects of ANDAs. An ANDA is designed to provide data that show the new product to be equivalent to the existing product, the method of manufacture to be reliable, and the information in the ANDA to be reliable. However, an NDA is needed if the route of administration is changed for a previously approved drug. For example, if the proposed product is a nasal spray and the previous product was an orally administered tablet, an NDA is needed.

With the increasingly sophisticated technology now available, there are a growing number of products that are combinations of drugs and devices. In these drug-device combinations, both the drug and the device may contribute to medical benefit. The FDA evaluates these drug-device combinations on a case-by-case basis to determine whether the product should be classified as a drug or a device. It is recommended that the manufacturer obtain a classification as a drug or device from the FDA as early in development of the drug-device combination as possible.

II. REGULATIONS, FORMS, AND GUIDANCES

The forms, regulations, and guidelines needed for assembling an NDA are available from the FDA's website on the internet, www.FDA.gov. The regulations, Title 21 of the Code of Federal Regulations (21 CRF), can also be purchased from government bookstores located in major cities or from the Government Printing Office; however, recently the bookstores have been closing due to the ability to order books online from the Government Printing Office. Copies of the various guidelines are available from the FDA Drug Information Branch, 5600 Fishers Lane, Rockville, MD 20857; phone (301) 827-4573.

Form FDA 356h, "Application to Market a New Drug, Biologic, or an Antibiotic Drug for Human Use," is the form that needs to accompany an NDA, a BLA, or an ANDA. Form FDA 356h and Form FDA 3397, "User Fee Cover Sheet," are available from the Forms Distribution Page of the CDER part of the FDA website. Both forms request the name, address, and phone number of the applicant or owner of the NDA. If the applicant is a foreign corporation or other entity, it is necessary to list an agent in the United States with legal authority to represent the foreign applicant. Product information such as the generic name, chemical or biochemical name, dosage form, strengths, route of administration, and proposed indications for use are to be entered on Form FDA 356h. For new drugs, a name approved by USAN is needed.

The regulations governing NDAs for new drugs are in 21 CRF Part 314, and those for biologicals are in 21 CRF Part 601. These describe the content of an NDA and also the legal and administrative procedures connected with an NDA. The regulations describing the bioavailability and bioequivalency testing needed for approval of an NDA are in 21 CFR Part 320. The proposed labeling for the new drug needs to be included in the NDA, and 21 CFR Part 201 contains these regulations. The manufacturing facilities for the new drug product and for the active pharmaceutical ingredient (API) need to be in compliance with GMP regulations, 21 CFR Parts 210 and 211. For non-clinical safety studies, the GLP regulations are in 21 CFR Part 58. For clinical studies in the NDA, the applicable regulations are those for informed consent,

21 CFR Part 50, institutional review boards, 21 CFR Part 56, the Declaration of Helsinki, 21 CFR Part 312.120, investigational new drug exemptions, 21 CFR Part 312, and the financial disclosure by clinical investigators, 21 CFR Part 54. An NDA also requires an environmental impact statement covering the manufacture of the proposed product, and the regulations covering this are in 21 CFR Part 25.

The FDA has issued a series of guidance documents for the preparation and assembly of an NDA [1–7]. A complete list of available guidance documents covering all aspects of drug development is available at the FDA website. Guidelines do not have the same force as regulations, so it is not absolutely necessary to follow them. However, it is recommended that guidelines be followed, if possible. If there is a deviation from a guideline, a clear explanation of the reason for the deviation should be provided.

The FDA has issued specifications for the color-coded binders that are needed for the volumes of an NDA [6]. The binders can be ordered from the U.S. Government Printing Office, Washington, DC 20404-0001 [Phone (202) 512-1800]. Alternatively, applicants can have the binders made and printed according to the FDA specifications. The specifications for the binders for NDAs, including specifications for IND and Drug Master File binders, can be found on the FDA website. The binders for an NDA have been asssigned form numbers, Form FDA 2626 and Forms FDA 2626a through h. These numbers are useful for ordering from the Government Printing Office.

III. INCORPORATION OF THE COMMON TECHNICAL DOCUMENT

At the present time (2003), the FDA is requesting that sponsors switch from using the traditional NDA to an NDA that incorporates the Common Technical Document (CTD). From the perspective of the organization and format of an NDA, this switch is the most fundamental change since 1963. However, the changes in organization and format do not affect the regulations governing an NDA, and it is still necessary to provide information on medical benefit, acceptability of risks, reliability of manufacturing, and quality assurance of the data in the NDA. The development of the CTD is the culmination of work by the International Conference on Harmonization since 1990. The main purpose of the ICH was to harmonize the regulatory requirements for pharmaceuticals that are to be marketed in the European Union, the United States, and Japan. Initially, the ICH issued guidelines that dealt with the design or reporting of specific types of studies. The CTD is the framework for organizing the reports and summary documents into a marketing application that will be acceptable in all three regions.

The organization of a traditional NDA was essentially linear. A volume containing proposed labeling, summaries, and administrative documents was followed by volumes containing all manufacturing and controls information, then volumes with all nonclinical information, volumes with microbiology information, if applicable, and volumes with biopharmaceutical, clinical, and statistical information. The organization of a CTD is more of a multidimensional matrix. The representation in the CTD guideline [1] is a triangle (Fig. 1). Module 1 is not technically part of the CTD, since it will vary with the administrative region and will contain the official forms and information to comply with region-specific regulations. Modules 2 through 5 make up the CTD and are to be identical for submissions to all regions. In the CTD, chemistry, manufacturing, and control information is known as quality information and appears in Modules 2 and 3. Nonclinical information will appear in Modules 2 and 4, and clinical, biopharmaceutical, and statistical information will appear in Modules 2 and 5.

For the US, Module 1 should contain the index for the entire submission, Form FDA 356h, annotated package insert and other labeling, patent information, patent certification, debarment certification, field copy certification, user fee cover sheet, and financial disclosure information. Information on United States patents related to the drug or drug product is to be included in Module 1 of the NDA. If there were waivers for bioquivalency studies or the environmental assessment, these would go in Module 1, since they would refer to specific US regulations. An environmental assessment would be part of

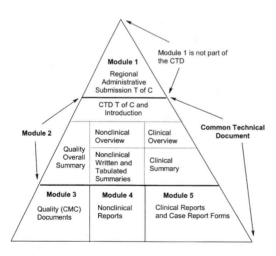

Figure 1

Module 1 but should be in a separate volume. The relevant types of patents are the composition-of-matter patent for the API, patents related to the formulation or composition of the drug product, and use patents that are applicable to the clinical indications claimed in the NDA. Process patents for any of the manufacturing processes used for the API or drug product need not be included. The applicant must certify the validity of each patent listed in the NDA. The proper wording for these certifications is in the regulations (21 CRF Part 314).

Because of instances of fraud, the FDA has instituted procedures for the debarment of individuals. Module 1 of the NDA needs to contain a certification that the applicant has not and will not use the services of any debarred individual in any capacity [6]. Notices of the debarment of individuals are published in the Federal Register, and the entire list can be found at www.FDA.org/ORA/compliance, the Office of Regulatory Affairs section of the FDA website. Note that the certification includes the statement that the applicant will not use any debarred person in the future. Thus it is recommended that the list be checked periodically, especially before letting any contracts. The FDA has been interpreting the phrase "in any capacity" to include jobs that are not involved with drug development, such landscaper or accountant.

Module 2 starts with a table of contents for the CTD, e.g., the table of contents for Modules 2 through 5, but does not include Module 1. A major organizational difference between a traditional NDA and a CTD-based NDA is that the CTD-based NDA relies on the use of divider tabs for locating documents rather than page numbers. This is a decided improvement in that it avoids the last-minute hassle of numbering pages and then going back and filling in the various tables of contents. On the other hand, the placement and labeling of the divider tabs becomes critical. The table of contents will refer to each document in the CTD by volume number and divider tab label. The tab label should be either the name of the document or the section heading according to the CTD format. Each document will have a covering divider tab and a single set of page numbers. Many toxicology laboratories and other contract laboratories use a system in which the cover page and all sequential pages are numbered in Arabic numerals starting at 1. The sponsor may find it useful to request that all parties providing reports or documents for the NDA use the same system (instead of an unnumbered cover page and of lowercase Roman numerals for introductory material). If a protocol or other document needs to accompany a study report, the document should be placed as an appendix with a divider tab identifying the document, such as "Protocol" or "CV Jones, MD" or "Appendix A" [6].

Module 2 also contains an introduction and two levels of summaries. The guidelines do not specify the content of the introduction, but it is recommended that this contain any background information that the sponsor would like the reviewers to consider, such as pharmacological class, prior marketing history, or medical need for the product. The first level of summaries is the Quality Overall Summary (chemistry, manufacturing, and controls), the Nonclinical Overview (pharmacology, drug metabolism and pharmacokinetics, and toxicology), and the Clinical Overview. The Quality Overall Summary provides brief descriptions of the information in Module 3 with a synthetic flow diagram, discussion of choice of controls, summary of stability results, and the postapproval stability protocol, and should not exceed 40 pages [2]. The Nonclinical Overview is an integrated, critical assessment of the results of the nonclinical studies, and should not exceed 30 pages [3]. The Clinical Overview should describe the approach to clinical development and the critical design decisions, evaluate the quality of the studies, provide an overview of the findings, discuss the limitations of the findings, discuss the risks and benefits, explain any unresolved issues in relation to approval, and explain any unusual prescribing information within about 30 pages [4]. The Overviews should be unbiased, balanced evaluations of the data, since they are replacements for the European expert reports that were traditionally written by experts who were independent from the sponsor. Module 2 should also include the more detailed Nonclinical Written and Tabulated Summaries and the Clinical Summary with the Synopses of Individual Studies. The Nonclinical Tabulated Summaries are extensive for the toxicology studies and have a format prescribed by the guidelines. The Synopses of the clinical studies are the synopses in the format described by the ICH guideline for clinical reports.

Module 3 will contain the documents related to chemistry, manufacturing, and the quality control of the manufacturing procedures. Since the manufacturing section usually consists of a myriad of relatively small documents, many being only one or two pages, a draft guidance has been issued that addresses where in Module 3 single documents (each starting at page 1) are needed and where it is optional for combining small documents into a single document. Once a sponsor has chosen a system for manufacturing documents for either Module 2 (Quality Overall Summary) or Module 3, any subsequent amendments to the NDA should follow the same system [2,7]. In addition to sending the NDA to the FDA central office in Rockville, MD, the sponsor needs to send a field copy of the Quality Overall Summary from Module 2 and all of Module 3 to the local district FDA office (21 CRF Part 314.50). The field copy should also contain a copy of form FDA 356h and a letter certifying that the field copy is an exact copy of the appropriate sections of the entire NDA.

Modules 4 and 5 will contain the reports of the nonclinical studies and the clinical studies, respectively. The order for the nonclinical reports is pharmacology, pharmacokinetics, then toxicology. Copies of all literature references for the nonclinical disciplines are to be combined at the end of Module 4. For the publications, the page numbers used by the journal suffice for the numbering of the document [3,6]. The order for the clinical reports is biopharmaceutic studies, studies of pharmacokinetics using human bioma- terials (usually in vitro studies such as protein binding), pharmacokinetic studies in humans, pharmacodynamic studies, safety and efficacy studies, and reports of postmarketing experience. The case report forms and individual patient data listings that are appendices 16.3 and 16.4 of clinical reports written in the ICH format are to be combined and placed in a separate section in Module 5. The order of the case report forms and individual patient data listings should be the same as the order of presentation of the reports. Copies of all literature references used in the Clinical Overview, Clinical Summary, or individual reports should be included at the end of Module 5 or should be available immediately upon request [4,6]. If the NDA would have had a microbiology section under the traditional format, the same reports should be incorporated into Module 5 [6].

IV. THE ELECTRONIC CTD AND NDA

In addition to the incorporation of the CTD into an NDA, the second major change is the ability to make electronic submissions. The ICH has issued a draft guidance with the specifications for electronic filing of CTDs, known as eCTDs [8]. The guidance acknowledges that it will need to change based on changes in technology and in the CTD requirements, and a procedure for change is described. One component of the eCTD is the electronic files of the individual documents described above for a paper CTD. These files are arranged in directories and subdirectories corresponding to the modules, sections, and subsections of the CTD. Tying the files together is a file written in Extensible Markup Language (XML) that serves as a backbone and table of contents providing hyperlinks to the individual files. Within the files for the individual documents there should also be hyperlinks to all tables, figures, and appendices. The individual documents should be formatted so that they can be printed on either A4 or 8.5 × 11″ paper without losing any information.

The submission should be completely electronic unless there are regional forms that require written signatures. Any cover letter should also be scanned and included electronically. Since NDAs are viable documents for the marketing life of a drug and perhaps beyond, the format should be as neutral and standard as possible, which was the reason for choosing XML. At this time, the submission should be sent to the FDA on a medium that is appropriately sized for the submission. A large submission (>7 GB) would need to be on digital tape, whereas a small amendment (<10 MB) could be sent on floppy discs. Submissions of intermediate size would be sent on CD-ROMs [8]. Since eCTDs will be encouraged in the future, it is advisable to start producing individual documents that meet the requirements for format and with the appropriate hyperlinks or bookmarks.

V. NDA REVIEW PROCESS

Before an NDA is submitted to the FDA, the applicant usually meets with the reviewing division in a pre-NDA meeting. The applicant presents a summary of the clinical studies, the proposed format for the organization of the NDA, and any other information the applicant considers relevant. The purpose of the meeting is to uncover any major unresolved issues and to help the reviewers become acquainted with the information to be included in the NDA. By this time, the classification of the NDA for the priority of the review should be known. A standard review (S) is used for drugs with therapeutic benefits similar to currently available drugs. A priority review (P) is used for drugs that represent significant advances over existing treatments.

Upon receipt of an NDA, the FDA conducts a review of the application to determine its completeness. Within 60 days, the FDA either accepts the filing or sends the applicant a refusal-to-file letter [9]. If the applicant receives a refusal-to-file letter, they can request a conference with the FDA. Grounds for refusing to file the application include

Form FDA 356h has not been completed.
The format of the application is not correct (21 CFR Part 314.50).
One or more items are missing from the content as described in the regulations (21 CFR Part 314.50).
The manufacturing facilities are not ready for inspection.
The environmental assessment is incomplete or there is insufficient information for consideration of a waiver.
Complete and accurate translations of all parts of the application not in English are not included.
There are no statements regarding compliance with IRB and informed consent regulations for each of the clinical studies.
The drug product is already covered by an approved NDA or ANDA.

After the NDA is accepted for filing, the various sections undergo concurrent review. The clinical information is reviewed by a medical officer, usually a physician. The nonclinical information on pharmacology, toxicology, and drug metabolism is reviewed by a pharmacologist. The information on the chemistry, manufacturing, and controls for both the API and the drug product are reviewed by a chemist. A statistician evaluates the relevance of the statistical methodology used and provides the medical officer with an assessment of the power of the findings and their extrapolation to the entire patient population. For an anti-infective drug, a microbiologist will review the effect of the drug on the target microorganisms and will assess any microbiology test that may be needed for clinical isolates. The biopharmaceutics section is reviewed by a clinical pharmacologist or pharmacokineticist who determines if there is sufficient information on the metabolism and elimination of the drug, and if the bioavailability and bioequivalency studies support the clinical data and the dissolution specifications. The medical officer takes the lead in integrating the results of the findings of the other reviewers with the clinical information.

When easily correctable deficiencies are found during the review, the FDA will notify the applicant, usually by phone or fax, and the applicant should send the additional information as soon as possible. At the end of the review, there may be more substantial scientific or medical issues, which would be discussed with the applicant and may also be presented to an advisory committee. An advisory committee for a reviewing division of the FDA includes medical experts in the therapeutic area and other relevant experts such as a statistician. The opinions of an advisory committee are not binding on the FDA; however, the FDA is very unlikely to override a negative advisory committee opinion. If scientific and medical issues remain after both discussions and an advisory committee, the FDA may request that additional information or revisions be submitted as an amendment to the NDA [10].

The applicant will be asked to submit safety reports four months after the initial submission and at other times requested by the FDA (21 CFR Part 314.50). These safety reports will include any animal or clinical safety data that were not available at the time of the initial submission.

When the scientific and medical issues are resolved, the CDER reviewing division will verify that the inspections of the manufacturing sites and selected clinical sites were satisfactory. Based on the medical and scientific reviews, the proposed labeling for the drug product will be reviewed. At this stage, the FDA will send one of three possible action letters to the applicant. One possibility is a Not Approvable Letter, which will list the deficiencies in the NDA and explain why it cannot be approved (21 CFR Part 314.120). The second possibility is an Approvable Letter, which indicates that ultimately the drug product should be approved, but lists minor deficiencies and labeling changes that are needed before approval (21 CFR Part 314.110). Requests for commitments for postapproval studies may be included. The sponsor needs to respond within 10 days of receipt of the Not Approvable Letter or the Approvable Letter with an amendment to the NDA or a letter of intent. The third possible letter is an Approval Letter (21 CFR Part 314.105). An applicant may receive both an Approvable Letter and an Approval Letter at a later date.

VI. APPROVAL TIMES

Since the implementation of the PDUFA, the review times for NDAs for new molecular entities have dropped. In 1993, the median total approval time was 23 months, of which 21 months were used by the FDA, and 25 new molecular entities were approved. By 1996, the median time had dropped to 14.3 months for total time, with a median of 12 months for FDA review, and 53 new molecular entities were approved [11]. In 2001, seven new molecular entities that were classified as priority were approved with a median review time of 6.0 months, and 17 new molecular entities that were classified as standard were approved with a median FDA review time of 15.7 months [12]. The lower number of approvals in 2001 versus 1996 is probably a reflection of a lower number of applications in 2000 and 2001 than in 1995 and 1996.

      Since the NDA process is in transition between traditional NDAs and CTD-based NDAs, it is strongly recommended that a sponsor submit a draft table of contents for discussion at the pre-NDA meeting. Any questions regarding the location of various documents within the CTD-based NDA should be asked at the meeting. The format and construction discussed above is based on current information and guidelines and may change as the agency gains experience with the CTD-based NDA.

ACKNOWLEDGMENT

The author would like to thank Dr. Randy Levin of the FDA for answering questions about the CTD.

REFERENCES

1. Guidance for Industry. M4: Organization of the CTD. U.S. Department of Health and Human Services, Food and Drug Administration. August 2001 ICH.
2. Guidance for Industry. M4Q: The CTD—Quality. U.S. Department of Health and Human Services, Food and Drug Administration. August 2001 ICH.
3. Guidance for Industry. M4S: The CTD—Safety. U.S. Department of Health and Human Services, Food and Drug Administration. August 2001 ICH.
4. Guidance for Industry. M4S: The CTD—Safety Appendices. U.S. Department

of Health and Human Services, Food and Drug Administration. August 2001 ICH.

5. Guidance for Industry. M4E: The CTD—Efficacy. U.S. Department of Health and Human Services, Food and Drug Administration. August 2001 ICH.

6. Guidance for Industry. Submitting Marketing Applications According to the ICH-CTD Format—General Considerations. Draft Guidance. U.S. Department of Health and Human Services, Food and Drug Administration. August 2001.

7. Draft Guidance. Common Technical Document—Quality: Questions and Answers/Location Issues Washington D.C. September 12, 2002.

8. Electronic Common Technical Document Specification. ICH M2EWG. Draft Guidance. International Conference on Harmonization of Technical Requirements for Registration of Pharmaceuticals for Human Use. ICH eCTD Specification V 2.0. February 12, 2002.

9. New Drug Evaluation Guidance Document: Refusal to File. Food and Drug Administration, July 12, 1993.

10. CDER Handbook. Department of Health and Human Services, Food and Drug Administration, Center for Drug Evaluation and Research. March 16, 1998.

11. CDER 1997 Report to the Nation. U.S. Department of Health and Human Services, Food and Drug Administration, Center for Drug Evaluation and Research. May 1, 1998.

12. Center for Drug Evaluation and Research 2001 Report to the Nation. Improving Public Health Through Human Drugs. U.S. Department of Health and Human Services, Food and Drug Administration, May 14, 2002.

5

The New Drug Application, Content and Format

Richard A. Guarino
Oxford Pharmaceutical Resources, Inc., Totowa, New Jersey, U.S.A.

I. INTRODUCTION

Submitting a New Drug Application (NDA) to the FDA requires a meticulous, well indexed, comprehensive, and readable prepared document. This chapter will describe the specifics needed to format, assemble, and submit an NDA that follows FDA regulations and ICH guidelines. It is the applicant's responsibility to submit data that will satisfy the requirements of the Food, Drug, and Cosmetic Act and the Code of Federal Regulations (CFR) used by the FDA in the review and approval of safe and effective drug products in the United States. The ICH guidelines on safety and efficacy used for international submissions are very similar to FDA regulations for new product approval, having only slight differences according to each country's requirements where the New Drug Application is submitted.

As one plans the formatting, there must be a clear understanding of how to separate the most essential data from supporting material. The FDA regulations and ICH guidelines, meetings with the FDA during the development stages, i.e., particularly the pre-NDA submission conference, are all invaluable to the applicant, especially if unforeseen problems arise owing to the nature of the product or data.

This chapter will detail a description of each specific section of the Code of Federal Regulations, Title 21, Section 314 (21 CFR 314) and will help the reader identify the purpose of each item of the NDA and how best to present the item, particularly for those with no prior knowledge of the format and content of an NDA.

II. GENERAL OVERVIEW OF AN NDA

All New Drug Applications (NDAs), including abbreviated NDAs (ANDAs) and supplemental NDAs (SNDAs), must contain the information required in 21 CFR 314.50. Two copies of the application are needed: an archival copy and a review copy. An application for a new chemical entity, an NDA, will generally contain a signed FDA 356h form, an index, a summary, five or six technical sections, case report tabulations of subject data, case report forms, drug samples, and labeling. ANDAs and SNDAs usually contain only some of the above items, and the information will be limited to what is needed to support that particular application. A field copy should be supplied upon request from the FDA. This is used for infield inspection of GMPs, GLPs, and GCPs. (See chapters 3 and 19).

A. Review and Archival Copies

Both the review copy and the archival copy should include a cover letter that confirms agreements or understandings between the FDA and the applicant. The letter should cite any relevant correspondence or meetings by date and topic, and identify one or more persons the FDA may contact regarding the application. The letter may include any other important information the applicant wishes to convey to the FDA about the application.

These copies are required to contain the following: *Application Form (FDA 356h)*. The application form, which serves as a cover sheet for the application, contains basic identifying information about the applicant and the drug product. Importantly, it obligates the applicant to comply with applicable laws and regulations. These include GMPs (21 CFR 210 and 211); *labeling regulations* (21 CFR 201); *prescription drug advertising regulations* (21 CFR 202); *regulations on making changes in an application* (21 CFR 314.70, 314.71, and 314.72); *regulations on reports* (21 CFR 314.80 and 314.81); *and local, state,* and *federal environmental impact laws*. In addition, FDA Form 3397—User fee cover sheet, should be included in this first volume (user fee ID number can be obtained from FDA Central Document Room). Financial Disclosure Forms 3454 (no financial interest) and 3455 (financial interest) must be completed and included. Also, the Debarment Certification Statement should be included.

If the person signing the application does not reside or have a place of business within the United States, the application must contain the name and address of, and be countersigned by, an attorney, agent, or other authorized official who resides or maintains a place of business within the United States (many CROs act as the legal agent for foreign pharmaceutical companies not having an established office in the United States).

The application form, as well as the index and the summary (items 1, 2, and 3 in FDA 356h), should be bound together in a single volume. Items 4 to 12 *should be submitted in separately bound volumes in the order in which they are listed. Patent information on the applicant's drug (item 13) and a patent certification with respect to the drug (item 14)* should be submitted on a separate piece of paper attached to the application form itself.

All Investigational New Drug Applications (INDs), Drug Master Files (DMFs), and any other applications that are referenced in an NDA must be identified in the space provided on the application form. It is recommended that the applicant use the following format:

Type of Document
(IND, NDA, DMF)

Document No.

Title or Subject
of Document

Document Holder
Vol., Page No.
Dates, etc.

An applicant may obtain copies of the application form (FDA 356h) by writing to Forms and Publication Distribution (HFD-268), 12100 Parklawn Drive, Rockville, Maryland 20852 or by downloading them from the Internet.

III. FORMATTING, ASSEMBLING, AND SUBMITTING NEW DRUG AND ANTIBIOTIC APPLICATIONS

With the development of new NDA regulations implemented in 1985 to improve the NDA process, the FDA designed an application format more amenable to an efficient review, the NDA rewrite [1]. The changes included requiring fewer copies (two as opposed to the previously required three) of the NDA, allowing a parallel review of all the technical data, eliminating the need for submission of all case report forms (except in certain cases), and permitting submission of certain segments on microfiche. This rewrite is expected to reduce the volume of the previously large submissions considerably, thereby improving review time and resulting in more approvals in a shorter period of time.

However, there are no shortcuts in the preparation of an NDA. The items highlighted in this chapter encompass information that can take literally thousands of pages of detailed explanation. To help prevent delays until approval is granted, the sponsor of a new drug must meticulously organize the NDA, check and recheck every fact, explain all omissions, and summarize all relevant information in an accurate, clear, concise, and complete manner. One author experienced in submitting NDAs has stated, "Every NDA is a learning experience. A trial that was sophisticated when planned 3 years ago may seem less than adequate when subjected to the harsh glare of tomorrow's advisory committee review" [2]. It is of extreme importance for a sponsor to anticipate and minimize time-consuming problems.

A. General Format of NDA

Index. The comprehensive index will contain the volume and page number for the summary, the technical sections, and any supporting information. The index serves as a detailed table of contents for the entire application. It is prudent for the sponsor to keep additional copies of the index and have them available if drug regulatory personnel are contacted by a reviewer. If microfiche is used for portions of an application, the fiche number should also be noted.

Each technical review section should have a copy of the overall index and an individualized table of contents based on the relevant portions of the application index.

The NDA regulations (21 CFR 314.50) require the submission of an archival copy and a review copy.

1. Archival Copy

This is a complete copy of an application submission and is intended to serve as a reference source for FDA reviewers to locate information not contained in the section of the review copy assigned to them. It serves as a reference source for other FDA officials, and as the repository of the copies of tabulations and clinical trial case report forms.

After approval, the archival copy is retained by the FDA and serves as the sole file copy of the approved application. Certain parts of the archival copy will be accepted on microfiche, another suitable microform system, or by electronic (computer) means. (It behooves the applicant to check with the FDA division that will be reviewing the NDA on the acceptability of the format the applicant chooses.)

2. Review Copy

The review copy of an application is divided into five (or six) sections containing the technical and scientific information required by FDA reviewers. Each of the technical sections of the review copy is separately bound and will go the reviewer in charge of that specific section, i.e., pharmacology, statistics, etc. Each section of the review copy should also contain a copy of Volume 1.1 with the following:

1. A copy of the FDA cover letter
2. A copy of the application form (FDA 356h)
3. A copy of the index to the entire application
4. A copy of the overall summary
5. A copy of a letter of reference or authorization to access NDAs, DMFs, etc.

Because of the procedures used at the FDA to file and retrieve material from the document rooms where applications are kept, it is necessary that applicants use the colored folders (or "jackets") to bind the specific sections of the review copy. The folder colors and form numbers are listed in the table.

Document	Folder color	Form number
Archival copy	Light blue	FD 2626
Chemistry, manufacturing, and controls section	(CMC) Red	FD 2626a
Nonclinical pharmacology and toxicology section	Yellow	FD 2626b
Human pharmacokinetics and bioavailability section	Orange	FD 2626c
Microbiology section	White	FD 2626d
Clinical data section	Light brown	FD 2626e
Statistical section	Green	FD 2626f
Field copy	Maroon	FD 2626h

The cover of each folder should bear the NDA number (if known), the name of the applicant, and the name of the drug product. It should also identify the kind of submission by the headings shown above.

Applicants may purchase these folders from the FDA (4). Requests should be made on company letterhead and specify the color(s) of the folder, the FD form number(s), the quantities required, the location where the shipment should be sent, and the name and telephone number of a contact person in case additional information about the order is needed.

3. Paper Size and Binding

All applications must be bound on the left side of the page using the United States standard size loose-leaf page ($8\frac{1}{2} \times 11''$).

Both sides of the page may be used for the presentation of information and data, provided

1. Information and data on both sides are not obscured in the binding
2. Legibility is not impaired because of bleeding of the copy through the page
3. Pages are in correct order and accurately numbered

4. Pagination

Any method of pagination may be used, as long as the paging and indexing permit rapid access to the entire submission. It is important that all pages in the application be numbered and that the numbering of the review copy pages be the same as the numbering of the corresponding pages in the archival copy.

If the archival copy is submitted on microfiche, the page numbers on the microfiche page image should correspond to the page numbers in the review copy.

5. Volume Size and Identification

Volumes submitted in hard copy form should be no more than 2 inches thick. As previously discussed, the front cover of each volume should have the proper information: name of applicant, drug, and NDA number, which can be obtained from the FDA's central document room (if not previously assigned), clearly written in waterproof marking pen or on typed stick-on labels. The volume number should be preprinted in the right upper corner, and in the lower right-hand corner of each jacket cover is the legend, "THIS SUB-MISSION: VOL. ___ OF ___ VOLS." The blanks should be filled in by the applicant to identify the specific volume and the total number of volumes submitted. For example, the first volume of a 50-volume submission would be, "VOL. *1* OF *50* VOLS." See the sample label below.

Labeling

                                                                    Volume _____

                                    NDA #

                                    Drug Name

                              Sponsor Name Address

                                                            This Submission
                                                            Vol. 1 of 100 Vols.

Numbering of the volumes for the technical sections of the review copy should be the same as that used for the volumes of the archival copy.

Preprinted on the upper right-hand corner of each jacket is "VOLUME ___." This section should be filled in for original applications and for chemistry presubmissions only. This section should be filled in with two numbers, the first giving the order in which the submission has been made and the second identifying the specific volume of the total number in that submission.

Microfiche corresponding to more than one volume of the paper (hard copy) application may be bound together if a clear physical separation is made between each "volume" of microfiche. This can be accomplished if one or more empty slots is left between the last microfiche sheet of one volume and the first microfiche sheet of the next. New drug application numbers for applications submitted in microfiche will be preassigned. For more information and details on the use of microfiche, the FDA has prepared a guideline for the submission in microfiche of the archival copy of the application. Contact the Office of Management (HFN-42) at the FDA for this information.

6. Packing Carton

The box size of $14 \times 12 \times 9\frac{1}{2}''$ is recommended for shipment of applications to FDA. Because ANDAs are handled and stored separately, smaller boxes may be appropriate for them. An exterior label should indicate the contents by applicant's name, drug name, and volume numbers; it is also important to identify which cartons contain the archival copy and which the review copy.

Full applications should be sent to

> Food and Drug Administration
> Office of Drug Evaluation and Review
> Central Document Room
> Park Building, Room 214
> 12420 Parklawn Drive
> Rockville, MD 20852

B. Abbreviated Applications Should be Sent to the Division of Generic Drug Products at

> Office of Generic Drugs (HFD-600)
> Center for Drug Evaluation and Research (CDER)
> Food and Drug Administration
> Metro Park North II, Room 150
> 7500 Standish Place
> Rockville, MD 20855

C. Supplements, Amendments, and Postmarketing Reports

The submission format for amendments to pending applications and supplements to approved applications will be the same as in an original application. Each submission will consist of two copies: a complete archival copy and an appropriately segmented review copy.

Amendments, supplements, resubmissions, annual reports, and other correspondence concerning full applications should be addressed to the appropriate FDA reviewing divisions.

Postmarketing reports of adverse drug experience, including the 15-day "alert reports" and the periodic drug experience reports, should be submitted, unbound, in duplicate, to

> Food and Drug Administration
> Office of Drug Evaluation and Review
> Central Document Room
> Park Building, Room 214
> 12420 Parklawn Drive
> Rockville, MD 20852

IV. NDA FORMAT [FDA 356h #3, 21CFR 314.50 (c)]

The Format of a New Drug Application (NDA) may follow FDA Form 356h. The items listed below are the ones widely used by industry and this format is recommended as the FDA is accustomed to following this sequence. Each item will be discussed in detail. The applicant will have to customize their NDA according to the information developed for the product being submitted for approval.

New Drug Application
Form 356h

Index

Volume/Page

Cover letter
A. Application Form
    List of INDs, NDAs, and DMFs
    referenced in the Application
B. Patent Certification
C. Application Summary
D. Technical Data Sections

    (1) Chemistry, Manufacturing
         and Controls Section
    (2) Nonclinical Pharmacology
         and Toxicology Section
    (3) Human Pharmacokinetics
         and Bioavailability Section
    (4) Microbiology Section
    (5) Clinical Data Section
         a. List of Investigators
         b. Background/Overview of
            Clinical Investigations
         c. Clinical Pharmacology Trials
         d. Controlled Clinical Trials
            (i) Table of Controlled Clinical Trials
            (ii) Reports of Controlled Clinical Trials
         e. Uncontrolled Clinical Trials
            (i) Table of Uncontrolled Clinical Trials
            (ii) Reports of Uncontrolled Clinical Trials
         f. Other Trials and Information
            (i) Table of Other Clinical Trials
            (ii) Reports of Other Clinical Trials
         g. Integrated Summary of Efficacy
         h. Integrated Summary of Safety
         i. Drug Abuse and Overdosage Information
         j. Integrated Summary of Benefits and Risks
         k. GCP Statement
         l. Transfer of Obligations
         m. List of Audited Trials
    (6) Statistical Data Section
         a. Controlled Clinical Trials
            (i) Table of Controlled Clinical Trials
            (ii) Table of Contents—Reports of Controlled Clinical
                Trials
         b. Integrated Summary of Efficacy
         c. Integrated Summary of Safety
         d. Risk Benefit Assessment
  E. Samples and Labeling
  F. Case Report Forms and Tabulations
         a. Case Report Form Tabulations
            Table of Contents
         b. Case Report Forms for Subjects Who Died
            or Discontinued

V. THE NDA APPLICATION

Items A and B in the above outline have been previously discussed as to their content and listings. Items C through F are the essential parts of the NDA that will be reviewed, questioned, and scrutinized by the FDA and its advisors, as this information and data will be the deciding factor for an approved or not approved NDA. Therefore the content of the Application Summary must be done with precision and clarity and contain only scientific data that can be substantiated.

The Application Summary (Item C on form 356h)

The summary should present in a comprehensive way the most important information about the drug product and the conclusions that can be drawn from the presentation. It must reflect a factual review of, and a neutral analysis of, the safety and effectiveness data. The summary should contain an annotated copy of the proposed labeling, a discussion of the benefits and risks of the drug, a discussion of the non–United States marketing history of the drug, and a summary of each technical section. In general, the summary should be as concise as possible—according to the guidelines, from 50 to 200 pages in length. One should also keep in mind that this will be the most widely distributed portion of the NDA at the FDA and will also serve as the basis for drafting the summary basis for approval for the product. The NDA Summary provides the FDA with a good general understanding of the specific drug product. It must state conclusions that can be derived from the most important data within the NDA submission. The information should be written as required for a publication in a medical journal with the results, where possible, reported in graphic and tabular form and must never be promotional in nature. The components of the summary are as follows:

A. Annotated Package Insert

This section should include the proposed text of the labeling for the product, with each statement made referenced back to the data in the technical sections that support the statement. For each statement, claim, caution, or related group of statements, the proposed text of the package labeling must be annotated by reference to volume and page number to the information in the summary and in the technical sections of the application in support of the statements. The format of labeling must follow that described in 21 CFR 201.57 and will form the basis for the advertising and promotion of the drug product. The labeling also serves as a minisummary of the NDA, and any omissions must be explained. This applies to information and to any section or subsection of the labeling format. Adverse experiences that appear in the nonclinical and clinical data sections but are not reflected in the labeling must be explained and must take into account the pharmacology of related drugs.

B. Pharmacological Class, Scientific Rationale, Intended Use, and Potential Clinical Benefits

A brief statement should be included to identify the pharmacological class of the drug, the scientific rationale for the drug, the mechanics of action, if it is identified, its intended use, the subject population being targeted, and its potential clinical benefit(s). Again, the development of the labeling should provide a basis for supplying the above information on the basis of the clinical pharmacology and indications for use.

C. Foreign Marketing History

If the product is marketed outside the United States, regardless of the dosage form, strength, salt, ester, or complex of the drug, the marketing history should be provided. This should include a list of the countries in which the product is marketed, with dates of marketing, if known, and a list of any countries in which the drug has been withdrawn for any reason related to safety or effectiveness. Specific reasons for withdrawal should be given.

D. Chemistry, Manufacturing, and Controls

The chemistry, manufacturing, and controls summary must provide a general overview of the drug substance and the drug product.

1. Drug Substance: Description Including Physical and Chemical Characteristics and Stability.

Names. Indicate the established (generic) name, synonym(s), code designation(s), proprietary (brand name or trademark) name, identification number [e.g., chemical abstract service (CAS) registry number], and chemical name. The applicant should not designate a drug or ingredient by a proprietary name that, because of a similarity in spelling or pronunciation, may be confused with the proprietary name or the established name of a different drug already available in the United States marketplace.

> *Note:* The FDA discourages the use of fanciful proprietary names for a drug or any ingredient that might imply that the drug or ingredient has some unique effectiveness or composition when, in fact, the drug or

ingredient is a common substance, the limitations of which are readily recognized when the drug or ingredient is listed by its established name.

Physical and Chemical Characteristics. The physical and chemical properties of the drug substance must be described in detail, including appearance, physical form, solubility, melting and/or boiling points, molecular weight, structural and molecular formulas, and Wisswesser line notation (WLN). Where applicable, provide information on isomers, polymorphs, pKa values, and pH. Include, in brief, the data obtained and the reference standard(s) used to elucidate the structure of the drug substance.

Stability. Summarize the results of all stability trials. Stability data should be submitted for the drug substance in the container in which it is packaged.

    i. Manufacturer. Provide the name and address of the manufacturer, i.e., the person(s) who performs the manufacturing, processing, packaging, labeling, and control operations on the drug substance. If more than one person is involved in any of these operations, describe the responsibilities of each.

    ii. Method of Manufacture. Describe the methods of synthesis or isolation and purification. Flow charts may be used to present this information.

    iii. Specifications and Analytical Methods. Describe the acceptance specifications and test methods used to assure the identity, strength, quality, and purity of the drug substance and the bioavailability of the drug products made from the drug substance. Any actual or potential impurities, by-products, or degradation products should be indicated. When test methods and specifications are established by an official compendium or other public standard, cite the standard used.

2. Drug Product

Composition and Dosage Form. State the composition: the name and amount of each active and inactive ingredient in the drug product in the form in which it is to be distributed (e.g., amount per tablet). Describe the dosage form: full details as to type and physical characteristics (e.g., shape, color, coating, hardness).

Manufacture. State the name and address of the manufacturer of the drug product. If more than one entity is involved in any part of the process, describe the responsibilities of each. Describe the manufacturing and packaging process for the finished dosage form.

Specifications and Analytical Methods. Describe, as with the drug substance, the acceptable specifications for the drug product and the test methods used to assure the specifications. Cite any official compendia.

Container/Closure System. Describe the proposed container/closure system(s) in which the drug product is to be marketed. Safety closure systems should be detailed.

Stability. State the proposed expiration dating period and storage conditions. Summarize the stability trials justifying the expiration dating period. Stability data should be submitted for the drug product in the container in which it will be marketed.

Investigational Formulations. Provide the quantitative composition and lot number of each finished dosage form used in each clinical trial, bioavailability and pharmacokinetic trial, clinical pharmacology trial, and dose tolerance trial conducted during the investigational phases of the drug product. Cross-reference each formulation to the trial report in the application and explain any differences in formulation.

E. Nonclinical Pharmacology and Toxicology Summary

In the nonclinical pharmacology and toxicology summary, all applicable trials must be listed. Provide an overview of the data from these trials with emphasis on notable adverse effects and dose relationships, species similarities and differences, and identified mechanisms for effects. The discussion should center on the appropriateness and adequacy of the data in support of the drug's proposed therapeutic uses.

Tabular summaries should be used that permit identification and comparison of the pertinent observations.

It is recommended that the trials for this section be presented as follows:

1.   Pharmacology trials. Further subgroup by type of test with trials that support the pharmacologic activity of the drug first, followed by secondary trials and safety pharmacology trials.

2.   Acute toxicity trials. Tabulate species, sex, age, dose range, pharmacological actions and interactions with other drugs, routes of administration, vehicle, toxic signs, lethal dose, time of death, etc.

3.   Multidose toxicity trials (subchronic, carcinogenicity, pharmacological, and interactions with other drugs). Provide a table of trials including species and strain, number of animals, sex, age, dose, dose schedule, and route of administration. Notable treatment and dose-related changes in survival, percent weight gain, toxic signs, hematology, clinical chemistries, organ weight, and pathology should be provided.

4.   *Carcinogenicity* trials. The following information should be included:

(a) For each treatment group, the number of animals entered and surviving 12, 15, 18, 21, and 24 months.

(b) A summary table of tumor occurrences with deaths and sacrifices combined, organized by body system, tumor type, and dose level.

(c) In the above table, each tumor shown to have a statistically significant dose response (positive or negative) at the $P = 0.05$ level (one-sided) using a mortality-adjusted statistical test of dose response over the entire trial time unadjusted for multiple comparisons or multiple testing should be indicated. Calculated P values for the significant dose–response test for each of these tumors should be included.

5. Special toxicity trials.
6. Reproduction trials.
7. Mutagenicity trials.
8. ADME (absorption, distribution, metabolism, excretion) trials. Animal species should be presented under each group by smallest (mouse) up to largest (monkey or other mammals). The route of administration should be presented under each species tested and the treatment group under each route of administration. For special toxicity trials, such as irritation and hemolysis trials, tabulate data as appropriate. An example of the format would be

Acute toxicity trials

A. Mouse
  (1) Oral
    (a) Untreated control
    (b) Vehicle control
    (c) Etc.
  (2) I.V.
    (a) Untreated control
    (b) Vehicle control
    (c) Etc.
B. Rat
  (1) Oral
    (a) Untreated control
    (b) Vehicle control
    (c) Etc.
  (2) I.V.
    (a) Untreated control
    (b) Vehicle control
    (c) Etc.

9. For *reproduction* trials, tabulate fertility and reproductive performance trials (segment I) and perinatal and postnatal trials (segment III) if differences are observed from controls. Teratology trial data (segment II) should be tabulated showing differences and similarities in gross viscera and skeletal anomalies.

10. For *mutagenicity* trials, data should be presented in the following order:

A. In vitro nonmammalian cell system
B. In vitro mammalian cell system
C. In vivo nonmammalian system
D. In vivo mammalian system

In summarizing the ADME trials, tabulate species, strain, and dose comparison data by the following:

Peak level, half-life, and so forth
Plasma protein binding
Tissue distribution/accumulation
Enzyme induction or inhibition
Metabolites
Excretion pattern and characteristics

The absorption, distribution, metabolism, and excretion in the species used in the toxicology trials should be discussed. Quantitative or notable qualitative differences in ADME between the various animal species and humans should be discussed, as well as any references to observed species' differences in toxicity and extrapolation of the findings to humans. The significance of these findings to the interpretation of the results of the carcinogenicity, bioassay, and other preclinical toxicity trials should be considered.

F. Human Pharmacokinetics and Bioavailability Summary

The human pharmacokinetic and bioavailability summary should include the following:

1. A brief description of each bioavailability trial of the drug in humans, by type, objective, design, analytical and statistical method used, and results.

2. A brief description of the pharmacokinetic characteristics of the active ingredient(s) and the performance of the dosage form, integrating conclusions from the bioavailability and pharmacokinetic trials and from clinical trials performed. Information on volume of distribution, half-life, routes and rates of excretion, and metabolism of each dosage form trials, and the proportionality of absorption over the therapeutic dose range should be included. If pertinent, a comparison with the bioavailability of other dosage forms should be provided. Any identified differences in pharmacokinetics among subject subgroups should be cited (age, renal status, etc.).

3. A description of the dissolution profile of the drug.

G. Microbiology Summary

For anti-infective and antiviral drugs, provide a summary of the results of the microbiology trials conducted with the drug. This should include the following:

1. A brief description of the known mechanisms of action together with structural or other similarities to known families of antimicrobial drugs.

2. A brief description of the antimicrobial spectrum of action and a summary of the results of in vitro susceptibility testing demonstrating the concentrations of the drug required for effective use.

3. A brief description of known mechanisms of resistance to the drug and results of any in vitro trials regarding resistance or any known epidemiological trials that demonstrate the prevalence of resistance factors.

4. A brief description of the clinical microbiology laboratory test method needed for effective use of the drug.

H. Clinical Data Summary and Results of Statistical Analysis

The clinical data summary and results of statistical analyses are divided into several parts as presented below. This section is probably the most scrutinized by the FDA's clinical reviewer. It is the basis of efficacy and safety that will determine an NDA approval.

1. Clinical Pharmacology

Describe the phase 1 trials that establish human tolerance to the drug, absorption, distribution, and elimination kinetics, blood concentrations as a function of time after dosing, the metabolic profile, drug interactions, dependence, and pharmacological effects at various doses. Although it is usual to test the drug during phase 1 trials in normal (healthy) subjects, if a drug has dramatic biochemical or pharmacological effects tailored to address a specific disease state, phase 1 trials are conducted only in individuals with such a disease state. A careful explanation in this section should be prepared. Information may be formatted as follows:

a. A tabular presentation of trials by protocol, investigator, trial design (e.g., randomized, double-blind, open, parallel, crossover), drug or other treatment used for comparison (if any), number of subjects, age, sex, dose, and duration of dosing. Location of trial report and CRFs (if submitted) should also be included.

b. A short narrative description of the design and results of each trial.

c. Conclusions drawn from this group of trials. A summary should provide the critical findings, especially those relevant to the clinical use of the drug (e.g., dose–response or blood level–response data, duration of action, and any specific potential problems associated with metabolism or excretion). There should be a complete discussion of data pertinent to other common important pharmacological properties, including cardiac electrophysiological effects, hemodynamic effects, anticholinergic effects, and effects on the central nervous system. Any effects related to age or sex should be highlighted.

2. Overview of Clinical Trials

The objective of all clinical trials is to produce clear and well-documented evidence that a new drug candidate is effective and safe when used in the manner intended. The clinical experience that the sponsor is submitting (see GCP Chap. 19) must provide assurance of the care taken in the evaluation of the drug product. This assurance must be passed on to the FDA reviewer in the summary of the clinical evaluation.

The overview should reference any specific FDA guidelines used and any FDA–sponsor discussions held on major issues, such as an end-of-phase-2 conference. The critical features of the trials should be explained, including duration, trial design, and particular advantages or potential problems examined. If there is pertinent clinical literature (controlled or uncontrolled clinical trials or reports on subjects), a review may be helpful. (The sponsor may want to comment on literature pertaining to closely related drugs that provide insight into potential problems or areas of special interest.)

It is important to comment on all trials of the drug, even those not completed or ongoing, or trials of claims other than those for which approval is sought.

3. Controlled Clinical Trials

All controlled trials, whether they provide positive, equivocal, or negative evidence, should be included. The recommended sequence for presentation, for each indication, is as follows:

a. A table of all completed trials sponsored by the applicant, including domestic trials and foreign trials, as well as those from published or unpublished papers or other sources. Provide the protocol number (where available), reference to any published report, investigator(s), trial design (e.g., double-blind, open, parallel, crossover), the formulation and dosage used, number of subjects, demographics of subjects, dose and duration of therapy, and location of the clinical report and CRFs.

b. A short narrative of each trial, including trial design, conduct, and analysis. This section should be of sufficient detail to allow the reader to understand what the dose was and what data were collected and analyzed for efficacy and safety determinations. Quantitative results should be provided, and the statistical methodologies, specific end points used, and any subject inclusion and exclusions should be described.

c. An analysis of each trial and all the trials as a whole to demonstrate how they relate to each claim of effectiveness. If some trials are considered more important than others, this should be noted and an explanation given. Any pooled analyses should be explained and presented. Any major inconsistencies or areas needing further exploration should be identified. Dose–response and dose-duration/dose-frequency information as well as any differences in response among subgroups should be included.

4. Uncontrolled Clinical Trials

This section should include the following:

a. A table of trials similar to that included in the controlled clinical trials section of the summary. The information should include the protocol number or other identifier, conditions studied, formulation and dosage, number of subjects, age and sex, duration of therapy, and location of the full report in the clinical data section.

b. A brief narrative description of the design and results of each trial, including effectiveness results and adverse experiences.

c. An overall analyses of these trials and the conclusions reached from them.

5. Other Trials and Information

A brief description of any trials not included in the clinical pharmacology, controlled clinical trials, or uncontrolled clinical trials sections should be included here. These may include trials and publications not directly related to the claims sought in the application but that provide pertinent safety information. Analyses of marketing experience or epidemiological data may also be included in this section.

6. Safety Summary—General Safety Conclusions

This section will include the following information:

Extent of Exposure. The extent of drug exposure and the number of subjects exposed to the drug for various periods and at various doses. These should include all subjects or patients.

Adverse Experiences. Data from controlled and uncontrolled trials should be integrated to provide estimated rates of adverse experiences. The tables of adverse experience rates, including the more serious or frequent experiences, should be compiled (see Chap. 11 on ADR reporting). It is useful to analyze results from controlled and open trials separately and distinguish short-term use from longer term trials. Any differences in rates related to dose, duration of therapy, and subject characteristics should be identified. Data related to drug–drug interactions should also be included. An analysis of subjects who left the trial prematurely because of an adverse experience or who died while on this trial drug should be included. For potentially serious adverse experiences that have not been established as drug related, the data should be discussed along with additional steps in premarketing or postmarketing, to determine whether the drug is associated with this effect.

Clinical Laboratory Data. Provide a short summary of these data, noting clinically significant trends and statistically significant changes. The summary should compare the active control drug with placebo and should show the numbers of subjects receiving each test. Also identify and evaluate those subjects who leave a trial because of clinical laboratory abnormalities.

Summary of Other Safety Assessments. If there were any special safety examinations performed (e.g., audiometric, electrocardiographic, or ophthalmologic examinations), these should be summarized here. Include any comparisons with active control drugs and placebo, if available, and the numbers of subjects receiving each test.

Overdosage. Any information available on the treatment of overdosage should be included.

Drug Abuse. If the drug is subject to abuse, provide a summary of the trials or other relevant information. If the drug is not considered abusable but is a member of a class of drugs known to have abuse potential, and if trials of its abuse potential have not been performed, then the reasons these trials were considered unnecessary should be discussed.

I. Discussion of Benefit/Risk Relationship and Proposed Postmarketing trials

On the basis of the results of effectiveness trials and the toxicity of the drug in human and animal trials, a benefit-to-risk assessment of the drug should be formulated and presented. The assessment should consider the risks and benefits of alternative treatment(s) for the target population identified in the labeling.

The applicant should also describe any proposed postmarketing clinical trials and the reasons for doing such trials, e.g., to trial further a suspected adverse reaction, or to do trials in children if there is a potential for use in this group.

VI. NDA TECHNICAL SECTIONS

The guidelines for the format and content of each relevant technical section should be reviewed for specific information. Included below are brief general descriptions and outlines of the NDA technical sections.

A. Chemistry, Manufacturing, and Controls

This section of the NDA, called the CMC section, requires extreme attention and precision in its presentation. Therefore these requirements and applicable guidelines for the chemistry, manufacturing, and controls section of an NDA submission are discussed in detail in Chap. 14 of this book.

B. Nonclinical Pharmacology and Toxicology

In this section, it is useful to include a summary of the preclinical trials as well as complete reports. A table of contents with the volume and page numbers for the location of each report should also be included. New trials or final reports not previously submitted to the IND or to a previous NDA submission for the drug under review should be identified in a consistent and conspicuous manner in the table of contents.

The FDA guidelines specifying the order in which the nonclinical pharmacology and toxicology trials should be presented in an NDA submission, are as follows:

1. Pharmacology trials
2. Acute toxicity trials
3. Multidose toxicity trials
4. Special toxicity trials
5. Reproduction trials
6. Mutagenicity trials
7. Absorption, distribution, metabolism, and excretion (ADME) trials

When more than one species is used, the following order of presentation is recommended, with males preceding females:

1. Mouse
2. Rat
3. Hamster
4. Other rodent(s)
5. Rabbit
6. Dog

7. Monkey
8. Other nonrodent mammal(s)
9. Nonmammals

Data for typical adult animals should precede that of infant, geriatric, or disease-model animals. Age and weight ranges, strains, and animal suppliers should be specified in each trial.

Regarding route of administration, the one that represents the intended route in humans should be presented first, followed by data from other routes in the following relative order:

1. Oral
2. Intravenous
3. Intramuscular
4. Intraperitoneal
5. Subcutaneous
6. Inhalation
7. Topical
8. Other in vivo
9. In vitro

Multiple-dose data should be displayed from lowest to highest dose as shown below:

1. Untreated control
2. Vehicle control
3. Low dose
4. Middle dose(s)
5. High dose
6. Positive or comparative control(s)

Dose should be based on the active moiety component and should be expressed on a body-weight basis if possible. When the drug is administered in diet or drinking water, the daily dose, calculated periodically from actual body weight and food or water consumption data, should be included in the report as the dose range per sex for each group at the beginning and end of the trial and at designated intervals throughout a chronic trial. Doses should not be expressed solely as a concentration in food or drinking water. One should also obtain blood level data to confirm that the drug is being absorbed by the animals.

C. Pharmacology Trials

Pharmacology trials related to the therapeutic indication should be presented first, followed by those related to possible adverse reactions and interactions with other drugs. Within the three categories listed above, the data should be grouped in the following order:

1. Gastrointestinal
2. Genitourinary
3. Endocrine
4. Anti-inflammatory
5. Immunoactive
6. Chemotherapeutic
7. Enzyme effects
8. Other

Where possible, data should be summarized in tabular form, with the various trials within each category grouped to present a coherent pharmacological profile of the drug.

D. Acute Toxicity Trials

The pretest conditioning and age of the animals, dosing procedures, vehicle used, and dosage volumes should be specified. The description of the results should include the types and severity of toxic signs and their onset and progression or reversal in relationship to dosage and time after dosing. The lethal dose data should be tabulated, including the total number dosed and mortality incidence with time of death for each sex at each dose.

E. Subchronic/Chronic/Carcinogenicity Trials

At the beginning of this subsection, all trials should be listed and briefly described in a table. trials should be grouped by species, order of increasing duration of treatment, and route of administration. The table should include animal species and strain, initial group size per sex, dosing route and mode of drug administration, dose groups, duration of the trial in weeks, week of any scheduled interim sacrifices, the name of the laboratory performing the trial, and the report number.

Within each individual trial report, there should be a description of the protocol, followed by trial results.

In the section of the report that describes how the trial was conducted, the following information should be included:

1. Species, strain, source, age
2. Sex, number at beginning and end of the trial
3. Route and mode of administration
4. Calculated dosage levels and ranges

 5. Rationale for dose selection
 6. Administration of vehicle or control treatment
 7. Drug batch or lot number
 8. Duration of treatment
 9. Duration of trial
10. Interim sacrifice

The results of the trial should include the following:

 1. Observed effects
 2. Mortality
 3. Body weight
 4. Food/water consumption
 5. Physical examination
 6. Hematology/bone marrow/coagulation
 7. Blood chemistry/urinalysis/ADME data
 8. Organ weights
 9. Gross pathology
10. Histopathology

For *carcinogenicity* trials, tumor data for male and female animals should be presented separately. A chronologic listing should be prepared showing the period in which each tumor was discovered, the dose group of the animal, the animal number, whether the animal was sacrificed or died, the site of the tumor, the tumor type, and an assessment of the malignancy of the tumor.

A summary table should be prepared for each period in which a death or sacrifice occurred, and for each dose group the number dying, the number sacrificed, the number of animals necropsied completely, and the number necropsied to any extent. This section should also include a summary table of tumor occurrences with deaths and sacrifices combined, organized by body system, organ, tumor type, and dose level. The number of animals with tumors of the stated type should also be included.

For each tumor found to be statistically significant at the $P = 0.05$ level (one sided) by use of a statistical test of dose response over the entire trial that is adjusted for mortality as appropriate and that is not adjusted for multiple comparisons or multiple testing, the following information should be included:

1. The estimated incidence rate of fatal tumors in each time period and the prevalence rate of nonfatal tumors in each time period.

2. The statistical test used and the calculated *P*-value should be included. Results for both statistically significant positive and statistically negative dose–response findings should be reported.

F. Special Toxicity Trials

This section includes trials appropriate to a particular formulation or route of administration, such as in vitro hemolysis or irritation at the injection site. In vivo results should be tabulated to show group comparison and time-related or progressive effects within each group. For in vitro trials, the data should be tabulated by type of test or test system, dose range, and effects related to dose.

G. Reproduction Trials

This section should include a summary table similar to that included in the subchronic/chronic/carcinogenicity trials section.

Segment I trials of fertility and reproductive performance should be presented first, followed by segment II teratology and segment III perinatal and postnatal; any other trials such as multigeneration trials should be presented last. Observations and their incidence in relationship to dosage or time should be presented in the following relative order. Maternal effects and day of parturition/necropsy (and paternal effects in segment I). Maternal necropsy.

1. Corpora lutea
2. Uterine contents
3. Implantation
4. Dead fetuses
5. Fetuses (grouped by litter)
6. Sex ratio
7. Weight
8. Viability
9. Gross observations
10. Visceral abnormalities
11. Skeletal abnormalities
12. Neonates to weaning
13. Sex ratio
14. Viability
15. Growth
16. Behavior and performance
17. Anatomical abnormalities

H. Mutagenicity Trials

The results of these trials should be tabulated by type of trial methods used, dose range, and effect at each dose. trials should be presented in the following order:

1. In vitro nonmammalian cell system

2. In vitro mammalian cell system
3. In vivo mammalian system
4. In vivo nonmammalian system

I. ADME Trials

These trials should be summarized in the following sequence:

1. Absorption, pharmacokinetics, serum half-life, etc.
2. Protein binding
3. Tissue distribution/accumulation
4. Enzyme induction or inhibition
5. Metabolism characteristics and metabolites
6. Excretion pattern

If possible, ADME data should be generated on the same species used in the toxicology trials.

J. Human Pharmacokinetics and Bioavailability Section

Included in the first portion of this section should be an overall tabulated summary of all in vivo biopharmaceutical trials carried out on the drug grouped by type of trial. The trial number, route of administration, dosage form, batch number, plant and date of manufacture, number of subjects, IND or NDA number under which the trial was conducted or submitted, date of submission, conclusions regarding the trial, and previous agency response on the trial or the protocol together with the date of the correspondence should be included.

Following this information is a summary of the bioavailability/pharmacokinetic data and the overall conclusions. The summary should include a table with the following pharmacokinetic parameters: peak concentration (C_{max}), AUC, time to reach peak concentration (T_{max}), elimination constant (k_{el}), distribution volume (V_d), plasma and renal clearance, and urinary excretion. Overall conclusions as well as any unresolved problems should be discussed.

In the third section, a list of all formulations used in clinical trials and in vivo bioavailability/pharmacokinetic trials together with the trials in which each formulation was used should be provided. For batches used in bioavailability/pharmacokinetic trials, significant manufacturing and formulation changes for the drug product over the course of its evaluation should be identified.

The fourth section relates to the analytical methods used to measure the levels of the drug and major metabolites in body fluids. A table should be included in this section listing the trial number, submission date, type of biological fluid, method used, sensitivity, and range of the method and specificity of the method for the parent compound and metabolites.

Dissolution data on each strength and dosage form for which approval is being sought should be provided in the fifth portion of this technical section. A comparative dissolution trial with the lot(s) used for in vivo biopharmaceutic trials should also be included. The date of the trials, dosage form and strength, lot number, dissolution apparatus, media/temperature, speed of rotation/flow, collection times, number of units tested, range, and mean percent dissolved should all be included in the table. A summary of the dissolution method and specification for the product should be provided.

The last portion of this technical section includes the reports for each of the trials referenced in this section. Each report should include the following information:

1. Objective
2. Dosage form studied
3. Investigator
4. Clinical facilities
5. Analytical facilities
6. Individual subject/patient data including demographics, concomitant medication, blood/urine levels, laboratory tests, and adverse reactions
7. Documentation on the sensitivity, linearity, specificity, and reproducibility of the analytical methods

The data analyses should include appropriate statistical analysis usually involving analysis of variance, calculations of power analysis, 95% confidence intervals, and ratio analysis. The details of pharmacokinetic parameter calculations, including pharmacokinetic models and equations used, should be adequately described and referenced. A brief summary of trial conclusions should be provided.

K. Microbiology

New drug applications for anti-infective and antiviral drugs require a technical section on microbiological data. This section should include the biochemical basis of the drug's action on microbial or viral physiology, the antimicrobial or antiviral spectrum of the drug including results of in vitro preclinical trials demonstrating concentrations of the drug required for effective use. Any known mechanisms of resistance to the drug including the results of any known epidemiological trials demonstrating prevalence of resistance factors and clinical microbiology laboratory methods to evaluate the effective use of the drug also should be included. This section is divided into the following 11 sections.

1. Mechanism of Action

The mode of action of the drug, together with its chemical structure and any structural or other similarities to known antimicrobial drugs should be included.

2. Pharmacokinetics

In this section, the pharmacokinetics for systemic dosage forms should be described, including absorption, routes of excretion, protein binding, metabolic changes to compounds of lesser or greater activity, and distribution into various pharmacokinetic compartments. References to the locations in the NDA of the full reports of the pharmacokinetics trials should be provided.

3. Antimicrobial Activity

A description of the antimicrobial spectrum of the drug and a summary table of the major in vitro susceptibility trials should be included.

4. Enzyme Hydrolysis Rates

The stability of the drug in the presence of enzymes produced by microorganisms should be summarized.

5. Miscellaneous trials

If applicable, any miscellaneous trials, such as those showing bacterial effects, activity of major metabolites, or relationships to known drugs, should be summarized.

6. Assessment of Resistance

A brief summary of the resistance to the drug should be included. A detailed discussion of the trials of resistant microorganisms as well as any resistance known to occur among normally susceptible species is also required. It is suggested that a table be prepared including each species or type of microorganism tested, antimicrobial drugs to which each microorganism is resistant, number of microorganisms tested, and percentage of microorganisms susceptible to the drug at each level of resistance.

7. Clinical Laboratory Susceptibility Test Methods

A detailed discussion of the development of clinical laboratory susceptibility test methods should be provided.

8. In Vivo Animal Protection trials

The results of any efficacy trials in experimentally infected animals should be summarized.

9. In Vitro trials Conducted During the Clinical Trials

The susceptibility testing of clinical isolates obtained in the clinical investigations should be summarized.

10. Conclusions

A brief narrative summary of the overall results and any conclusions about the drug must be included in this section.

11. Published Literature

Included in this section is a bibliography and copies of all published reports of trials used in support of the data and information contained in the microbiology section.

L. Clinical Data Section

The clinical data section is probably the most important and most complicated section of an NDA. It is the part that provides the safety and efficacy data on the drug for its intended use. In the *Guidelines for the Format and Content of the Clinical and Statistical Sections of an Application*, the FDA has outlined how it would like to see this section of the NDA organized. This outline is provided here.

M. Outline of the Clinical Section

    A. List of investigators, list of INDs and NDAs
    B. Background/overview of clinical investigations
    C. Clinical pharmacology
       1. Table of all trials, grouped by trial type

    2. ADME trials
- a. Synopsis of each trial
- b. Full report of each trial
- c. Summary and evaluation of all trials

    3. Early dose–tolerance trials a, b, c, as above

    4. Short-term trials of therapeutic response or of a pharmacodynamic effect thought to relate to therapeutic response, including dose–response and blood level–response trials a, b, c, as above

    5. Trials of pharmacodynamic properties other than the property thought to be related to clinical effectiveness a, b, c, as above

    6. "Special" trials a, b, c, as above

    7. Overall summary of clinical pharmacology

D. Controlled clinical trials

    1. Table of trials, grouped by indication, trial design, completion status, location, and availability of case reports. If more than one indication is included in the NDA, each section should be divided by indication.

    2. Indication 1
- a. Placebo-controlled trials
  - 1) Completed trials
    - a) Domestic, full case reports available
      - (1) For each trial, information should be provided as follows:
        - i. Brief synopsis
        - ii. Protocol
        - iii. Related publication
        - iv. List of investigators
        - v. Integrated clinical and statistical report
    - b) Foreign, full case reports available
      - (1) Data for each trial should be provided as in i–v above
    - c) Published reports and other reports lacking full case reports
      - (1) Again, data for each trial should be provided (as appropriate) as in i–v above
  - 2) Ongoing trials with interim results (a–c) as above
  - 3) Incomplete trials no longer active (a–c) as above
- b. Dose comparison concurrent control trials (1–3) as above
- c. No-treatment concurrent control trials (1–3) as above
- d. Active treatment concurrent control trials (1–3) as above
- e. Explicit historical control trials (1–3) as above

    3. Any additional indications should be organized as in Indication 1, above

    4. Optional overall summary and evaluation of data from controlled trials

E. Uncontrolled clinical trials

    1. Table of all trials, grouped by indication, completion status, location, and availability of case reports

    2. Indication 1

        a. Completed trials

           1) Domestic, full case reports available

              a) For each trial, information should be provided as listed below:

                  (1) Brief synopsis

                  (2) Protocol

                  (3) Related publication

                  (4) List of investigators

                  (5) Report of the trial

           2) Foreign, full case reports available

              a) As above

           3) Published reports and other reports lacking full case reports

              a) Complete trials as above

              b) Incomplete trials (1–3) as above

    3. Any additional indications should be organized as in Indication 1, above

F. Other trials and information

    1. Table of all trials

    2. Controlled trials of uses other than those claimed in the application, any trial design, complete or incomplete

        a. trials with case reports available

           1) For each trial, information should be provided as outlined below

              a) Brief synopsis

              b) Protocol

              c) Related publication

              d) List of investigators

              e) Report of the trial

        b. trials without case reports available

           1) As above

    3. Uncontrolled trials of uses other than those claimed in the application

        a. trials with case reports available

   1) For each trial, information should be provided as outlined below:

    a) Brief synopsis

    b) Protocol

    c) Related publication

    d) List of investigators

    e) Report of the trial

  b. Trials without case reports available

   1) As above

 4. Commercial marketing experience

  a. List of countries in which drug has been approved

  b. Reports from regulatory authorities

  c. Epidemiological trials

  d. Spontaneous reports from foreign marketing experience of serious adverse experiences

 5. Reports from literature or elsewhere not otherwise reported

  a. Published case reports, letters, etc.

  b. Other information

G. Integrated summary of effectiveness data

 1. Identification of trials fulfilling the statutory requirements for adequate and well-controlled trials showing that the drug has its intended effect

 2. Comparison and analysis of all controlled trials

 3. Results of uncontrolled trials

 4. Analysis of dose–response or blood level–response information

 5. Analysis of response in subsets of the overall population: drug–demographic, drug–drug, and drug–disease interactions

 6. Evidence of long-term effectiveness, tolerance, and withdrawal effects

H. Integrated summary of safety data

 1. Table of all investigations pertinent to safety, identified by protocol number and principal investigator, grouped by trial type

 2. Overall extent of exposure

 3. Demographic and other characteristics of the trial population

 4. Adverse experiences in clinical trials

  a. Narrative summary of adverse experiences

  b. Display of adverse experiences and occurrence rates

  c. Analysis of adverse experience rates

  d. Display and analysis of deaths, dropouts due to adverse experiences, and other serious or potentially serious adverse experiences

    5. Clinical laboratory evaluation
    6. Adverse experiences, including laboratory abnormalities, from sources other than clinical trials
    7. Animal data
    8. Analysis of dose–response information
    9. Drug–drug interactions
   10. Drug–demographic and drug–disease interactions
   11. Pharmacologic properties other than the property of principal interest
   12. Long-term adverse effects
   13. Withdrawal effects
  I. Drug abuse and overdosage
  J. Integrated summary of benefits and risks of the drug

Parts of the clinical data section are discussed in greater detail below.

1. Listing of IND and NDA Investigators

This section should contain a complete alphabetical list of all the names and addresses of all known investigators that the applicant supplied with the drug substance or product. In addition, all dosage forms used by these investigators should be stated. This list should also include the kinds of trials carried out, trial identifier, location of each report, case report tabulations, and case report forms. In addition, a list of all known INDs under which the drug was studied and any other NDAs submitted for the same drug substance should be included.

2. Background/Overview of Clinical Investigations

This is a very important part of the clinical data section of an NDA. It provides the medical reviewer with a summary of how the drug was developed. Because of the time required for the clinical development of a product, many times the FDA reviewers assigned to the project have changed. As a result, the NDA may be reviewed by a new set of individuals who are unfamiliar with the history of the development of the project. It is also possible that the standards for research in the particular field may have changed and what was standard clinical practice when the clinical trials were initiated is no longer the method of choice for trialing the particular class of drugs. In this section, one is given the opportunity to describe the general approach and rationale used in developing the clinical data. This discussion should include how information derived from clinical pharmacology trials led to critical features of the clinical trials. The basis for the critical design features of the clinical trials as well as their suitability and selection of major clinical end points also should be discussed. Any FDA drug-class or other guidelines used in designing the trials, and the rationale for any deviations from the guidelines, should be discussed.

Food and Drug Administration/Sponsor discussions concerning issues related to the clinical program, the major agreements reached, and any important differences between these agreements and the ultimate conduct of the clinical trials must be referenced. The selection of areas of special interest for trial and analysis, and effectiveness or safety issues raised by drugs of the same pharmacological or therapeutic class warrant discussion. Any specific questions raised by the results of the clinical trials or by experience with related drugs and not answered by the clinical trials should be cited, together with an explanation of how the sponsor plans to handle these issues. Any planned trials in support of an additional indication also should be noted here.

3. Clinical Pharmacology

As noted in the outline of the clinical data section of an NDA, this section is divided into five parts. It should also include a table of all trials grouped by type and an overall summary of the clinical pharmacology trials. The table should list investigators, trial identifiers, starting date of the trial, and location of the trial report, tabulations, and case report forms. Other information, including number of subjects, trial design, formulation and dosage strength used, control treatment, dose range, dose regimen, and duration of dosing should also be included. For each group of trials, there should be a 1- to 2-page synopsis of the results of each trial, followed by the complete report of the trial. At the end of each of the five sections, there should be an overall summary and evaluation, including a narrative or tabular comparison of the human trials with the animal pharmacology and toxicology data.

An overall summary of the clinical pharmacology data should be included. In this summary, findings relevant to the clinical use of the drug, such as dose–response or blood level–response data, duration of action data, and potential problems that can be associated with the observed patterns of metabolism or excretion must be discussed.

4. Controlled Clinical trials

Before a detailed discussion of the information to be included in this section is given, it is useful to review the definition of adequate and well-controlled trials. Approval of a new drug requires substantial evidence of effectiveness. Substantial evidence is defined under the Federal Food, Drug and Cosmetic Act as

> evidence consisting of adequate and well-controlled investigations by experts qualified by scientific training and experience to evaluate the effectiveness of the drug involved, on the basis of which it could fairly and responsibly be concluded by such experts that the drug will have the effect it purports or is represented to have under the conditions of use prescribed, recommended, or suggested in the proposed labeling. The requirement for well-controlled investigations has been interpreted to mean that the effectiveness of a drug should be supported by more than one well-controlled trial and carried out by independent investigators.

Recently, there has been active lobbying to accept a single pivotal clinical trial as the basis for approval. This thrust is based on the FDA Modernization Act (FDAMA) of 1997. Section 115 of the FDAMA states that the "substantial evidence" of efficacy requirement may be satisfied by *one* adequate and well-controlled clinical investigation supported by confirmatory evidence. The FDA issued a guidance on when one phase 3 trial would suffice in May 1997.

In this section of the NDA, all controlled trials including those that were incomplete and abandoned must be provided. For trials intended to support effectiveness, full reports are required; for others, an abbreviated report may be acceptable.

A table of all trials grouped by indication and type of control, as shown in the outline, should be included. The table lists investigators, trial identifiers, starting date of the trial, location of the report, tabulations, and case report forms. The number, age, and sex of the subjects, trial design, formulation, dosage form and strength, control, doses, and duration of dosing also should be provided. The order of presentation of the trials should be as indicated in the outline. Completed trials should be presented before ongoing trials with interim results, followed by incomplete trials.

Reports of individual trials should include a 1- to 2-page synopsis, a copy of the protocol, any publications on the data, a list of all investigators and other persons whose participation materially affected the conduct of the trial, and a brief description of their training and role in the trial. A statement regarding compliance with the IRB regulations in 21 CFR Part 56 and the informed consent regulations 21 CFR Part 50 is also required.

In a presentation, Dr. Robert Temple, Director of the Office of Drug Research and Review at the FDA [1], suggested the following approach to the presentation of individual trials in the clinical data section:

Synopsis: prepare a brief (1-page) summary of the trial.

Manuscript: provide a short summary (about 10 pages) for major trials.
Comprehensive summary: for all trials, present a detailed description of
the trial design and results, including the following:

   a. Investigator
   b. trial objectives
   c. Detailed design
   d. Subject selection criteria
   e. Clinical observations and laboratory measurements
   f. Evaluation criteria
   g. Planned statistical analyses
   h. Method of eliciting adverse experiences
   i. Comparability of treatment groups for demographic and other
      variables
   j. Analysis of effectiveness results
   k. Detailed accounting of subjects entered/excluded from the trial
   l. The dosage and duration of treatment

This critical section should include individual subject data in a tabulated
form. Demographic values (age, sex, race, etc.), subject inclusion and exclusion criteria, and relevant clinical measures for the particular trial must
also be included. Special clinical and laboratory measures used for the trial
must have a rationale for these tests as well as an explanation for the significance of the results. All concomitant medications used during the clinical
trial must be listed for each subject admitted into the trial. Other clinical
observations of less relevance should be addressed.

5. Safety Information

Safety information should be presented as a summary of adverse experiences
by frequency and body system, except for subjects who died or who left the
trial prematurely because of an adverse experience. These should be described
in detail, and the role of the drug should be evaluated for each reaction. The
safety analysis should consider abnormal laboratory values as well as adverse
experiences, and the following points should be kept in mind:

   a. Is the subject receiving several different medications simultane-
      ously?
   b. Are the subject's complaints totally subjective, e.g., headache,
      nausea, dizziness? Many of these often appear in healthy
      volunteers taking placebo.
   c. The evaluation of adverse experiences is dependent in great part
      on the extent of the control of the trial.

    d. The effect of the environment in which the trial was conducted—
acute medical ward vs. outpatient sample.

    e. Examination of subject's history and careful follow-up of subject;
authentication of facts.

An applicant may provide an overall summary of data from controlled trials. This section is optional and many firms do not include it because the results of the trials are presented in the integrated summaries of efficacy and safety, which will be discussed later in this chapter. The *Guidelines for the Clinical and Statistical Sections of a New Drug Application* also address the format and content of an integrated clinical/statistical report for a clinical trial; this too will be discussed later.

6. Uncontrolled Clinical trials

Uncontrolled trials will not, in general, be useful in contributing to substantial evidence of effectiveness of a drug, but they can provide support for controlled clinical trials and provide safety information. The format for this section is the same as that contained in the outline. As in the controlled clinical trials section, this section should begin with a table, followed by the reports for the trials. Data should be provided in the same manner as that discussed in the controlled clinical trials section.

7. Other trials and Information

In this section, a description and analysis of any additional information obtained by the applicant from any source, foreign or domestic, that is relevant to the evaluation of the efficacy and safety of the product should be included. It may include results of controlled or uncontrolled clinical trials of uses of the drug other than those claimed in the application, commercial marketing experience, and reports in the literature or otherwise obtained, other than those cited in the controlled trials and uncontrolled trials sections of the clinical data section.

    This first part of this section is a table of all the trials listing the same information contained in the tables in the controlled clinical trials and uncontrolled clinical trials sections of the clinical data section. Reports of the trials should be presented as shown in the outline. The content of the reports for the trials should be the same as those discussed in the other sections.

    The next portion of this section deals with commercial marketing experience and foreign regulatory actions. This part should contain the following information:

    a. A list of the countries in which the drug has been approved with
dates of approval and a list of the countries in which approval has
been applied for with the dates of the applications.

b. All reports from foreign regulatory authorities or foreign affiliates, licensors, or licensees of the applicant, including reports and analyses of adverse effects, warning letters sent to physicians, and major changes in marketing status or labeling information resulting from marketing or other experience.

  A copy of any letter from a foreign regulatory body that refuses drug approval on safety grounds should also be included. It is requested that copies of approved labeling from European countries, Canada, Australia, New Zealand, and Japan be included together with English translations. Important differences between these and the proposed United States labeling with respect to contraindications, warnings, precautions, adverse reactions, or dosing instructions should be identified and explained.

c. Epidemiology trials.

d. Spontaneous reports from foreign marketing experiences of serious adverse experiences.

  Reports from the literature that are not included in other sections of the NDA should be provided in this section.

8. Integrated Summary of Efficacy (ISE)

This section should provide an integrated summary of the data demonstrating substantial evidence of effectiveness for each claimed indication. It should also include a summary of the evidence supporting the dosage and administration section of the labeling, including the dose and dose interval recommended.

  An overview of the results should show that the regulatory requirements for approval have been met by adequate and well-controlled trials that support the claimed effect. This is especially important if results are inconsistent or marginal. An examination of trial-to-trial differences in results, effects in subsets of the treated population, dose–response information, and comparisons with alternative drugs should be addressed. A description of the information to be included in this section is contained in the outline provided earlier in this chapter.

  The first portion of this section is an identification of those trials that fulfill the requirements for adequate and well-controlled trials showing that the drug has its intended effect. This is followed by a discussion of those trials as well as the data from all controlled clinical trials. Any differences in outcome between trials of similar design should be explained where possible. Tables showing major trial design features, numbers of subjects, numbers of dropouts, and major outcomes are sometimes useful.

  The results of uncontrolled trials should be discussed to the extent that they provide supportive evidence of effectiveness. This is followed by an analysis of dose–response or blood level–response information. This section should include (a) an integrated summary and analysis of all data, from animal, pharmacokinetic, pharmacodynamic, and other clinical pharmacology trials, and from controlled and uncontrolled clinical trials that bear a dose–response or blood level–response relationship to effectiveness, (b) the method of dose selection, and (c) the choice of dose interval. Data that support the dosing recommendation proposed in labeling, including the recommended starting and maximal doses, the method of dose titration, and other methods regarding individualization of dosage also should be discussed. Any deviations from relatively simple dose–response or blood level–response relationships due to nonlinearity of pharmacokinetics, delayed effects, tolerance, etc., as well as limitations of the data, should be described.

If dosing recommendations are different from those in other countries, the differences should be explained along with the reasons for using different dosages and different delivery systems, if applicable.

Differences in dose–response relationship in age, sex, disease, or other subpopulations should be described. The gnawing concern that FDA drug developers and the scientific community have about drug response in different populations need to be addressed in this section. Any data regarding subsets of the population receiving the drug should be clearly presented. Adequate information about the effects of the drug in women should be clarified in an analysis capable of identifying potential gender differences in drug efficacy and safety. Considerations should entail differences of age, ethnic background, metabolic phenotype, body fat content and distribution, and body size.

An analysis of responses in subsets of the overall population is required. The extent of this part of the integrated summary of efficacy will depend to a large extent on the drug and its intended subject population. Subsets of interest may include sex, race, age, disease severity, concomitant illness, concomitant drugs, smoking and alcoholism, and prior therapy.

9. Integrated Summary of Safety (ISS)

This section integrates safety information from all sources, including pertinent animal data, clinical pharmacology trials, controlled and uncontrolled trials, foreign marketing experience (if any), and epidemiologic trials related to any use of the drug. Dose–response and blood level–response relationships for adverse effects should be identified, as should drug–drug or drug–disease interactions, and any demographic or clinical features that predispose to adverse effects. A description of any statistical analyses not included under the individual trial reports should be provided. In this section, the safety analyses should examine all trials together, as well as possible safety concerns in different subsets of subjects, which would be impossible in individual summaries because of the limited number of subjects in each trial. This also permits detection of more serious adverse experiences that were too rare to be seen in individual trials.

The format of the integrated summary of safety is provided in the following outline.

A table of all trials that provide safety information identified by protocol number, principal investigator, and indication, and divided by type of trial, is required. This table should include the following information:

a. Type of trial
b. Status (complete, continuing, discontinued)
c. Location of full clinical/statistical report
d. Availability of CRFs
e. Number of subjects in each treatment group
f. Indications studied
g. Age range of subjects in each trial and sex/race distribution
h. Duration of drug exposure in the trial
i. Dose range in the trial
j. Frequency of dosing

The extent of exposure to the drug should be described in tables. This should include the number of subjects exposed to the drug for specific periods, for example, 1 day or less, more than 1 day to 1 week, more than 1 week to 1 month, or more than 1 month. The numbers should be broken down by sex and other relevant demographic subgroups. Subjects included in more than one trial should be counted only once. If it cannot be determined whether the same subject appears in more than one trial, this should be indicated.

The number of subjects exposed to various doses for defined periods should be presented. Because many times this can be difficult to display, one possible way to approach this section is to attribute to each subject the dose he or she was given/or the longest time, providing a crude but reasonable picture of exposure. An alternative is to count each dose-duration segment for each subject exposed to several doses.

10. Demographic Data

The relevant demographic, baseline, and other characteristics of the trial population are addressed. These usually include the following:

a. Age
b. Sex
c. Race
d. Body weight

   e. Primary diagnosis
   f. Secondary diagnosis
   g. Concomitant therapy taken during the trial
   h. Smoking status and history
   i. Use of alcohol
   j. Relevant prognostic variables

These should be presented for the entire drug-exposed population and for logical groups of trials, such as all controlled trials, short-term trials, long-term trials, etc. It is preferable that the same groupings be used in displaying adverse experiences.

11. Adverse Experiences and Adverse Reactions

The adverse experience section of the integrated summary of safety is divided into four sections as provided in the following outline.

   a. The first section is a narrative of the overall adverse experience in all trials. The conclusions should be supported by the data and tabulations provided for the following three groupings.

     1. A display of adverse experiences and occurrence rates. All new adverse experiences should be summarized in tables listing each experience, the number of subjects in whom the experience occurred, and the occurrence rate. Although this information can be provided for all trials, excluding short-term trials (pooled together, in many cases), it is better to perform separate analyses of those trials for which case report forms are available and those without case report forms. One may also consider grouping controlled trials, all trials excluding short-term trials in normal volunteers, or trials of similar duration together. Trials in which adverse experiences were reported by checklist or direct questioning versus those in which they were volunteered may also be handled separately. One may want to consider separating foreign and domestic trials. Which groupings are most appropriate will depend on the drug and the nature of the trials conducted.

     2. Adverse experiences should be grouped by body system and arranged in decreasing frequency as well as divided into severity categories. They may also be further divided into those that are considered related and not related to trial drug treatment. An explanation of how the relationship to the trial drug was obtained should be included. Analysis of rates of adverse reactions is required. The most common adverse experiences that appear to be drug-related should be analyzed for relationship to dosage, dose interval, and duration of treatment, as well as to demographic characteristics. A final display of adverse reaction rates should be developed for use in labeling.

3. A display and analysis of deaths, dropouts due to adverse experiences, and other serious or potentially serious adverse experiences should be generated. The listing should include a subject identifier, trial identification, location of the report, and location of the narrative description of the experience. A table giving the rate of these experiences is also useful.

b. The second section should cover the following categories.

1. Clinical Laboratory Evaluation in Clinical Trials. In this section, data from individual trials should be combined and analyzed. Relationships between laboratory tests and clinically relevant subsets of subjects as well as particular adverse experiences and laboratory abnormalities should be assessed. The relationship of drug-related abnormalities to dose, duration of treatment, and subject demographic characteristics should be explored where applicable.

2. Adverse Experiences, Including Laboratory Abnormalities, from Sources Other than Clinical trials. All sources of adverse experiences other than clinical trials, including foreign marketing experience and epidemiologic trials, should be summarized. The procedures used to obtain this information should be described.

3. Animal Data. Summarize the animal data that are relevant to human safety. Any additional trials that are planned should be described, and the implications of any important findings for labeling should be discussed.

4. Analysis of Adverse Effect Dose–Response Information. An integrated analysis of all data from animal and human trials that affect the dose–response and blood level–response relationships of adverse experiences, the method of dose selection, the choice of dose interval, and dosing recommendations in the package insert should be performed. The effect of demographics and other subject characteristics on the dose–response relationships should be explored.

c. Drug–Drug Interactions.

1. Interactions that are predictable on the basis of the pharmacological activity of the drug, and potential interactions with drugs that are likely to be coadministered with the drug should be identified.

2. All data regarding drug–drug interactions should be summarized, including those obtained from formal pharmacokinetic and pharmacodynamic trials and clinical trials. Listings of the number of subjects exposed to each concomitant drug should be developed and each of these groups examined for any unusual adverse experiences.

3. Drug–Demographic and Drug–Disease Interactions. The information from pharmacokinetic and pharmacodynamic trials as well as clinical trials should be analyzed in the same way as were done to determine drug–drug interactions.

4. Pharmacologic Properties Other than the Property of Principal Interest. The available preclinical and clinical data that describe other pharmacological properties of the drug should be discussed with emphasis placed on those actions that are related to unwanted effects and drug–drug interactions.

5. Long-Term Adverse Effects. Available long-term data (6 months or more) should be summarized, and any delayed adverse effects should be noted.

d. Withdrawal Effects.

Specific trials of withdrawal effects, and any data concerning withdrawal effects observed in the clinical trials should be summarized.

12. Drug Abuse and Overdose Information

For drugs with a potential for abuse, information relating to the abuse of the drug as well as a proposal for scheduling under the Controlled Substances Act should be included. If the drug is structurally or pharmacologically related to a drug with abuse potential, but no trials have been done, the reasons why these trials are considered unnecessary should be included. Information related to overdose, as well as antidotes, other treatments, and measures to be taken in the case of overdose, must also be provided.

13. Integrated Summary of Benefits and Risks of the Drugs

Generally, the integrated summary of benefits and risks is a brief summary of the main evidence for effectiveness and the main adverse experiences noted during the clinical program. These data should show that under the conditions of the labeling, the benefits of the drug exceed the risks. In some situations, such as the ones listed below, a more detailed discussion is warranted.

    a. Presence of a severe known or potential human toxicity
    b. A positive carcinogenicity finding
    c. Marginal effectiveness or inconsistent results
    d. A limited data base
    e. Use of a surrogate end point

N. Other NDA Requirements

1. Safety Updates

After the NDA application has been filed with the FDA, sponsors are required to update their submissions at regular intervals with safety data that may affect the contraindications, warnings, precautions, and adverse reactions sections of the labeling.

These updates must be submitted 4 months after the original NDA submission, after receipt of an approval letter, and at other times when requested by the FDA. The exact content of these filings will depend on the number and types of trials conducted after the NDA filing. The information to be in the safety update may include the following.

a. Table of new investigators organized in the same manner as the list of investigators in the clinical data section of the NDA.

b. Additional extent of exposure. If the total exposure has changed substantially, it may need to be reanalyzed.

c. Demographies of additional exposure. The demographics of the additional subjects exposed to the drug should be provided. Again if the total exposure has substantially changed, demographics may have to be reanalyzed.

d. The adverse experiences reported in the new investigations should be analyzed and displayed as outlined in the integrated summary of safety. If the extent of exposure has increased substantially, the analyses should be performed including both the new data and the data submitted in the NDA. If the new data lead to conclusions that are different from those in the original NDA submission, possible causes of the differences should be examined, and complete reports of the safety aspects of the trials should be provided.

e. Clinical laboratory data should be provided in the same manner as was discussed for the adverse experiences.

f. Adverse experience data from other sources including the world literature should be included.

g. If new data are extensive and improve the ability to conduct analyses of drug–response, drug–drug, drug–demographic, or drug–disease interactions, they should be provided, along with any relevant information on pharmacological properties, long-term adverse effects, or withdrawal effects.

O. The Integrated Clinical/Statistical Report

The clinical and statistical information and analyses from a clinical trial should be integrated into a single report. For uncontrolled trials, trials of conditions for which no claim is made in the application, or other trials being provided in the application in support of safety only, the effectiveness results may be presented more briefly than described here; complete safety analyses should always be performed. For all analyses, tables, and figures, the subject population from which these data were generated should be clearly identified.

The contents of a fully integrated clinical/statistical report should include the following information.

1. Title Page. This includes the protocol numbers of other trial identifiers, the title of the trial, name and address(s) of the investigator(s),

identification of the individuals who prepared the report, dates of initiation and completion of the trial, as well as the date of the final report.

2. Table of Contents

3. Identity of Test Materials, Lot Numbers, etc.

4. Introduction. This is a brief statement of the purpose and design of the trial. Background information on the drug and any special features or aims of the trial should be described.

5. trial Objectives. The specific objectives of the trial, including any secondary objectives and subgroup hypotheses, should be explained; whether the objectives were preplanned or formulated during or after completion of the trial should be stated.

6. The Investigational Plan. (a) Overall Design and Plan of the trial. In this section, the overall trial plan and design as well as the organization of the trial are discussed. This should include the subject populations, methods of blinding, assignment of subjects to treatment groups, duration of trial periods, and other pertinent information; any changes in the protocol or conduct of the trial after the trial was initiated should also be described. (b) Description and Discussion of the Design and Choice of Control Group(s). Discuss specific control(s) chosen; any known or potential problems associated with the trial design as well as its suitability for the support of specific claims should be included. (c) trial Population. In this section, the trial population together with the inclusion and exclusion criteria should be discussed. Information to support the suitability of the population for use in the trial, as well as a rationale for the sample size, should be provided. (d) Method of Assigning Subjects to Treatment. The means for assigning subjects to treatment should be described. A copy of the randomization schedule should also be provided as an appendix to the trial. (e) Dose Selection. The procedures for assigning the doses of the test drug and control agent(s) should be described. (f) Blinding. The specific procedures used for blinding should be described, including the circumstances under which the blind can be broken, and the person who has access to the subject codes. If blinding was found to be unnecessary or unfeasible, this as well as the implications should be discussed. (g) Effectiveness and Safety Variables Recorded and Data Quality Assurance. The specific efficacy and safety parameters measured in the trial and when they were conducted should be discussed. Describe the means for obtaining adverse experience data. If a rating scale is used for assessing efficacy or safety, the criteria for point assignments should be provided. (h) Compliance with Dosing Regimens. (i) Appropriateness and Consistency of Measurements. (j) Criteria for Effectiveness. The primary measurements and end points used to determine effectiveness should be clearly specified. (k) Concomitant Therapy. (l) Removal of Subjects from the trial or Analysis. Predetermined reasons for removing subjects from therapy should be described along with follow-up

procedures. If decisions about evaluability are made after blinding is broken, this should be noted and any potential bias discussed.

7. Statistical Methods. The planned sample size and the formula for sample size and power calculations should be provided. (a) Statistical and Analytical Plans. Discuss the planned statistical analyses and any changes made while the trial was conducted. Emphasis should be placed on which analyses and comparisons are planned, not on the specific statistical techniques to be used. (b) Interim Analyses. The frequency and nature of any planned interim analyses and any circumstances under which the trial may be terminated should be discussed. Include any statistical adjustments to be used because of interim analyses.

8. Disposition of Subjects Entered. All subjects who entered the trial should be provided for. Reasons for discontinuation of those who did not complete the trial and information on whether the blind was broken at the time the subject left the trial should be included.

9. Data Sets Analyzed. (a) Which subjects are included in the efficacy and safety analyses should be precisely defined. If the analyses are based on a subset of the subjects with data, an intent-to-treat analysis of all randomized subjects should also be performed. (b) Demographic and Baseline Features of Individual Subjects and Comparability of Treatment Groups. Critical demographic and baseline characteristics of the subject population and any other factors that might affect response should be presented; comparability of treatment groups for each relevant characteristic should be documented. If there is an effectiveness subset of subjects as well as an intent-to-treat population, this should be done for both groups. In a multicenter trial, comparability should be assessed by center, and the centers should be compared.

10. Efficacy Results. (a) Analysis of Measures of Effectiveness. The treatment groups should be compared by use of the analyses that were outlined in the protocol. For multicenter trials, the information presented should give a clear picture of the results at each site. (b) Statistical/Analytical Issues. Important features of the analysis, including adjustments for interim analyses, handling of dropouts, and missing data, should be included. Information on the selection and adjustments for covariate or prognostic factors such as baseline measurements, demographics, and concomitant therapy, together with the results of analyses, should be included. (c) Multicenter trials. In a multicenter trial, the results from the individual centers should be presented, and tests for treatment-by-center interactions should be performed. (d) Multiple End Points. (e) Use of an "Efficacy Subset" of Subjects. One should be careful to assess the effects of dropping subjects with available data from analyses. An intent-to-treat analysis including all available data from all subjects should be performed. (f) Active-Controlled trials. When an active control is used, the data should be compared with previous trials of

similar design that included a placebo and the active control to document the response of the active control. Confidence limits for the difference between the drug and the active control and/or power to detect a difference between the treatments also should be included to document the capability of the trial to distinguish between the two treatment groups. (g) Examination of Subgroups. (h) Tabulation of Individual Response Groups. Individual response and other relevant trial information should be tabulated and included in the appendix. (i) Analysis of doses administered and, if possible, dose–response and blood level–response relationships. (j) Analysis of Drug–Drug and Drug–Disease Interactions. (k) Depending on the nature of the trial, by-subject displays of data may also be useful to include in the appendix.

11. Safety Results. (a) Extent of Exposure. The extent of exposure of subjects to the trial medications should be described. Generally, this is presented in categories such as 1 day or less, 2 days to 1 week, 1 week to 1 month, etc. The duration of posttreatment follow-up should also be included. Generally, all subjects who received at least one dose of trial medication are included in the safety analysis. If this is not the case, an explanation should be provided. (b) Adverse Experiences. (i) The overall adverse experiences in the trial should be discussed in a narrative form and supported by tabulation and analyses. Information on both the test drug and the control should be presented. (ii) All new adverse experiences should be displayed and analyzed in tables listing each reported experience, number of subjects in each treatment group experiencing the experience, and rates of occurrence. These may be divided by body system, severity, and relationship to trial drug. (iii) Adverse experiences that are related should be grouped together by means of a standard adverse reaction dictionary such as WHO or COSTART. (iv) The analysis of adverse experience rates should be used to compare rates in treatment and control groups. For the more common adverse experiences, one also may want to look at the relationship to dose, duration of treatment, demographics, or other baseline features. (v) Listings of all adverse experiences for each subject by investigator and treatment group should be provided in an appendix. It is suggested that this information include the following:

Subject identifier
Age, sex, race, weight
Treatment and dose
Onset
Duration
Intensity
Action taken

Outcome

Relationship to test drug

(vi) Display and analysis of deaths and dropouts due to adverse experiences that are serious or potentially serious should be included. All subjects who left the trial prematurely because of adverse experiences (including laboratory abnormalities) should be listed. All deaths and potentially serious adverse experiences also should be listed, and a description of the experience and relationship to the trial drug should be included. Summary information and narrative discussions of the data should be included in the report, and the listings should be provided in an appendix. (c) Clinical Laboratory Evaluation. A narrative discussion and summary tables should be included in the report, and the data listings should be provided in an appendix. (i) Tabular listings should be provided for all safety-related laboratory tests carried out on each subject. Abnormal values should be identified. (ii) List each abnormal value. (iii) Evaluate each laboratory parameter. This section should include mean or median values over time as well as individual subject changes. Individual marked abnormalities should be highlighted.

12. Summary and Conclusions. The efficacy and safety data should be briefly summarized. Any inconsistencies or limitations of the trial should also be addressed.

13. Appendices. The appendices generally include the following information:

a. Cross references of all pertinent materials
b. Protocol, sample case report form, and amendments
c. Publication
d. Investigator's(s') curriculum(a) vita(e)
e. Randomization scheme and codes
f. Documentation of statistical analyses
g. Subject data listings

P. Samples, Methods Validation, and Labeling

The *Guidelines for Submitting Supportive Analytical Data for Methods Validation in New Drug Applications* provides specific directions for this section.

Samples should not be submitted to the FDA with the application. The reviewing chemist will contact the applicant and provide the laboratory address(es) where the samples should be sent. The applicant should prepare four representative samples in sufficient quantity to permit the FDA to perform each test described in the application three times to determine whether the drug substance and the drug product meet the specifications given in the application and whether the assay methodologies work in the FDA's hands. The four samples are

1. Drug product proposed for marketing
2. Drug substance used in the drug product
3. Reference standards and blanks
4. Samples of the finished market package, if requested by the FDA

Depending on the product, the FDA may also request samples of impurities and degradation products.

The archival copy of an application is required to contain copies of the label and all labeling proposed for the drug product: for draft labeling, the applicant must submit four copies; for final printed labeling, 12 copies should be submitted. When draft labeling is submitted, one copy should be placed in the archival copy. Single copies should be placed in the chemistry, pharmacology, and clinical review sections of the application. When final printed labeling and carton labeling is submitted, one copy should be mounted, bound, and inserted in the archival copy. The remaining 11 copies should be mounted, bound, and submitted in a separate jacket clearly labeled "Final Printed Labeling."

Well-prepared draft labeling can go a long way toward hastening NDA approval. The FDA, if satisfied with the draft labeling, sometimes will bypass the "approvable" letter if the labeling is the only document needed for final NDA approval. This will be done only if editorial or minor modifications, not substantive changes, need to be made in the labeling.

Q. Case Report Forms and Tabulations

The FDA places a great deal of importance on tabulations of subject data, data elements within tables, and CRFs. It is recommended that applicants meet with the FDA personnel of the division that will receive the application to discuss the extent to which tabulations are needed. Alternative modes of data presentation should be reviewed, along with the requirement for special supporting information in selected cases (e.g., the need for ECGs, x-rays, or pathology slides).

Case report forms should be kept as simple as possible by use of checklists, fill-ins, or the recording of specific measurements. Detailed narratives should be used for an investigator's written summary of the trial. Complicated CRFs make the preparation of good tabulations more difficult. Where abbreviations or little-used terms are used on tables or graphs, explanations or definitions should be provided for ease of review.

1. Case Report Tabulations

Tabulations of data on individual subjects are required from

The initial clinical pharmacology (phase 1) trials
The "adequate and well-controlled" (phase 2 and 3) trials
The safety data, e.g., side effects, adverse reactions, and laboratory data from all other trials (phase 2 or 3 trials that are not considered adequate or well controlled).

Efficacy data on subjects from trials that are not adequate and well controlled need not be tabulated. Applicants should resist the temptation of combining uncontrolled with controlled trials because it "strengthens" the statistics of the data. trials should be grouped by design, not outcome.

Upon request, the FDA will discuss with the applicant in a pre-NDA conference those tabulations the FDA agrees may be deleted because they are not considered pertinent to a review of the drug's safety and effectiveness. If a circumstance arises in which previously agreed-to deleted material is requested in a tabulation, the request will come from the director of the FDA division responsible for reviewing the application. Any additional tabulations requested by the FDA should be submitted by the applicant within 30 days after receipt of the request.

2. Case Report Forms

The routine submission of copies of all CRFs for each clinical trial is no longer required. Unless waived by the FDA, CRFs are required only for

All subjects who died during a clinical trial.
Subjects who did not complete a trial because of any adverse experience, whether or not the adverse experience is considered drug related by the investigator or sponsor. This includes subjects receiving reference drugs or placebo.

Generally, the FDA also requires complete sets of CRFs for trials the sponsor has designated as adequate and well controlled. It is suggested that this be discussed at the pre-NDA meeting and CRFs for those trials be included in the NDA if requested by the FDA.

It should be clearly understood that for certain drug classes or therapeutic areas, the FDA may request additional CRFs to conduct a proper review. The FDA will designate the critical trials for which CRFs will be required. The director of the FDA division responsible for the review will make any requests to the applicant. In addition, CRFs may be requested if data tabulations are not adequate to convey important information contained in CRFs. All requests for CRFs must be compiled by the applicant within 30 days after receipt of the request.

3. Information Incorporated by References

Applicants may incorporate by reference any information previously submitted in DMFs or other applications. An incorporation by reference should be made in that segment of the application in which the information referenced would ordinarily appear.

References should be identified by name, reference number, volume, and page number in the FDA's records where the information can be found. If an applicant incorporates by reference information to the FDA by another person, the applicant should obtain and include in the application a written statement from that person authorizing the reference.

N.B.: Each of the technical sections in the review copy must be separately bound in its own particular color folder as previously discussed. Each technical section should include an index (table of contents) for the section, a copy of the application form (FDA 356h), a copy of the cover letter, any letters of authorization, and a copy of the application summary. These items should be separated by tabs clearly marked as to the information being submitted.

VII. SUMMARY

This and the preceding chapters are merely a guide to the preparation of an NDA. All sponsors and applicants must become familiar with the rules and procedures the FDA follows in reviewing highly detailed, complex, and voluminous documents. It takes the collective efforts of many talented people in a drug company to compile the data necessary to fulfill the requirements of an NDA and to put them together in a package that can be reviewed. It then takes the skills of FDA personnel to examine, review, and rule on the submitted data to ensure that the NDA meets all the requirements of the Federal Food, Drug and Cosmetic Act. It is hoped that the NDA format and the publication of guidelines delineating content requirements will help produce more consistently high-quality applications by providing guidance in new areas, especially those that have proved to be problems in the past.

APPENDIX A.   NDA REVIEW GUIDE

1. General Information

The name of the drug and the associated descriptive features, especially if changes occurred during the investigational process.

2. Chemistry, Manufacturing, and Controls

Review any problems with clinical implications, especially if a variety of dosage forms were used.

3. Pharmacology

Pharmacodynamics, pharmacokinetics, and toxicology should be reviewed thoroughly, especially where equivocal results occurred.

4. Clinical Background

Prior history of similar human trials and results
Literature references (pertinent to the drug studied)
Related INDs and NDAs

5. Clinical trials

Controlled trials
Review trials for objective of the trial.—Rationale for the trial
Experimental design, especially designs that may be considered novel
or unusual
Procedures
Safety considerations (and comparative safety considerations)
Efficacy considerations (and comparative efficacy considerations)
Results of statistical consultation
Results of the trial

6. Scientific Conclusions

What will the trials support?
What claims for labeling and advertising?
What are the deficiencies/problems in any trial that may need to be
reflected in the labeling?

7. Regulatory Conclusions

Impact on proposal labeling, especially comparative claims
Side effects
Alert reports
Adverse experiences; comparison to placebo or competitive products
Warnings; any severe or life-threatening (boxed)
Uncontrolled trials; safety data
An accounting for investigators

Need for postmarketing trials—for duration, for specialty groups (e.g., children, the elderly)

Labeling review with a careful evaluation of each section for basic content, clarity, and full disclosure (review 21 CFR 201.56 and 201.57)

REFERENCES

1. Temple R. The NDA rewrite. Presentation at the Fifth Annual Arnold Schwartz Memorial Program. New York, 1984.
2. Lavy NW. Factors influencing clinical research success. In: Finkel M.J., ed. Principles and Techniques of Human Research and Therapeutics. Vol. XI. Mount Kisco, NY: Futura, 1976:133–142.
3. FDA/Center for Drug Evaluation and Research, Last updated: February 13. 2003. Originator: OTCOM/DML, HTML by SJW.
4. US GOP, Washington, DC 20404-0001.

APPENDIX B. DATA FOR THE NDA

Tables 1 through 4 provide lists of the types of information that must be gathered, evaluated, categorized, and tabulated for use in preparing the NDA. By no means all-inclusive, the references should help the reader respond to the

Table 1 Data for NDA

Chemistry	Quality control and process engineering
Subject situation	Drug substance
Analogs	Reference substance
Choice of salt or form	Development of tentative/final assay
Contract manufacturer of chemical	methods
Development of laboratory process	Chemical and physical stability testing
Preparation of bulk	Supply methods/IND
Process description-IND	Feasibility run/clinical supplies
Develop process phase 1 & 2 bulk	Manufacturing data/NDA
Product bulk phase 1 & 2	Contol data/NDA
Preparation of tagged materials	Quality assurance in place
Develop manufacturing process	
Produce bulk phase 3	Manufacturing
Process description-NDA	Engineering of production lines
	Routine production/drug product

Table 2 Data for NDA

Nonclinical pharmacology	Toxicology and biopharmaceutics
Pre-IND trial	Acute toxicity
Screening	Range Finding
cardiovascular	Subacute toxicity
respiratory-visceral	Pre-IND trials
CNS	Microbiology
endocrinology	Immunology
Summary	Chemotherapy
Publication	Biochemistry
Phase 1 & 2 clinical support	Data/IND
Update summary	Reproduction (seg. I, II, III)
Support phase 3 Clinical	Chronic toxicity
Clinical feedback	Carcinogenicity data
Summary reports/NDA kinetics	Metabolism (animal, human)
Labelling information	Interaction trials
	Summary reports/NDA

intricacies of the application and help confirm the review and examination of all items that may be of interest in the development of the NDA.

Because each therapeutic or diagnostic situation is different, there can be no predetermined measure of the amount of data that must be submitted with each application. Therefore an NDA should be submitted only when the sponsor is convinced and satisfied that the safety and efficacy of the drug product have been established to the degree required by the FDA to permit appropriate use by medical practitioners for the prevention or alleviation of human suffering.

Table 3 Data for NDA

Pharmacy and packaging	Medical research
Pre-IND information	Preclinical brochure
Phase 1	Prepare phase 1 & 2
Dosage forms	plans
Laboratory formula sheets	protocols
Processing instructions	case report forms
Short-term stability for IND	Demonstrate safety
Clinical trials phase 1 & 2 dosage forms	Demonstrate effectiveness
Phase 2 dosage forms	FDA contact
Packaging	Clinical biopharmaceutical trials
Clinical supplies phase 3	Summary phase 1 & 2
Long-term stability	Select dosage
Scale-up and production	Update brochure
Feasibility run	Phase 3
Stability report/data	plans
Summary report/NDA	protocols
	case report forms
	FDA contact-end of phase 2 meeting
	Phase 3 trials
	Summary report/NDA
	First draft of package insert
	Pre-NDA review
	Monitor summaries
	Review investigator summaries

Table 4 Data for NDA

Science information, regulatory affairs, information monitor	Statistical and science information sciences
Review investigator brochure	Prepare case report form
Review phase 1 & 2	Format for tabulations
plans	Automation of data handling
protocols	methodology
case report forms	Statistics phase 1 & 2
Regulatory compliance	Statistics phase 3
Labeling preparation	Special statistical analysis
FDA contact-end of phase 2 meeting	Special printouts
Review protocols	adverse experiences
Review summary	subject summaries
Review brochure/update	investigator summaries
FDA contact-pre-NDA meeting	laboratory summaries
Review statistical evaluation phase 3	Literature summaries and reprints
Assemble and integrate NDA-archival and review copies	Translation of foreign materials
Final NDA summary and package insert	
Advertising and promotion review	

DEPARTMENT OF HEALTH AND HUMAN SERVICES FOOD AND DRUG ADMINISTRATION **APPLICATION TO MARKET A NEW DRUG, BIOLOGIC, OR AN ANTIBIOTIC DRUG FOR HUMAN USE** *(Title 21, Code of Federal Regulations, Parts 314 & 601)*	*Form Approved: OMB No. 0910-0338* *Expiration Date: August 31, 2005* *See OMB Statement on page 2.*
	FOR FDA USE ONLY APPLICATION NUMBER

APPLICANT INFORMATION

NAME OF APPLICANT	DATE OF SUBMISSION
TELEPHONE NO. *(Include Area Code)*	FACSIMILE *(FAX) Number (Include Area Code)*
APPLICANT ADDRESS *(Number, Street, City, State, Country, ZIP Code or Mail Code, and U.S. License number if previously issued):*	AUTHORIZED U.S. AGENT NAME & ADDRESS *(Number, Street, City, State, ZIP Code, telephone & FAX number)* IF APPLICABLE

PRODUCT DESCRIPTION

NEW DRUG OR ANTIBIOTIC APPLICATION NUMBER, OR BIOLOGICS LICENSE APPLICATION NUMBER *(If previously issued)*

ESTABLISHED NAME *(e.g., Proper name, USP/USAN name)*	PROPRIETARY NAME *(trade name)* IF ANY
CHEMICAL/BIOCHEMICAL/BLOOD PRODUCT NAME *(If any)*	CODE NAME *(If any)*
DOSAGE FORM:	STRENGTHS:	ROUTE OF ADMINISTRATION:

(PROPOSED) INDICATION(S) FOR USE:

PRODUCT DESCRIPTION

APPLICATION TYPE
(check one)   ☐ NEW DRUG APPLICATION (21 CFR 314.50)   ☐ ABBREVIATED NEW DRUG APPLICATION (ANDA, 21 CFR 314.94)
                              ☐ BIOLOGICS LICENSE APPLICATION (21 CFR Part 601)

IF AN NDA, IDENTIFY THE APPROPRIATE TYPE   ☐ 505 (b)(1)   ☐ 505 (b)(2)

IF AN ANDA, OR 505(b)(2), IDENTIFY THE REFERENCE LISTED DRUG PRODUCT THAT IS THE BASIS FOR THE SUBMISSION

Name of Drug _____   Holder of Approved Application _____

TYPE OF SUBMISSION *(check one)*   ☐ ORIGINAL APPLICATION   ☐ AMENDMENT TO A PENDING APPLICATION   ☐ RESUBMISSION
          ☐ PRESUBMISSION   ☐ ANNUAL REPORT   ☐ ESTABLISHMENT DESCRIPTION SUPPLEMENT   ☐ EFFICACY SUPPLEMENT
          ☐ LABELING SUPPLEMENT   ☐ CHEMISTRY MANUFACTURING AND CONTROLS SUPPLEMENT   ☐ OTHER

IF A SUBMISSION OF PARTIAL APPLICATION, PROVIDE LETTER DATE OF AGREEMENT TO PARTIAL SUBMISSION: _____

IF A SUPPLEMENT, IDENTIFY THE APPROPRIATE CATEGORY   ☐ CBE   ☐ CBE-30   ☐ Prior Approval (PA)

REASON FOR SUBMISSION

PROPOSED MARKETING STATUS *(check one)*   ☐ PRESCRIPTION PRODUCT (Rx)   ☐ OVER THE COUNTER PRODUCT (OTC)

NUMBER OF VOLUMES SUBMITTED _____   THIS APPLICATION IS   ☐ PAPER   ☐ PAPER AND ELECTRONIC   ☐ ELECTRONIC

ESTABLISHMENT INFORMATION (Full establishment information should be provided in the body of the Application.)
Provide locations of all manufacturing, packaging and control sites for drug substance and drug product (continuation sheets may be used if necessary). Include name, address, contact, telephone number, registration number (CFN), DMF number, and manufacturing steps and/or type of testing (e.g. Final dosage form, Stability testing) conducted at the site. Please indicate whether the site is ready for inspection or, if not, when it will be ready.

Cross References (list related License Applications, INDs, NDAs, PMAs, 510(k)s, IDEs, BMFs, and DMFs referenced in the current application)

	This application contains the following items: *(Check all that apply)*
☐	1. Index
☐	2. Labeling *(check one)*　　☐ Draft Labeling　　☐ Final Printed Labeling
☐	3. Summary (21 CFR 314.50 (c))
☐	4. Chemistry section
☐	A. Chemistry, manufacturing, and controls information (e.g., 21 CFR 314.50(d)(1); 21 CFR 601.2)
☐	B. Samples (21 CFR 314.50 (e)(1); 21 CFR 601.2 (a)) (Submit only upon FDA's request)
☐	C. Methods validation package (e.g., 21 CFR 314.50(e)(2)(i); 21 CFR 601.2)
☐	5. Nonclinical pharmacology and toxicology section (e.g., 21 CFR 314.50(d)(2); 21 CFR 601.2)
☐	6. Human pharmacokinetics and bioavailability section (e.g., 21 CFR 314.50(d)(3); 21 CFR 601.2)
☐	7. Clinical Microbiology (e.g., 21 CFR 314.50(d)(4))
☐	8. Clinical data section (e.g., 21 CFR 314.50(d)(5); 21 CFR 601.2)
☐	9. Safety update report (e.g., 21 CFR 314.50(d)(5)(vi)(b); 21 CFR 601.2)
☐	10. Statistical section (e.g., 21 CFR 314.50(d)(6); 21 CFR 601.2)
☐	11. Case report tabulations (e.g., 21 CFR 314.50(f)(1); 21 CFR 601.2)
☐	12. Case report forms (e.g., 21 CFR 314.50 (f)(2); 21 CFR 601.2)
☐	13. Patent information on any patent which claims the drug (21 U.S.C. 355(b) or (c))
☐	14. A patent certification with respect to any patent which claims the drug (21 U.S.C. 355 (b)(2) or (j)(2)(A))
☐	15. Establishment description (21 CFR Part 600, if applicable)
☐	16. Debarment certification (FD&C Act 306 (k)(1))
☐	17. Field copy certification (21 CFR 314.50 (l)(3))
☐	18. User Fee Cover Sheet (Form FDA 3397)
☐	19. Financial Information (21 CFR Part 54)
☐	20. OTHER *(Specify)*

CERTIFICATION

I agree to update this application with new safety information about the product that may reasonably affect the statement of contraindications, warnings, precautions, or adverse reactions in the draft labeling. I agree to submit safety update reports as provided for by regulation or as requested by FDA. If this application is approved, I agree to comply with all applicable laws and regulations that apply to approved applications, including, but not limited to the following:

1. Good manufacturing practice regulations in 21 CFR Parts 210, 211 or applicable regulations, Parts 606, and/or 820.
2. Biological establishment standards in 21 CFR Part 600.
3. Labeling regulations in 21 CFR Parts 201, 606, 610, 660, and/or 809.
4. In the case of a prescription drug or biological product, prescription drug advertising regulations in 21 CFR Part 202.
5. Regulations on making changes in application in FD&C Section 506A, 21 CFR 314.71, 314.72, 314.97, 314.99, and 601.12.
6. Regulations on Reports in 21 CFR 314.80, 314.81, 600.80, and 600.81.
7. Local, state and Federal environmental impact laws.

If this application applies to a drug product that FDA has proposed for scheduling under the Controlled Substances Act, I agree not to market the product until the Drug Enforcement Administration makes a final scheduling decision.
The data and information in this submission have been reviewed and, to the best of my knowledge are certified to be true and accurate.
Warning: A willfully false statement is a criminal offense, U.S. Code, title 18, section 1001.

SIGNATURE OF RESPONSIBLE OFFICIAL OR AGENT	TYPED NAME AND TITLE	DATE:

ADDRESS *(Street, City, State, and ZIP Code)*	Telephone Number (　　　)

Public reporting burden for this collection of information is estimated to average 24 hours per response, including the time for reviewing instructions, searching existing data sources, gathering and maintaining the data needed, and completing and reviewing the collection of information. Send comments regarding this burden estimate or any other aspect of this collection of information, including suggestions for reducing this burden to:

Department of Health and Human Services Food and Drug Administration CDER, HFD-99 1401 Rockville Pike Rockville, MD 20852-1448	Food and Drug Administration CDER (HFD-94) 12229 Wilkins Avenue Rockville, MD 20852	An agency may not conduct or sponsor, and a person is not required to respond to, a collection of information unless it displays a currently valid OMB control number.

INSTRUCTIONS FOR FILLING OUT FORM FDA 356h

APPLICANT INFORMATION This section should include the name, street address, telephone and facsimile numbers of the legal person or entity submitting the application in the appropriate areas. Note that, in the case of biological products, this is the name of the legal entity or person to whom the license will be issued. The name, street address and telephone number of the legal person or entity authorized to represent a non-U.S. Applicant should be entered in the indicated area. Only one person should sign the form.

PRODUCT DESCRIPTION This section should include all of the information necessary to identify the product that is the subject of this submission. For new applications, the proposed indication should be given. For supplements to an approved application, please give the approved indications for use.

APPLICATION INFORMATION If this submission is an ANDA or 505(b)(2), this section should include the name of the approved drug that is the basis of the application and identify the holder of the approved application in the indicated areas.

TYPE OF SUBMISSION should be indicated by checking the appropriate box:

Original Application = a complete new application that has never before been submitted;

Amendment to a Pending Application = all submissions to pending original applications, or pending supplements to approved applications, including responses to Information Request Letters;

Resubmission = a complete response to an action letter, or submission of an application that has been the subject of a withdrawal or a refusal to file action;

Presubmission = information submitted prior to the submission of a complete new application;

Annual Report = periodic reports for licensed biological products (for NDAs Form FDA-2252 should be used as required in 21 CFR 314.81 (b)(2));

Establishment Description Supplement = supplements to the information contained in the Establishment Description section (#15) for biological products;

Efficacy Supplement = submissions for such changes as a new indication or dosage regimen for an approved product, a comparative efficacy claim naming another product, or a significant alteration in the patient population; e.g., prescription to Over-The-Counter switch;

Labeling Supplement = all label change supplements required under 21 CFR 314.70 and 21 CFR 601.12 that do not qualify as efficacy supplements;

Chemistry, Manufacturing and Controls Supplement = manufacturing change supplement submissions as provided in 21 CFR 314.70, 21 CFR 314.71, 21 CFR 314.72 and 21 CFR 601.12;

Other = any submission that does not fit in one of the other categories (e.g., Phase IV response). If this box is checked the type of submission can be explained in the **REASON FOR SUBMISSION** block.

Submission of Partial Application Letter date of agreement to partial submission should be provided. Also, provide copy of scheduled plan.

CBE "Supplement-Changes Being Effected" supplement submission for certain moderate changes for which distribution can occur when FDA receives the supplement as provided in 21 CFR 314.70 and 21 CFR 601.12.

CBE-30 "Supplement-Changes Being Effected in 30 Days" supplement submission for certain moderate changes for which FDA receives at least 30 days before the distribution of the product made using the change as provided in 21 CFR 314.70 and 21 CFR 601.12.

Prior Approval (PA) "Prior Approval Supplements" supplement submission for a major change for which distribution of the product made using the change cannot occur prior to FDA approval as provided in 21 CFR 314.70 and 21 CFR 601.12.

REASON FOR SUBMISSION This section should contain a brief explanation of the submission, e.g., "manufacturing change from roller bottle to cell factory" or "response to Information Request Letter of 1/9/97" or "Pediatric exclusivity determination request" or "to satisfy a subpart H postmarketing commitment".

NUMBER OF VOLUMES SUBMITTED Please enter the number of volumes, including and identifying electronic media, contained in the archival copy of this submission.

This application is
☐ Paper   ☐ Paper and Electronic   ☐ Electronic
Please check the appropriate box to indicate whether this submission contains only paper, both paper and electronic media, or only electronic media.

ESTABLISHMENT INFORMATION This section should include information on the locations of all manufacturing, packaging and control sites for both drug substance and drug product. If continuation sheets are used, please indicate where in the submission they may be found. For each site please include the name, address, telephone number, registration number (Central File Number), Drug Master File number, and the name of a contact at the site. The manufacturing steps and/or type of testing (e.g. final dosage form, stability testing) conducted at the site should also be included. Please indicate whether the site is ready for inspection or, if not, when it will be ready. Please note that, when applicable, the complete establishment description is requested under item 15.

CROSS REFERENCES This section should contain a list of all License Applications, INDs, NDAs, PMAs, 510(k)s, IDEs, BMFs and DMFs that are referenced in the current application.

Items 1 through 20 on the reverse side of the form constitute a check list that should be used to indicate the types of information contained within a particular submission. Please check all that apply. The numbering of the items on the checklist is not intended to specify a particular order for the inclusion of those sections into the submission. The applicant may include sections in any order, but the location of those sections within the submission should be clearly indicated in the Index. It is therefore recommended that, particularly for large submissions, the Index immediately follows the Form FDA 356h and, if applicable, the User Fee Cover Sheet (Form FDA 3397).

The CFR references are provided for most items in order to indicate what type of information should be submitted in each section. For further information, the applicant may consult the guidance documents that are available from the Agency.

Signature The form must be signed and dated. Ordinarily only one person should sign the form, i.e., the applicant, or the applicant's attorney, agent, or other authorized official. However, if the person signing the application does not reside or have a place of business within the United States, the application should be countersigned by an attorney, agent, or other authorized official who resides or maintains a place of business within the United States.

6
Abbreviated and Supplemental New Drug Applications

Richard A. Guarino
Oxford Pharmaceutical Resources, Totowa, New Jersey, U.S.A.

An Abbreviated New Drug Application (ANDA) is specifically designed for an approval of a generic drug product. When data within an ANDA are submitted to the Food and Drug Administration's Center for Drug Evaluation and Research (CDER), Office of Generic Drugs, the applications are reviewed and approved from that division. On approval of the application the applicant may manufacture and market the generic drug product with the purpose of providing consumers with a safe, effective, and low cost alternative of the generic form of a brand name drug.

A generic drug must be a drug product that is comparable to an innovator drug product in dosage form, strength, route of administration, quality, performance characteristic, and intended use [1].

I. BACKGROUND HISTORY

The Waxman–Hatch Act, also known as the Drug Price Competition and Patent Term Restoration Act of 1984, established bioequivalence as the basis for approving generic copies of drug products. This act permits the FDA to approve ANDAs submitted to market generic versions of brand-name drugs without conducting costly and duplicative preclinical and clinical trials. To access additional information on the bioequivalence review of generic products, the Office of Generic Drugs provides a home page to generic drug developers including an interactive flowchart presentation of an ANDA focusing on how CDER determines the safety and bioequivalence of generic drug products prior to an approval for marketing.

II. ANDA CONTENT

A. General

The term *abbreviated* is used in generic drug applications because, as stated above, they are usually not required to include preclinical and clinical data to establish safety and efficacy. However, a sponsor of a generic drug must scientifically demonstrate that the product is bioequivalent. Bioequivalent, for the purpose of this submission, refers to having the generic product perform in the same manner as the innovator drug. A way scientists demonstrate bioequivalence is to measure the time it takes the generic drug, to reach the bloodstream in 24 to 36 healthy volunteers. The rate of absorption is determined or the bioavailability of the generic drug, which then can be compared to the innovator drug. It must be shown that the generic drug version delivers the same amount of active ingredients into a subject's bloodstream in the same amount of time as the innovative drug.

B. Legal Requirements and Guidance Documents

Guidance documents are prepared for FDA review staff and applicants or sponsors to provide guidelines for the processing, content, evaluation, and approval of an application. In addition they also provide design, production, manufacturing, and testing of regulated products. The policies emanating from guidelines are intended to achieve consistency in the FDA's regulatory approach and establish inspection and enforcement procedures. It must be remembered that guidance documents are not regulations or laws and as a result are not enforceable either through administrative actions or through the courts. However, it is prudent for the applicant to consider these guidelines and review them before the final submission of each ANDA.

The detailed components described in this chapter, Specific Requirements, Content, and Format of an NDA, detail how the content of the ANDA might be approached. With the exception of the preclinical and nonclinical sections and the clinical section, an ANDA should follow the items in Application Form 356h (see chapter 5, p. 168). The guidance documents that have been developed by the FDA to assist applicants in preparing ANDAs are listed together on CDER's Guidance Document Index webpage. The guidelines to assist in preparing ANDAs include

1. Format and content for

   a. Application summary
   b. Chemistry, manufacturing, and controls section
   c. Nonclinical pharmacology and toxicology section
   d. Human pharmacokinetics and bioavailability section
   e. Clinical and statistical section
   f. Microbiology section

2. Guideline for postmarketing reporting of adverse reactions
3. Guideline for the submission in microfiche of the archival copy of an application
4. Guideline for submitting supporting documentation for the manufacture of drug substance
5. Guideline for submitting supporting documentation for the manufacture of finished dosage forms
6. Guideline for submitting supportive analytical data for methods validation in new drug applications
7. Guideline for submitting supporting documentation for stability studies of human drugs and biologics
8. Guideline for packaging

III. ANDA CHECK LIST

The following ANDA checklist provides the applicant with an itemization of all the necessary components for an ANDA submission.

ANDA CHECKLIST
FOR COMPLETENESS and ACCEPTABILITY of an APPLICATION

ANDA#_____   FIRM NAME

RELATED APPLICATIONS(s)   FIRST GENERIC?

DRUG NAME: _____

DOSAGE FORM:

Electronic submission:	E-mail notification sent:	Comments:
Random assignment queue:	Chem team leader:	PM:

Labeling reviewer: _____ Micro review: _____ PD study (Med Ofcr): _____

Letter date   **Received date**

Comments   On cards   Therapeutic code

Methods validation package (3 copies)
(Required for non-USP drugs)

Archival and review copies
Field copy certification (original signature)

Cover letter

Table of contents

                                                                                    ACCEPTABLE

Sec. I	**Signed and completed application form (356h)** (Statement regarding Rx/OTC status)	☐
Sec. II	**Basis for submission** **NDA:** RLD: Firm: ANDA suitability petition required? If yes, consultation needed for pediatric study requirement.	☐
Sec. III	**Patent certification** 1. Paragraph: 2. Expiration of patent: A. Pediatric exclusivity submitted? B. Pediatric exclusivity tracking system checked? **Exclusivity statement**	☐
Sec. IV	**Comparison between generic drug and RLD-505(j)(2)(A)** 1. Conditions of use 2. Active ingredients 3. Route of administration 4. Dosage form 5. Strength	☐
Sec. V	**Labeling** 1. 4 copies of draft (each strength and container) or 12 copies of FPL 2. 1 RLD label and 1 RLD container label 3. 1 side by side labeling comparison with all differences annotated and explained	☐

Sec. VI Bioavailability/bioequivalence ☐
1. **Financial certification** (Form FDA 3454) **and Disclosure statement** (Form 3455)
2. **Request for waiver of in-vivo study(ies)**:
3. **Formulation data same?** (Comparison of all strengths) (ophthalmicals, otics, topicals parenterals)
4. **Lot numbers of products used in BE study(ies)**:
5. **Study type:** (Continue with the appropriate study type box below)

Study type **IN-VIVO PK STUDY(IES)** (i.e., fasting/fed/sprinkle) ☐
a. Study(ies) meets BE criteria (90% CI or 80–125, Cmax, AUC)
b. Data files (computer media) submitted
c. In-vitro dissolution

Study type **IN-VIVO BE STUDY with CLINICAL ENDPOINTS** ☐
a. Properly defined BE endpoints (eval. by clinical team)
b. Summary results meet BE criteria (90% CI within $+/- 20\%$ or 80–120)
c. Summary results indicate superiority of active treatments (test & reference) over vehicle/placebo ($P < 0.05$) (eval. by clinical team)
d. Data files (computer media) submitted

Study type **TRANSDERMAL DELIVERY SYSTEMS** ☐
a. *In-vivo PK study*
1. Study(ies) meet BE criteria (90% CI or 80–125, Cmax, AUC)
2. In-vitro dissolution
3. Data files (computer media) submitted
b. *Adhesion study*
c. *Skin irritation/sensitization study*

Study type **NASALLY ADMINISTERED DRUG PRODUCTS** ☐
a. *Solutions* (Q1/Q2 sameness):
1. **In-vitro studies (dose/spray content uniformity, droplet/drug particle size distrib., spray pattern, plume geometry, priming & repriming, tail off profile)**
b. *Suspensions* (Q1/Q2 sameness):
1. In-vivo PK study
a. Study(ies) meets BE criteria (90% CI or 80–125, Cmax, AUC)
b. Data files (computer media) submitted

2. In-vivo BE study with clinical endpoints
   a. Properly defined BE endpoints (eval. by clinical team)1
   b. Summary results meet BE criteria (90% CI within $+/-$ 20% or 80–120)
   c. Summary results indicate superiority of active treatments (test & reference) over vehicle/ placebo ($p < 0.05$) (eval. by clinical team)
   d. Data files (computer media) submitted
3. **In-vitro studies (dose/spray content uniformity, droplet/drug particle size distrib., spray pattern, plume geometry, priming & repriming, tail off profile)**

Study type | **TOPICAL CORTICOSTEROIDS (VASOCONSTRICTOR STUDIES)** □
a. Pilot study (determination of ED50)
b. Pivotal study (study meets BE criteria 90% CI or 80–125)

Sec. VII | **Components and composition statements** □
1. Unit composition and batch formulation
2. Inactive ingredients as appropriate

Sec. VIII | **Raw material controls** □
1. **Active ingredients**
   a. Addresses of bulk manufacturers
   b. Type II DMF authorization letters or synthesis
   c. COA(s) specifications and test results from drug substance mfgr(s)
   d. Applicant certificate of analysis
   e. Testing specifications and data from product manufacturer(s)
   f. Spectra and chromatograms for reference standards and test samples
   g. CFN numbers
2. **Inactive ingredients**
   a. Source of inactive ingredients identified
   b. Testing specifications (including identification and characterization)
   c. Suppliers' COA (specifications and test results)
   d. Applicant certificate of analysis

Sec. IX | **Description of manufacturing facility** □
1. Full address(es) of the facility(ies)
2. CGMP certification
3. CFN numbers

Sec. X   **Outside firms including contract testing laboratories**   ☐
1. Full address
2. Functions
3. CGMP certification/GLP
4. CFN numbers

Sec. XI   **Manufacturing and processing instructions**   ☐
1. Description of the manufacturing process (including microbiological validation, if appropriate)
2. Master production batch record(s) for largest intended production runs (no more than 10x pilot batch) with equipment specified
3. If sterile product: aseptic fill/Terminal sterilization
4. Filter validation (if aseptic fill)
5. Reprocessing statement

Sec. XII   **In-process controls**   ☐
1. Copy of executed batch record (antibiotics/ 3 batches if bulk product produced by fermentation) with equipment specified, including packaging records (packaging and labeling procedures), batch reconciliation and label reconciliation
2. In-process controls—specifications and data

Sec. XIII   **Container**   ☐
1. Summary of container/closure system (if new resin, provide data)
2. Components specification and test data (type III DMF references)
3. Packaging configuration and sizes
4. Container/closure testing
5. Source of supply and supplier's address

Sec. XIV   **Controls for the finished dosage form**   ☐
1. Testing specifications and data
2. Certificate of analysis for finished dosage form

Sec. XV   **Stability of finished dosage form**   ☐
1. Protocol submitted
2. Post approval commitments
3. Expiration dating period
4. Stability data submitted
   a. 3 month accelerated stability data
   b. Batch numbers on stability records the same as the test batch

Sec. XVI **Samples** – statement of availability and identification of   ☐
1. Drug substance
2. Finished dosage form
3. Same lot numbers

Sec. XVII **Environmental impact analysis statement**   ☐

Sec. XVIII **GDEA (generic drug enforcement act)/other**   ☐
1. Letter of authorization (U.S. agent [if needed, countersignature on 356h])
2. Debarment certificate (original signature)
3. List of convictions statement (original signature)

Reviewing
CSO/CST
   Date   **Recommendation:**
                                ☐**FILE**   ☐**REFUSE TO RECEIVE**

Supervisory Concurrence/Date: _____   **Date:**

Duplicate copy sent to bio: (Hold if RF and send when acceptable)

Duplicate copy to **HFD-**   for consult: Type:

IV. ADDITIONAL COMMENTS REGARDING THE ANDA

Each component and section of the checklist should be carefully reviewed for content and completeness. Every precaution must be taken so that the applicant does not receive a letter of Refusal to Receive that clarifies the CDER's decision to refuse to receive an incomplete application. The specific copies i.e., archival, review, and field, to be submitted in the ANDA, outlined in the beginning of the checklist, should follow the NDA format as stated below.

A. Archival Copy

Cover letter
Application Form (356h) 21 CFR 314.50(a) 21 CFR 314.50(b)
ANDA suitability statement
Chemistry, manufacturing, and controls 21 CFR 314.50(d) (1)
Human pharmacokinetics and bioavailability 21CFR 314.50(d) (3)
Samples and labeling section 21 CFR 314.50(e)
Other information 21 CFR 314.50(g)

B. Review Copy

Each of the technical sections in the review copy of the ANDA must be separately bound in its own particular color folder as previously discussed in the format of an NDA, and a copy of the application form (FDA 356h) must also be included. Although an integrated summary is not required, a summary that would help the reviewing chemist may expedite the ANDA approval.

C. Field Copy

A field copy certification with an original signature of the chemistry, manufacturing, and controls, with a copy of the application form and any references to DMFs, should be clearly explained.

D. Summary

ANDAs are specifically designed to help the manufacturers of generics to provide these products rapidly to the consumer at lower cost than those of brand names. The sponsors of these applicants must prepare these applications with the mission of the FDA in the forefront, *to enforce laws enacted by the U.S. Congress and regulations established by the agency to protect the consumer's health, safety, and pocketbook.* They must assure consumers that generic drugs and devices are safe and effective for their intended uses, and that all labeling and packaging is truthful, informative, and not deceptive. Bearing this in mind, the preparation of an ANDA and the review of the same will be as intensively examined and scrutinized as if it were a new drug, device, or biologic product.

V. SUPPLEMENTAL APPLICATIONS (SNDAS)

A Supplemental New Drug Application (SNDA) is for the most part submitted to the FDA by holders of New Drug Applications. These submissions usually occur after approval of NDAs. The most frequently submitted supplements usually fall in one of the following categories:

Components and composition of products
Manufacturing site changes
Manufacturing process changes
Specification changes in drug products
Packaging changes
Labeling changes

Miscellaneous changes
Multiple related changes
SNDAs fall into one of three categories,

A. Major Changes

These are changes that may have a substantial effect on adverse experiences and may reflect a change related to identity, strength, quality, purity, or potency. As these changes may relate to the safety or effectiveness of the product, an expedited review might be requested. If so, the FDA will give this type of supplement immediate attention. Submission in this category of a supplement is usually labeled.

> *REQUESTED A PRIOR APPROVAL*
> *SUPPLEMENT EXPEDITED REVIEW*

B. Moderate Change

A moderate change supplemental request is often based on the potential of the product to cause an adverse experience. This type of change may also reflect a change in identity, strength, quality, purity, or potency of a product. As these changes may relate to safety or efficacy but may not require immediate attention, they are placed into two categories.

> *CHANGES BEING EFFECTED*
> *IN 30 DAYS*

> *CHANGES BEING EFFECTED*

C. Minor Changes

These SNDAs are considered to be minor changes and are categorized as having a minimal potential to cause any adverse experience. This type also reflects a change in identity, strength, quality, purity, or potency of a product. However, as these changes have a minimal effect on the safety or efficacy of the subject they are described in the next Annual Report.

In some instances there may be supplements submitted proposing to add a new use of an approved drug to the product labeling. This type of supplemental submission can be categorized as a standard efficacy supplement or as a *priority supplement*.

Under the Food and Drug Administration Modernization Act of 1997 the FDA is required to publish in the Federal Register standards for the prompt review of supplemental applications submitted for approved articles. This legislative act indicated that this provision was directed at certain types of efficacy supplements such as supplement applications proposing to add a new use for an approved drug to the product labeling. According to the statistics reported since 1998, Standard Efficacy Supplements under the Modernization Act can take an average of 10 to 12 months to review. The supplements falling under the PRIORITY REVIEW are taking 6 months to review. A supplement eligible for PRIORITY REVIEW for the Center for Drug Evaluation and Research (CDER) and the Center for Biologics Evaluation and Research (CBER) would fall in the category that "would be a significant improvement, compared to marketed products, including non-drug products and therapies in the treatment, diagnosis, or prevention of a disease."

Supplemental New Drug Applications must be done with careful consideration as to the type of supplement, the importance of it, and the urgency for approval. Caution must be given to each submission as the Prescription Drug User Fee Act (PDUFA) (www.fda.gov/cber/pdufa.htm).

7

The Biologic License Application (BLA)

Albert A. Ghignone
AAG, Inc., Easton, Pennsylvania, U.S.A.

I. INTRODUCTION

The 1990s have brought us the era of FDA regulatory reform. The law, the regulations, and the agency itself have undergone a tremendous change. The Center for Biologic Evaluation and Research (CBER) has undergone some of the most significant changes. As former FDA Commissioner David Kessler, M.D., had wanted, the drug and biologic approval processes have become very similar. Gone forever is the two-license system, the responsible head designation, and all the many other things that had made the biological approval process so unique and distinct and so different from drugs.

All this change has brought us to the new CBER and the single application and single license era. The Biologic License Application (BLA) has replaced the Product License Application (PLA) and the Establishment License Application (ELA). Gone are many CBER regulations, replaced now by CDER regulations. This is not so foreign considering that in the early 1970s, the FDA had declared and defined all biological products as drugs, thus allowing the FDA to regulate biological products under two laws: the Federal Food, Drug and Cosmetic Act and the Public Health Service Act.

In the BLA, a biological product sponsor submits thousands of pages of nonclinical and clinical data, chemical and biological information, and product manufacturing descriptions. The submission must allow CBER reviewers to make three principal determinations:

1. Whether the biological is safe and effective in its indicated use, and whether the benefits of using the product outweigh the risks.
2. Whether the biological's proposed labeling is appropriate.
3. Whether the methods used in manufacturing and quality control are adequate to preserve the biological's identity, strength, quality, potency, and purity.

II. A SHORT HISTORY OF THE LICENSING PROCESS FOR BIOLOGICALS

Given that government regulation of biologicals has historically focused on the product manufacturing process, it is not surprising that the ELA has a considerably longer history than the PLA. Congress was first spurred to regulate the biological industry in 1901, when 10 children died after being treated with diphtheria antitoxin that had been contaminated with tetanus.

But in establishing regulatory controls to prevent the contamination of the biological products of that day—essentially vaccines and antitoxins—Congress had to work within the limitations of existing scientific knowledge and technology. At that time, it was difficult, and in many cases impossible, to identify the component parts of any biological product or to detect the presence of pathogens and other contaminants. The absence of sensitive assays for identifying, and purification processes for separating, biological contaminants left researchers to use crude immunological and in vivo tests.

This situation was complicated by the fact that the production processes for traditional biologicals, usually involving human or animal extracts, were highly susceptible to contamination. The reality that contaminants were often infectious materials or toxins amplified the threat.

At that time, regulating production facilities seemed to be the only mechanism likely to control the quality of biological products. Consequently, Congress passed the Biological Control Act of 1902, which required that biologicals in interstate commerce be manufactured in facilities holding a valid establishment license. Interestingly, the statute failed to mandate government review or sanction of the products themselves, only that the establishments manufacturing and preparing the products meet specific criteria and permit the inspection of their facilities.

Not until 1944, when Congress modified the statute, did federal law require the licensure of products as well. Under the revision, both establishments and products must "meet standards designed to insure the continued safety, purity, and potency of such products, prescribed in regulation."

For the next 52 years, the dual licensure procedure was the centerpiece of biologicals regulation in the United States. Because biological products are difficult to characterize structurally, complete descriptions of the production processes and manufacturing facility have been regarded as essential to the control of product manufacture. Thus the difficulty in biological product characterization has been the most important scientific reason for CBER's continuing reliance on the ELA.

In 1994, the FDA began to look for ways to lesson regulatory burdens on industry. Because of this initiative, CBER took steps to modernize its regulatory program to reflect scientific and technological advances. Although these reforms affected virtually every aspect of biologicals regulation, they signaled the end of CBER's dual licensing system.

In 1996, CBER began to consolidate the dual licensing system that had been in place since 1944. Specifically, with a final regulation published in May 1996, CBER established that categories of highly characterized products would require only the submission of a single license application, a BLA, and the granting of a single license for marketing. In justifying this change, CBER stated "that technical advances have greatly increased the ability of manufacturers to control and analyze the manufacture of many biologic/biotechnology-derived products. Methodologies are now available to characterize these products, allowing the product to be more clearly evaluated by end-product testing." The end of the dual licensing era had arrived, at least for certain categories of products. For these products, gone forever was the ELA. In November of 1997, President Clinton signed the Federal Food, Drug and Cosmetic Modernization Act of 1997. One section of this law required that all biological products be licensed under the single licensing system. With his signature, President Clinton put an end to the CBER's dual licensing system. Since the signing of this law, CBER has issued guidances for the submission of the "Chemistry, Manufacturing, and Control Information and Establishment Description" for all categories of biological products. By the end of 1999, the single licensing system was to be fully implemented. As all these changes are being implemented, CBER is also preparing for the next-phase computerized license applications. Numerous guidance documents already have been issued by CBER to address the computerized format.

III. INTRODUCTION TO BLAs: CONTENT AND FORMATTING REQUIREMENTS

The Center for Biologics Evaluation and Research had established no specific formatting requirements for PLAs. This was in sharp contrast to new drug applications, for which the agency has detailed formatting standards.

Although the lack of a uniform PLA format has caused industry concern in the past, significant differences between various license applications, and biological products themselves, had slowed efforts to standardize PLA formats.

However, CBER did make available a series of PLA application forms that identify basic PLA submission requirements for different types of products. Most of these PLA forms applied to blood products, vaccines, and other, more traditional, biological products. The center has not yet developed forms for many of the more advanced biological products, including new therapeutic products.

In most cases, PLA forms identified submission requirements by posing a series of questions that the sponsor had to answer in the application. Essentially, the lack of a standard format was a function of the diversity of questions posed by different PLA forms. Often, applicants based the formats of their applications on the sequence of questions specified in the PLA form.

Given the absence of a standard PLA format and the advent of the new single license system, CBER in 1996 published a new draft BLA form (Form FDA-3439). Subsequent to this, during 1997, CBER and CDER issued the harmonized application form—Form FDA 356(h). This form represented a standard format for all drug, biological, antibiotic, and generic drug products. Hence the harmonized form. The form is titled "Application to Market a New Drug, Biologic, or an Antibiotic Drug for Human Use" (see p. 168).

The Form FDA 356(h) is a one-page form that is two-sided. The first side is administrative, providing information on the applicant as well as the product. The back side identifies the content requirements for a BLA application. However, because the form is to be used for generic drug and antibiotic products also, not all 19 sections are applicable to BLAs. In addition to the BLA application form, federal regulations, CBER guidelines, and points-to-consider documents developed for specific product classes also offer information on BLA application submission requirements. In general terms, the BLA consists of reports of all investigations sponsored by the applicant, and all other information pertinent to an evaluation of the product's safety, effectiveness, potency, and purity.

IV. THE CONTENTS OF THE BLA

As stated above, the 356(h) form is a one-page, two-sided document; the front side contains administrative information about the applicant and product, and the back side includes content and format requirements for the BLA application. In addition to this form, a cover letter should always accompany any FDA submission. Addressed in the following pages are the Form

FDA 356(h), the cover letter, and all 19 sections of the BLA application (see p. 168).

Cover letter
Application form—Form FDA 356(h)
Section 1—Index
Section 2—Labeling
Section 3—Summary
Section 4—Chemistry section
Section 4a—Chemistry, manufacturing, and controls information
Section 4b—Samples
Section 4c—Methods validation package
Section 5—Nonclinical pharmacology and toxicology
Section 6—Human pharmacokinetics and bioavailability
Section 7—Clinical microbiology
Section 8—Clinical data section
Section 9—Safety update report
Section 10—Statistical section
Section 11—Case report tabulations
Section 12—Case report forms
Section 13—Patent information
Section 14—Patent certification
Section 15—Establishment description
Section 16—Debarment certification
Section 17—Field copy certification
Section 18—User fee cover sheet
Section 19—Other

Before each section is addressed individually, it is worth emphasizing the importance of the application form [Form FDA 356(h)], the cover letter, and the first three sections. Applicants frequently overlook their significance, perhaps because they are not technical sections or because they often are not seen as critical. For several reasons, this is unfortunate. First, these items and sections are among the few in the entire application that each member of the BLA licensing committee receives for review. Additionally, because these sections, particularly the cover letter and the summary, provide information in an abridged form, they are also likely to be read thoroughly by each committee member. The sections are also important because they represent, in some ways, the applicant's "opening argument" for its product. In the summary section, for instance, the sponsor is granted what some view as a greater editorial license not available in any of the BLA's other sections. Such views aside, the sponsor must use these sections to frame and build its case for the new biological's safety and effectiveness.

A. Cover Letter

Although not required by regulation, the cover letter is requested by the FDA to accompany all FDA submissions. In the cover letter, sponsors often supply the FDA with much of the basic administrative information requested about the BLA application (e.g., sponsor name and address, etc.). The cover letter should provide at least seven types of information:

1. Name and Address of Sponsor and Others

The cover letter should provide the name and address of the sponsor. If the sponsor is using outside contractors or manufacturing sites at other locations, the cover letter should provide their addresses and identify their functions.

2. Product Name

The sponsor should provide the trade and generic names of the product in the cover letter.

3. Reason for the Submission

The cover letter should identify the type of application being submitted (e.g., original submission, supplement, amendment, etc.).

4. Information Contained in the Submission

In the cover letter, the sponsor should identify what information is contained in the submission. Identify the total number of volumes being submitted and the contents of each volume (e.g., volumes 50–150 contain clinical information).

5. Agreements with the FDA

If the sponsor has reached any agreements with CBER relevant to the BLA, this information should be included in the cover letter. Given the quantity of applications under review within CBER and the fact that such agreements often are made months in advance, reviewers might not recall the existence or details of such agreements. Reviewer turnover is another factor that makes recounting these agreements good working practice.

6. Other Documents Relating to the Submission

To alert CBER reviewers to other documentation that must be referenced during the BLA review, the sponsor should note in the cover letter other documents associated with the application, such as INDs, BLAs, and master files.

7. Special Circumstances

Alert CBER to any special circumstances surrounding the product. For example, the product may be an orphan drug product. Because of the circumstances relating to the product, CBER may pay special attention to the submission and shepherd it through the licensure process more quickly.

8. Priority Review

If your product has been classified for priority review, remind CBER of the fact in the cover letter.

B. Application Form FDA 356(h)

The application form [Form FDA 356(h)] serves several functions. First, it is an administrative document providing CBER with information on the applicant, product, and application. Second, it is a legal contract binding the applicant, contractors, suppliers, and physicians to FDA laws and regulations. The applicant is already bound by FDA laws and regulations, but many contractors, suppliers, and physicians are not. Contrary to what many believe, physicians are not regulated by the FDA or FDA laws and regulations. Physicians are licensed by states and controlled in this manner. The Food and Drug Administration will not accept an application unless the application form is signed.

C. Item 1—Index

Perhaps the single most important factor in a BLA's "user friendliness" is the speed and ease with which a reviewer can find information during the review process. Because it can influence the speed and efficiency of the review as well, the manner in which the applicant indexes BLA information is of central importance. Applicants can use this format for indexing the BLA:

Item	Description	Volume/page
2	Labeling	1.010

The "Item" column refers to the item number listed on the back of the Form FDA 356(h) application. The "Description" column identifies the subject of the item number listed on the back of Form FDA 356(h). In the "Volume/page" column, the number to the left of the decimal point represents the application's volume number, whereas the number to the right refers to the page within that volume containing the relevant section. In practice, the index is typically far more detailed, with each item broken down into specific subparts.

D. Item 2—Labeling Section

This section encompasses the initial draft labeling submitted with the BLA and the final printed labeling that is submitted just prior to licensure. Labeling includes the immediate container label, carton label, insert, and user instructions. The container and package labels should permit accurate identification of the contents, whereas the package insert should summarize the essential information required for the product's safe and effective use. These data should be accurate, balanced, informative, and nonpromotional. When possible, the information should be based on data obtained from the product's use in humans.

E. Item 3—Summary Section

In many ways, the BLA summary is a condensed version of the entire application. The summary serves as a guide to the full application, explaining the application's intent-to-establish the biological's safety and effectiveness for a particular indication, and highlighting the studies and evidence supporting the biological's safety and effectiveness.

The summary's importance cannot be overstated. In this section, the sponsor can state and argue its case for the product's approval. A well-prepared summary includes a straightforward description of the product and its manufacturing technology, testing data, nonclinical data, clinical data, and adverse and beneficial effects.

Such a summary can build CBER's confidence in the applicant, the validity of the BLA's information, and the product itself. In addition, because the summary is one of the few sections reviewed by all members of the BLA licensing committee, it can be pivotal in establishing a foundation for product approval.

The summary, ordinarily 50–200 pages in length, provides reviewers in each review area, and other agency officials, with a good general understanding of the product and of the application. The summary should discuss all aspects of the application and should be written with about the same level of detail required for publication in refereed scientific and medical journals and should meet the editorial standards generally applied by these journals. To the extent possible, data in the summary should be presented in tabular and graphic forms. The summary should comprehensively present the most important information about the product and the conclusions to be drawn from this information.

The summary should avoid any editorial promotion of the product, i.e., it should be a factual summary of safety and effectiveness data and a neutral analysis of these data. The summary should include an annotated copy of the proposed labeling, a discussion of the product's benefits and risks, a description of the foreign marketing history of the drug (if any), and a summary of each technical section.

1. Summary Format

Description of Drug and Formulation
Annotated draft insert
Product pharmacological class
Scientific rationale for use of product
Clinical benefits
Foreign marketing history
CMC summary
7a. Drug substance
7b. Drug product
7c. Stability
7d. Investigational summary (listing of batches used in the clinical studies)
Nonclinical summary
8a. Pharmacology
8b. Toxicology
Human pharmacokinetics and bioavailability
Microbiological summary
Clinical summary
Benefit/risk relationship

F. Item 4—Chemistry Section

The BLA's chemistry section is composed of three parts:

1. Chemistry, manufacturing, and controls information
2. Samples
3. Methods validation package

In most aspects, the BLA is essentially a PLA that features a new chemistry section in which the sponsor provides some, but not nearly all, of the data and information previously submitted in the PLA/ELA. The remaining information formerly provided in the PLA/ELA will be reviewed during CBER's preapproval inspection.

The Center for Biologics Evaluation and Research has issued guidance documents identifying the CMC information that will be required in BLAs for each class of product.

1. Chemistry, Manufacturing, and Controls Information

This section is composed of five parts:

Drug Substance
Drug Product
Investigational Formulation
Environmental Assessment
Method Validation

Drug Substance. Many of CBER's guidelines address the information required for the drug substance. This indeed does make a lot of sense, because the drug substance is the active moiety, the item that produces the pharmacological response in humans. The information required by CBER for the drug substance is identified below.

Description and Characterization. This section should provide a clear description of the physical and chemical properties of the synthetic drug substance, including the chemical structure, primary and subunit structure, molecular weight, and molecular formula. If the product is cellular based, the source of the cell line and all the pertinent physical and chemical properties necessary to characterize the cell line should be listed. The biological name or chemical name, including the USAN name, should also be provided. A description and the results of all the analytical testing performed on the manufacturer's reference standard lot and qualifying lots to characterize the drug substance should be included. The section should provide information from specific tests regarding the identity, purity, stability, and consistency of manufacture of the drug substance. All test methods should be fully described and the results provided.

A description and results of all relevant in vivo and in vitro biological testing performed on the manufacturer's reference standard lot to show the potency and activity of the drug substance should be included. Results of relevant testing performed on lots other than the reference standard lot and that might have been used in establishing the product's biological activity should also be provided.

Manufacturer. The application should include the name, address, FDA registration number, and other pertinent organizational information for each manufacturer performing any portion of the manufacture or testing operations for the drug substance. A brief description of the operations performed at each location, the responsibilities conferred upon each party by the applicant, and a description of how the applicant will ensure that each party fulfills its responsibilities should be included.

For each manufacturing location, the BLA should include a floor diagram that indicates the general facility layout. This diagram need not be a detailed engineering schematic, but should be a simple drawing that depicts the relationship of the subject manufacturing areas, suites, or rooms to one another, and should indicate other uses made of adjacent areas that are not the subject of the application. This diagram should be clear enough to permit the reviewer to visualize the flow of the drug substance's production and to identify areas or room "proximities" that may be of concern for particular operations (e.g., segregation of animal facilities).

This section should provide a comprehensive list of all additional products to be manufactured or manipulated in the areas used for the product. The applicant should indicate the rooms in which the additional products will be introduced and the manufacturing steps that will take place in the room. An explanation should be given as to whether these additional products will be introduced on a campaign basis or concurrently during production of the product under review.

For all areas in which operations for the preparation of cell banks and product manufacturing are performed, including areas for the handling of animals used in production, the following information regarding precautions taken to prevent contamination or cross-contamination should be provided:

Air quality classification of rooms or areas in which an operation is performed, as validated and measured during operations

A brief narrative description of the procedures and facility design features for the control of contamination, cross-contamination, and containment (air-pressure cascades, segregation of operations and products, etc.)

General equipment design description (e.g., does design represent an open or a closed system or provide for a sterile or nonsterile operation?)

A description of the in-process controls performed to prevent or to identify contamination or cross-contamination

Method(s) of Manufacture. This subsection should include the following information on raw materials and reagents: (1) a list of all components used in the manufacture of the drug substance, and their tests and specifications, or a reference to official compendia, (2) a list with tests and specifications of all special reagents and materials used in the manufacture of the drug (e.g., culture media, buffers, sera, antibiotics, monoclonal antibodies, preservatives), and (3) a description of the tests and specifications for materials of human and animal source that may be contaminated with adventitious agents (mycoplasma, bovine spongiform encephalopathy [BSE] agent for bovine-derived products, and other adventitious agents of human origin).

A complete visual representation of the manufacturing process in flow chart format should be included. This flow chart should indicate the step in the process, the equipment and materials used, and the room where the operation is performed, and it should provide a complete list of the in-process controls and tests performed on the product at each step. The diagram should also include information, including a descriptive narrative, on the methods used to transfer the product between steps (i.e., sterile, SIP connection, sanitary connection, open transfers under laminar flow units, etc.).

If animals are used in the production process, the subsection should include descriptions of the sources of animals, the method of creating and the genetic stability of transgenic animals, adventitious agent screening and quarantine procedures used to assure that the animals are appropriate for use in manufacturing, animal husbandry procedures, and veterinary oversight. For more guidance, use the appropriate CBER guidelines and "Points to Consider" documents.

For monoclonal antibodies, the submission should include a detailed description of the development of the monoclonal antibody, including characterization of the parent cells, donor history for human cells, immunogen, immortalization procedures, and cell cloning procedures.

For recombinant DNA products, including rDNA-derived monoclonal antibodies produced from cellular sources, the guideline states that the submission should include a detailed description of the host cell and the expression vector systems and their preparation, including the following:

1. *Host Cells.* A description of the source, relevant phenotype, and the genotype for the host cell used to construct the biological production system. The results of the characterization of the host cell for phenotypic and genotypic markers, including those that will be monitored for cell stability, purity, and selection, should be included.

2. *Gene Construct.* A detailed description of the gene that was introduced into the host cells, including both the cell type and the origin of the source material, should be provided, along with a description of the method(s) used to prepare the gene construct and a restriction enzyme digestion map of the construct. The complete nucleotide sequence of the coding region and regulatory elements of the expression construct, with translated amino acid sequence, should be provided, including annotations designating all important sequence features.

3. *Vector.* Detailed information regarding the vector and genetic elements should be provided, including a description of the source and function of the component parts of the vector.

4. *Final Gene Construct.* A detailed description should be provided of the cloning process that resulted in the final recombinant gene construct.

5. *Cloning and Establishment of the Recombinant Cell Lines.* Depending on the methods to be used to transfer a final gene construct or isolated gene fragments into its host, the mechanism of transfer, the copy number, and the physical state of the final construct inside the host cell should be provided. In addition, the amplification of the gene construct, if applicable, the selection of the recombinant cell clone, and the establishment of the seed should be completely described.

The method of manufacture section should also include a subsection on the cell seed lot system, which should address three items:

6. *Master Cell Bank.* In most cases, the cell bank used to manufacture the biological will derive from a larger group of cells called the master cell bank, or MCB. A detailed description of its preparation and testing as outlined in the ICH guideline should be provided. The MCB should be described in detail, including the methods, materials, reagents, and media used, date of creation, quantity of the MCB, in-process controls, and storage conditions. This section should also provide the results of the characterization of the MCB for identity and purity using phenotypic markers and the testing of the MCB for endogenous and adventitious agents.

7. *Master Working Cell Bank.* A detailed description of the working cell bank, or WCB, and the cell line used to produce the biological product must be provided. The production of the WCB should be described in detail.

8. *End of Production Cells.* A detailed description of the end of production cell's (EPC's) characterization that demonstrates that the biological production system is consistent during growth should be included. This section should also include test results showing that the EPC is free from contamination by adventitious agents.

Lastly, the cellular sources subsection of the methods of manufacture section must include a detailed description of the process of inoculation, cell growth, and harvesting. The stages of cell growth should be described carefully, including the selection of the inoculum, scale-up for propagation, and established and proposed (if different) production batch size.

The CMC section of the BLA must also provide details of the purification and downstream processing, including a rationale for the chosen methods. In addition, the precautions taken to ensure the containment and prevention of contamination or cross-contamination should be identified. If applicable, the section should indicate the multiuse nature of areas and equipment (e.g., campaigning versus concurrent manufacture; dedicated versus shared equipment) used for these procedures.

Finally, the methods of manufacture section must provide a completed (executed) representative batch record of the drug substance's production process.

Process Controls. This CMC subsection should provide information in two key areas:

1. *In-Process Controls.* A description of the methods used for in-process controls (e.g., those involved in fermentation, harvesting, and downstream processing) should be included. A brief description of the sampling procedures and test methods used should be provided. For testing performed at significant phases of production, the criteria for accepting or rejecting an in-process batch should be specified.

2. *Process Validation.* A description and documentation of the validation studies should be included. If the process was changed or scaled up for commercial production and this involved changes in the fermentation steps, the revalidation of cell line stability during growth should be described, as in the previous section, and the data and results provided. A description and documentation of the validation studies for the cell growth and harvesting process that identify critical parameters of routine products should be submitted. Similarly, description and documentation of the validation of the purification process should be included. Finally, the subsection should describe and document the validation studies or any processes used for media sterilization and inactivation of cells prior to their release to the environment (if such inactivation is required).

A summary report, including protocols and results, should be provided for the validation studies of each critical process or factor that affects the drug substance specifications for

Propagation
Harvest
Purification
Inactivation
Microbiology
Aseptic processing

3. *Reference Standard.* If an international reference standard (WHO, NIBSC) or compendial reference standard (USP) is used, the applicant should submit the citation for the standard and a certificate of analysis. If an in-house working reference standard is used, a description of the preparation, characterization, specifications, and testing and results should he provided.

4. *Specifications/Analytical Methods.* The specifications and tests sufficient to assure the identity, purity, strength, and potency of the drug substance, as well as its lot-to-lot consistency, should be submitted. Certificates of analysis and analytical results for at least three consecutive qualification lots of the drug substance should be provided. Lastly, this subsection should include a discussion of the impurity profiles, with supporting analytical data, as well as profiles of variants of the protein drug substance (e.g., cleaved, aggregated, deamidated, oxidized forms) and non–product-related impurities (e.g., process reagents and cell-culture components).

5. *Container/Closure System.* A description of the container and closure system and its compatibility with the drug substance should be submitted. The section should include detailed information concerning the supplier and the results of compatibility, toxicity, and biological tests. Alternatively, a drug master file (DMF) may be referenced for this information.

6. *Drug Substance Stability.* This subsection should include a description of the storage conditions, study protocols, and results supporting the stability of the drug substance. For more specific information, the FDA guideline "Stability Testing for Drug Substances and Drug Products" should be consulted.

Drug Product. Although less detailed than those for the drug substance, the requirements of the guideline for the drug product are also grouped into eight areas.

Composition. This subsection should include a tabulated list of all components with their unit dose and batch quantities for the drug product or diluent in accordance with the "Guideline for Submitted Documentation for the Manufacture of and Controls for Drug Products." The compositions of all ancillary products that might be included in the final product should be provided.

Specifications and Methods for Drug Product Ingredients. If the information is not specified in the drug substance section, this section should include a description of tests and specifications for all active ingredients. The specifications for all ancillary products included in the drug product should be provided as well. Information on all excipients, including process gases and water, should be included and should include a list of compendial excipients (and their citations) and tests and specifications for noncompendial excipients.

Manufacturer. The names and addresses of all manufacturers involved in the manufacture and testing of the drug product, including contractors, and a description of their respective responsibilities should be included. A list of all other products (i.e., research and development, clinical, or approved) made in the same rooms should be provided as well.

Methods of Manufacture and Packaging. A complete description of the manufacturing process of the formulated bulk and finished drug product, including a description of sterilization operations, aseptic processing procedures, lyophilization, and packaging procedures. Along with this narrative, the subsection should include a flow chart indicating each production step, the equipment and materials used, the room or area where the operation is performed, and a listing of the in-process controls and tests performed on the product at each step. This flow diagram or narrative should also include information on the methods for transferring the product between steps.

Specifications and Test Methods for Drug Product. This subsection should include the sampling procedures for monitoring a batch of finished drug product. The specifications used for the drug product and a description of all test methods selected to assure the identity, purity, strength, or potency, as well as the lot-to-lot consistency of the finished product, should be provided.

Container/Closure System. A description of the container and closure system and its compatibility with the drug product should be submitted. Detailed information concerning the suppliers, their addresses, and the results of compatibility, toxicity, and biological tests should be included. Alternatively, a DMF can be referenced for this information.

Microbiology. Information should be submitted as described in the FDA's "Guidance for Industry in the Submission of Documentation for Sterilization Process Validation in Applications for Human and Veterinary Drug Products."

Drug Product Stability. A description of the stability protocols and results supporting the product's stability (expiration date and storage condition) should be provided. Stability data supporting the proposed shelf-life of reconstituted drug products and for all labeled dilutions also should be included. The stability protocol provided should include the following:

Potency
Physiochemical measurements that are potency-indicating
Moisture, if applicable
pH, if applicable
Sterility or control of bioburden
Viability of cells
Pyrogenicity
General safety

A plan for an ongoing stability program should be included. This should comprise the protocol to be used, the number of lots to be entered each year, and an indication of how the lots will be selected.

Investigational Product/Formulation. This section should consist of a discussion of any differences in formulation, manufacturing process, or site between the clinical trial materials and commercial production batches of the drug substance and drug product.

Environmental Assessment. If an environmental assessment is required, it should be prepared as outlined in the federal regulations (21 CFR 25). It should include a description of the action being considered and address all components involved in the manufacture and disposal of the product. A statement of exemption under a categorical exclusion may be provided if applicable.

Method Validation. Although the guideline states that the CMC section must include a method validation section, it does not specify submission requirements. Rather, the guideline refers applicants to the FDA's "Guideline for Submitting Samples and Analytical Data for Methods Validation."

As noted above, the CMC subsection is only one of three elements in the BLA's chemistry section. The other two subsections address samples and the methods validation package.

Samples. Before a biological product is marketed, the FDA will want to validate the sponsor's characterization methods for both the biological substance and the finished product. Therefore, at some point during the review process, CBER may request any or all of the following: a biological substance sample, a finished product sample, and the sponsor's reference standards. According to FDA regulations, the sponsor must submit "four representative samples of each sample in sufficient quantity to permit FDA to perform three times each test described in the application to determine whether the drug substance and drug product meet the specifications given in the application."

Methods Validation Package. The methods validation package provides information that allows FDA laboratories to validate all of the analytical methods for both the drug substance and the drug product. Specifically, the package consists of three copies of the analytical methods and related descriptive information in the CMC section for the drug substance and drug product.

According to the FDA's "Guideline for Submitting Samples and Analytical Data for Methods Validation," the methods validation package should include a statement of composition, new drug substance and product specifications, certificates of analysis for each sample submitted, and the regulatory analytical methods. Detailed information in the package should include a tabular listing (lot, identity, etc.) of all samples to be submitted, a listing of all proposed regulatory specifications, information supporting the integrity of the reference standard, a detailed description of each method of analysis, and information supporting the suitability of the methodology for the new drug substance and the dosage form.

G. Item 5—Nonclinical Pharmacology and Toxicology Section

The BLA must describe all nonclinical pharmacology and toxicology studies conducted on the biological product. These nonclinical laboratory studies include those submitted in the IND, those submitted during clinical investigations, and new nonclinical studies not previously submitted. The Center for Biologics Evaluation and Research reviews these studies to evaluate their adequacy and comprehensiveness and to ensure that there are no inconsistencies or inadequately characterized toxic effects. The application also should include information on studies not performed by the sponsor but of which the sponsor has become aware (e.g., studies in published literature).

Content requirements for the nonclinical pharmacology and toxicology section of license applications are not defined specifically in CBER regulations or guidelines. As it does in many other instances, the BLA form refers biologicals' sponsors to regulations for the pharmacology/toxicology section of an NDA. These regulations ask for descriptions, with the aid of graphs and tables, of animal and in vitro studies with the drug, including the following:

1. Studies of the pharmacological actions of the drug in relation to its proposed therapeutic indication and studies that otherwise define the pharmacological properties of the drug or are pertinent to possible adverse effects.

2. Studies of the toxicologic effects of the drug as they relate to the product's intended clinical uses, including, as appropriate, studies assessing the product's acute, subchronic, and chronic toxicity, and studies of toxicities related to the product's particular mode of administration or conditions of use.

3. Studies, as appropriate, of the effects of the drug on reproduction and on the developing fetus.

4. Any studies of the absorption, distribution, metabolism, and excretion of the drug in animals.

5. For each nonclinical laboratory study subject to good laboratory practice (GLP) regulations, a statement that it was conducted in compliance with such regulations or, if not conducted in compliance with those regulations, a brief statement of the reason for the noncompliance.

For each study identified above, the applicant should include a summary, followed by a full report including data and statistical analyses. Summaries assist FDA reviewers in obtaining a brief analysis of the study. Along with the summaries and full reports, the applicant should provide an integrated report. Such a report integrates results from all pharmacology studies in a single, comprehensive analysis. Sponsors should provide a similar report for the toxicology information.

H. Item 6—Human Pharmacokinetics and Bioavailability Section

Although few biological products will have bioavailability data, most will have pharmacokinetics data that must be provided in the BLA. As it does for the pharmacology and toxicology section, Form 356(h) refers biologicals' applicants to the regulatory requirements specified for an NDA human pharmacokinetics and bioavailability section, as follows:

1. A description of each of the bioavailability and pharmacokinetic studies of the drug in humans, including a description of the analytical and statistical methods used in each study and a statement with respect to each study that it either was conducted in compliance with IRB regulations or was not subject to the regulations, and that it was conducted in compliance with the informed consent regulations.

2. If the application describes in the chemistry, manufacturing, and controls section specifications or analytical methods needed to assure the bioavailability of the drug product or drug substance, or both, a statement in this section of the rationale for establishing the specifications or analytical methods including data and information supporting the rationale.

3. A summary discussion and analysis of the pharmacokinetics and metabolism of the active ingredients and the bioavailability or bioequivalence, or both, of the drug product.

More detailed recommendations on the development and presentation of this section are available from CDER's guidelines.

I. Item 7—Clinical Microbiology

This section is required only for anti-infective products. Because these products affect microbial, rather than clinical, physiology, reports relevant to the product's in vivo and in vitro effects on the target microorganisms are critical for establishing product effectiveness.

Current regulations require that an application's anti-infective section include microbiology data characterizing (a) the biochemical basis of the drug's action on microbial physiology, (b) the antimicrobial spectra of the drug, including the results of in vitro nonclinical studies to demonstrate concentrations of the drug required for effective use, (c) any known mechanisms of resistance to the drug, including the results of any known epidemiological studies to demonstrate prevalence of resistance factors, and (d) clinical microbiology laboratory methods (for example, in vitro sensitivity discs) needed for effective use of the product.

More specific guidance on developing the microbiology component of the BLA is available from a CDER guideline entitled "Guideline for the Format and Content of the Microbiology Section of an Application."

J. Item 8—Clinical Data Section

The applicant's clinical data section is a particularly critical element of the filing. Included in this section are the safety and effectiveness data pivotal to the FDA's decision-making process. The clinical data section is also likely to be the applicant's most complex and voluminous section.

The clinical data section of a BLA should consist of the following basic elements:

1. A description and analysis of each clinical pharmacology study of the biological, including a brief comparison of the results of the human studies with the animal pharmacology and toxicology data.

2. A description and analysis of each controlled clinical study pertinent to the biological's proposed use, including the protocol and a description of the statistical analyses used to evaluate the study. If the study report is an interim analysis, this must be noted and a projected completion date provided. Controlled clinical studies that have not been analyzed in detail for any reason (e.g., because they have been discontinued or are incomplete) should be provided, including a copy of the protocol and a brief description of the results and status of the study.

3. A description of each uncontrolled clinical study, a summary of the results, and a brief statement explaining why the study is classified as uncontrolled.

4. A description and analysis of any other data or information relevant to an evaluation of the product's safety and effectiveness obtained or otherwise received by the applicant from any foreign or domestic source. This should include information derived from clinical investigations (i.e., including controlled and uncontrolled trials of uses of the product other than those proposed in the application), commercial marketing experience, reports in the scientific literature, and unpublished scientific papers.

5. An integrated summary of the data providing substantial evidence of effectiveness for the clinical indications. Evidence is also required to support the dosage and administration section of the labeling, including the dosage and dose interval recommended and modifications for specific subgroups of patients (e.g., pediatrics, geriatrics, patients with renal failure).

6. An integrated summary of all available information about product safety, including pertinent animal data, demonstrated or potential adverse effects of the drug, clinically significant drug–drug interactions, and other safety considerations, such as data from epidemiological studies of related drugs. This subsection should also include a description of any statistical analyses performed in reviewing safety data, unless it is included elsewhere in the clinical section.

7. If the drug has the potential for abuse, a description and analysis of studies or information related to abuse of the drug, including a proposal for scheduling under the Controlled Substances Act. A description of any studies related to overdosage is also required, including information on dialysis, antidotes, or other treatments, if known.

8. An integrated summary of benefits and risks of the biological, including a discussion of why the benefits exceed the risks under the conditions stated in the labeling.

9. A statement noting that each human clinical study was conducted in compliance with IRB and informed consent regulations. If the study was not conducted according to these regulations, the applicant must state this fact and the reasons for noncompliance.

10. If a sponsor has transferred any obligations for the conduct of a clinical study to a contract research organization (CRO), a statement providing the name and address of the CRO, identifying the clinical study, and providing a list of the obligations transferred. If all obligations regarding the conduct of the study have been transferred, a general statement of this transfer—in lieu of a listing of the specific obligations transferred—may be submitted.

11. If original subject records were audited or reviewed by the sponsor in the course of monitoring any clinical study to verify the accuracy of the case reports submitted to the sponsor, a list identifying each clinical study so audited or reviewed.

Although there is no required format for the clinical section, I recommend formatting the section in the following manner:

1. Integrated summary of benefits and risks
2. Integrated summary of safety
3. Integrated summary of effectiveness
4. Phase 3 adequate and well-controlled studies used for the determination of product safety and effectiveness
5. All other phase 3 studies
6. Phase 2 studies
7. Human pharmacology studies not included in item 6
8. Other information

This format allows CBER to review the most important information first.

K. Item 9—Safety Update Report

As implied by its title, the safety update report is not submitted with the original BLA but is submitted in the form of updates at specific points in the application review process. Applicants must submit safety update reports 4 months after the BLA submission, after receipt of a complete response letter, and at other times requested by CBER. In these reports, the sponsor must update the pending BLA with new safety information learned about the product that may reasonably affect the labeling statements in the contraindications, warnings, precautions, and adverse reactions sections. The updates must include the same types of information from clinical studies, animal studies, and other sources and must be submitted in the same format as the BLA's integrated safety summary. They must also include case report forms for each patient who died during a clinical study or who did not complete the study because of an adverse event.

L. Item 10—Statistical Section

The statistical section of the BLA is essentially the same as the clinical data section, inasmuch as the clinical reports include all the statistical analyses. With this information, the statisticians can assess the validity of key analyses and evidence supporting the biological's safety and efficacy.

The statistical section is composed of the following information:

1. A list of investigators supplied with the drug or known to have investigated the drug, INDs under which the drug was studied, and NDAs submitted for the same drug substance
2. An overview of the clinical studies conducted
3. Item 8, the clinical data section
4. Statistics used for the integrated summaries of benefits/risks, safety and effectiveness, and the rationale for the use of such statistical methods

M. Item 11—Case Report Tabulations Section

During the the FDA's most recent revision of its NDA regulations, the agency declared that "an efficient agency review of individual patient data should be based primarily on well-organized, concise data tabulations. Reviews of the more detailed patient case report forms should be reserved for those instances where a more complete review is necessary."

The agency advises sponsors to meet with the FDA to discuss the extent to which tabulations of patient data in clinical studies, data elements within tables, and case report forms are needed. Such discussions can also cover alternative modes of data presentation and the need for special supporting information (for example, ECGs, x-rays, or pathology slides).

According to agency regulations and guidelines, the case report tabulations section must provide

1. Tabulations of the data from each adequate and well-controlled study (phase 2 and phase 3)
2. Tabulations of the data from the earliest clinical study
3. Pharmacology studies (phase 1)
4. Tabulations of the safety data from all other clinical studies

Federal regulations add that these tabulations should include the data on each patient in each study, except that the applicant may delete those tabulations that the agency agrees, in advance, are not pertinent to a review of the drug's safety or effectiveness.

N. Item 12—Case Report Forms (CRF) Section

As stated above, the FDA does not require the routine submission of patient CRFs. The forms are required only for (a) patients who died during a clinical study, and (b) patients who did not complete a study because of any adverse event, whether or not the adverse event is considered drug related by the investigator or the sponsor.

The FDA may request that the sponsor submit additional CRFs that the agency views as important to the drug's review. Typically, the agency will request all CRFs for the pivotal studies. In doing so, the agency's reviewers will attempt to designate the critical studies for which CRFs are required about 30 days after the application's receipt. If a sponsor fails to submit the CRFs within 30 days of the FDA's request, the agency may view the eventual submission as a major amendment and extend the review period as appropriate.

O. Item 13—Patent Information Section

Applicants must provide information on any patent(s) on the product for which approval is sought or on a method of using the product. Such information is included in the "Orange Book" (*Approved Drug Products with Therapeutic Equivalence Evaluations*). All approved (licensed) drug products are listed in this book.

P. Item 14—Patent Certification Section

Applicants must provide a patent certification or statement regarding any relevant patents that claim the listed drug or any other drugs on which investigators seeking approval of the application relied, or that claim a use for the listed or other drug.

According to the FDA's "Guideline on Formatting, Assembling, and Submitting New Drug and Antibiotic Applications," the patent certification and patent information should be attached to the application form in the submission.

Q. Item 15—Establishment Description Section

The CBER guidance documents state that item 15 of the BLA should be composed of three principal sections that provide information describing establishment standards and good manufacturing practices (GMP) controls in place for the manufacture of the product. The three principal sections are (a) General Information, (b) Specific Systems, and (c) Contamination/Cross-Contamination Issues.

1. General Information

For each manufacturing location, the BLA should include a floor diagram indicating the general production facility layout. Each diagram or accompanying narrative should include product, personnel, equipment, waste, and air flow for production areas; an illustration or indication of which areas are served by each air-handling unit; and air pressure differentials between adjacent areas.

2. Specific Systems

Water Systems. The BLA should include information for systems used in the production of water for manufacturing and rinsing of product-contact equipment. This subsection should include a general description of water system(s), a validation summary, and information on the routine monitoring program.

Heating, Ventilation, and Air Conditioning (HVAC) Systems. This subsection must also include a general system description, a validation summary, and information on the routine monitoring system.

Computer Systems. This section should contain information on computer systems that control critical manufacturing processes. The developer of the system should be identified, and information provided also should include a brief description of procedures for changes to the computer system. This section also should contain a validation summary for each of these systems and a certification that an IQ and an OQ have been completed.

3. Contamination/Cross-Contamination Issues

For dedicated equipment, the sponsor must provide a brief description of the cleaning procedures and reagents used, as well as certification that cleaning validation for removal of product residuals and cleaning agents has been successfully completed. For shared equipment, including that used for processing the cells of more than one patient, BLA sponsors must provide a description of the cleaning procedures and reagents used, the rationale for the chosen procedures, and a report describing validation procedures, sampling methods, and analytical methods. The section must also provide information on containment features, including segregation and containment procedures for areas, manufacturing operations, personnel, equipment, and waste materials designed to prevent product contamination.

In general, the BLA must provide CBER reviewers with an overview of the manufacturing facility and its operations regarding the product.

R. Item 16—Debarment Certification Section

Since mid-1992, the FDA has required that all NDAs and BLAs include a certification that the applicant did not and will not use the services of individuals or firms that have been debarred by the FDA. Under the Generic Drug Enforcement Act of 1992, the FDA is authorized to debar individuals convicted of crimes relating to the development, approval, or regulation of drugs or biologicals from providing any services to applicants. The statute requires that applications for drug products (including biological products) include a certification that the applicant did not and will not use in any capacity the services of any person debarred in connection with such application.

S. Item 17—Field Copy Certification Section

Since 1993, United States–based NDA sponsors have been required to submit a "field" copy of the NDA's chemistry, manufacturing, and controls section, application form, and summary directly to the relevant FDA district office for use during the preapproval manufacturing inspection. The applicant has also been required to certify in its NDA that an exact copy of the chemistry, manufacturing, and controls contained in the application has been forwarded to the relevant FDA district office. In the past, CBER itself conducted preapproval biologicals' inspections, and no such certification was required in the BLA. With the advent of Team Biologics and the introduction of the field force to biological inspections, it is now advisable to talk to the application division the sponsor is dealing with to get the current requirements.

T. Item 18—User Fee Cover Sheet Section (Form FDA 3397)

Since January 1994, the FDA has required every new drug application and biological license application to include a copy of the User Fee Cover Sheet. This form provides information that permits the FDA to determine whether the application is subject to user fees and, if so, whether the appropriate fee for the application has been submitted. The FDA will not start a review of an application unless verification of receipt of the user fee has been obtained.

U. Item 19—Other Information Section

The BLA applicant may provide in this section any other information that may help the agency evaluate the safety and effectiveness of the product.

V. AMENDING THE LICENSE APPLICATION

During the review of the BLA, the FDA is likely to request additional information to address unresolved issues regarding the original submission. A response to such a request is generally referred to as an amendment. A change to any unapproved application is called an amendment (IND, BLA, NDA). The content of a BLA amendment will depend on the nature of CBER's information request. The format used in this submission is similar to that used for the original BLA submission. The cover letter for the amendment should be titled: "Amendment to BLA _____." In the cover letter, the applicant should clearly identify the purpose of the amendment and the contents of the submission. The amendment should be paginated in a manner that will allow CBER to locate the section of the BLA in which the amendment should be incorporated.

VI. SUPPLEMENT TO THE ORIGINAL BLA

Although amendments are submitted to update or modify an unapproved BLA, supplements are submitted to modify approved license applications. The holder of an approved BLA may seek to change its manufacturing methods, expand the product's indication, or make other changes that reflect new technology or make its product or processes more competitive. Compared with companies holding approved NDAs for drug products, biological licensees traditionally have had considerably less latitude in making minor changes to labeling or manufacturing processes without first obtaining FDA approval through a supplemental application.

In April 1995, however, CBER implemented a new policy creating a three-tier reporting and approval mechanism for postapproval manufacturing and facility changes. Under this policy, only significant changes—those in categories II and III—will require the submission of a supplement. Only category III changes—important proposed changes in manufacturing methods—will require FDA preclearance before implementation.

Because category II and III changes can be expected throughout a product's life cycle, supplementing the BLA becomes an ongoing process. Supplement-related activity is particularly high as a company refines, scales up, and streamlines its manufacturing operation. Content requirements for supplemental BLAs will depend on the nature of the proposed change. In general, the applicant provides new data and information sufficient to support the modification.

VII. ASSEMBLING AND SUBMITTING THE BLA

Whether submitting an original BLA, an amendment, or a supplement, the applicant should follow these requirements:

1. The BLA should be properly indexed and paginated for ease of review. Each volume should be no more than 2 inches thick, bound on the left side of the page, and printed on standard U.S. paper (8.5 × 11″). The front cover of each volume should specify the name of the applicant, the name of the product, and the BLA number (if known). The lower right-hand corner of each volume should read, "This submission: 'Volume _ of _ volumes.'" The upper right-hand corner should read "Volume _."

2. Applicants must submit two copies of the BLA to CBER (most likely the CBER division will ask for additional copies). The copies may be hand-delivered or mailed. If the applicant hand-delivers the BLA, the sponsor should bring an extra copy of the cover letter with the shipment so that the letter may be date-stamped upon delivery to the FDA's Document Control Center. This letter provides evidence that the document was submitted to the FDA. If forwarded by standard mail service, the BLA shipment should include a letter of instructions with a document stating that the BLA submission has been received by the FDA. The FDA document control person will sign the document, place it in a stamped return envelope provided by the sponsor, and return it to the company. This document also serves as proof that the BLA was submitted.

Sponsors mailing the BLA should forward the application and all related submissions to the following address:

Center for Biologics Evaluation and Research
Food and Drug Administration
1401 Rockville Pike
Suite 200N, HFM-99
Rockville, MD 20852-1448

If the applicant forwards the BLA using a commercial overnight service, a return receipt is provided. In this case, the receipt provides evidence of the BLA's delivery.

8

Device Legislation and Application

Max Sherman
Sherman Consulting Services, Warsaw, Indiana, U.S.A.

I. NEW MEDICAL DEVICE APPROVAL PROCESS IN THE UNITED STATES

There is the long-standing belief that the approval process for medical devices is much faster than the IND/NDA drug method. This is certainly true for Class I, Class II, and some preenactment Class III devices—products that can be cleared through Premarket Notification or 510(k) submissions. Such products are often approved for commercialization in 90 days or less. However, the difference in time is less apparent for manufacturers of new Class III products, where preclinical studies, clinical trials, and the premarket approval process is required. Statistics with respect to time of inception through time to market for new Class III devices are not readily available, but in the author's opinion it would be similar to that required for a new drug.

A medical device is defined as an instrument, apparatus, implement, machine, contrivance, implant, in vitro reagent, or other similar or related article, including any component, part, or accessory, which is recognized in the official National Formulary or the United States Pharmacopeia or any supplement to them, intended for use in the diagnosis of disease or other conditions, or in the cure, mitigation, treatment, or prevention of disease in man or other animals, or intended to affect the structure or any function of the body of man or other animals, and which does not achieve any of its primary intended purposes through chemical action, and which is not dependent upon being metabolized for the achievement of any of its primary intended purposes. The primary difference between drugs and devices relates to whether there is a chemical or metabolic action to achieve the intended purpose.

Medical devices were included in the 1938 Federal Food, Drug and Cosmetic Act [1] (the act), but only in terms of prohibited actions related to adulteration or misbranding. Following passage of the Medical Device Amendments on May 28, 1976, a host of new provisions were added [2]. Included among others were regulations pertaining to registration, device listing, classification, performance standards, labeling, good manufacturing practices, premarket notification, and premarket approval. Classification is unique to medical devices—it provides a risk-based system for regulating these products. There are three categories of regulatory control. Class I represents products of lowest risk, subject only to general control provisions. Class II devices are subject to general and special controls. The latter can include performance standards, postmarket surveillance, patient registries, certain guidelines (including guidelines for the submission of clinical data), and other information such as special labeling. Class III devices cannot be adequately regulated under either Class I or II, they have the potential for higher risk. They are thus subjected to the strictest type of regulatory requirement. Manufacturers of Class III products must submit a premarket approval application (PMA) containing valid scientific evidence of their safety and efficacy. To understand today's requirements for marketing medical devices that require clinical studies it would be prudent to review a capsuled history of device legislation. The provisions listed here for the most part are limited to those required to achieve product approvals.

1976   Medical Device Amendments were passed May 28 (1) to assure safety and effectiveness of medical devices, including certain diagnostic and laboratory products, and (2) to upgrade the regulatory authority over such devices. In addition, the amendments required the classification of all devices with graded regulatory requirements, establishment registration, device listing, premarket notification or 510(k), premarket approval, investigational device exemptions, good manufacturing practice regulations, records and reporting requirements, performance standards, and preemption of state and local regulation of devices.

1990   The Safe Medical Devices Act (SMDA), signed into law on November 28, amended the federal Food, Drug and Cosmetic Act to add new requirements and provisions concerning the regulation of medical devices [3]. Some provisions went into effect upon enactment of the SMDA, while others had different effective dates or required implementing regulations. New provisions included user facility reporting, distributor reports, Medical Device Reports (MDRs), certification, device tracking, reports of removals and corrective actions, postmarket surveillance, civil penalties, recall authority, temporary suspension of premarket approval, design validation, new provisions related to 510(k)s, use of premarket approval data, reclassification of Class III preamendment devices, transitional devices, Class II redefinition, Humanitarian Device Exemptions, combination products, repair, replacement, or refund, and establishment of the Office of International Relations.

1992 Medical Device Amendments of 1992 signed into law on June 16, included changes to some of the provisions of the SMDA [4]. The amendments (1) provided for a broader definition of "serious injury" for MDR reports, (2) deemed failure to comply with Postmarket Surveillance requirements as misbranding under the FD&C Act, and (3) changed the provision for repair, replacement, and refund. Prior to passage of the 1992 Amendments, for the FDA to issue an order under section 518 of the act, the FDA would have to show, among other things, that the device was not "designed *and* manufactured" in accordance with the state of the art at the time of design and manufacture. Under the 1992 Amendments, the FDA would only have to show that the device was not "designed *or* manufactured" in accordance with the state of the art at that time.

1997 The FDA Modernization Act (FDAMA) was signed into law on November 21 [5]. With certain provisions noted in the act itself, most of the law's provisions became effective on February 19, 1998. The act complemented and built on the FDA's measures to focus its resources on medical devices that present the greatest risks to patients. The FDAMA also added a number of provisions affecting clinical studies and premarket approval. Under Section 201, sponsors who intend to perform clinical studies of any Class III or implantable devices were given an opportunity to have their investigational plan discussed with FDA to reach an agreement on its contents before applying for an Investigational Device Exemption (IDE). A written request to the FDA is required prior to FDA review. The request shall include a detailed description of the device, proposed conditions of use, and a proposed investigational plan (including the clinical protocol). The FDA has 30 days to meet with the sponsor after receipt of the written request. An official record is made of any agreement reached between the sponsor and the FDA. Agreements reached at these pre-IDE meetings are binding and not subject to change except (1) with written agreement of the sponsor or (2) if the sponsor has been notified by the FDA that a substantial scientific issue essential to determining the safety or effectiveness of the device involved has been identified.

Under Section 205 of FDAMA, sponsors planning to submit a Premarket Approval Application can submit a written request to the FDA for a meeting to determine the type of information (valid scientific evidence) that is necessary to support the effectiveness of a device. The request must include a detailed description of the device, proposed conditions of use, an investigational plan, and if available, information regarding the device's expected performance. The FDA must meet with the requester and communicate the agency's determination of the type of data that will be necessary to demonstrate effectiveness in writing within 30 days after the meeting. When making this determination the FDA must assure that the information they have specified is necessary to provide a reasonable assurance that the device is effective and that the agency has considered the method of evaluation that is least burdensome. The FDA's decision will be binding and not subject to change unless the agency determines that the decision could be contrary to the public health.

Section 209(b) of the FDAMA states that the FDA must, upon written request of the applicant, meet with that party within 100 days of receipt of the filed PMA application to discuss the review status of the application. Prior to this meeting, the FDA must inform the applicant in writing of any identified deficiencies and what information is required to correct these deficiencies. The FDA must also promptly notify the applicant if the FDA identifies additional deficiencies or any additional information required to complete the agency's review. Sections 201(a), 205(a), and 209(b) provide early collaboration and allow for frequent interaction between the applicant and the FDA to address deficiencies.

Section 205(c) deals with labeling claims for Premarket Approval Applications. The FDA must rely solely on the conditions of use submitted as proposed labeling in the PMA application, so long as the proposed labeling is neither false nor misleading. In this determination, the FDA shall fairly evaluate all material facts pertinent to the proposed labeling.

There are a host of other provisions incorporated into the FDAMA, and many reflect the agency's new philosophical approach, which redefines and broadens the FDA's original character as a self-reliant public health law enforcement agency [6].

2002 The Medical Device User Fee and Modernization Act (MDUFMA) amended the Federal Food, Drug and Cosmetic Act to provide the FDA with important new responsibilities, resources, and challenges [7]. The MDUFMA has three significant provisions: (1) Premarket Approval Applications (PMAs), Product Development Protocols (PDPs), Biological License Applications (BLAs), certain supplements, and 510(k)s are now subject to fees. (2) Establishment inspections may be conducted by accredited persons (third parties), under carefully prescribed conditions. (3) There are now new regulatory requirements for reprocessed single use devices.

The standard fee in 2003 for PMAs, PDPs, BLAs, Premarket reports, panel track supplements, and efficacy supplements is $154,000. Small businesses (ones with gross sales or receipts of no more than $30 million) are charged $58,520. For 180 day supplements, the standard fee is $33,110; small businesses pay $12,582. For real-time supplements the fee is $11,088; small businesses pay $4,213. The fee for 510(k)s is $2187 for any size business.

II. PREMARKET NOTIFICATION

Premarket Notification or a 510(k) is required before a manufacturer can commercialize a nonexempt Class I, a Class II, or a preamendment Class III device. (Preamendment refers to the period before May 28, 1976.) A 510(k) submission is a marketing application submitted to the FDA to demonstrate that a medical device is as safe and as effective or substantially equivalent to a legally marketed device that was or is currently on the U.S. market and that does not require premarket approval. The premarket notification requirements are found in 21 CFR Part 807, Subpart E. A device is substantially equivalent if, in comparison to a legally marketed device, it has the same intended use, and has the same technological characteristics as the legally marketed device or has different technological characteristics, and submitted information does not raise new questions of safety and effectiveness, and demonstrates that the device is as safe and as effective as the legally marketed device. All 510(k) applications must include descriptive information and labeling and may require performance and effectiveness testing depending upon the technological characteristics of the device and the risks associated with its application. Performance and effectiveness information may include mechanical bench testing, biocompatibility, animal testing, and clinical evaluation. (Clinical data are required in less than 10 percent of all 510(k) submissions.) Devices in contact with the human body must be biocompatible [8], and most implanted and life-supporting devices require clinical evaluation in support of a 510(k) application. If the FDA determines the device to be substantially equivalent (SE), it can be marketed. If the FDA determines the device is not substantially equivalent (NSE), the manufacturer may resubmit another 510(k) with new data, file a petition to reclassify the device, or submit a premarket approval application.

To streamline the evaluation of premarket notifications for certain Class I devices, Class II devices subject to premarket notification, and preamendments Class III devices for which FDA has not yet called for PMAs, the agency has developed "The New 510(k) Paradigm." The new paradigm presents device manufacturers with two new optional approaches for obtaining marketing clearance for devices subject to 510(k) requirements. While the new paradigm maintains the traditional method of demonstrating substantial equivalence, it also presents the "Special 510(k) Device Modification" option, which utilizes certain aspects of the Quality System Regulation, and the "Abbreviated 510(k)" option, which relies on the use of guidance documents, special controls, and recognized standards to facilitate 510(k) review. (See The New 510(k) Paradigm: Alternate Approaches to Demonstrating Substantial Equivalence in Premarket Notifications, issued March 20, 1998.)

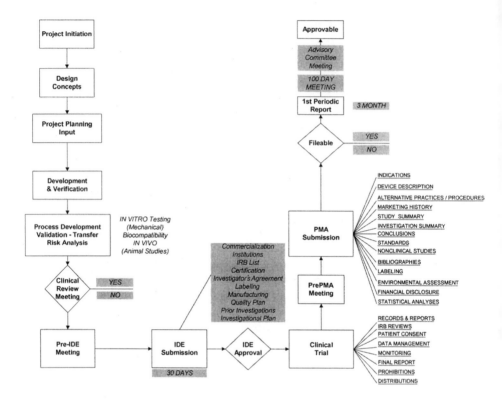

Figure 1 IDE/PMA flow chart.

The premarket approval process must in most cases begin with a clinical trial, and its requirements are included in the following sections on Investigational Device Exemptions. The Investigational Device Exemption/Premarket Approval process is not a trivial undertaking. It will likely take three to five years to complete (see Fig. 1).

III. CLINICAL DATA

Clinical data are required in all premarket approval applications. The PMA applicant must provide a cogent demonstration of the safety and effectiveness for all diagnostic and/or therapeutic medical claims for the device based on laboratory, animal, and clinical data.

Regardless of the type of marketing application, the clinical data must be based on sound scientific principles to demonstrate the endpoint of substantial equivalence or safety and effectiveness. These principles consist of a proper study design, including controls and the adequate number of patients, monitoring of the study to assure the protocol is followed by the investigators, and proper analysis of results.

A PMA based solely on foreign clinical data and otherwise meeting the criteria for approval may be approved if the foreign data are applicable to the United States population, medical practice, and the requirements for informed consent in conformance with the Declaration of Helsinki; if the studies have been performed by clinical investigators of recognized competence; and if the data may be considered valid with the need for an on-site inspection by the FDA, or, if the FDA considers such an inspection to be necessary, the FDA can validate the data through an on-site inspection or other appropriate means. Applicants who seek approval based solely on foreign data should meet with FDA officials in a "presubmission" meeting.

All clinical studies performed in the U.S. in support of a 510(k) or PMA must be conducted in accordance with the Investigational Device Exemption (IDE) regulation (21 CFR Part 812).

IV. INVESTIGATIONAL DEVICE EXEMPTIONS

The final rule for the IDE regulation was published on January 18, 1980. Devices being evaluated under IDEs were exempted from the original current good manufacturing practices regulation (cGMPs) because it was believed that it was not reasonable to expect sponsors of clinical investigations to ensure compliance with cGMPs for devices that may never be approved for commercial distribution. However, sponsors of IDE studies were required to ensure that investigational devices were manufactured under a state of control. When the new Quality System regulation was passed, the Commissioner made it clear that investigational devices must follow design control procedures found in Section 820.30 [9]. To allow manufacturers of devices intended solely for investigational use to ship devices for use on human subjects, the act authorizes the FDA to exempt these devices from certain requirements of the act that would apply to devices in commercial distribution. Clinical evaluation of devices not cleared for marketing, unless exempt, requires an approved Investigational Device Exemption (IDE) either by an institutional review board (IRB) or an IRB and the FDA, and informed consent for all patients, adequate monitoring, and necessary records and reports. The exemptions from the act include misbranding under Section 502, registration, listing and premarket notification under Section 510, performance standards under Section 514, premarket approval under Section 515, banned devices under Section 516, records and reports under Section 519, restricted device requirements under Section 520(e), current good manufacturing practice requirements with the exception of Design Controls, and color additive requirements under Section 721.

The five primary regulations regarding clinical studies included in the Code of Federal Regulations, Title 21 (21CFR 21), are Part 812, which provides the procedures for the conduct of clinical studies with medical devices; Part 50, which provides the requirements and general elements of informed consent; Part 54, which provides the requirements for financial disclosure by clinical investigators; Part 56, which provides the procedures and responsibilities for the institutional review board; and Part 11, Electronic Records and Signatures. The latter has become an integral element in all FDA inspections. A paper that excels in demystifying the records process and compliance issues with Part 11 should be reviewed prior to initiating a clinical study [10].

There are other regulations that affect clinical research. These relate to patient privacy, and are included in 45 CFR Parts 160 and 164. They set forth guidelines for the protection of patient health information. 45 CFR Part 142 provides guidance for the security of such information. The regulations are collectively referred to as HIPAA or Health Insurance Portability and Accountability Act [11]. HIPAA has definitions for the organizations it covers. These organizations are termed Covered Entities and Business Associates. HIPAA defines Covered Entities as health care providers, health care plans, and health care clearinghouses. These organizations are required to comply with the regulations. However, there is another type of relation entitled business associates that covers organizations with access to protected health information (PHI) for legitimate reasons. Business associates must have legal contacts in place in order to receive PHI. These agreements cover the business associate's responsibilities when receiving PHI. Organizations participating in clinical research must have HIPAA-compliant informed patient consents and/or data use agreements for any research study. Specific language must inform the patient of the following rights:

The purpose for collecting patient information
Who will see the information
How the information will be used
The patient's ability to cancel permission to use the information

For specific language and details concerning the informed patient consent and data use agreement, sponsors should review the information available from the Department of Health and Human Services Centers for Medicare and Medicaid Services or their privacy officers. (See http://www. cms. hhs.gov/hipaa.) Another useful link to a guidance document specifically related to research under the HIPAA privacy regulations can be accessed at http://www.hhs.gov/ocr/hipaa/guidelines/research.pdf. (See Chaps. 20 and 24.)

All clinical investigations for devices must have an approved IDE or be exempt from the IDE regulations. Exemptions are listed in 21CFR 812 (c). They (1) include exceptions for devices, other than transitional devices, in commercial distribution before May 28, 1976, when used or investigated in accordance with the labeling in effect at that time, (2) exceptions for diagnostic devices if the testing is noninvasive, does not require an invasive sampling procedure that presents significant risk, does not by design or intention introduce energy into a subject, and is not used as a diagnostic procedure without confirmation of the diagnosis by another medically established diagnostic product or procedure, (3) a device undergoing consumer preference testing, testing of a modification, or testing of a combination of two or more devices in commercial distribution, if the testing is not for the purpose of determining safety or effectiveness and does not put subjects at risk, (4) a device intended solely for veterinary use, (5) a device shipped solely for research on or with laboratory animals and specially labeled (812.5(c); and (6) exceptions for custom devices, unless the device is being used to determine safety or effectiveness for commercial distribution.

Investigations that are not exempt from the IDE regulation are subject to differing levels of regulatory control depending on the level of risk. The IDE regulation distinguishes between *significant risk* (SR) and *nonsignificant risk* (NSR) device studies and the procedures for obtaining an IDE differ accordingly. The determination of whether a study presents a significant risk is initially made by the sponsor of the device. A proposed study is then submitted to an IRB for review. If the IRB agrees with the sponsor that the device study presents a nonsignificant risk, no IDE submission to FDA is necessary. A sponsor of a significant risk study must obtain both IRB and FDA approval before starting a study. A SR device study is defined [21 CFR 812.3(m)] as a study of a device that presents a potential for serious risk to the health, safety, or welfare of a subject and (1) is an implant or (2) is used in supporting or sustaining human life; or (3) is of substantial importance in diagnosing, curing, mitigating, or treating disease, or otherwise prevents impairment to human health; or (4) otherwise presents a potential for serious risk to the health, safety, or welfare of a subject. An NSR device investigation is one that does not meet the definition of a significant risk study. (There is a blue book memorandum or FDA Information Sheet #D86-1 that further clarifies the difference between significant and nonsignificant risk medical device studies.)

V. AN IDE SUBMISSION

In order to conduct a significant risk device study a sponsor must

> Submit the investigational plan and report of prior investigations to an IRB for review and approval
>
> Submit a complete IDE application to the FDA for review (see application section below) and obtain FDA approval of the IDE
>
> Select qualified investigators, provide them with necessary information on the investigational plan and report of prior investigations, and obtain signed agreements from them

The following information must be included in an IDE application for a significant risk device investigation. A sponsor cannot begin a study until FDA and IRB approval are granted. Three copies of a signed application are required, and the application shall include

> Name and address of sponsor
>
> A complete report of prior investigations
>
> An accurate summary or a complete investigational plan
>
> A description of the methods, facilities, and controls used for the manufacture, processing, packing, storage, and installation of the device
>
> An example of the agreements to be signed by the investigators and a list of the names and addresses of all investigators
>
> Certification that all investigators have signed the agreement, that the list of investigators includes all investigators participating in the study, and that new investigators will sign the agreement before being added to the study
>
> A list of the names, addresses and chairpersons of all IRBs that have or will be asked to review the investigation and a certification of IRB action concerning the investigation
>
> The name and address of any institution (other than those above) where a part of the investigation may be conducted
>
> The amount, if any, charged for the device and an explanation of why sale does not constitute commercialization
>
> A claim for categorical exclusion (for example, by stating "Devices shipped under the IDE are intended to be used for clinical studies in which waste will be controlled or the amount of waste expected to enter the environment may reasonably be expected to be nontoxic")

or provision for an environmental assessment, as provided for in 21 CFR 25.31

Copies of all labeling for the device

Copies of all informed consent forms and all related information materials to be provided to subjects

Any other relevant information that the FDA requests for review of the IDE application

An investigational plan shall include the following items and in the following order:

1. Purpose (the name and intended use of the device and the objectives and duration of the investigation)
2. Protocol (a written protocol describing the methodology to be used and an analysis of the protocol demonstrating its scientific soundness)
3. Risk analysis (a description and analysis of all increased risks to the research subjects and how these risks will be minimized; a justification for the investigation; and a description of the patient population including the number, age, sex, and condition of each subject)
4. Description of this device (a description of each important component, ingredient, property, and principle of operation of the device and any anticipated changes in the device during the investigation)
5. Monitoring procedures (the sponsor's written procedures for monitoring the investigation and the name and address of each monitor)
6. Labeling (copies of all labeling for the device)
7. Consent materials (copies of all forms and materials given to subjects to obtain informed consents)
8. IRB information (a list of the names, addresses, and chairpersons of all IRBs that will review the investigation and a certification of any action taken by them)
9. Other institutions (the name and address of any other institution not previously identified at which a part of the investigation may be conducted)
10. Additional records and reports (a description of any records or reports of the investigation other than those required in Subpart G of the IDE regulation)

As mentioned above under the FDAMA of 1997, a manufacturer should schedule a pre-IDE meeting to discuss its proposed investigational plan prior to submitting an IDE.

A report of prior investigations is also required in an IDE application. It must include reports of all prior clinical, animal, and laboratory testing of the device. It should be comprehensive and adequate to justify the proposed investigation. Specific contents of the report must include

A bibliography of all publications, whether adverse or supportive, that are relevant to an evaluation of the safety and effectiveness of the device

Copies of all published and unpublished adverse information

Copies of other significant publications if requested by an IRB or by the FDA

A summary of all other unpublished information (whether adverse or supportive) that is relevant to an evaluation of the safety and effectiveness of the device

If nonclinical laboratory data are provided, a statement that such studies have been conducted in compliance with the good laboratory practice (GLP) regulation in 21 CFR Part 58. If the study was not conducted in compliance with GLPs, include a brief statement of the reason(s) for noncompliance.

VI. SUBMITTING AN IDE

There are no preprinted forms for an IDE application, but an IDE application must include all of the information described in 21 CFR 812.20(b). The FDA will not review an incomplete submission. The sponsor must demonstrate that there is reason to believe that the risks to human subjects from the proposed investigation are outweighed by the anticipated benefits to subjects and the importance of the knowledge to be gained, that the investigation is scientifically sound, and that there is reason to believe that the device as proposed for use will be effective. A suggested format and checklist for preparing IDE applications is included in HHS Publication FDA 96-4159, Investigational Device Exemptions Manual, available on the FDA's website: www.fda.gov/ cdrh. Sponsors can also receive information from the Division of Small Manufacturers Assistance (DSMA) by calling toll free 800 638-2041 or by fax at 301 443-8818. All submissions, in triplicate, should be addressed to Food and Drug Administration, Center for Devices and Radiological Health, IDE Document Mail Center (HFZ-401), 9200 Corporate Boulevard, Rockville, MD 20850.

VII. FDA ACTION ON APPLICATIONS

The FDA will notify the sponsor in writing of the date it receives an IDE. The FDA may approve, approve with modification, or disapprove. An investigation may not begin until 30 days after the FDA receives the IDE application for the investigation of a device unless the FDA notifies the sponsor that the investigation may not begin, or until the FDA approves by order an IDE for the investigation. The FDA may disapprove or withdraw approval of an IDE if FDA finds that

> The sponsor has not complied with the applicable requirements of the IDE regulation, other applicable regulations, statutes, or any condition of approval imposed by an IRB or FDA.
>
> The application or report contains untrue statements or omits required material or information.
>
> The sponsor fails to respond to a request for additional information within the time prescribed by FDA.
>
> There is reason to believe that the risks to the research subjects are not outweighed by the anticipated benefits or the importance of knowledge to be gained; that the informed consent is inadequate; that the investigation is scientifically unsound; or that the device as used is ineffective.
>
> It is unreasonable to begin or continue the investigation because of the way the device is used, or the inadequacy of the investigational plans; the reports of prior investigations; the methods, facilities, and controls used for the manufacturing, processing, packaging, storage, and installation of the device; or the monitoring and review of the investigation.

If the FDA disapproves an IDE application or proposes to withdraw approval, it will notify the sponsor in writing. A disapproval order will contain a complete statement of the reasons for disapproval and will advise the sponsor of the right to request a regulatory hearing under 21 CFR Part 16. The FDA will provide an opportunity for a hearing before withdrawal or approval unless the FDA determines that there is an unreasonable risk to the public health if testing continues.

When the FDA grants approval, the sponsor will be notified and the study can commence with due consideration to a host of responsibilities. The study will be granted a unique identifier beginning with the letter G, i.e., G03XXXX. The number 03 is used for 2003, the XXXX is a sequential number supplied by Document Management. The FDA often grants Conditional Approval, allowing the study to start, pending correction of minor deficiencies. The FDA considers the existence of an IDE as confidential and it will not disclose its existence unless the FDA determines that the information had been previously disclosed to the public; or that the FDA approved a PMA for a device subject to an IDE, or the device has in effect a Product Development Protocol notice of completion. *Note:* Product Development Protocols will not be included in this section as they have been rarely employed.

VIII. RESPONSIBILITIES OF SPONSORS

Sponsors are responsible for selecting qualified investigators and providing them with the information they need to conduct an investigation properly. Proper monitoring of the investigation, ensuring IRB review and approval, and informing the IRB and the FDA promptly of any significant new information are also responsibilities of the sponsor. Sponsors must ensure that investigators are qualified by training and experience. Control of the device is of critical importance. A sponsor shall ship investigational devices only to qualified investigators participating in the investigation. Sponsors should review 21 CFR 812.43 to ascertain all of the requirements for an investigator's agreement, and sponsors should supply all investigators with copies of the investigational plan and the report of prior investigations of the device. A sponsor who discovers that an investigator is not complying with the signed agreement, the investigational plan, the requirements of Part 812, or other applicable FDA regulations, or any conditions of approval imposed by the reviewing IRB or the FDA shall promptly either secure compliance or discontinue shipments of the device to the investigator and terminate the investigator's participation. A sponsor shall also require that an investigator dispose of or return the device, unless this action would jeopardize the rights, safety, or welfare of a subject.

Once the study begins, sponsors shall immediately conduct an evaluation of any unanticipated adverse device effect. An unanticipated adverse device effect means any serious adverse effect on health or safety or any life-threatening problem or death caused by, or associated with, a device, if that effect, problem, or death was not previously identified in nature, severity, or degree of incidence in the investigational plan or application, or any other unanticipated serious problem associated with a device that relates to the rights, safety, or welfare of subjects. On a practical note, adverse effects that appear in a study that are not included in the package insert may be considered "unanticipated."

To demonstrate further that IDE studies are not trivial matters, there are a number of records and reports for which sponsors are responsible. The following records must be maintained:

> All correspondence including required reports
> Records of shipment and disposition
> Signed investigator's agreements
> Records concerning adverse device defects whether anticipated or not
> Any other records that the FDA requires to be maintained by regulation or by specific requirement for a particular device or category of devices

The following reports must also be prepared:

Unanticipated adverse device defects—within 10 working days after receiving notice of the adverse effect, and submitted to the FDA and all reviewing IRBs and investigators.

Withdrawal of IRB approval—within 5 working days of receipt of the withdrawal of IRB approval, and submitted to the FDA and all reviewing IRBs and participating investigators.

Withdrawal of FDA approval—within 5 working days after receipt of the notice of withdrawal of FDA approval, and submitted to all reviewing IRBs and participating investigators.

Current list of investigators and addresses—every 6 months, and submitted to the FDA for a significant risk device study.

Progress reports—at regular intervals and at least yearly, and submitted to all reviewing IRBs. For a significant risk device, the sponsor shall also submit the progress report to the FDA.

Recalls and device disposition—within 30 working days after receipt of a request to return, repair, or dispose of any investigational device, and submitted to the FDA and all reviewing IRBs.

A final report—the sponsor shall notify the FDA and all reviewing IRBs within 30 working days of the completion or termination of a significant risk device investigation, and submit a final report to the FDA and all reviewing IRBs and participating investigators within 6 months after the completion or termination of the investigation. For a nonsignificant risk device, the sponsor must submit a final report to all reviewing IRBs within 6 months after the completion or termination.

Use of a device without informed consent—within 5 working days after receipt of notice of such use, and submitted to the FDA.

Significant risk device determination—within 5 working days of an IRB determination that the device is a significant risk device and not a nonsignificant risk device as proposed, and submitted to FDA.

Other reports—accurate, complete, and current information about any aspect of the investigation that the FDA or the reviewing IRB may request.

IX. RETENTION PERIOD

Sponsors shall maintain the records listed above during the investigation and for a period of 2 years after the later of the following two dates: the date on which the investigation is terminated or completed, or the date that the records are no longer required for purposes of supporting a premarket approval application or a notice of completion of a PDP.

X. INSPECTION

The FDA has the authority to inspect facilities at which investigational devices are being held, including any establishments where devices are manufactured, packed, installed, used, implanted, or where records of use are kept. Sponsors, IRBs, and investigators are required to permit authorized FDA employees reasonable access at reasonable times to inspect and copy all records of an investigation. Upon notice, the FDA may inspect and copy records that identify subjects.

XI. RESPONSIBILITIES OF INVESTIGATORS AND IRBs

Subpart D in Part 812 covers the responsibilities of IRBs as specified in Part 56 (the IRB regulation). Subparts E and G include responsibilities for investigators including compliance, device disposition, informed consent, and records and reports.

XII. IDE GUIDANCE

The FDA's Office of Device Evaluation, Center for Devices and Radiological Health, has developed a number of information sheets and guidance policies to help sponsors conduct clinical trials. IDE Memorandum #D94-1 is particularly helpful. It contains an IDE Checklist for Administrative Review that sponsors can use to ensure that their IDE is administratively complete. Another important document is entitled "Implementation of the FDA/ HCFA Intragency Agreement Regarding Reimbursement Categorization of Investigational Devices—IDE Memorandum #D95-2. This memo establishes procedures pertaining to the reimbursement of investigational devices. The Health Care Financing Administration (HCFA), now the Center for Medicare and Medicaid Services (CMS), governs payment for Medicare and Medicaid Services. Sponsors should be aware of the category their investigational device is assigned to, A or B. Category A is reserved for innovative devices believed to be in Class III for which "absolute risk" of the device type has not been established. Category B includes those device types known to be safe and effective because, for example, other manufacturers have obtained

FDA approval/clearance for that device type. For purposes of determining Medicare coverage, medical devices classed as Category B could be viewed as "reasonable and necessary" if they also meet all other Medicare coverage requirements. Companies that consider embarking on clinical trials would be wise to investigate whether there are reimbursement issues to consider, including coding, coverage, and payment. Clinical Utility should be part of the decision process. The study must demonstrate that the subject device has a beneficial therapeutic effect, or that as a diagnostic tool, it provides information that measurably contributes to a diagnosis of a disease or condition. (See FDA Guidance #P91-1, 5/3/91.)

XIII. LABELING

Special labeling is required for investigational devices. (See 21 CFR 812.5.)

An investigational device or its immediate package shall bear a label with the following information: the name and place of business of the manufacturer, packer, or distributor, the quantity of contents, if appropriate, and the statement "CAUTION—Investigational Device. Limited by Federal (or United States) law to investigational use." The label or other labeling shall describe all relevant contraindications, hazards, adverse effects, interfering substances or devices, warnings, and precautions.

XIV. PROHIBITION OF PROMOTION AND OTHER PRACTICES

A sponsor, investigator, or any person acting for or on behalf of a sponsor or investigator shall not (a) promote or test market an investigational device until after the FDA has approved the device for commercial distribution, (b) commercialize an investigational device by charging the subjects or investigators for a device a price larger than that necessary to recover costs of manufacture, research, development, and handling, (c) unduly prolong an investigation, or (d) represent that an investigational device is safe or effective for the purposes for which it is being investigated. (See 21 CFR 812.7.)

XV. IMPORT AND EXPORT REQUIREMENTS

In addition to complying with other sections of the IDE requirements, a person who *imports* or offers for importation an investigational device shall be the agent of the foreign exporter with respect to investigations of the device and shall act as the sponsor of the clinical investigation, or ensure that another person acts as the agent of the foreign exporter and the sponsor of the investigation. A person *exporting* an investigational device shall obtain the FDA's prior approval, as required by section 801(e) of the act, and comply with section 802 of the Act.

XVI. PREMARKET APPROVAL

Premarket Approval (PMA) is the FDA process to evaluate the safety and effectiveness of all Class III devices. Due to the level of risk associated with Class III devices, the FDA has determined that general and special controls alone are insufficient to assure their safety and effectiveness. Therefore these devices require a premarket approval (PMA) application under section 515 of the act, in order to obtain marketing clearance.

Under section 515 of the act, all devices placed into Class III are subject to premarket approval requirements. Premarket approval is the process of scientific and regulatory review to ensure the safety and effectiveness of Class III devices. An approved PMA is, in effect, a private license (some would say a regulatory patent) granted to the applicant for marketing a particular medical device. A Class III device that fails to meet PMA requirements is considered to be adulterated under section 501(f) of the act and cannot be marketed. Premarket approval requirements apply differently to preamendment devices, postamendment devices, and transitional Class III devices.

Manufacturers of Class III preamendment devices, devices that were in commercial distribution before May 28, 1976, are not required to submit a PMA until 30 months after the promulgation of a final classification regulation or until 90 days after the promulgation of a final regulation requiring the submission of a PMA, whichever period is later. The FDA may allow more than 90 days after promulgation of a final rule for the submission of a PMA.

A postamendment device is one that was first distributed commercially on or after May 28, 1976. Postamendment devices that the FDA determines are substantially equivalent to preamendment device Class III devices are subject to the same requirements as the preamendment devices. The FDA determines substantial equivalence after reviewing an applicant's premarket notification 510(k). Postamendment devices determined by the FDA to be not substantially equivalent to either pre- or postamendment devices classified into Class I or II are "new" devices and fall automatically into Class III. Before such devices can be marketed, they must have an approved premarket approval application or be reclassified into Class I or II.

Class III transitional devices, i.e., devices considered to be a new drug or antibiotic drug before May 28, 1976, and "new" devices are automatically classified into Class III by statute and require premarket approval by FDA before they may be commercially distributed. Applicants may either submit a PMA or PDP, or they may petition FDA to reclassify the devices into Class I or II. Clinical studies in support of a PMA, PDP, or a reclassification petition are subject to the Investigational Device Exemption application.

The PMA requirements are found in 21 CFR Part 814. Not all Class III devices require an approved PMA to be marketed at this time. Class III devices that are substantially equivalent to devices legally marketed through May 28, 1976, and do not currently require premarket approval may be marketed through the 510(k) process until the FDA publishes a regulation requiring the submission of a premarket approval (PMA) application process for those Class III devices.

XVII. THE PMA SUBMISSION

Section 515(c) of the act specifies the required contents of PMA applications to be as follows:

(A) Full reports of all information, published or known to, or which should reasonably be known to, the applicant, concerning investigations that have been made to show whether or not such device is safe and effective.

(B) A full statement of the components, ingredients, and properties and of the principle or principles of operation, of such device.

(C) A full description of the methods used in, and the facilities and controls used for, the manufacture, processing, and, when relevant, packing and installation of such device.*

(D) An identifying reference to any performance standard under section 514 that would be applicable to any aspect of such device if it were Class II, and either adequate information to show that such aspect of such device fully meets such performance standard or adequate information to justify any deviation from such standards.

(E) Such samples of such device and of components thereof as the Secretary may reasonably require, except that where the submission of such samples is impractical or unduly burdensome, the requirement of this subparagraph may be met by the submission of complete information concerning the location of one or more such devices readily available for examination and testing.

(F) Specimens of the labeling proposed to be used for such device.

(G) Such other information relevant to the subject matter of the application as the Secretary, with the concurrence of the appropriate panel under section 513, may require.

*Guidance is available to assist manufacturers in preparing the quality system information required in the PMA application. This is particularly valuable for companies who elect a modular review. If the company elects to use this method, the FDA suggests that the design control information and manufacturing information be submitted in modules that are separate from other information. (See Quality System Information for Certain Premarket Application Reviews; Guidance for Industry and FDA Staff, issued February 3, 2003.)

XVIII. FORMAT

To facilitate the FDA's handling of PMA applications, the following recommendations are offered:

Use paper with dimensions of $8\frac{1}{2}$ by 11".

Use at least a $1\frac{1}{2}$ "wide left margin to allow for binding into jackets."

Use 3-holed punched paper.

If the submission exceeds 2" in thickness, separate into volumes and identify volume number.

Clearly and prominently identify the submission as an original PMA application or, for additional submissions to a PMA application, clearly identify the FDA assigned document number (e.g., P030000) and type of submission (amendment, supplement, or report), and the type of submission (e.g., Response to an FDA letter dated _____).

All copies of each submission must be identical.

Sequentially number the pages, providing a detailed table of contents, and use tabs to identify each section.

Send six copies of an original PMA and three copies of amendments and supplements (except as specified below) directly to

Food and Drug Administration
Center for Devices and Radiological Health
PMA Document Mail Center (HFZ-401)
9200 Corporate Blvd.
Rockville, MD 20850

If an amendment or supplement refers to more than one PMA, three copies of the submission must be submitted for each PMA. If more than one PMA is affected by the submission, the applicant may wish to submit three complete copies to one of the PMAs and cover letters to the other PMAs that incorporate by reference that complete copy and identify all affected PMAs. All copies of the first volume of each submission must include a signed and dated cover letter.

Do not combine PMAs, IDEs, and 510(k)s together. They must be separate submissions.

Only the PMA applicant on record with the FDA may amend, supplement, or submit reports to their PMA, unless the PMA includes the original and not a copy of an appropriate letter of authorization from the applicant permitting another person to submit information on behalf of the applicant.

To facilitate review of a PMA, FDA suggests the following information be submitted in separate volumes.

MANUFACTURING INFORMATION. Manufacturing information should be submitted in a separate volume of which only five copies are needed for FDA review.

ENVIRONMENTAL ASSESSMENT (21 CFR 25.31). If an applicant believes that the device qualifies for an exemption, they must provide information that establishes to the FDA's satisfaction that the device meets the criteria for a categorical exclusion (21 CFR 25.24). The majority of PMA applications have been granted categorical exclusion. The submission of an environmental assessment in a separate volume will expedite FDA review. Three copies are needed.

COLOR ADDITIVES. Applicants may have responsibilities to demonstrate that color additives remaining in or on the device are safe. The addition of any additive to the device requires biocompatibility information, which includes chemical identification and toxic potential determination for all residues remaining in or on the device. Manufacturers may use color additive regulations in 21 CFR Parts 70 to 82 as a reference to get more information, but toxicity of color additives for food may not be relevant to devices. If a color additive has not been previously listed, manufacturers may need to submit a color additive petition. (See HHS Publication FDA-97-4214— Premarket Approval Manual, January 1998.)

INDIVIDUAL SUBJECT REPORT FORMS. A PMA or PMA supplement, if applicable, is required by 21 CFR 814.20(b)(6)(ii) to include copies of individual case report forms for each subject who died during a clinical investigation or who did not complete the investigation. Before submitting the PMA, the applicant should consult with the Office of Device Evaluation (ODE) reviewing division to determine the information to be included in these report forms, how many copies are required, and whether these forms will be required for other subjects enrolled in the study (e.g., subjects experiencing specified adverse effects or complications).

XIX. PREMARKET APPROVAL APPLICATION FILING REVIEW

Once the manufacturer files the PMA application, the FDA must make a threshold determination about whether the application is sufficiently complete for the agency to undertake a substantive review. The PMA regulation [21 CFR 814.42(e)] states that the FDA may refuse to file a PMA if *any* of the following applies:

1. The PMA is incomplete because it does not on its face contain all of the information required under section 515(c)(1)(A–G) of the act.

2. The PMA does not contain each of the items required under section 814.20, and justification for the omission of any item is inadequate.

3. The applicant has a pending premarket notification under section 510(k) of the act with respect to the same device, and the FDA has not determined whether the device falls within the scope of section 814.1(c).

4. The PMA contains a false statement of material fact.

5. The PMA is not accompanied by a statement of either certification or disclosure as required by 21 CFR Part 54 Financial Disclosure by Clinical Investigators.

Section 814.20 of the regulation further specifies that PMAs must include, among other things, "*technical sections which shall contain data and information in sufficient detail to permit FDA to determine whether to approve or deny approval of the application* [21 CFR 814.20(b)(6)]. The key issue here is that the phrase "data and information in sufficient detail" sometimes leads to subjective interpretations. Because of this, CDRH has frequently expressed the need for more specific guidance in applying this regulatory standard to the PMA application filing decision-making process.

XX. PRESUBMISSION INTERACTION

Before submitting a PMA, applicants are encouraged to interact with CDRH review staff. Such presubmission interaction is an important way of improving the quality and completeness of a PMA and thus increases the likelihood of fileability. Applicants are also encouraged to meet face-to-face with CDRH staff before preparing the PMA to discuss issues related to their specific device and PMA. The CDRH PMA Manual (mentioned earlier) as well as other applicable CDRH device-specific guidance documents provide valuable information for preparing PMAs; all of which are available on the Internet. See http://www.fda.gov/cdrh/guidance.html. Excellent guidance with regard to filing review is now available on the Internet. The document issued on May 1, 2003 is entitled "Premarket Approval Application Filing Review;" it supersedes PMA Filing Decisions (P-90-2), dated May 18, 1990, and PMA Refuse to File Procedures (P94-1), dated May 2, 1994.

XXI. FDA ACTION ON A PMA

The FDA must review a PMA within 180 days after receiving an application that is accepted for filing and to which the applicant does not submit a major amendment. The FDA will review the PMA and the requirements of 814.39(e) after receiving the recommendation of the appropriate advisory committee; then it will send the applicant one of the following: an order approving the PMA, an approval letter, a not-approvable letter, or an order denying approval. The approvable letter and the not-approvable letter will provide an opportunity for the applicant to amend or withdraw the application, or to consider the letter to be a denial of the PMA. The applicant may request administrative review under 515(d)(3) and (g) of the act.

XXII. FDA STEPS IN THE PMA APPLICATION PROCESS

From the FDA's perspective, the review of a PMA is time and resource intensive (see Fig. 2). The review involves a number of offices and divisions. The following constitutes all of their responsibilities:

Office of Device Evaluation (ODE) Filing Review
Office of Surveillance and Biometrics Statistical Review for Filing
Office of Compliance (OC) Review of Manufacturing Information for GMP Inspection Anytime After PMA filing
PMA Filing Decision
GMP Inspection(s) by the Field
Bioresearch Monitoring (BIMO) Audit of several investigational sites
Substantive Review Coordination and Completion in Areas such as

Preparation of FDA Summary of Safety and Effectiveness Data (SSED)
Nonclinical Studies
Microbiological
Toxicological
Immunological
Biocompatibility
Shelf Life
Analytical (For In Vitro Diagnostics)
Animal Studies

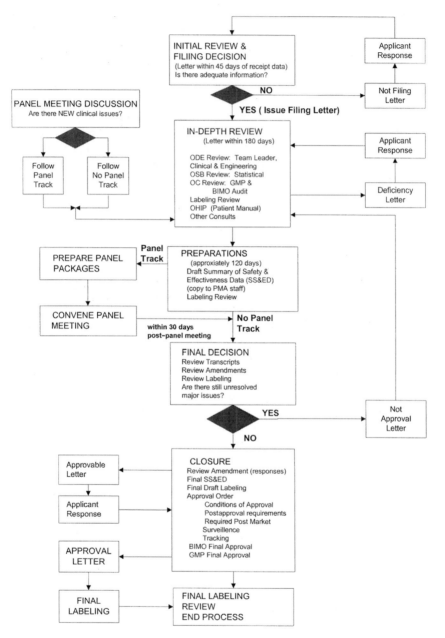

Figure 2 Original PMA (premarket approval) application review and approval decision process.

Engineering (Stress, Wear, Fatigue Testing, etc.)
Clinical Studies
Panel Meeting Decision and Mailing (if Panel Meeting Is Appropriate)
Panel Date
Transcripts Received, Reviewed, and Placed in Administrative Record
GMP Clearance
Final Response from OC for GMP/BIMO
Final ODE Decision Memo
Approval Package—Action Memo, Approval Order, Federal Register
Notice, SSED, Final Draft Labeling

XXIII. PANEL REVIEW

Unless the device meets the criteria for a "me too" product, panel review will be required. Section 512(c)(2) of the act requires that a premarket approval application be referred to an appropriate FDA Advisory Panel "for study and for submission of a report and recommendation respecting approval of the application." The definition of a "me too" device can be found in FDA Guidance #P86-6, 7/25/86.

XXIV. CONDITIONS OF APPROVAL

Whenever the manufacturer has completed all the requirements for the PMA, and the FDA has completed its favorable review, the agency will issue standard postapproval conditions. These "Conditions of Approval" are applicable to all original PMAs and PMA supplements. Applicants should carefully read the conditions of approval enclosed with the FDA approval letter. Conditions of approval include submission of final printed labeling; advertising requirements whereby a brief statement of the intended uses, relevant warnings, precautions, side effects, and contraindications must be provided; supplemental submissions whenever changes are made to the device; postapproval reports; adverse reaction and device defect reporting; and reporting under the Medical Device Reporting (MDR) Regulation.

XXV. AVAILABILITY OF SAFETY AND EFFECTIVENESS SUMMARIES FOR PREMARKET APPROVAL APPLICATIONS

The FDA publishes a list of PMAs that have been approved. The list is intended to inform the public of the availability of safety and effectiveness summaries of approved PMAs through the Internet and the agency's Dockets Management Branch. Persons with access to the Internet may obtain the documents at http://frwebgate.access.gpo.gov/cgi-bin/leaving.cgi?from = -leavingFR.html&log = linklog. Copies are also available from the Dockets Management Branch. Submit written requests for copies to the Dockets Management Branch (HFA-305), Food and Drug Administration, 5630 Fishers Lane, Room 1061, Rockville, MD 20852. Cite the appropriate docket number [12].

REFERENCES

1. Public Law No. 75-717, 52 Stat 1040, 1938.
2. Pub. L. No. 94-295, 90 Stat 540, 1976.
3. Pub. L. 101-629, 104 Stat 4511, 1990.
4. Pub. L. 102—300, 106 Stat 238, 1992.
5. Pub. L. No. 105-115, 111 Stat 2296, 1997.
6. Suydam LA, Kubic MJ. FDA's implementation of FDAMA: an interim balance sheet. Food Drug Law J 2000; 56:131–135.
7. Pub. L. No. 107-250, 2002.
8. Biological Evaluation of Medical Devices—Use of ISO 10993 (FDA Guidance #G95-1, 5/1/95).
9. 61 Federal Register 52654, October 7, 1996.
10. Wood D. The Management of 21 CFR 11 Compliance in Clinical Trials Monitor. Summer 2003; 39–43.
11. Pub. L No. 104-191, 110 Stat 1936, 1996.
12. 67 Federal Register 67629, November 6, 2002.

9
Orphan Drugs

John T. Zenno
Regulatory Services, Inc., Yardley, Pennsylvania, U.S.A.

Richard A. Guarino
Oxford Pharmaceutical Resources, Inc., Totowa, New Jersey, U.S.A.

I. INTRODUCTION

When one hears the word "orphan," it may conjure up something out of a Dickens novel—a picture of a homeless, ragged urchin cowering in a doorway in a cold, deserted alley. Unfortunately, relative to orphan diseases and the drugs to treat them, the metaphor has been all too close to the reality of the situation. Many diseases have gone wanting for treatment simply because it is not economically feasible to develop drugs for them. The federal government, however, has the means to make it more attractive to develop drugs for this lonesome group of diseases. In 1983, the Orphan Drug Act created much-needed changes to provide resources that will develop products to treat diseases and conditions. It has had worldwide impact; orphan drug legislation has been enacted in Japan and is being considered in the European Union [1]. Interestingly, although the FDA has an orphan drugs directorate and advisory body, one will not find the term "orphan drugs" in any Act of the United States, even though, as noted below, these entities are covered.

There are several benefits of the Orphan Drug Act. First, it provides for the development of drugs that ordinarily would not generate enough revenue to render it worthwhile for a company to make, thus benefiting society. Second, it provides tax incentives and product exclusivity to the firms that do provide the drugs. This is important. Currently, there are more than 5,000 rare diseases that, although they affect millions of people, do not represent significant commercial market opportunity to warrant development of drugs for them by many manufacturers.

Several points should be noted. First, an orphan designation does not provide any immunity from producing a valid NDA. The orphan's NDA will be reviewed as rigorously as any NDA. Second, all orphan designated drugs must be studied under an IND, which will be reviewed as rigorously as any other IND. If the product provides treatment for a life-threatening disease and warrants accelerated development, like any other product under development, it will be treated according to the standards for reviewing such diseases, including review under accelerated development in partnership with the FDA.

It also should be noted that often the disease entities involve such a small population of subjects that they do not require manufacture under an NDA; rather, these conditions often are treated under an IND. Filing of such an IND is done with the knowledge of the FDA, and often the FDA will note that the IND is granted with its knowledge and acceptance that no new drug application will be filed as a result of the trials performed under the IND. However, this is a unique situation reserved for orphan drugs. Often, there are few resources to pursue a full NDA. Often, the sponsor is unable to create appropriate protocols. As will be discussed, the FDA encourages the writing of special protocols to cover the orphan disease and is willing to help write the protocols and help fund the trials. In addition, once an NDA is filed, there are additional incentives that assist the company that is pursuing an orphan drug application.

A. Incentives of the Orphan Drug Act

The Orphan Drug Act (P.L. 97-414, as amended) includes various incentives that have stimulated a considerable amount of interest in the development of orphan drug and biological products. These incentives include tax credits for clinical research undertaken by a sponsor to generate required data for marketing approval, and seven years of marketing exclusivity for a designated drug or biological product approved by the FDA.

Section 527 of the Orphan Drug Act provides a seven-year period of exclusive marketing to the first sponsor who obtains marketing approval for a designated orphan drug or biological product. Exclusivity begins on the date that the marketing application is approved by FDA for the designated orphan drug, and it applies only to the indication for which the drug has been designated and approved. A second application for the same drug for a different use could be approved by FDA.

Final regulations on the tax credits were published in the Federal Register on October 3, 1988 (53 FR 38708), and the current version of these regulations are in Title 26, Code of Federal Regulations, Section 45c. The

Internal Revenue Service administers the tax credit provisions, and specific questions about the interpretation of the law or regulations affecting the applicability of the tax credit provision of the Act should be directed to the IRS. If more information on tax credits is needed, contact Pass Through and Special Industries Division, Office of the Chief Counsel, Internal Revenue Service, 1111 Constitution Avenue, NW, Washington, DC 20224; telephone (202) 622-3120.

Section 525 of the Orphan Drug Act provides for formal protocol assistance when requested by the sponsors of drugs for rare diseases or conditions. The formal review of a request for protocol assistance is the direct responsibility of the Center for Drug Evaluation and Research (CDER) or the Center for Biologic Evaluation and Research (CBER), depending on which Center has the authority for the review of the product. The Office of Orphan Products Development (OOPD) is responsible for ensuring that the request qualifies for consideration under section 525 of the FFDCA. This includes determining "whether there is reason to believe the sponsor's drug is a drug for a disease or condition that is rare in the United States." A sponsor need not have obtained an orphan drug designation to receive protocol assistance.

Once the OOPD determines that the proposed compound is for a disease or condition that is rare in the U.S., the request will be forwarded to the responsible division for formal review and direct response. The OOPD monitors the review process within the respective CDER/CBER reviewing division and, where possible, assists in resolving specific issues that may arise during the review process. It should be understood that protocol assistance provided under the Act does not waive the necessity for the submission of an Investigational New Drug Application (IND) by sponsors planning to conduct clinical trials with the product.

B. Research Grants

The FDA, through the OOPD, funds the development of orphan products through its grants program for clinical trials. The Request for Applications (RFA) announcing the availability of funds is published in the Federal Register each year, usually in June. Eligibility for grant funding is extended to medical devices and medical foods for which there is no reasonable expectation of development without such assistance. Applications are reviewed by panels of outside experts and are funded by priority score.

In the Food, Drug, and Cosmetic Act of 1938, as amended, the location of what we affectionately refer to as orphan drugs is "Subchapter B—Drugs for Rare Diseases or Conditions." The original parts of the subchapter were added in 1983, with amendments made in 1984, 1985, and 1988. The Orphan Drug Final Regulations were published in the Federal Register on December 29, 1992 and became effective 30 days thereafter.

C. Orphan Drug Designation

In order for a sponsor to obtain orphan designation for a drug or biologic product, an application must be submitted to Office of Orphan Products Development (OOPD) and the designation approved. The approval of an application for orphan designation is based upon the information submitted by the sponsor. A drug that has obtained orphan designation is said to have "orphan status." Each designation request must stand on its own merit. Sponsors requesting designation of the same drug for the same indication as a previously designated product must submit their own data in support of their designation request. The approval of an orphan designation request does not alter the standard regulatory requirements or process for obtaining marketing approval. Safety and efficacy of a compound must be established through adequate and well-controlled trials.

II. RECOMMENDATIONS FOR INVESTIGATIONS OF DRUGS FOR RARE DISEASES OR CONDITIONS

In Section 525(a), the FDA notes that the sponsor of a drug for a disease or condition that is rare may request the Secretary to provide written recommendations for the nonclinical and clinical investigations that must be conducted with the drug before it may be approved for such disease or condition under Section 505. This is important, because often the complexity of the disease requires more specialization in protocol writing than the sponsor can muster. In addition, having the FDA help with the protocols will assure speedier review further along in the NDA process.

A. Designation

The Act describes how a firm can provide proof to the agency that a drug is to be considered for such designation. Section 526(a)(2) states,

> For purposes of paragraph (1), the term "rare disease or condition" means any disease or condition which (A) affects less than 200,000 persons in the United States, or (B) affects more than 200,000 in the United States and for which there is no reasonable expectation that the cost of developing and making available in the United States a drug for such disease or condition will be recovered from sales in the United States of such drug. Determinations under the preceding sentence with respect to any drug shall be made on the basis of the facts and circumstances as of the date the request for designation of the drug under this subsection is made.

There are a number of caveats that the FDA adds when approving drugs for rare diseases or conditions. Section 526(b) notes,

A designation of a drug under subsection (a) shall be subject to the condition that (1) if an application was approved for the drug under section 505(b), a certificate was issued for the drug under section 507, or a license was issued for the drug under section 351 of the Public Health Service Act, the manufacturer of the drug will notify the Secretary of any discontinuance of the production of the drug at least one year before discontinuance, and (2) if an application has not been approved for the drug under section 505(b), a certificate has not been issued for the drug under section 507, or a license has not been issued for the drug under section 351 of the Public Health Service Act and if preclinical investigations or investigations under section 505(i) are being conducted with the drug, the manufacturer or sponsor of the drug will notify the Secretary of any decision to discontinue active pursuit of approval of an application under section 505(b) . . . or approval of a license under section 351 of the Public Health Service Act.

B. Protection for Drugs for Rare Diseases or Conditions

One of the key provisions the FDA worked into the regulations was the protection of the holder of the application. For holders of NDAs that have been approved under these provisions, the FDA will grant 7 years market exclusivity. Section 527 of the Act notes,

Except as provided in subsection (b), if the Secretary—(1) approves an application filed pursuant to section 505(b), (2) issues a certification under section 507 [*Ed. note*: This was repealed in 1997], (3) issues a license under section 351 of the Public Health Service Act for a drug designated under section 526 for a rare disease or condition, the Secretary may not approve another application under section 505(b) . . . or issue another license under section 351 of the Public Health Service Act for such drug for such disease or condition for a person who is not the holder of such approved application . . . or of such license until the expiration of seven years from the date of the approval of the approved application . . . or the issuance of the license. Section 505(c)(2) does not apply to the refusal to approve an application under the preceding sentence.

The FDA goes on to note that although there is market exclusivity of 7 years, if the applicant is unable to meet demand, the Secretary may approve another product to meet such demand. Section 527(b) notes,

If an application filed pursuant to section 505(b) is approved for a drug designated under section 526 for a rare disease or condition . . . or if a license is issued under section 351 of the Public Health Service Act for such a drug, the Secretary may, during the seven-year period beginning on the date of the application approval . . . or of the issuance of the license, approve another application under section 505(b) . . . or issue a license under section 351 of the Public Health Service Act, for such drug for such disease or condition for a person who is not the holder of such approved application . . . or of such license if—(1) The Secretary finds, after providing the holder notice and opportunity for the submission of views, that in such period the holder of the approved application . . . or of the license cannot assure the availability of sufficient quantities of the drug to meet the needs of persons with the disease or condition for which the drug was designated; or (2) such holder provides the Secretary in writing the consent of such holder for the approval of other applications, issuance of other certifications, or the issuance of other licenses before the expiration of such seven-year period.

1. Open Protocols for Investigations of Drugs for Rare Diseases or Conditions

As noted earlier, an IND needs to be filed for any orphan indication. To meet the needs of an NDA, many different types of trials are needed, as noted in other chapters in this book. The FDA specifically encourages the preparation of protocols to trial the rare disease and condition preparatory to filing an NDA. Section 528 of the Act states,

If a drug is designated under section 526 as a drug for a rare disease or condition and if notice of a claimed exemption under section 505(i) or regulations issued thereunder is filed for such drug, the Secretary shall encourage the sponsor of such drug to design protocols for clinical investigations of the drug which may be conducted under the exemption to permit the addition to the investigations of persons with the disease or condition who need the drug to treat the disease or condition and who cannot be satisfactorily treated by available alternative drugs.

To discuss briefly the incentives available to the industry,

1. The sponsor receives 7 years' exclusivity if its NDA remains unique for the product, and if no significant improvements are instituted by a competitor.
2. If requested, the sponsor can have help with protocol assistance from the FDA during development.
3. An orphan product manufacturer is entitled to tax credits up to 50% of qualified clinical research expenses incurred in developing the product. This tax credit was permanently extended by Congress and signed by the President in August of 1997 [2].

4. Researchers may apply for grant funds to support pivotal clinical trials. As noted later on, this may be for up to $200,000 for a phase II or III trial.

2. Steps in Obtaining Orphan Product Designation

As discussed earlier, the first step in orphan product development is the determination that the product is indeed entitled to orphan designation. The government gives one criterion as a *prevalence* of 200,000 individuals in the United States (not *incidence*). Extensive research into the disease must be conducted. The object of this chapter is not to discuss research techniques; there are numerous government sources or national foundations that may be enlisted to help research the disease with appropriate demographic data. All such data should be carefully compiled and tabulated for presentation to the government.

Careful analysis must be made to assure proper presentation of the specific aspects of the disease and of the product itself in relation to the disease. Presentation of the product is very important. Sponsors of orphan products that cannot prove their product's individuality in the treatment of the disease might find themselves competing with another similar product, which has also earned an orphan designation. One thing to remember is that although there may be exclusivity to an orphan product granted an NDA, there is no exclusivity to the orphan designation itself; thus two competitors may be pursuing an NDA for the same indication. If the products are sufficiently similar, the first one with an NDA will be the one with exclusivity. Unless the competitor can show that his product is unique and different from the other product, he will be denied an NDA. If the two products can be shown to be significantly different from each other, both will be granted an NDA, assuming they both pass the government's scrutiny on review.

With regard to the scope of orphan drug exclusivity, the FDA notes the following in 21 CFR 316.31—Scope of orphan drug exclusive approval:

(a) After approval of a sponsor's marketing application for a designated orphan drug product for treatment of the rare disease or condition concerning which orphan drug designation was granted, FDA will not approve another sponsor's marketing application for the same drug before the expiration of 7 years from the date of such approval as stated in the approval letter from FDA, except that such a marketing application can be approved sooner if, and such time as, any of the following occurs:

(1) Withdrawal of exclusive approval or revocation of orphan drug designation by FDA under any provision of this part; or

(2) Withdrawal for any reason of the marketing application for the drug in question; or

(3) Consent by the holder of exclusive approval to permit another marketing application to gain approval; or

(4) Failure of the holder of exclusive approval to assure a sufficient quantity of the drug under section 527 of the act and Sec. 316.36.

(b) If a sponsor's marketing application for a drug product is determined not to be approvable because approval is barred under section 527 of the act until the expiration of the period of exclusive marketing of another drug product, FDA will so notify the sponsor in writing.

It should also be noted that if the sponsor receives NDA approval and then is not able to provide sufficient supply, he might lose exclusivity. He can either consent to let other applications be filed, or the director may decide to grant approval to other applications. FDA may withdraw exclusivity even if other applications are not pending. Once withdrawn, exclusive approval may not be reinstated for the drug [3].

There are a number of applications that can be filed in relation to orphan products. The first is a request for orphan drug designation. An institutional sponsor who wishes a designation in order to perform trials in support of an NDA would file one of these. Another is a request for a grant to conduct a clinical trial of safety and effectiveness of an orphan product. A corporate sponsor with limited funds, or an investigator who is conducting research into a disease with an orphan designation or which is eligible for an orphan designation, would file this application. A number of products have been approved from trials given grants.

In keeping with section 316.40—Treatment use of a designated orphan drug—prospective investigators seeking to obtain treatment use of designated orphan drugs may do so as provided in 21 CFR 312.24.

3. Content and Format of a Request for Orphan Drug Designation

Title 21 of the Code of Federal Regulations, Section 316.20, describes the means by which a company can actually file an application for an orphan drug designation. It is in this section that the government indicates that "More than one sponsor may receive orphan drug designation of the same drug for the same rare disease or condition, but each sponsor seeking orphan drug designation must file a complete request for designation as provided in paragraph (b) of this section."

The regulations require that a permanent resident of the United States act as the sponsor's agent upon whom service of all processes, notices, orders, decisions, requirements and other communications may be made on behalf of the sponsor. The name of the agent must be provided to

> Office of Orphan Products
> Development (HF-35), Food and Drug Administration
> 5600 Fishers Lane
> Rockville, MD 20857 [4]

It must also be noted that one may apply for orphan drug designation at any time in the drug development process prior to the submission of a marketing application for the drug product for the orphan indication. A sponsor may request designation of an already approved drug product for an unapproved use without regard to whether the prior marketing approval was for an orphan drug indication [5].

The format of the application is straightforward [6].

The sponsor must submit two copies of a completed, dated, and signed request for designation that contains the following:

1. A statement that the sponsor requests orphan drug designation for a rare disease or condition, which shall be identified with specificity.

2. The name and address of the sponsor.

   a. The name of the sponsor's primary contact person and/or resident agent
   b. The title, address, and telephone number of the contact person/ resident agent
   c. Generic and trade name, if any, of the drug
   d. The name and address of the source of the drug if it is not manufactured by the sponsor

3. A description of the rare disease or condition for which the drug is being or will be investigated, the proposed indication or indications for use of the drug, and the reasons why such therapy is needed.

(Note that it is not necessary in this part to deliver volumes of information. The information provided should be factual and concise. Tabulations of statistical data are helpful in describing the subject demographics. The content of the text should be that of a peer-reviewed journal article, about 30 to 40 pages at most. If the volume of data is such that a brief presentation is not thought possible, it is suggested that the agency be contacted to discuss with them the acceptability of providing longer presentations.)

4. A description of the drug and a discussion of the scientific rationale for the use of the drug for the rare disease or condition, including all data from nonclinical laboratory trials, clinical investigations, and other relevant data that are available to the sponsor, whether positive, negative, or inconclusive. Copies of pertinent unpublished and published papers are also required.

(Note that if there are massive amounts of nonclinical data to be provided, it is wise to discuss the submission of large numbers of volumes to the orphan product review division. Large volumes of information must be submitted with an IND or NDA. Tabular summaries of data, with comprehensive summaries of data, are better suited for the orphan designation application.)

5.   If the sponsor of a drug that is otherwise the same as an already approved orphan drug seeks orphan drug designation for the subsequent drug for the same rare disease or condition, an explanation of why the proposed variation may be clinically superior to the first drug is required. (This is extremely important. The differences alone will not guarantee that the government will grant another application. One must show definitive superiority. Price is not a consideration, unfortunately, in this aspect. Considerable reduction in adverse experiences, superior availability, superior activity, etc., must be considered parts of this process.)

6.   Where a drug is under development for only a subset of persons with a particular disease or condition, a demonstration that the subset is medically plausible.

7.   A summary of the regulatory status and marketing history of the drug in the United States and in foreign countries, for example, IND and marketing application status and dispositions, what uses are under investigation and in what countries; for what indication is the drug approved in foreign countries; what adverse regulatory actions have been taken against the drug in any country.

8.   Documentation, with appended authoritative references to demonstrate that

a.   The disease or condition for which the drug is intended affects fewer than 200,000 people in the United States or, if the drug is a vaccine, diagnostic drug, or preventive drug, the persons to whom the drug will be administered in the United States are fewer than 200,000 per year as specified in 21 CFR 316.21(b).
b.   For a drug intended for diseases or conditions affecting 200,000 or more people, or for a vaccine, diagnostic drug, or preventive drug to be administered to 200,000 or more persons per year in the United States, there is no reasonable expectation that costs of research and development of the drug for the indication can be recovered by sales of the drug in the United States as specified in section 316.21(c).

9.   A statement as to whether the sponsor submitting the request is the real party interested in the development and the intended or actual production and sales of the product.

Any of the information previously provided by the sponsor to the FDA under subpart B of 21 CFR may be referenced by specific page or location if it duplicates information required elsewhere in section 316.20.

4. Clinical Trials of Safety and Effectiveness of Orphan Products

One way in which orphan products are made available is for the OPD to support clinical research to determine whether the products are safe and effective. All funded trials are subject to the requirements of the FD&C Act and the corresponding Code of Federal Regulations. The goal is the clinical development of products for use in rare diseases or conditions in which either no current therapy exists or current therapy could be improved. Grants are offered for trials intended to provide data acceptable to the agency that will either result in or substantially contribute to approval of these products. The FDA asks applicants to keep this in mind. It requires an explanation in the "Background and Significance" section of the application of how their proposed trial will either facilitate product approval or provide essential data needed for product development.

In fiscal year 1999, grants awarded to support clinical trials on the safety and effectiveness of products for a rare disease or condition were anticipated to be in the range of $11.3 million,of which $8.8 million will be for non-competing continuation awards. This will leave $2.5 million for funding approximately 10 new applications. Any phase clinical trial is eligible for up to $100,000 in direct costs per year plus applicable indirect costs for up to 3 years.Phase II and III clinical trials are eligible for up to $200,000 in direct costs per year plus applicable indirect costs for up to 3 years. The FDA supports trials covered by this notice under section 301 of the Public Health Service Act. Work plans submitted under the application should comply with "Healthy People 2000," a copy of which may be obtained through the Superintendent of Documents, the Government Printing Office, Washington, DC 20402-9325 (stock no. 017-001-00474-0).

The FDA will consider awarding grants only to support clinical trials for determining whether the products are safe and effective for either premarket approval (devices) or in support of an IND for drugs or biologics. Investigations of approved products to evaluate new orphan indications are also acceptable; however, these are also required to be conducted under an IND or IDE to support a change in official labeling. Trials that are submitted for the larger grants ($200,000)must continue in phase 2 or phase 3 of investigation.Those that are submitted for the smaller grants (100,000) may be phase 1, 2, or 3. The various phases of clinical investigations are discussed in other chapters in this volume. Annual reports must be made on an annual financial status report (FSR) (SF-269) form. The original and two copies of this report must be submitted to the grants management officer within 90 days of the budget expiration date.

Applications must propose a clinical trial of one therapy for one indication. The applicant must provide supporting evidence that a sufficient quantity of the product to be investigated is available to the applicant in the form needed for the clinical trial. The applicant must also provide supporting evidence that the subject population has been surveyed and that there is reasonable assurance that the necessary number of eligible subjects is available for the trial. In addition, subjects must provide informed consent, and the trials must be conducted in accordance with GCP under the oversight of a duly constituted IRB.

Applications are accepted at designated times during the year. The announcements for this are published in the *Federal Register*, usually mid-year. The most recent version was published in August 1998; another should be published about the same time in 1999.

Application forms are available from, and completed applications should be submitted to, the Grants Management Officer, Division of Contracts and Procurement Management (HFA-522), Food and Drug Administration, 5600 Fishers Lane, Park Bldg., Room 2129, Rockville, MD 20857, telephone 301-827-7185. Applications hand-carried or commercially delivered should be addressed to 5630 Fishers Lane, Room 2129, Rockville, MD 20852.

Applications will be evaluated for responsiveness to the application requirements; those deemed unresponsive will be returned. Responsiveness will be based on the following criteria:

1. The application must propose a clinical trial intended to provide safety or efficacy data of one therapy for one orphan indication. Additionally, there must be an explanation in the "Background and Significance" section of how the proposed trial will either facilitate product approval or provide essential data needed for product development.

2. The prevalence, *not incidence*, of the population to be served by the product must be fewer than 200,000 individuals in the United States. The applicant should include, in the "Background and Significance" section, a detailed explanation supplemented by authoritative references in support of the prevalence figure. If the product has been designated by the FDA as an orphan product for the proposed indication, a statement of that fact will suffice. Diagnostic tests and vaccines will qualify only if the population of intended use is fewer than 200,000 persons per year.

3. The number assigned to the IND/IDE for the proposed trial should appear on the front page of the application with the title of the project. Only

medical foods not requiring premarket approval are exempt. The IND/IDE must be in active status and in compliance with all regulatory requirements of the FDA at the time of the submission of the application. To meet this requirement, the original IND/IDE application, pertinent amendments, and the protocol for the proposed trial must have been received by the appropriate FDA reviewing division at least 30 days prior to the due date of the grant application. Trials of already approved products, evaluating new orphan indications, also must have an active IND. Exempt INDs must have their status changed to active to be eligible for this program. If the sponsor of the IND/IDE is other than the principal investigator listed on the application, a letter from the sponsor verifying access to the IND/IDEs required, and both the application's principal investigator and the trial protocol must have been submitted to the IND/IDE.

    4. The requested budget should be within the limits as stated in the application.

    5. Consent and/or assent forms and any additional information to be given to a subject should be included in the grant application.

    6. All applicants should follow guidelines specified in the PHS 398 grant application kit.

5. Scientific/Technical Review Criteria

To provide the first level of review, the FDA will convene an ad hoc expert panel. The applicant will be apprised of the makeup of the panel and will have the opportunity to discuss its makeup to assure that there will be no one sitting on the panel with a conflict of interest.

    The application will be judged on the following scientific and technical merit criteria:

1. The soundness of the rationale for the proposed trial
2. The quality and appropriateness of the trial design, including the rationale for the statistical procedures
3. The statistical justification for the number of subjects chosen for the trial, based on the proposed outcome measures and the appropriateness of the statistical procedures to be used in analysis of the results
4. The adequacy of the evidence that the proposed number of eligible subjects can be recruited in the requested time frame
5. The qualifications of the investigator and support staff, and the resources available to them
6. The adequacy of the justification for the request for financial support

7. The adequacy of plans for complying with regulations for protection of human subjects
8. The ability of the applicant to complete the proposed trial within both its budget and the time limitations stated in the RFA

A priority score will be given, based on the scientific and technical review criteria noted above.

6. Submission Requirements

Note: Do not send applications to the Division of Research Grants, National Institutes of Health (NIH). Any application sent to NIH which is sent to FDA by them after the due date will be deemed unresponsive and returned to the applicant. However, instructions for completing the forms can be found on the NIH home page on the Internet at http://www.nih.gov/grants/funding/phs398/ phs398.html. Forms may be found at http://www.nih.gov/grants/funding/phs398/ forms_toc.html. The FDA *does not* adhere to the page limitations or the type size and line spacing requirements imposed by the NIH on its applications. Applications must be submitted by mail delivery as stated above. The FDA is unable to receive applications through the Internet.

Submission of the application must be on grant application form PHS 398, as noted above. An excellent guide entitled "How to Write a Research Grant Application" has been prepared by the government and is available on request. The FDA has indicated that guidelines will be maintained and a request for the list or for any guideline should be directed to the Office of Orphan Products Development (HF 35), Food and Drug Administration, 5600 Fishers Lane, Rockville, MD 20857 [7].

7. FDA Review and Actions

The FDA will review the applications and make recommendations as to the completeness of the submission and what else may be needed.

In section 316.12, Providing written recommendations, the FDA notes,

(a) FDA will provide the sponsor with written recommendations concerning the nonclinical laboratory trials and clinical investigations necessary for approval of a marketing application if none of the reasons described in Sec. 316.14 for refusing to do so applies.

(b) When a sponsor seeks written recommendations at a stage of drug development at which advice on any clinical investigations, or on particular investigations would be premature, FDA's response may be limited to written recommendations concerning only nonclinical laboratory trials, or only certain of the clinical trials (e.g., Phase 1 trials as described in Sec 312.21 of this chapter). Prior to providing written recommendations for the clinical investigations required to achieve marketing approval, FDA may require that the results of the nonclinical laboratory trials or completed early clinical trials be submitted to FDA for agency review.

As noted above, the FDA may refuse to provide written recommendations for various reasons, such as incompleteness or absence of required information in section 316.10(b). Insufficient information about the drug to identify the active moiety and its physical and chemical properties are cause for refusal to provide recommendations as is, insufficient evidence that the disease is indeed of sufficient incidence to warrant orphan designation, among others. Such refusal will be in writing. The FDA will describe the information or material it requires or the conditions the sponsor must meet for the FDA to provide recommendations [8].

Once an orphan designation is granted, it is transferable, provided the owner of the designation informs the FDA in writing of the name of the transferee, and what rights to the designation have been transferred (not all rights need to be transferred). In addition, the new owner must submit a letter accepting orphan drug designation and the date the change is effective, stating that he or she has a complete copy of the request for orphan designation including amendments and supplements and all relevant correspondence. A list of the rights assigned should also be provided. The new owner of the designation should provide a new contact name, including a United States agent if the new owner is a foreign company. The FDA notes that no sponsor may relieve itself of responsibilities under the ODA by assigning rights to another without assuring that the sponsor will carry out its responsibilities, or without obtaining prior permission from the FDA [9].

As with other submissions to the FDA, the recipient of orphan designation must provide a report to the FDA within 14 months and annually thereafter until marketing approval to indicate progress, stated in 21 CFR 316.30 as follows:

(a) A short account of the progress of drug development including a review of preclinical and clinical trials initiated, ongoing, and completed and a short summary of the status or results of such trials.

(b) A description of the investigational plan for the coming year, as well as any anticipated difficulties in development, testing, and marketing; and

(c) A brief discussion of any changes that may affect the orphan drug status of the product. For example, for products nearing the end of the approval process, sponsors should discuss any disparity between the probable marketing indication and the designated indication as related to the need for an amendment to the orphan drug designation pursuant to Sec. 316.26.

The FDA will not publicly disclose the existence of a request for orphan designation, but there are certain conditions that apply, including whether the sponsor has made it publicly known he has orphan designation. The FDA will determine whether the disclosure can be made in accordance with confidentiality requirements of INDAs and NDAs. Once public availability eligibility has been determined, FDA will publish a list in accord with part 20 and section 314.430 of the CFR and other applicable statutes and regulations [10].

III. FINAL NOTES

To recap, to receive an orphan drug designation for a product, a sponsor must file an application (two copies) with the FDA, according to the prescribed format in 21 CFR 316.20. If the disease affects fewer than 200,000 persons per year (or, in the case of a vaccine, the administration will be to fewer than 200,000 persons per year), the agency may grant an orphan designation. Once so designated, a proper INDA must be filed, which will need to contain a full description of the product, its synthesis and method of manufacture as a drug product, its preclinical pharmacology and toxicology, and clinical protocols for the trials to be conducted. If the sponsor is unable to write the protocols, the FDA will assist in the writing and will even fund the trials if the sponsor has insufficient funds. Orphan designation is assignable, provided the sponsor assures that the new owner will act responsibly in developing the drug. If an NDA is filed and approved, there will be 7 years of market exclusivity granted, as well as tax benefits. The biggest benefit is to the subjects who receive much needed help in the treatment of their disease.

It is clear that the Orphan Drug Act, as implemented by existing administrative practices, has significantly increased the rate at which new orphan drugs are marketed. While two or three drugs that might be eligible as orphan drugs were approved annually prior to the Orphan Drug Act, an average of eight designated orphan drugs have been approved per year and marketed since 1984. Moreover, orphan drug designation has been granted to an average of 41 drugs per year since 1984. Thus the Orphan Drug Act, as implemented since 1983, has provided an effective stimulus for the development and marketing of drugs for diseases or conditions that are rare in the United States.

In debating the need for orphan drug exclusive marketing, Congress weighed the potential dangers of granting orphan drug exclusive marketing, which would limit competition, against the benefits to be gained by encouraging sponsors to develop drugs of marginal commercial value. In passing the law, Congress determined that the benefits exceeded the dangers.

Any form of exclusive marketing may have negative consequences, such as noncompetitive pricing. To date, however, there has been insufficient experience with the implementation of the statute to judge whether an optimal be benefit–cost balance has been attained. It is clear, nonetheless, that these incentives have been highly successful in contributing to the development and approval of orphan drugs that would not otherwise have been developed. Thus, in the FDA's view, the essential benefit–cost considerations of Executive Order 12291 have been satisfied in favor of the rule as here published.

The agency also recognizes that changes in the statutory incentive structure would theoretically produce corresponding changes in the level of benefits, i.e., the number of orphan drugs developed. The FDA, however, concludes that further incremental analysis of the statutory provisions would be highly conjectural and beyond the availability of meaningful data from experience to date.

The Regulatory Flexibility Act requires that the agency consider the impact of the regulation on small entities. The FDA believes that these rules benefit, rather than disadvantage, most affected small businesses. Prior to the enactment of the Orphan Drug Act, few small businesses could afford to devote resources to the discovery of new treatments for rare diseases, because the small market for such products severely limited the profitability of this research. Subsequent to enactment, the combined stimulus of research grants, tax credits, and exclusive marketing influenced many small firms to develop new products for formerly inaccessible markets. The FDA finds therefore that, in general, the incentives provided under the act will serve to enhance the viability and competitiveness of small entities.

REFERENCES

1. Haffner M.E. Orphan drug development—International program and trial design issues. Drug Information Journal 1998; 32:93–99.
2. 26 CFR 1.28-1. (These are the IRS regulations on rare disease research tax credit.)
3. 21 CFR 316.36 Insufficient quantities of orphan drugs.
4. 21 CFR 316.22. Permanent-resident agent for foreign sponsor.
5. 21 CFR 316.23. Timing of requests for orphan-drug designation.
6. 21 CFR 316.10. Content and format of a request for written recommendations.
7. 21 CFR 316.50. Guidelines.
8. 21 CFR 316.14. Refusal to provide written recommendations.
9. 21 CFR 316.27. Change in ownership of orphan-drug designation.
10. 21 CFR 316.52. Availability for public disclosure of data and information in requests.

10
Clinical Research Protocols

Richard A. Guarino
Oxford Pharmaceutical Resources, Inc., Totowa, New Jersey, U.S.A.

I. INTRODUCTION

The practice of clinical research—to establish safety and efficacy for new drugs, devices, and biologicals—is considered the most important part of the new drug approval process by many individuals in the FDA, sponsor companies, and users of pharmaceutical products. Accomplishing this task requires careful strategic planning to meet research objectives, an available subject population that meets the criteria of trial requirements, and experienced well trained clinical investigators who can evaluate the trial subjects following the protocol design.

Clinical research protocols are key to assuring successful approvals of new products in the health care industry. The protocol becomes the Bible for each research program. It must be followed exactly, without deviations, and must be the reference for any discussions that arise during the course of the investigation. This chapter will give instructions on how to write a clinical protocol for all phases of clinical research. It will include all necessary FDA requirements for confirming safety and efficacy for products marketed for human use. The format for protocol development is recommended on the basis of its successful use in clinical research. The recommendations throughout this chapter may not always be applicable to all clinical programs.

The objective of most clinical trials is to record scientific data concerning the efficacy and safety of a treatment for a specific disease on which valid conclusions can be drawn. The degree of success in achieving this objective depends largely, but not entirely, on the quality of the basic trial design. Faulty execution, due either to sloppiness or (in rare instances) dishonesty, can undermine the validity and usefulness of the data generated from a particular trial site. All investigators and their staffs must be meticulous in observing and reporting their clinical observations. On the other hand, even if a lengthy trial is carried out with the utmost care, the data generated will be useless if the protocol has not been designed intelligently. Overall, it must include all the necessary ingredients so that the eventual clinical results will support IND and NDA submissions.

Because the framework of every clinical research trial relies on a number of interdependent disciplines, the development of a clinical trial protocol is ideally a multidisciplinary task. Teamwork, coordinated by one experienced person in clinical research with good knowledge of the regulatory requirements for new drug development, is essential. The protocol design team should also include input, recommendations, and review by the following:

A chemist who is fully conversant with the physical and chemical properties of the investigational drug

A pharmacologist and/or toxicologist with a full understanding of the pharmacology and toxicology of the drug in animals and the expected effective dose, therapeutic effects, and possible adverse experiences in humans

A medical monitor, preferably one who specializes in the condition or illness to be studied, and who is experienced in the logistics and practicalities of clinical trials

A statistician who will address those aspects of trial design that determine the form the trial data will take for analysis and the types of analyses that will be applied to the data

A data management person who will be both involved in coding and in charge of data entry

A potential investigator or consultant who understands the indication to be researched and the objectives of the protocol and procedures to be followed

A capable program manager who can coordinate the multidisciplinary effort to form a final protocol and effect practical execution in the clinical setting straight through to data analysis and final write-up

Together, these specialists can provide both the criteria for all aspects of the trial and the rationale used to develop them. Once the specific objectives of the protocol have been established, it is customary for a protocol introduction to summarize these objectives, give a brief overview of the information found in the Investigator's Brochure (referencing the Brochure), and state the purpose of conducting the trial. The rationale for the criteria to be used for subject selection, exclusion, and randomization (if any) and the clinical variables to be monitored during the trial should also be stated.

II. TRIAL OBJECTIVE

A common fault in trial design is to have too many objectives in a single trial. Objective(s) should be clearly and concisely stated. If a trial has more than one objective, the objectives should be listed in order of priority. The fewer the questions to be answered in one trial, the greater the likelihood that they will be answered conclusively. The key to successful trial design is simplicity.

III. GENERAL CONSIDERATIONS IN PROTOCOL DESIGN

The trial protocol is the end point of research design. It is the blueprint that displays the elements of the trial plan and provides explicit instructions as to how the plan should be executed.

The protocol designers should approach the subject by first organizing a checklist similar to the one presented later in this chapter (see Elements of a Protocol: A Checklist). This list will serve in protocol design much as an outline helps a writer or a speaker touch on all salient points in an article or speech. Judging from the number of NDAs that are returned to their sponsors for more clinical information (time-consuming revisions) by the FDA, one might assume that there are tricks to the art of a successful filing. No secret ingredients are needed for the successful preparation of a clinical protocol or its presentation within an IND and ultimately the NDA—just logic, completeness, and a practical understanding of the disease under investigation.

In drug development, time is of the essence. Clinical protocols should be concise, straightforward, and logical. The demands upon the investigators, their staffs, and the subjects must be reasonable. The FDA's guidelines for drug development by disease must be considered in order to expedite the final NDA review and approval. The objective to remember throughout protocol development, and execution and presentation of the acquired data, is to demonstrate efficacy and safety to fulfill the FDA's requirements for NDA approval.

IV. DIFFERENT TRIAL DESIGNS

Conventionally, phase 1, 2, 3, 3b, and 4 trials refer to the successive stages of the clinical investigation of a drug or the continued experiment of the same. Although the objectives of all of the phases are different, they are not entirely separate entities because the information obtained from one phase provides the basis for the next. In broad terms, the objective of phase 1 is a demonstration of safety based on dose tolerance; phase 2 is for dose tolerance and safety balanced with efficacy (probably the most important phase in clinical research development); phase 3 reconfirms efficacy and safety in a larger subject population for a specified dose and indication in a target subject population; phase 3b is designed for large-scale safety. Phase 4 trials are usually classified as marketing trials and are designed to demonstrate how similar drugs, prescribed for the same indications, may show one having certain advantages over another. The basic principles of good scientific methods of trial design apply equally to all five phases. The major tenets of all scientific experimentation should be regarded as fundamentals of the design: the possibility of coincidence as well as bias should be ruled out, and the results produced by the trial design should be as conclusive as possible. In other words, the trial should be controlled, designed, and analyzed for optimum statistical reliability and specificity.

V. CONTROLLED TRIALS

A trial drug can be compared with a placebo or with an active drug. If active medication is used as a control group, it should be a standard drug accepted in medical practice for the specific indication(s) under investigation. Double-blind trials are usually indicated to assure that the data obtained from these trials, when evaluated statistically, will support judgments regarding the safety and the efficacy of the investigational drug without bias. Because of ethical considerations, however, there are many drugs that cannot be evaluated under double-blind conditions. In these cases, a sponsor should review the situation with the FDA and establish the acceptability of data to be obtained from a trial of alternate design before the trial has begun. It is not unusual, however, for phase 1 trials to be open-label (not blinded), because the objective is to observe the response to the investigational substance primarily in terms of safety.

Double-blinded, controlled trials that are well designed yield the most valid results. In the majority of investigations, test agents are blinded against placebo controls. The FDA's NDA approvals, in most cases, are based on the following: two clinical trials proving that a drug versus placebo shows statistically significant difference. These are termed pivotal trials. Rare exceptions are made, with active agents used as controls assumed to exert similar therapeutic conditions.

Very rigid criteria are established to preclude investigator or subject bias. Impressions of drug efficacy or lack of the same based on previous evaluations of reported efficacy must be avoided. In a trial comparing the effects of two or more treatments, if the investigator or the subjects are aware of the treatments administered, the preconceptions and prejudices of both toward the treatments can have a significant biasing influence on the accuracy with which assessments of the effects of the treatments are made. This extraneous variable of bias can be minimized by suitable blinding techniques. The single-blind method, as the name implies, ensures that only the subject is unaware of the distribution of treatments during the trial. The double-blind method, which is now accepted as the standard blinding procedure in comparative drug trials, ensures that the investigators, their staffs, and the subject are unaware of the type of treatments that are being prescribed and administered.

A. Blinding Techniques

Attaining and maintaining double-blind conditions in a clinical trial requires strict attention to a number of details. A drug form identical to the test drug is necessary for double-blind conditions. Pharmaceutical manufacturers can usually supply their products, placebo, and comparison drugs in forms that meet these requirements. Comparative evaluation trials cannot be done on drugs in dissimilar formulations, such as tablets versus syrups, ampules versus suppositories, or liquid concentrates versus capsules. Additional blinding problems are presented by variations in physical characteristics including color, taste, texture, viscosity, shape, or size. If a trial calls for the comparison of two treatments with formulations that make physical matching impossible, the problem can be solved by the double-placebo (double-dummy) method, which establishes manifest equality of product characteristics. It consists of simultaneously administering to each subject an active test agent and a placebo of the other active agent that is being evaluated (Table 1).

Inasmuch as the two agents (whatever their forms) are administered simultaneously to each subject at all times during the trial, there is no way of

Table 1 Double-Placebo Method

Group 1 subjects	Group 2 subjects
Active Drug A tablets	Active Drug B liquid
+	+
Placebo B liquid	Placebo A tablets

telling the difference between active drug and placebo. In all cases, the assigned placebo is physically identical to the test agent and is administered through an identical route. In addition, the method can be adapted to compare a suppository with a liquid concentrate or a syrup with a capsule. Any two drugs with different routes of administration, or different forms, can be effectively blinded in this manner and can satisfy all the rigid requirements of classical double-blind clinical research trials.

The procedure also can accommodate the double-blind evaluation of two active agents that must be administered at different times of the day because of their dissimilar modes of actions. Table 2 demonstrates how all subjects receive an active agent and placebo or two placebos at the same time.

Active drug and placebo are administered twice a day to all subjects in both groups: 4:00 P.M. and 8:00 P.M. for group 1 subjects, and 7:30 A.M. and 4:00 P.M. for group 2 subjects. During each day, subjects in both groups receive a total of two doses of drug A or drug B, but at different times of the day.

The double-placebo method can help overcome the problem of blinding drugs that are dissimilar with regard to color, taste, viscosity, volume, dosage equivalency, or dosage regimen. It can only prove successful under good clinical management conditions and meticulous monitoring of the trial to assure full compliance. Double-blind, double-placebo techniques depend on reliable research coordinators who consistently check on drug administration and accountability, and in turn, close monitoring is required.

No matter how rigorous the enforcement of blinding techniques, circumstances may arise that threaten the integrity of the blindness of a clinical trial. For example, a larger number of adverse reactions in one treatment group compared with another may provide a clue as to which treatment is

Table 2 Delivery of Two Active Agents with Different Administration Regimens

Time of Administration	Group 1 Subjects Drug A (tablets)	Group 2 Subjects Drug B (capsules)
7:30 AM	Drug A Placebo +	Drug A Placebo +
	Drug B Placebo	Drug B Active
4:00 PM	Drug A Active +	Drug A Placebo +
	Drug B Placebo	Drug B Active
8:00 PM	Drug A Active +	Drug A Placebo +
	Drug B Placebo	Drug B Placebo

involved, particularly in placebo-controlled trials. Likewise, different patterns of symptom response in treatment groups may suggest the treatment involved.

Blindness can also be destroyed by accidental breaking of the randomization code. With good design and adequate safeguards, however, this should not occur.

The only circumstance under which the identity of trial materials should be deliberately known is when a subject has an adverse reaction that makes it imperative for the investigator to know which treatment the subject received. However, the method of labeling the trial drugs should allow for this to be done without revealing the randomization code for the entire trial. One such technique is for each medication container to have a two-part label, one of which is a sealed tear-off section containing the identity of the drug. At the time the subject begins treatment, the tear-off section is detached and affixed to the subject's case report form and can be opened in an emergency.

VI. UNCONTROLLED TRIALS

Most regulatory bodies, concerned with the approval of new drugs for clinical use, do not accept the results of uncontrolled trials as stand-alone evidence of efficacy. There are, however, circumstances under which data from uncontrolled trials can provide acceptable evidence of efficacy: (a) the treatment results in consistent and clinically significant improvement in a disease with a well-established natural course and remission rate; (b) the treatment consistently results in significant improvement in all or almost all subjects.

Apart from the limited value of uncontrolled trials for the demonstration of efficacy, they may be helpful in obtaining an early indication of the optimum dose, the adverse reaction potential, and the preferred route of administration of a drug. As a general rule, it is best to confine clinical drug trials in phases 1, 2, 3, and 4 to those that use adequate controls and unbiased techniques.

VII. PARALLEL AND CROSSOVER TRIAL DESIGNS

Controlled trials can be conducted under matched pairs, parallel, crossover, group comparisons, or mixed design conditions. Parallel and crossover trial designs each have advantages and disadvantages. Both can be used to compare two or more treatments, one of which may be placebo. In a crossover trial, all treatments to be compared are administered to every enrolled subject in a carefully designed and blinded sequence with an interim drug washout period. Each subject receives all treatments and thus serves as his or her own control.

In a trial using parallel groups, subjects are randomly assigned to one of the treatments (which might be placebo). In spite of adequate selection criteria and random assignment, the treatment groups in a parallel group trial may indeed differ. Fewer subjects are required in a crossover trial than in a parallel group trial. Although the desired duration of exposure to each treatment can be achieved, subjects have to participate in a crossover trial for at least twice as long as in a parallel group trial. This makes it especially necessary that the clinicians selected have good rapport with the subjects, therefore demonstrating the ability to maintain a low subject attrition rate, as well as protocol compliance. In addition to this potential source of difficulty, another drawback of the crossover method should be noted: if two active drugs are being compared, all subjects are exposed to the possible safety hazards of both drugs, or in the case of a placebo, the risk of allowing the pathology to go untreated. For the results of a crossover trial to be valid, each subject must be in the same clinical condition at the beginning of the second treatment period as at the initiation of the first treatment period. In practice, this is frequently difficult to achieve because the pharmacological and psychological effects of the first treatment often have a carryover effect on the response to the second treatment. This is especially true if the drug administered during the first treatment period has a long biological half-life. Theoretically, these objections can be minimized by imposing a sufficiently long washout period between treatments. The theory, however, is often more easily prescribed than achieved.

There are certain obvious caveats concerning the use of the crossover design. It should not be used in drug trials involving self-limiting diseases of short duration, or with treatments that result in rapid relief or cures because of the likelihood of the illness being resolved and symptoms alleviated before the crossover takes place. Parallel group trials are more popular than crossover comparisons because they present fewer problems. The parallel group trial is probably a less complicated and expeditious way to double-blind and complete a trial in a much shorter period.

A. Elements of a Protocol: A Checklist

The following items provide an outline of the factors that must be addressed in planning a protocol for all phases of clinical research (including bioavailability trials). Although some of the headings cited below may seem obvious, often they are completely overlooked or taken for granted by protocol designers/administrators.

1. Title Page

Provide the full title of the trial, including, if possible, a precise description of the trial objective. (If you feel that it would aid FDA reviewers in identifying the trial, give the full name, including initials, of the investigator and, where applicable, co-investigators.) Many protocols are identified by a trial number assigned by the sponsor; this number should be cited throughout the protocol where necessary, particularly if there is the possibility of confusion with similar trials being conducted at the same time and location. It is sound practice to have the sponsor's name and address listed on the title page. More than one sponsor may be using the same teaching hospital or institution to conduct other clinical trials on other drugs. The following is an example of a protocol title page:

A PHASE 2 DOUBLE-BLIND PARALLEL TRIAL OF DOSE
TOLERANCE, SAFETY, AND EFFICACY COMPARING DRUG
A TO PLACEBO IN CONTROLLING SYMPTOMS OF MILD TO
MODERATE HYPERTENSION

Chief Investigator:

Co-investigator(s):

Trial Number:

Sponsor (Name and Address):

Date:

2. Table of Contents

An interested investigator should read the entire protocol to understand the objective(s) of the trial. However, sometimes certain sections of the protocol are of more interest than others to different participants conducting the clinical trial. A protocol may, for example, contain separate sections devoted to the interests of the project coordinator, a nurse, a psychologist, a cardiologist, and others. When one or more individuals have to refer quickly to a section of the protocol to clarify points concerning a particular procedure or method, they should be able to do so easily with the aid of a table of contents and its main headings, subheadings, and appropriate page numbers.

3. Introduction

The main point to cover in the introduction is the purpose of the investigation. Each clinical trial should have a significant purpose that will be fulfilled at the conclusion of the trial. No clinical trial should ever use a subject population without the specific goal of knowing more about a product and its benefit to the subject. Also included in the introduction is a description of the specific diagnosis and special subject characteristics for each disease to be investigated.

An optional part of the introduction can include all significant past research and literature references on the drug being investigated; this should be carefully reviewed, summarized, and incorporated into the introduction. This section should include the following: all relevant published materials; preclinical information from the Investigator's Brochure; and any previously conducted, comparable clinical trials (with appropriate comment on the methods of observation and qualitative evaluations used in the other trials [i.e., design, placebo controls, active controls, and methods of data analysis]). Other points that should be considered for inclusion in the introduction include identity and potency of the drug(s) being used, trial setting (nursing homes, psychiatric wards, outpatient clinics, etc.) and the rationale for using that setting. This should not be a repeat of a clinical brochure but a summary of any knowledge about the drug based on completed evaluations. Many protocol writers consider the clinical brochure an adequate introduction to the protocol and the product being developed. However, it is always a concern that investigators don't always take the time to read voluminous clinical brochures, but they will read the introduction of a protocol. One of the critical areas considered by the FDA in reviewing a clinical protocol is the merit of a clinical research investigation. The introduction should satisfy the reviewer that this trial will attempt to produce a reliable solution to a scientific question about the drug being tested.

4. Bibliography

All interpretive commentary should be referenced in a bibliography, together with all of the citations of previous research. This will help the investigators feel comfortable using an experimental drug, especially when they have need for more detailed information.

5. Objective

The objective is the essence of a protocol. It should state explicitly the purpose of the clinical research project. One short statement should describe the type of trial (i.e., open, double-blind, crossover) and why the trial is being conducted. In addition, a brief description of the medications to be used, the indication(s) for effectiveness, and the type of subject population to be evaluated should be included. The objective should be stated succinctly, as in the following example: "The objective of this controlled, double-blind, parallel trial is to evaluate the efficacy and safety of medication X versus medication Y in (diagnosis of disease) as found in an outpatient (or other) population." In one simple statement, the purpose of the trial, the controls, the diagnosis of the subject population, and the setting where these subjects will be observed have been presented. Objectives should reflect the phase or type of clinical research that will be conducted.

A phase 1 trial with safety evaluations based on dose tolerance as its major objective would not necessarily be double-blinded; phase 2, 3, and 4 trials, on the other hand, would concentrate on dose tolerance and safety, as well as efficacy, and should always (when possible) be conducted using double-blind standards to guard against bias.

6. General

This section usually contains a condensed summary of the protocol. It can prove helpful to personnel charged with recruiting clinical research investigators and their staffs. In many cases, the first contact with a prospective investigator is by telephone. Initial reactions—interest or no interest—can be elicited by a reading of the general section of the protocol. It should offer a brief description of the trial objective, the trial design, the trial duration, the evaluations needed for efficacy and safety, and the estimated amount of time required from the investigator and his or her staff. More importantly, it should answer the question as to whether the investigator has the subject population that meets the inclusion and exclusion criteria of the trial design. The preparation of a succinct general section can save hours of needless conversation describing protocol design and responsibilities of the investigator and staff.

7. Risks

Whereas risk is always a factor in all medical intervention, the relatively unknown magnitude of risk entailed in the use of a new investigational substance is the focus of much of the FDA's concern. The burden of proof for justifying the experimental use of an investigational drug lies with the sponsor. Documentation within the IND must be presented in an argument that makes it seem probable. This is heavily based on preclinical research in animals: the pharmacology and toxicology of the investigational drug that affirm that the drug is probably safe at a specified dose in the defined human population. It is sometimes appropriate to weigh the relative risks of untreated disease with the projected risks with use of the investigational drug. In any event, the methodology of the trial should minimize risks to the subjects so that potentially the benefits will outweigh the risks.

8. Confidentiality

The doctor–patient relationship has traditionally entailed the right of the subject to complete confidentiality; enrollment in a clinical trial should not compromise this right. Just as the staff in a physician's office is trained to understand that they must not breach a subject's right to confidentiality, any additional staff working with files of subjects enrolled in clinical trials must also respect this confidentiality. Procedures by which subjects can be numbered or identified by their initials and site number should be spelled out to ensure that there is no unnecessary disclosure of the identity of the participants in the trial.

9. Materials and Methods

Under this heading, the following points should be listed and described:

Subject Sample. Provide a statement describing the total number of subjects expected to complete the trial; this number can include an estimate of treatment failures but should not include administrative dropouts. (If subjects are transferred from inpatient clinics, if they relocate, or if they do not complete the trial for any other reason [not drug related], they should not be included in the total.) Establish the number of subjects that must complete the trial and be part of the final statistical analysis. Additional subjects should always be enrolled in a clinical trial to make certain that, minus trial dropouts, the required number of subjects needed for meaningful statistical analyses is still available, and that administrative dropouts will not jeopardize numbers needed for the final statistical analysis.

Age Range. Include a precise age range for the trial subjects. Do not allow an investigator to amend the age range during the course of the investigations; it should be established before the trial is initiated and strictly adhered to. The age range for subjects should be carefully selected according to the disease being investigated. It would not be advisable, for example, to trial schizophrenia in subjects aged 65 years or older; nor should mononucleosis be studied in subjects' 40 years of age or older, inasmuch as the disease is more prevalent in young adults. However, it should be noted that the age range in the final clinical trials for an NDA is the one that will eventually be included in the package insert.

Gender. Indicate whether males, females, or both sexes will be used in the trial.

Subject Inclusion Criteria. This is one of the most important parts of protocol development. Describe the type of subject to be admitted into the trial. The criteria for selecting subjects must be clearly and accurately stated, whether the trial calls for a specific diagnosis or a diagnostic profile of a symptom cluster; in either case, the diagnosis must be well established. (The FDA favors a protocol with a specific diagnosis.) Specifically state the symptoms to be rated for subjects meeting the criteria of the trial. It is up to the investigator to confirm and document the diagnosis with an accurate account of the medical history and a complete medical examination.

And finally, the following statement must be included in this section of the protocol: "Each subject enrolled should be fully eligible according to the protocol criteria. Each subject should also give every clinical and personal indication that he or she can be expected to complete the full course of the investigation." Otherwise they should not be enrolled. Nothing is more frustrating to a sponsor—or to the designer of a protocol—than to have subjects drop or be dropped from a trial because they do not meet criteria for entry, or they fall into categories that disqualify them from receiving the trial medications, or they simply do not wish to continue in the trial because their obligations for participation in the trial were not clearly spelled out. Obviously, any subject has the right to withdraw from a clinical trial at any time, but it is up to the investigators to select trial subjects they feel are most likely to complete the trial and to avoid entering those with doubt.

Subject Exclusion Criteria. This part of the protocol must be very explicit. Any subject who by every reasonable expectation would be incapable of responding to a trial drug or does not meet inclusion criteria must be ruled out. Subjects with existing ailments that would prevent the trial medication from showing its maximum therapeutic effect must be excluded from participation, as should any subject who is hypersensitive to the medications under investigation. The criteria should also exclude any subject whose medical history, physical condition, concomitant medications, or personal habits (e.g., smoking) might compromise the integrity of the data to be gathered during the clinical trial or might pose a safety concern. It must be remembered constantly when designing a protocol that this is an investigational trial, not a routine medical visit!

The protocol designer must pay particular attention to the number of exclusions listed in the protocol; too many can make it extremely difficult to enter enough subjects in the trial, and too few can lead to compromised data.

Trial Procedures. It is essential to the protocol to give the relative sequence of events that each subject will be expected to complete and to define each event thoroughly. Screening visits, baseline laboratory evaluations, day 1 of dosing, washout periods, postdosing evaluations, etc. should all be discussed and mapped out. A table or flowchart is usually helpful so that, at a glance, the events during the course of an investigational trial can be seen in relation to each other and at the same time keep the investigators and the research staff on course.

Drug-free and washout intervals must be defined. Washout, dryout, predrug, run-in, and other similar periods must be carefully noted. They must be long enough to assure that any previous medications that might interfere or interact with the trial drug will be eliminated from the subject's system before trial drug administration. Washout periods are critical to the success of a trial. They must be observed before a baseline evaluation is made and the trial medication is administered. (Placebo responders must also be considered during the predrug evaluation period.) There are, however, exceptions to the washout period conditions. For example, if a subject exhibits symptoms of sufficient severity to warrant not withholding treatment, this subject may be entered into the trial even though the washout period is less than that specified. If a note to this effect is included in the protocol, the investigator should provide ample justification in the comment section of the case report form. In the monitoring of a trial, subject records should be carefully checked for validity (acceptability) of the reasons for exemption from the full washout period.

Note: If a predrug symptom rating falls into the category of mild or moderate and a subject is entered into an investigation before the washout period is terminated, this predrug rating will not justify the subject's exemption from the medication-free period unless a valid reason is given by the investigator or is stated in the protocol.

10. Trial Drugs

Include a complete description of the medication, including the lot number, to be used in the trial. The generic as well as the trade name (if available) should be stated. Describe the form of the drug and placebo (i.e., capsules, tablets, injectable). Also provide the methods of preparation, especially for the placebo (lactose or sucrose fillers, for example). Detail as well the way the trial medication will be blinded. In addition, the strength of the trial medication must be stated in milligrams, grams, cubic centimeters, etc. The details that would be stated in a package insert should be provided. If a marketed drug is used as a control, the package insert for that medication should be included in an appendix to the protocol. The dose of each drug must be listed (e.g., "capsules containing 10 mg of drug X"). Medication used in a clinical trial must have all of its components completely listed by name and quantities.

11. Assignment of Trial Drugs

In this section, it is important to do two things: outline the method of randomization so that the procedure is clear and is set out as a standard for all sites (in the case of multicenter trials); and make certain that the method of randomization is shown to be truly random and thus supportive of scientifically valid conclusions and equitable to the subjects.

Prepare an explicit description of the actual assignment of the type or types of medication(s) used in the trial. The opening statement could read, for example, numbers 01 to 100 will be assigned to the trial medication bottles on a random basis, as determined by the use of a table of random numbers. Subjects will then be assigned to bottles 01 to 100 in sequence, that is, the first subject admitted into the trial will be assigned to the bottle marked 01, the second subject to the bottle marked 02, etc. (Numbers are assigned to bottles, and subjects are assigned to numbered bottles.) When each subject is to receive only one bottle, this should be stated: "Each subject will be assigned one bottle of trial medication. The bottle will contain a total of X capsules (or tablets, cc's, etc.) of trial medication—a quantity sufficient to meet the maximum medication requirement as required by this trial (X days or X weeks, etc.)." If medication is to be administered on a daily or weekly basis, for example, bottle numbers and the quantity in each bottle for that period should be specified. A reference to the type of randomization table used should be made and footnoted. The investigator should be aware of how the medications were randomized, for example, in blocks of 4, 6, 10, etc., so that he or she will strive to complete a block of subjects. A note should be added stating: "To allow for possible attrition, sufficient drugs will be provided for X subjects, a number beyond that required by the protocol." This point is important to explain, as it may not be immediately obvious why, if 50 subjects are required to complete a trial, the medication will be randomized for 70. This is necessary to allow for circumstantial attrition and subjects dropped for administrative reasons.

12. Dosage Range

Describe the dosage range to be used in the trial. If applicable, include daily minimum and maximum dosages; these should reflect recommendations in the manufacturer's package insert or the dose range established during the early phases of clinical research.

Be sure to correlate the phase of clinical research that is being conducted and the dosage range recommended; the range used in a phase 1 trial is often much broader than that used in a phase 2 or 3 trial.

Designed to measure dose tolerance and safety, phase 1 dose ranging should be initiated and augmented very conservatively. During phase 2, the suggested dose range will, for the most part, have been influenced by results derived from the phase 1 trials. The objectives of dose tolerance and safety in a phase 2 trial often allow a dose range different from that described for phase 1 trials. The phase 2 trials reflect responses of diseased subjects in contrast to those observed with normal subjects. Prior to the preparation of a phase 3 protocol, the minimum and maximum dosage(s) will have been determined from the phase 2 program. If not, it is almost invariably a sign that phase 2 clinical trials were not adequately conducted.

13. Dosage Schedule

This section addresses the question of when appropriate amounts of drug are to be administered: once daily (q.d.), twice daily (b.i.d.), every 4 hours (q4h), three times daily (t.i.d.), and so forth. If specific dosages are to be given in the morning or evening, or both, specific instructions should be provided.

14. Administration of Trial Drug

A statement should describe how the drug is to be administered to or taken by the subject: with meals, before or after meals, with liquids, or dissolved in specific juices, and so forth. These directions are extremely important, because they may affect dissolution and absorption rates, may cause gastric upset, or may interact with certain elements or foods.

15. Labeling of Trial Drugs

The proper labeling of all medications is imperative all of the time; however, during a clinical trial, it is essential that the blinding of the trial drugs be protected. Therefore, labels containing the code of trial drugs should be designed so that no one involved in the trial knows which medication is being administered or dispensed. The label having the code should bear the same subject identification as that appearing on the drug label on the bottle for the subject. The sealed labels contain decoding information and are to be opened only in the event of an emergency or an adverse experience necessitating identification of the drug.

Drug code labels come in many forms. One of the most reliable is the dual-labeled form, in which the code is covered by a mercury film that can be scratched off easily by a coin or similar blunt object to reveal the identity of the contents. Another effective type is the three-sided envelope: A B C in front and C B A in back. Section C contains the written code and is sealed to part B. If an emergency arises, the detached code label portion is immersed in warm water for 2 minutes and then peeled apart. If the A B C form is used, the investigator should remove and save the coded portion prior to dispensing the medication, and attach it to the case report form. These labels are to be returned to the sponsor at the conclusion of the trial. If a code label is missing from a subject evaluation form, the sponsor may not accept that subject's data for statistical analysis.

All unused trial drugs must be accounted for and returned to the sponsor at the completion of a trial. All unused trial drugs in unopened bottles should be checked by the investigator and the sponsor for an accurate count. This information should be recorded and kept in the investigator's file. While the investigator is responsible for drug accountability, it is unwise to rely solely on his or her calculations. It is recommended that the clinical research monitor either perform a drug count on-site or have the drugs returned to the sponsor's clinical pharmacy department for recounting.

16. Duration of Drug Treatment

During protocol design, it is important to determine how long a drug should be evaluated before it can be determined as safe and effective. This decision is usually based on previous research or a history of clinical experience of the disease under investigation. Drugs must be administered, monitored, and evaluated long enough to demonstrate optimum therapeutic response. However, diseases that have a short duration (e.g., a cold) should not be studied longer than necessary. Evaluating a short-acting drug such as an antihistamine for 2 weeks in treating a cold is impractical (if more than 3 days are required for this type of drug to show effectiveness, it is pointless to continue treatment). In contrast, the effect of tricyclic amine antidepressants takes at least 2 to 3 weeks, and therefore subjects should be observed for 3 to 6 months to judge the maximum efficacy of this type of medication. One of the most crucial determinations of how effective a drug can be relies on whether it is possible to administer the drug for the predetermined duration without dose-limiting adverse experiences occurring, while still achieving the maximum therapeutic effect on the disease being treated.

17. Concomitant Medications

The protocol should list all medications that subjects are allowed to receive simultaneously with the trial drug. Any contraindicated medications or those that are to be excluded during the investigation because they might interfere or interact with the trial drug also should be listed. It should be emphasized that subjects who receive any kind of concomitant medication not permitted in the protocol will be dropped from the trial, and their data will not qualify for inclusion in the final statistical analysis of efficacy.

Regarding other medications allowed during the trial, the following or a similar statement may be useful: "Other medications that are considered necessary for the subject's welfare and that will not interfere with the trial drug may be given at the discretion of the investigator. Administration of all concomitant medications must be recorded in the appropriate section of the case report form." If the investigator administers to a subject any drug that is determined to be similar to the one under investigation, that subject will be dropped from the trial and will not be entered in the data to be submitted at the conclusion of the investigation.

18. Case Report Forms

All the data gathered on an individual subject during the course of a clinical trial is recorded on a subject's CRF. Designing an easy-to-complete, accurate case report form containing all the essential data can be an arduous task. All of the details pertaining to the safety and efficacy of the drug under trial have to have a place on the CRF. Depending on the phase of clinical research, the trial design, the drug's indication(s), and the parameters being examined, a CRF can be anywhere from 5 to 10 pages to literally hundreds of pages in length. (*Note*: the more complicated the CRF, the more chance of data inconsistency.)

The case report form is the vital record of a clinical trial. It is necessary to design the CRF to collect all the data required by the protocol. Carefully designed CRFs are essential for the following reasons:

As a means of checking the logistics, design, and practicality of the protocol

For later processing, analysis, and interpretation of the trial data so that the results may be accurately reported

To record safety and efficacy data that are consistent from subject to subject or patient to patient

To check for protocol adherence and/or investigator compliance
To fulfill FDA requirements

The design of the CRF is a collaborative effort of the investigator, trial coordinator, clinical monitor, program manager, statisticians, and data management personnel.

Content of the Case Report Form

1. Have the questions on the CRF directly address those defined in the protocol. The data collected must support the questions that are to be answered by the statistical analysis.

2. Provide definitions for terminology and scales to obtain consistency in evaluations from CRF to CRF within a trial, as well as across trials. These definitions should appear directly on the case report forms to make them readily available to the investigator.

3. Do not include additional questions that address ancillary issues. The attempt to collect and record too much information often leads to carelessness and lack of enthusiasm by the trial participants. The more that is asked for, the more variability will occur in the answers.

4. Questions should be asked directly and unambiguously free from jargon.

5. In long-term trials, the CRF may be formatted in sections and used for each visit or group of visits. This helps to decrease the likelihood of ambiguity in recording when an event occurs, as well as to help expedite the flow of data in-house and through data processing.

6. Order the questions on the CRF logically, following the order in which a physician would ordinarily collect data. Separate questions that routinely would be asked by a trial nurse from those that would be asked by the clinical investigator.

7. Be clear on how precise answers should be—should a value be rounded or carried to one or more decimal places? Lack of clarity here creates some doubt in the trial recorder's mind; the resulting inconsistencies also increase the difficulties for the data processing staff. Collect direct numerical measurements, where possible, rather than broad categorical judgments. This usually improves overall consistency, especially across trials.

8. When questions include comparative terms, use positive terms such as better, bigger, and more, rather than negative terms such as worse, smaller, or less. Research has shown as much as a 20% difference in accuracy when positive terms are used.

9. Use design techniques that make the form easy to read and complete:

Balance white space with text. Make the form aesthetically pleasing, not cluttered.

Use check-off blocks (coded responses) wherever possible. Checking a block is less time-consuming and error prone than entering a value or term.

Block sections of the form to make them easy to locate and complete.

Use variations in size and attributes of type (e.g., bold, italics, underlining) for headings and for emphasis of important questions.

Highlight the areas of the form where the investigator is expected to make entries. This decreases the chance that the investigator will overlook a question and helps during the in-house review and processing of the data.

Keep calculations to a minimum.

Alphanumeric fields (such as for adverse experiences) should be sized to hold the largest possible response. Include instructions for filling out the CRF (e.g., use black ink, print, etc.).

19. Laboratory Assessments

Through laboratory determinations and the subsequent review of this data, the safety of a drug can be adequately assessed and, in some instances, the efficacy can be measured. Laboratories usually provide normal ranges with appropriate notations to highlight values outside the normal ranges. These are then reviewed to determine whether the abnormality or deviations are clinically significant or severe enough to cause concern for the safety of the subject taking the trial drug. Safety evaluation criteria can include such determinations as sequential multiple analysis computer (SMAC) tests, CBC, urinalysis, vital sign monitoring, EEGs, ECGs, CAT scans, MRI, and radiologic examinations, including barium enemas and endoscopies. Many other tests capable of providing objective safety measurements may be considered. These results, coupled with any signs and symptoms attributed to drug reactions, will help complete the overall picture of a drug's safety profile. Many of the safety parameters, in most instances, do not reflect the efficacy of a drug. Whereas drugs with a spotless safety profile may be more desirable, therapeutic efficacy, in balance with an acceptable safety profile, is, after all, the more realistic goal.

Safety and efficacy evaluations may be objective or subjective. Objective evaluations are simpler to record, because they represent true values of drug response for safety and efficacy.

Objective values (numerical, photographic documentation, etc.) are easily recorded; for example, blood pressure, pulse rate, measurements of lesions seen on endoscopy. It is more difficult accurately and consistently to measure subjective impressions of improvement of symptoms, such as a reduction in pain or psychiatric disorders, by measuring and rating cognitive functions or feelings of well being. Proper standardization of the symptoms to be evaluated is essential. Although there is some confidence in using certain subjective, validated evaluations to distinguish between improvement and deterioration, it is often difficult to have the results unanimously accepted. One approach to measuring subjective evaluations with unknown scales is to ascertain that there is an acceptable explanation for quantifying the severity or improvement that the investigator is evaluating. For example, if a symptom such as pain is being measured using a 7-point scale (from 0 = absent to 7 = extremely severe), the interim points may be designated as very mild, mild, moderate, moderately severe, and severe, each term being precisely defined. As an example, the type of definitions, listed below, are designed to reduce bias (variables) and increase accuracy in scoring the results. In other words, a numeric value is placed on a degree of pain that corresponds to a definition. By using this method to rate subjective symptoms, we gain consistency of data, especially when the trial is multicenter.

    1 = **Absent:** feels no pain

    2 = **Very Mild:** feels pain once a week

    3 = **Mild:** feels pain < three times per week

    4 = **Moderate:** feels pain every day, but not severe enough for medication

    5 = **Moderately Severe:** feels pain every day and needs mild pain medicine for relief

    6 = **Severe:** feels pain all the time and needs strong pain medicine for relief

    7 = **Extremely Severe:** feels pain all the time and gets no relief from pain medication

Of course, variations in defining degrees of severity of any subjective rating is totally dependent on the creator of the scale and the scope of the overall objective of the trial.

20. Adverse Experiences

The protocol should include an adverse experience statement, such as "All adverse experiences occurring during the trial must be reported on the drug reaction record provided in the subject case report forms." The drug reaction record is a complete questionnaire that covers all pertinent items concerning adverse experiences. (See Chap. 11.)

In addition, there should be a procedure for reporting serious, fatal, and life-threatening reactions expeditiously to the sponsor. This will enable the sponsor to make any changes in the protocol necessary for safety and to report the applicable adverse experiences to the FDA within the required time frame. This is discussed in Chap. 11, "Adverse Reactions and Interactions of

Drugs." Most protocols require that unexpected and severe, life-threatening, or fatal adverse experiences be reported immediately by telephone to the sponsor; a "24-hour" telephone number must be included in every protocol. The information provided on the drug reaction should be complete enough to enable the sponsor to provide the FDA with the proper and legal material necessary for reporting adverse experiences.

21. Statistical Handling of Data

The statistical handling section of the protocol must be finalized before an investigational trial begins. Draft protocols should be reviewed and discussed with a biostatistician before they are finalized and presented to clinical investigators. Early input from a biostatistician is vital in the planning and writing stage of a protocol and leads to the success of a clinical research project. The CRFs should be developed and coded with statisticians before printing; this will facilitate data entry and expedite data processing. Requirements set forth in the protocol require careful planning and adherence to procedures. This will generate the type and quantity of scientific data necessary to achieve statistically valid documentation that will confirm the safety and efficacy of a drug. The statistical handling of the data is an integral part of the research protocol and is designed in the early planning stages of the trial. It cannot be an afterthought when a mass of data has already been collected. The FDA will not accept the clinical data of any phase trial if the statistical analysis methodology is not incorporated into the protocol before the initiation of the trial.

22. Overall Duration of the Trial

The maximum allowable time required by an investigator to complete the evaluations of all subjects entered into the trial should be clearly stated. The agreed-upon schedule should be strictly observed. Be realistic in your expectations. If an investigator estimates that he or she can handle 50 subjects in 1 year, it may be safe to assume that it may take 2 years to complete the investigation. Some investigators do not realize how much work is required in completing the CRFs for the number of subjects necessary to conclude a clinical trial successfully. The timetable described in the protocol must be reviewed with the investigator so that the time commitment is fully understood. If a flow chart is created, use it to demonstrate how many evaluations have to be completed over a defined period. For example, if a trial calls for the entry of five subjects per week and four or five CRF pages for that subject's entry (e.g., a physical, a history, a laboratory examination, and baseline determinations) and, in subsequent weeks, the trial calls for two or three evaluations per week, by the third week an investigator will have 16 to 21 evaluations. In a 50-subject trial with each subject evaluated for 5 weeks, by the fifth week, the investigator will have 28 to 37 evaluations. It is apparent, then, that it is more practical for the primary investigator to enter fewer subjects over a longer period and to persevere in completing the trial rather than be faced with an impossible burden of work, deadline, and failure. It should be emphasized to the investigator that subjects meeting the criteria of the protocol are not the same as in clinical practice; scientific research and adherence to the protocol require a different discipline.

23. Institutional Review Board

A formally recognized and certified IRB must review the proposed clinical research protocol to determine whether the relative safety and anticipated benefits to subjects/patients are adequately and fairly represented in the protocol design. If the research is to be done at a large hospital or teaching institution, it is likely that there is an affiliated IRB. Independent, certified IRBs are used at sites that lack their own IRB. A protocol used for a multicenter trial must be reviewed by an IRB for each site participating in the program. All protocols used in clinical research must have an IRB approval before drugs may be administered to subjects entering a research trial.

No clinical trial plan is complete unless all the necessary precautions have been taken to protect the safety and rights of the subject. All trials conducted in the United States must be designed and carried out in accordance with Parts 50 and 56 of Title 21 of the Code of Federal Regulations (CFR), the regulations concerning the safety and rights of subjects. For foreign investigations, ICH guidelines must be followed.

It must be remembered that an IRB will consider the following principal ethical requirements of a clinical research trial before allowing the research program to start:

1. The risks to participants are minimized and are reasonable in relation to the anticipated benefits.
2. Selection of subjects is equitable.
3. Appropriately worded and documented informed consent is obtained from each prospective participant or from a legally authorized representative if the participant is considered unable to give such consent.
4. The research plan makes appropriate provisions for monitoring the safety of the participants.
5. The privacy of the participants and confidentiality of the data will be maintained.

6. The protocol objective will conclude a benefit for subjects suffering with the disease under investigation.

24. Informed Consent

Some institutions have a preferred format for the informed consent form to be executed by subjects within their own institution. The purpose of all such forms is to ensure that no experimentation is carried out on people who are unaware or unwilling to participate in an investigational clinical program. As this is a crucial tenet of modern investigational medicine, the protocol must specify that each subject must execute an informed consent document prior to enrollment in the trial, randomization, and administration of any drug. In the case of a participant who is considered incompetent, a legally authorized representative must execute the document. Children under the age of 18 must have a parent or guardian sign the informed consent. These consent forms become part of the permanent subject records to be kept available for FDA inspection (see Chap. 20).

25. Monitoring

The following statement should be included in all trial protocols: "At regular intervals throughout the trial, the investigator will allow a representative of the sponsor's monitoring team, or the sponsor's designate, or a representative of the FDA to inspect all case report forms and corresponding portions of an enrolled subject's original office and/or hospital medication records. These inspections are for the purpose of verifying adherence to the protocol and the completeness and exactness of the data being entered on the case report forms."

The monitor of a clinical trial (typically called a clinical research associate, or CRA, in the pharmaceutical industry) has to confirm that all of the necessary information requested on the CRF has been recorded. During a site visit, the monitor should be alert to the items on the CRF that are central to the trial objectives. In an anxiety–depression trial, for example, the most important symptoms are anxiety, tension, depression, or other anxiety–depression-related symptoms. These must be carefully noted and documented. The CRA should notice any changes recorded during the course of an investigation that indicate trends across the participating subject population. If there are significant rating changes after a certain number of weeks or after an assumed drug effect, these should be carefully documented and discussed with the investigator. A completed evaluation form for every subject in a clinical trial is of paramount importance.

It is also the monitor's responsibility to account for all concomitant medications. Unfamiliar drugs should be cross-checked in the *PDR* to determine if any component(s) of the medication taken concomitantly with the investigational drug violates the protocol. All brand and generic names of drugs should be legible and identifiable. Monitors must assure that every adverse experience has been reported and documented properly.

Other items, such as dosage titration information, should be examined, recorded, and (when applicable) reported with comments as to the reasons for these changes. Any incomplete item on a CRF must be explained, and a signed and dated statement from the investigator substantiating the reasons for the incomplete entry must be obtained. Any problems a monitor encounters during a clinical trial should be discussed as soon as possible after the trial has begun, and these should be expeditiously resolved and noted.

26. Location of Trial

List the investigator(s) name(s), address(es), and telephone number(s) where the trial is to be conducted. If more than one location is involved (institutions, universities, and other medical offices), provide their locations as well.

27. Location of Laboratory Testing Facilities

List the names, addresses, and telephone numbers for all test laboratories involved in the trial. An investigator must be able to contact laboratory personnel at all times. The protocol must include a record of where laboratory testing is being conducted. The laboratory director's CV and the laboratory's certification number have to be kept on file.

28. Investigator's Obligations

When agreeing to participate in the sponsor's clinical trial, an investigator is making several contractual agreements that must be clearly understood. The protocol must be adhered to, including the enrollment criteria, the blinding procedures, and the meticulous and timely record-keeping. A realistic estimate of the number of eligible subjects the investigator will be able to enroll and follow up will help to minimize the difficulties of conducting a rigorous clinical investigation. To the extent possible, the agreed-upon time frame for completion of the trial should be adhered to. It is also advisable to receive written assurance from the investigator that he or she agrees to conduct the trial according to the protocol design and will adhere to the GCP regulations (21 CFR Part 312).

In addition, the investigator must complete Financial Disclosure Forms, i.e., FDA Form 3454 (no financial interest) or FDA Form 3455 (financial interest). These forms will confirm any or no financial involvement of the investigator with the company or product they are investigating.

29. Signature Page

Allow space for the investigator's signature and the date the agreement is signed. The sponsor's clinician also should sign off on the protocol.

30. Amendments and Addenda

Amendments. Amendments to protocols have created a lot of controversy through the years. According to 312.30 in the CFR, any change in a phase 1 protocol that significantly affects the safety of subjects, or any change in a phase 2 or 3 protocol that significantly affects the safety of subjects, the scope of investigation, or the scientific quality of the trial requires an amendment to the protocol. Some examples of these changes are increase in drug dosage, duration of exposure of individual subjects to a drug beyond that stated in a protocol, or increase of trial population size. Other examples are adding or dropping a control group, adding a new test or procedure that is intended to improve the monitoring for, or reduce the risk of, adverse experiences or adverse reactions, or conversely dropping a test intended to monitor safety. Overall, any significant change in the design of a protocol that requires doing something that may affect the subject's safety requires an amendment.

Any change that would apply to any of the above-stated items must have approval from the FDA and should be submitted as an amendment to the FDA with written approval from an IRB before its implementation. At the same time, if there is a change in the protocol intended to eliminate an apparent hazard to subjects, it may be implemented immediately, provided that the FDA and the IRB are subsequently notified of a protocol amendment. It is important to remember that all protocol amendments to the FDA should be properly identified and labeled "Protocol Amendment: Change in Protocol." In the case of a change in a protocol, a brief description of the change in reference to the submission that contained the original protocol should be submitted with the amendment. In other instances, when new investigators are added to carry out a previously submitted protocol, the sponsor shall notify the FDA by an amendment within 30 days of the investigator's being added and await IRB approval.

Although amendments can be submitted at any time during a clinical investigation, it behooves the investigators not to amend the protocol unless it is absolutely necessity to expedite the acceptability of subjects entering into a trial, that is, the deletion or addition of significant requirements for subject eligibility. The reason is that statistically, it is very difficult to deal with changes made from the original protocol design in the final statistical analysis. The analysis of these data must reflect the results of the subject's evaluations before and after amendments. In the analysis of the results of all subjects in trials with or without amendments, it is difficult to conclude results based on different protocol designs, such as subjects previously admitted to the trial with no history of hepatic disease and subsequently, through an amendment, allowing subjects into a trial having a hepatic disease 1 year before entering the trial. It is imperative, therefore, to abide by the initial recommendation of this chapter, that is, whenever possible, do not change a protocol once it has been designed with diligence, intelligence, and expertise in meeting the original objectives of the clinical trial plan. Amendments should never be done after 49% of the subjects have entered the trial unless to ensure the safety of the subject.

Addenda. Often when protocol designers speak of addenda, they confuse them with amendments. There is a distinct difference from amendments, which are significant changes that can affect the safety of the subject, the implementation of procedures of a protocol, and the results obtained from a protocol. Addenda are simply additions to the protocol that do not change the safety measures of the subjects or the original trial protocol. For example, if specific quantities of blood are being drawn from a subject and another laboratory test is added using this same blood sample, this is an addendum. This typical addendum to the protocol does not change any procedures from the original protocol and does not affect the safety of the subject. It is usually an additional test that could be reported in the final statistical analysis and clinical report.

Addenda to the protocol do not have to be submitted to the FDA or IRB committees for approval.

VIII. SUMMARY

Many approaches and different styles are useful in the development and preparation of a sound clinical research trial protocol. The foregoing guidelines can be modified to suit the applicant's needs and objectives. No matter which path is mapped out, it is imperative that investigators abide by the final protocol. Strict adherence to a well-designed protocol will result in research projects that reflect the stated objectives in the required amount of time leading to successful and definitive conclusions.

ADDITIONAL REFERENCE MATERIAL

1. Armitage P. Controversies and achievements in clinical trials. Control Clin Trials 1984; 5:243–251.

2. Bradford Hill A. Principles of Medical Statistics. 9th ed. London: The Lancet, 1971.
3. Clinical trials: design and analysis. Semin Oncol 1981; 8:347–477.
4. Davey P. Comparative clinical trials of antimicrobial drugs. J Antimicrob Chemother 1984; 13:204–208.
5. Doongaji DR. Some problems in the conduct of psychotropic drug trials (a review). J Postgrad Med 1983; 29:67–74.
6. Feinstein AR. Current problems and future challenges in randomized clinical trials. Circulation 1984; 70:767–774.
7. Finkel M. General considerations for the clinical evaluation of drugs. HEW (FDA) 77–3040. Washington, D.C.: U.S. Government Printing Office, 1977.
8. Fischer-Cornelssen KA. Methods of multicenter trials in psychiatry, part I: a review. Prog Neuropsychopharmacol Biol Psychiatry 1980; 4:545–560.
9. Friedewald WT. Overview of recent clinical and methodological advances from clinical trials of cardiovascular disease. Control Clin Trials 1982; 3:259–270.
10. Grahame-Smith DG, Aronson JK, eds. Oxford Textbook of Clinical Pharmacology and Drug Therapy. London: Oxford University Press, 1984.
11. Guarino RA. Writing protocols for new drugs. Drug Cosmet Indus 1975; 117: 50.
12. Johnson FN, Johnson S, eds. Clinical Trials. Oxford, England: Blackwell Scientific, 1971.
13. Johnson FN, Johnson S. Clinical Trials. Oxford, England: Blackwell Scientific Publications, 1977.
14. Hadler NM. On the design of the phase III drug trial: the example of rheumatoid arthritis. Arthritis Rheum 1983; 26:1354–1361.
15. Haegerstam G. Placebo in clinical drug trials—a multidisciplinary review. Meth Find Exp Clin Pharmacol 1982; 4:261–278.
16. Lavori PW, et al. Designs for experiments—parallel comparisons of treatment. N Engl J Med 1983; 309:1291–1299.
17. Linden M. Phase IV clinical research: specifics, objectives and methodology. Pharmacopsychiatry 1984; 17:162–167.
18. Louis TA. Critical issues in the conduct and interpretation of clinical trials. Annu Rev Public Health 1983; 4:25–46.
19. Louis TA. Crossover and self-controlled designs in clinical research. N Engl J Med 1984; 310:24–31.
20. Maxwell C. Clinical Research for All. Cambridge: Cambridge Medical Publications, 1973.
21. Pocock TJ. Current issues in the design and interpretation of clinical trials. Br Med J 1985; 290:39–42.
22. Pollack AV. Review article: controlled clinical trials. Life Support Syst 1983; 1:7–233.
23. Proceedings of a Conference on the Recent History of Randomized Clinical Trials. Santa Ynez Valley, California: Kroc Foundation, November 1981.
24. Rossi AC. Discovery of adverse drug reactions. A comparison of selected phase IV trials with spontaneous reporting methods. JAMA 1983; 249:26–28.
25. Sachar DB. Placebo-controlled clinical trials in gastroenterology. A position

paper of the American College of Gastroenterology. Am J Gastroenterol 1984; 79:913–917.

26. Sackett DL, Haynes RB, eds. Compliance with Therapeutic Regimens. Baltimore: Johns Hopkins University Press, 1976.

27. Smith W. Randomization and optimal design. J Chronic Dis 1983; 36:609–615.

28. Spilker B. Practical considerations in planning clinical trials with investigational or marketed drugs. Clin Neuropharmacol 1983; 6:325–347.

29. Tallarida RI. A scale for assessing the severity of diseases and adverse drug reactions. Application to drug benefit and risk. Clin Pharmacol Ther 1979; 25: 381–390.

30. Venn RD. Experience with the collection and evaluation of drug adverse reaction data. Proceedings of the European Society for the Trial of Drug Toxicity. Vol. 10. Amsterdam: Foundation, Excerpta Medica, 1969.

31. Warrington SJ. Limitations of dose tolerance trials on predictability for phase III. Arzneimittel Forschung 1985; 35:781–783.

32. Wittenborn JR, ed. Guidelines for clinical trials of psychotropic drugs. Pharmacopsychiatry 1977; 10(3):207–231.

33. Wittenhorn JR. Reliability, validity and objectivity of symptom-rating scales. J Mental Nervous Dis 1972; 154:79–87.

34. Zelen M. A new design for randomized clinical trials. N Engl J Med 1979; 300: 1242–1245.

11
Adverse Experiences, Adverse Reactions, and Interactions of Drugs

Richard A. Guarino
Oxford Pharmaceutical Resources, Inc., Totowa, New Jersey, U.S.A.

I. INTRODUCTION

There is an old but nonetheless true dictum in pharmacology: no drug has a single action. Unfortunately, multiple actions of therapeutic drugs are not always in the best interest of the subject. In addition to the primary therapeutic effect for which a drug is prescribed, the likelihood exists for the emergence of concurrent or delayed, unwanted, and potentially harmful effects–adverse reactions—which may be due to other known pharmacological or toxic effects of the drug. Such reactions also may be attributed to some idiosyncrasy in certain individuals. Any active drug, therefore, may be a double-edged sword, doing good on one hand and perhaps harm on the other.

With the recent impressive advances in pharmacology and the ability to synthesize new, complex, and more potent drugs without commensurate knowledge of how and under what conditions they act in humans, the question of adverse reactions (ADRs) and the interactions of drugs has become an increasingly serious aspect of modern therapeutics. It is not surprising, therefore, that drug legislation in most countries is concerned as much with the safety of drugs and devices as with their efficacy. As a result, this aspect of drug evaluation is demanding more and more attention from those involved in drug, device, and vaccine research and development, particularly with respect to unwanted or toxic effects.

According to FDA regulations and the International Committee on Harmonization guidelines on Good Clinical Practices (ICH GCPs), in the preapproval clinical experience with a new medicinal product or its new usages, particularly as the therapeutic dose(s) may not be established, all noxious and unintended responses to a medicinal product related to any dose should be considered as adverse experiences (AEs). The phrase "responses to a medicinal product" means that a causal relationship between a medicinal product and an adverse experience is at least a reasonable possibility (i.e., the relationship cannot be ruled out). Regarding marketed medicinal products, an adverse reaction (ADR) is a response to a drug that is noxious and unintended and that occurs at doses normally used in humans for prophylaxis, diagnosis, or therapy of diseases or for modification of physiologic function [1].

Because of the difficulty in obtaining accurate records, the true incidence of adverse reactions to drugs in the population at large is unknown. In the April 15, 1998, issue of the *Journal of the American Medical Association*, Lazarou and colleagues [2] attempted to assess the incidence of serious and fatal ADRs in hospitalized subjects by searching four electronic databases and selecting 39 prospective trials from hospitals in the United States. The overall incidence of serious ADRs was 6.7% and of fatal ADRs, 0.32%. Indeed, ADRs were between the fourth and sixth leading cause of death in hospitalized subjects. The incidence of ADRs of all severities (including serious and nonserious) was 10.9%. Although the authors recommend that the results be reviewed with circumspection because of heterogenicity among trials and small biases in the samples, they concluded that ADRs represent an important clinical issue.

The necessity of a clear understanding of the total pharmacology of therapeutic drugs, particularly of their potential for inducing ADRs either alone or in concert with other drugs, needs no further emphasis. It has become a major concern for those responsible for developing, prescribing, and dispensing therapeutic agents.

II. CLASSIFICATION OF ADVERSE DRUG REACTIONS

In general, adverse reactions to a drug may be either dose dependent or dose independent. Although both types may be produced to a greater or lesser extent by the same drug, dose dependency is a convenient and satisfactory method for classification.

A. Dose–Dependent Adverse Reactions

If an active drug is administered in sufficiently large doses, eventually all individuals will manifest adverse reactions. The dosage level at which the reactions occur, however, may vary considerably from individual to individual. Dose-dependent adverse reactions are usually specific for the drug concerned. They can be categorized as follows: (1) known for unwanted pharmacologic effects (e.g., the anticholinergic effects of the phenothiazine tranquilizers); or (2) exaggerated therapeutic effects (e.g., orthostatic hypotension with antihypertensive drugs such as clonidine and guanethidine when these agents are taken at higher than usual doses); or (3) reactions unrelated to the therapeutic effects (e.g., ototoxicity produced by excessive doses of streptomycin).

Dose-dependent adverse reactions are influenced by a number of physiologic and pathologic factors that have little or no bearing on dose-independent reactions. Prominent among these factors are liver and kidney disease, enzyme abnormalities, and drug interactions that may affect absorption or involve competition for transport binding sites of action, certain physiological conditions altering drug excretion, and age. Dose-dependent ADRs are often more prominent at the chronological extremes of life. The fetus, the newborn infant, and the aged are more susceptible than young adults and the middle aged to the effects, good and bad, of many drugs.

1. Pregnant Women

The fetus is particularly susceptible to the toxic effects of certain drugs that pass the placental barrier. The ill effects of such drugs may vary according to the stage of pregnancy at which they are administered. Drugs with teratogenic properties, for example, given during the first trimester—the period of fetal organogenesis—may cause congenital abnormalities. Moreover, susceptibility of particular organs to drug-induced malformation depends on the time the drug is given during the first trimester. The critical teratogenic period for the nervous system is from gestation days 20–40, for the limbs, gestation days 24–36, and for the eye, gestation days 24–40. Drugs given to the mother after the first trimester may affect the growth or function of normally formed fetal tissues or organs [3]. The classic example of a drug with teratogenic activity in humans is thalidomide, which is associated with phocomelia; this stimulated the drug regulatory bodies in many countries, including the United States, to adopt more stringent controls on new drug development.

Antineoplastic drugs such as 6-mercaptopurine, methotrexate, cyclophosphamide, and aminopterin administered in early pregnancy have produced various congenital malformations. Cytotoxic drugs also have induced fetal malformation and early abortion of malformed fetuses [4–6].

Corticosteroids administered during the period of fetal organogenesis have been associated with anencephaly [7] and carry a high risk of inducing cleft palate. Lysergic acid diethylamide (LSD), among other hallucinogenic drugs, has been shown to produce chromosomal damage; on less certain evidence, its use during pregnancy may result in congenital anomalies.

The more frequently prescribed drugs that have been reported to affect growth and function of organs when given to the mother after the period of fetal organogenesis, or to the newborn infant, are discussed below.

Antibacterial and Antibiotic Drugs. Sulfonamides are extensively protein bound. If these drugs are administered to mothers immediately before delivery or to the premature or full-term infant while there is physiological hyperbilirubinemia, they may displace bilirubin from plasma protein, causing severe jaundice or kernicterus [8].

Chloramphenicol is not adequately detoxified and excreted by the fetus or the premature infant. Administration of this antibiotic to the mother shortly before parturition may produce gray coloration of the infant's skin with associated muscle hypotonia and circulatory collapse, known as "the gray baby syndrome" [9]. (This *adverse reaction* is more often noted in premature infants.)

Anticoagulants. Coumarin and indandione derivatives given during pregnancy cross the placental barrier. Even though the maternal prothrombin times remain normal, the use of these anticoagulant compounds may result in fetal death owing to hemorrhage in utero [10] or to intracranial bleeding caused by birth trauma [11].

Antithyroid Drugs. Congenital goiter and neonatal hypothyroidism may occur if thiouracil drugs are administered during pregnancy [12].

Oral Hypoglycemia Drugs. Intrauterine fetal death and prolonged symptomatic neonatal hypoglycemia have been reported after treatment of the mother with sulfonylurea drugs [13,14].

Cardiovascular Drugs. In general, cardiovascular drugs have the same but exaggerated effects on the fetus as on the mother. Beta-receptor stimulants (e.g., isoproterenol), and beta-receptor-blocking agents, such as propranolol, may respectively cause significant fetal tachycardia or bradycardia. Norepinephrine and other alpha-receptor stimulants given during pregnancy may induce constriction of the uterine vessels and thus indirectly result in fetal asphyxia.

Anesthetics, Analgesics, and Hypnotics. If anesthetics, analgesics, and hypnotics are given during labor, they can adversely affect the newborn child by inducing respiratory depression and neonatal asphyxia.

The appearance of typical withdrawal symptoms in the newborn infant of an opiate-addicted mother has been well documented.

So that the aforementioned teratogenic effects can be avoided, pregnant women should, in general, be excluded from clinical trials in which the drug is not intended for use in pregnancy. Before the inclusion of pregnant women in clinical trials, all the reproductive toxicity trials [15,16] and the standard battery of genotoxicity tests [17] should be conducted. In addition, safety data from previous human exposure are usually needed. If a subject becomes pregnant during administration of the drug, treatment should generally be discontinued if this can be done safely. Follow-up trials of the pregnancy, the fetus, and the child are very important. For clinical trials of a medicinal product for use during pregnancy, follow-up trials of the pregnancy, the fetus, and the child are important.

2. Nursing Women

In investigations in nursing women, excretion of the drug or its metabolites into human milk should be examined where applicable. When nursing mothers are enrolled in clinical trials, their infants should be monitored for the effects of the drug.

3. Women of Childbearing Potential

The subjects included in clinical trials should, in general, reflect the population that will receive the drug when it is marketed. For most drugs, therefore, representatives of both sexes should be included in clinical trials in numbers adequate to allow detection of clinically significant sex-related differences in drug response.

Appropriate precautions should be taken in clinical trials to guard against inadvertent exposure of fetuses to potentially toxic agents and to inform subjects of the potential risk and the need for precautions. In all cases, the informed consent document and the investigator's brochure should include all available information regarding the potential risk of fetal toxicity.

In general, it is expected that reproductive toxicity trials will be completed before there is large-scale exposure of women of childbearing potential (i.e., usually by the end of phase 2 and before any expanded access program is implemented).

Except in the case of trials intended for trial of drug effects during pregnancy, clinical protocols should also include measures that will minimize the possibility of fetal exposure to the investigational drug. These would ordinarily include provisions for the use of a reliable method of contraception (or abstinence) for the duration of drug exposure (which may exceed the length of the trial) and the use of pregnancy testing (beta human chorionic gonadotropin [HCG]) to detect unsuspected pregnancy before trial treatment begins.

4. Geriatric Population

The geriatric population is arbitrarily defined as comprising subjects 65 years or older. The older the population likely to use the drug, the more important it is to include the older age range, 75 years and older. For drugs used to treat diseases not unique to, but present in, the elderly, a minimum of 100 subjects usually would allow detection of clinically important differences between the elderly and younger subjects with respect to efficacy as well as adverse reactions.

Elderly individuals often develop adverse reactions to drugs at dosage levels well tolerated by younger persons. These reactions may be due to an age-related increase in sensitivity to drugs or impairment of detoxification (metabolism) and excretion functions.

Sedating, hypnotic, tranquilizing, and tricyclic antidepressant drugs are prone to precipitate confusional states in the elderly, particularly if there is preexisting evidence of impairment of cognitive function [18–21]. Extrapyramidal symptoms such as akathisia and parkinsonism are more common in the elderly than in younger subjects treated with phenothiazine tranquilizers, particularly piperazine derivatives, butyrophenones, and tricyclic antidepressants [22]. Furthermore, these psychotropic agents and other drugs with anti-intestinal motility effects in the elderly result in troublesome constipation, fecal impaction, and occasionally paralytic ileus [23,24].

Digitalis toxicity is not infrequently encountered in geriatric subjects given digitalizing doses considered normal for younger subjects. The elderly also are more likely to develop hypokalemia with the potassium-wasting diuretics. If these drugs are given concurrently with digitalis, the therapeutic regimen further increases the risk of digitalis toxicity.

It has also been reported that heparin administered to women older than age 60 renders them approximately 50% more susceptible to bleeding complications than men similarly treated [25].

5. Pediatric Population

The pediatric population consists of four pediatric subgroups: neonates (birth up to 1 month), infants (1 month to 2 years), children (2–12 years), and adolescents (13–16 years).

Many drugs labeled only for adult use are in fact widely used in pediatric subjects for the same indications. Less than half the drugs approved for treatment of HIV infection carry any pediatric safety or effectiveness information. Almost no information on use in subjects younger than 2 years of age is available for most drug classes [26].

Some ADRs occur in children because of inadvertent drug overdoses or other drug administration problems, such as inadequate treatment, that could have been avoided with better information on appropriate pediatric use. This is of particular concern in infants and neonates, because correct pediatric dosing cannot necessarily be extrapolated from adult dosing information using an equivalence based either on weight (mg/kg) or body surface area (mg/m^2). Potentially significant differences in pharmacokinetics may alter a drug's effect in pediatric subjects. The effects of growth and maturation of various organs, maturation of the immune system, alterations in metabolism throughout infancy and childhood, changes in body proportions, and other developmental changes may result in significant differences in the doses needed by pediatric subjects and adults. One of the earliest cases in which serious *adverse reaction* were observed in neonates after administration of a drug that had not been adequately studied in pediatric subjects was the development of "gray baby syndrome" from chloramphenicol, an antibiotic [27]. After an initial report of five deaths and a subsequent report of 18 deaths in neonates, it was learned that the immature livers of these infants were unable to clear chloramphenicol from the body, allowing toxic doses of the drug to accumulate. Other cases in which inadequately studied drugs have resulted in serious adverse effects in pediatric subjects include teeth staining from tetracycline, kernicterus from sulfa drugs, withdrawal symptoms after prolonged administration of fentanyl in infants and small children, seizures and cardiac arrest caused by bupivacaine toxicity, development of colonic strictures in pediatric cystic fibrosis subjects after exposure to high-dose pancreatic enzymes, and hazardous interactions between erythromycin and midazolam [26–37]. Many such adverse reactions could be avoided if pediatric trials were conducted before drugs were widely used in pediatric subjects.

In the future, the FDA will require pediatric trials if the drug product will be widely used in the claimed indication, and the absence of adequate pediatric labeling could pose significant risks to pediatric subjects. trials will also be required if the drug product is indicated for a very significant or life-threatening illness, but additional dosing or safety information is needed to permit its safe and effective use in pediatric subjects.

6. Enzyme Abnormalities

Enzyme abnormalities may be inherited or acquired. Some of the more important inherited enzyme abnormalities are discussed below. The acquired conditions are dealt with later in this chapter under Drug Interactions.

Inherited Enzyme Abnormalities. It is becoming increasingly evident that a number of adverse reactions to drugs are due to genetically transmitted inborn enzyme abnormalities or deficiencies. The best known example of this category is the hereditary relative deficiency of the enzyme glucose-6-phosphate-dehydrogenase (G-6-PD), which occurs in 5% to 10% of Mediterranean littoral races, blacks, Pakistanis, and Sephardic Jews. This condition renders affected individuals susceptible to acute hemolytic anemia when they are exposed to such drugs as primaquine, phenacetin, aspirin, chloramphenicol, nitrofurantoin, and sulfonamides, and to the fava bean.

Other hereditary enzyme deficiencies that may result in adverse reactions to certain drugs are comparatively rare, often familial, and of worldwide distribution. Examples of these conditions are pseudocholinesterase deficiencies in certain people who, when given succinylcholine or suxamethonium, develop a profound, general neuromuscular blockade with apnea [38].

Tuberculous subjects lacking in liver *N*-acetyl transferase who are treated with isoniazid are likely to develop polyneuritis [39]. An enzyme abnormality is also responsible for the precipitation of acute intermittent porphyria by the barbiturate drugs [40]. Likewise, the rare hereditary resistance to coumarin anticoagulant drugs is thought to be due to an enzyme deficiency [41].

7. Liver Disease

Biotransformation of most drugs takes place in the liver. A disease that affects liver function, therefore, may impair metabolism and inactivation of drugs. This will increase the degree and duration of action of a drug to the extent that exaggerated therapeutic effects and adverse reactions may occur at normal therapeutic dose levels. The list of therapeutic agents so affected is long and varied. It includes such widely used drug groups as phenothiazines, barbiturates, narcotic analgesics, corticosteroids, and oral anticoagulants. Also, subjects with markedly reduced liver function are especially prone to develop hepatic encephalopathy when given potassium-wasting diuretics, narcotic analgesics, and central depressant medications.

Drugs also may be the cause of impaired liver function. Direct hepatotoxicity is induced by known hepatotoxins that produce fatty infiltration, degeneration, and widespread necrosis of the liver cells. Carbon tetrachloride, arsenic, gold, mercury, iron, phosphorus, some insecticides, and industrial solvents all have a dose-dependent direct toxic effect on the liver. Fortunately, except perhaps when taken in massive overdoses for suicidal purposes (such as acetaminophen), direct hepatotoxicity with therapeutic drugs is rare. This sinister potential of hepatotoxicity is usually detected in preclinical animal trials, and the drug candidate is then rejected on this account. A dose-dependent form of drug-induced hepatitis, clinically similar to viral hepatitis, may be produced by halothane anesthesia, particularly after multiple exposures [42]. Cholestatic jaundice, the most common manifestation of drug-induced liver dysfunction, is essentially an allergic-type phenomenon and is discussed under dose-dependent reactions.

8. Renal Disease

If renal function is sufficiently impaired, unchanged drugs and their metabolites that are primarily excreted in the urine can be retained in the circulation to a greater or lesser degree. As a result, the therapeutic or adverse effects of the unchanged portion of the drug may be exaggerated and prolonged; additional adverse reactions due to accumulating metabolites may also appear. Impaired renal function markedly increases the likelihood of ototoxicity due to the administration of the aminoglycosides streptomycin, kanamycin, and gentamicin. The likelihood of toxic effects of normal doses of digitalis preparations on the heart is greatly increased in subjects with renal insufficiency.

B. Dose-Independent Adverse Reactions

Occurring less frequently than dose-dependent reactions, dose-independent incidents are largely confined to allergic reactions in persons sensitized by previous administration of the same drug, or by another drug with cross antigenicity with the original medication. Allergic responses also may occur in individuals who are uniquely susceptible to relatively weak antigens or who develop sensitivity on the first use of a drug—the so-called idiosyncratic reaction.

Allergic responses to drugs are mediated by the release of histamine or histamine-like substances, and they commonly present as skin rashes, particularly urticaria. More serious hypersensitivity responses include bronchospasm or the acute explosive anaphylactic reaction with cyanosis and cardiovascular collapse. A delayed reaction known as serum sickness, although more often associated with such drugs as the penicillins and cephalosporins rather than with serum, manifests clinically 7 to 10 days after receiving the drug or serum as fever, malaise, joint pains, and urticarial skin rashes.

Blood dyscrasias, mostly dose independent, are among the most important allergic-type adverse reactions to drugs. Aplastic anemia is a serious but rare (presumably) idiosyncratic reaction. It has been reported in association with chloramphenicol, quinacrine, phenylbutazone, mephenytoin, gold compounds, and potassium chlorate. Hemolytic anemia, thrombocytopenia, and agranulocytosis may result from an unusual acquired sensitivity to a variety of widely used drugs including aminopyrine, phenylbutazone, phenothiazines, propylthiouracil, diphenylhydantoin, penicillins, chloramphenicol, sulfisoxazole, and tolbutamide.

Certain collagen-like diseases are caused by hypersensitivity reactions to drugs. Hydralazine, and particularly procainamide, may produce a clinical picture similar to systemic lupus erythematosus [43]. A number of cases of polyarteritis nodosa have developed during treatment with guanethidine and after repeated exposure to the sulfonamides, penicillin, and iodides [44]. Nephropathy has been reported following high doses of methicillin and benzylpenicillin [45].

Dose-independent, drug-induced liver dysfunction (cholestatic jaundice) is not an unusual adverse reaction. Caused by a number of different commonly used drugs, cholestasis is a hypersensitivity reaction that primarily affects the biliary canaliculi, causing an intrahepatic obstructive jaundice. An alteration in bile secretion by the hepatocytes, however, may also be involved [46]. Among the drugs known to be responsible for the development of cholestatic jaundice are the phenothiazines, the tricyclic antidepressants, the benzodiazepines, phenylbutazone, erythromycin, chlorpropamide, methyltestosterone (dose dependent), and the oral contraceptives containing estrogens and progestins.

III. DRUG INTERACTIONS

Surveys in the United States have revealed the discomforting fact that subjects on the average receive as many as 10 to 14 different medications during hospitalization. This regrettable trend toward unnecessary "polypharmacy" has greatly increased the likelihood of drug interactions and has become a new and important professional responsibility for the pharmacist as well as the physician [47].

The number of documented adverse drug interactions is formidable. They should, however, be viewed in perspective. The prescribing physician needs to be aware of all serious drug interactions that may occur within the range of drugs prescribed. Many drug interactions, though of academic interest, may not be of sufficient clinical significance to justify withholding a drug's use. A number of drugs may offer therapeutic benefits in spite of adverse interactions with other medication.

No attempt will be made to list the major drug interactions. These are readily available in a large number of texts devoted to the subject. The general principles and typical samples of various types of drug interactions, however, which may be of interest in clinical drug research, are discussed below.

A. Mechanisms of Drug Interactions

The various factors that influence responses to single-drug therapy, including age, race, and physiological and pathological states, play an equally important role in drug interactions. The concurrent or close sequential administration of two or more drugs adds a further dimension to the mechanisms of action and the possible outcome of the therapeutic program. Two or more drugs may (1) act independently, (2) interact directly with one another, or (3) interact indirectly with one another—one drug acting on an intermediate endogenous substrate that in turn modifies the effects of the other drug. Whichever mechanism is involved, the therapeutic effect of one or both drugs may be either increased (additive or synergistic) or decreased (antagonistic), and a new and unexpected adverse reaction may emerge. Drugs also may interact with other therapeutic devices or their containers, including disposable plastic syringes, rubber stoppers, and plastic bottles [48,49]. This aspect of interaction is outside the scope and intent of this chapter.

B. Pharmacokinetic Pathways and Drug Interactions

Interactions may occur at one or more of the various states in the pharmacokinetic pathways of drugs in the body (i.e., during absorption, distribution, biotransformation [metabolism], sites of action, and excretion). Each of these states is considered separately.

1. Absorption

The extent and rate of absorption of drugs from the gastrointestinal tract is dependent on a number of factors such as bacterial flora, pH, motility, and the transport system involved in the absorptive process. Interaction of therapeutic agents in the gut may seriously impede absorption. Elevation of the pH of the stomach contents by antacids, for example, greatly delays absorption of acidic drugs such as aspirin and phenobarbital. Interaction of drugs forming poorly absorbed complexes, which occurs with tetracycline and antacids containing calcium, aluminum, and magnesium salts, may significantly decrease blood levels of the antibiotic [50].

2. Distribution-Competition for Transport Sites

The distribution of drugs is affected by the circulating plasma that transports them to sites of action, metabolism, and excretion. After absorption, most drugs are partially or almost totally bound to plasma and tissue proteins. The portion that is protein bound is pharmacologically inactive. It serves as a reservoir from which the usually much smaller unbound active fraction can be replenished as the free drug is metabolized and excreted [51].

When two drugs compete for a limited number of binding sites, the drug with the greater affinity for protein binding will displace a portion of the other drug. This increases the unbound active fraction of the other drug, thereby enhancing its pharmacological effect. Sodium warfarin, for example, is about 98% bound to plasma protein and 2% free. If phenylbutazone, which has a greater affinity for protein binding, is given concurrently, it displaces warfarin from its binding sites. As a result, the bound portion of warfarin may drop to 96%, thereby increasing the active unbound fraction to 4%. Consequently, there is twice the amount of active warfarin available, and evidence of overdosage, such as spontaneous hemorrhage, may result [52].

It is evident that displacement of even small amounts of extensively protein-bound drugs can result in a relatively large increase in the active fraction. This commensurate rise in the therapeutic effect often leads to an undesirable or even dangerous level. Competition for protein-binding sites is an example of one drug acting on an intermediate endogenous substrate, thus affecting the activity of another medication.

3.   Interference with Drug Metabolism

Biotransformation or metabolic inactivation of drugs occurs mainly in the liver and, to a lesser extent, in the plasma, kidney, and other tissues, depending on the enzyme system involved. In the liver, microsomal enzymes catalyze many of the metabolic processes involved in the biotransformation of drugs. These metabolic processes may involve nonsynthetic reactions such as oxidation, reduction, or hydrolysis, or synthetic reactions, including conjugation, whereby the drug is coupled with an endogenous substrate [53].

A number of different drugs, especially phenobarbital, have the capacity for enhancing synthesis and activity in the liver microsomes—a process known as enzyme induction. The increased amount of metabolizing enzymes induced by one drug results in the accelerated metabolism of a number of other drugs with metabolic inactivation pathways similar to that of the enzyme-inducing drug. Subjects receiving phenobarbital, for example, metabolize coumarin anticoagulants, steroid hormones, antihistamines, analgesics, anti-inflammatory agents, diphenylhydantoin, and many hypnotic drugs at a greater-than-normal rate. They consequently experience diminished therapeutic activity and duration of action [54].

Some drugs, such as glutethimide, phenylbutazone, probenecid, and tolbutamide, stimulate only their own metabolizing enzymes. This may explain the increasing tolerance to these drugs that often develops after prolonged administration. On the other hand, there are drugs that can slow down or even arrest the metabolism of other drugs, resulting in their prolonged and intensified action, presumably by enzyme inhibition. Diphenylhydantoin intoxication, for example, may occur if either bishydroxycoumarin or isoniazid are given concurrently, as both the latter drugs inhibit the metabolic inactivation of the former. Also, allopurinol, a xanthine oxidase inhibitor, is used to reduce the synthesis of uric acid in gout. But xanthine oxidase is also the enzyme responsible for the deactivation of two potentially toxic antileukemic and immunosuppressant drugs, mercaptopurine and azathioprine. Concomitant medication with allopurinol will therefore elevate the plasma levels of these two cytostatic drugs and greatly increase the risk of serious bone marrow depression [55]. More recently, cimetidine has been shown to inhibit the hepatic metabolism of theophylline, resulting in significant increases in serum concentrations of this drug [56]. Cimetidine also interacts with, and produces significant increases in, the bioavailability of propranolol, oral anticoagulants, and diazepam, probably by the same mechanism [57–59].

4. Modification of Drug Effect at Sites of Action

Apart from drug interactions that result in increasing or decreasing the amount of drug available to the target organs, there are interactions that can directly or indirectly alter the response of the receptors in the target organs. A classic example of this type of interaction is the hypertensive crisis produced in subjects concurrently receiving monoamine oxidase (MAO) inhibitors and an indirectly acting amine such as amphetamine or tyramine (found in cheese and fermented foods). The MAO inhibitors reduce the intraneuronal breakdown of norepinephrine, whereas the amines stimulate the release of the excess of norepinephrine from the adrenergic neurons, thus inducing the crisis.

An altered response of one drug on its target organ may be affected by the action of a concurrently administered drug on another organ. The hypokalemia produced by potassium-wasting diuretics, for example, may potentiate the action of digitalis on the heart to the point of toxicity.

5. Excretion

The kidney is the prime organ for excretion of drugs. Drugs may be eliminated from the body either unchanged or as metabolites of the parent drug. Excretion of one drug through the kidney may be affected by concurrent administration of another and may result in an increased or reduced rate of excretion of either one or both drugs. This mechanism of action can be used to therapeutic advantage. The blood level of penicillin, for example, can be maintained at a higher level for longer periods by the concomitant administration of probenecid, which inhibits the penicillin transport system. On the other hand, quinidine reduces the renal clearance of digoxin. It also may displace digoxin from tissue-binding sites, increasing the serum level of digoxin and enhancing the risk of digoxin cardiotoxicity [60].

Drugs that alter the pH of urine can significantly affect the renal excretion of other drugs. Acid urine increases the effectiveness of mercurial diuretics. It also accelerates the excretion of basic drugs such as meperidine, tricyclic antidepressants, amphetamines, and antihistamines. Acidic drugs, such as aspirin, streptomycin, phenobarbital, sulfonamides, nalidixic acid, and nitrofurantoin have been shown to increase renal clearance in alkaline urine [61]. The possible effects of urine pH on the renal excretion of drugs has been illustrated by the observation that if urine is rendered sufficiently alkaline, the excretion of amphetamine is markedly delayed, and effective blood levels, after a single dose, can be maintained for several days [62].

C. The Beneficial Effects of Drug Interactions

It is customary, and indeed prudent, to emphasize the possible hazards of drug interactions. A number of drug interactions, however, with demonstrable beneficial therapeutic effects have been used to advantage in clinical practice for many years. Well-known examples of these include the chelating effects of calcium disodium edetate, dimercaprol, and penicillamine in chronic poisoning with arsenic, bismuth, gold, and lead, and penicillamine in chronic poisoning with arsenic, bismuth, gold, lead, and mercury; the simple expedient of alkalinization of the urine to increase renal elimination in poisonings with acidic drugs such as barbiturates and aspirin; the use of protamine sulfate to bind with heparin, forming an inactive complex, thus counteracting the effects of overheparinization; and the synergistic antibacterial effect of trimethoprim and sulfamethoxazole in the urine when these drugs are administered together.

Paradoxically, the unpleasant effects of a toxic metabolite produced by a drug interaction can have therapeutic benefits, such as the administration of disulfiram in the treatment of alcoholism. Furthermore, interactions at receptor sites to block the effects of a drug may be used to advantage (e.g., nalorphine in morphine poisoning). It is common practice to use antiparkinsonian drugs such as benztropine to ameliorate extrapyramidal symptoms—the commonly occurring adverse reactions to psychotropic drugs such as the phenothiazines, butyrophenones, and thioxanthenes. Combination therapy with the potassium-wasting diuretics and spironolactone (an aldosterone antagonist) or triamterene can be used to reduce excessive potassium loss and avert hypokalemia.

Whereas these and other beneficial drug interactions are well known and often used in clinical practice, some interactions that are currently considered to be adverse also may be applied therapeutically. For example, the analgesic effects of meperidine and the opiates are augmented by the concurrent administration of MAO inhibitors. This interaction can be used to increase the desirable effects of the analgesics without having to increase the dose. The regimen may have a place in the relief of severe chronic pain in subjects with terminal malignant disease.

In spite of the well-known adverse reactions and dangers that attend the concomitant administration of many drugs, it is reassuring that the selective use of certain drug interactions has a positive place in pharmacotherapy; "sweet uses of adversity" as Hollister [63] has so aptly phrased it.

IV. COLLECTION, EVALUATION, AND REPORTING OF ADVERSE EXPERIENCES (AEs) AND ADVERSE REACTIONS (ADRs) TO DRUGS, DEVICES, AND BIOLOGICS

A. Collection of Adverse Experiences: Investigational Products

The adverse experience potential of an investigational new drug may to some extent be indicated by its molecular structural similarities to other drugs of known actions and by pharmacological and toxicological preclinical trials in appropriate species of laboratory animals. The full adverse reaction profile of a drug, however, can only be determined by human experience, and this not until the drug has been administered to a relatively large number of subjects of different ages, both sexes, and diverse ethnic groups, and for extended periods.

Phase 1, 2, and 3 clinical research programs required by the FDA and similar regulatory bodies in other countries are sufficient to define the more frequently occurring adverse experiences and to establish the safety of an investigational new drug. The safety evaluation during clinical drug development is not expected to characterize rare adverse reactions—for example, those occurring in less than 1 in 1,000 subjects—but is expected to characterize and quantify the safety profile of a drug over a reasonable duration of time consistent with the intended long-term use of the drug. The number of subjects treated for 6 months at dosage levels intended for clinical use should be adequate to characterize the pattern of AEs over time that can actually be claimed as adverse reactions only when the cause is a result of prescribing the experimental product. Usually from 300 to 600 subjects should be adequate.

There is concern that, although they are likely to be uncommon, some AEs may increase in frequency or severity with time, or that some serious AEs may occur only after drug treatment for more than 6 months. Therefore, some subjects should be treated with the drug for 12 months. In the absence of more information about the relationship of AEs to treatment duration, selection of a specific number of subjects to be monitored for 1 year is to a large extent a judgment based on the probability of detecting a given AE frequency level and practical considerations. One hundred subjects exposed for a minimum of 1 year is considered acceptable [64].

In response to a clinical trial in subjects with chronic hepatitis B infection, in which 5 of 15 subjects died of delayed hepatotoxicity after using fialuridine (FIAU), the FDA reviewed the requirements for the design of clinical trials, data analysis, and reporting. A task force recommended that a "worst-case" analysis be conducted in a semiannual report; a placebo control group should be included in early clinical trials when the underlying disease process is likely to produce AEs that might be confused with toxicity; the sponsor should estimate the expected incidence of death and serious AEs from the disease and should develop appropriate "stopping" rules; the length and type of the follow-up period should be described to detect delayed toxicities; and the sponsor should develop safety monitoring and evaluation programs [65].

B. Collection of Adverse Experiences: Postmarketing

It is only by continued close surveillance and tracking after a drug is available for general clinical administration, under an expanded variety of circumstances, that rare, sometimes severe, and even life-threatening adverse drug reactions or interactions are detected. Only then can the full adverse reaction spectrum of a drug be finally delineated. An example of a serious adverse reaction that was discovered postmarketing is the occurrence of serious regurgitant cardiac valvular disease during use of dexfenfluramine, an anti-obesity drug, especially when the drug is used in combination with phentermine (FEN/PHEN). It should be noted that use of the combination was not approved by the FDA.

C. Methods for Obtaining Adverse Experience Information From Subjects

There are three generally accepted methods by which adverse experiences may be elicited from trial subjects:

1. Systematic questioning using a checklist containing the adverse experiences considered most likely to occur with the particular drug being studied.
2. Direct questioning without the use of a formal checklist. Questions concerning untoward symptoms should be put to subjects in

such a way that they do not, by suggestion, lead the subject into giving invalid information.

3. Recording only those adverse experiences that are volunteered by the subjects or observed by the investigator or others involved in the trial.

Of the three methods, the first, or checklist technique, has the greatest tendency to make subjects introspective regarding their symptoms. Not surprisingly, this approach elicits the largest number of adverse experience reports. Regardless of the method used, however, it is imperative that the questions be applied in the same way at each subject assessment, preferably by the same person, for the duration of the trial. It is also recommended that subjects be carefully questioned *prior* to administration of investigational products. It is remarkable how many so-called adverse reactions are, in fact, symptoms of other conditions present before the trial treatment starts, and therefore the principle of collecting adverse experiences becomes even more valuable.

D. Reporting of Adverse Experiences and Adverse Reactions

Drug safety and adverse reactions are closely related in an inversely proportional manner. In the United States, drug safety is under strict legislative control mandated by the FDA. Federal regulations require a sponsor to report adverse experiences and reactions for an investigational product at both the investigational and the postmarketing stages.

1. Investigational Stage

A distinction should be made between an ADR and an AE. An AE is any untoward medical occurrence in a clinical investigation subject who has been given a pharmaceutical product, which does not necessarily have a causal relationship with this treatment. An AE can therefore be any unfavorable and unintended sign (including an abnormal laboratory finding), symptom, or disease temporally associated with the use of medicinal (investigational) product, whether or not related to the medicinal (investigational) product [1].

During the clinical investigation of a new drug (phases 1–3, and 3b) before FDA approval, it is the sponsor's responsibility to notify the FDA of all AEs as described in the chapter pertaining to the IND. The FDA has recently revised the regulations for expedited reporting of AEs and issued definitions of terms to comply with recent ICH Guidelines [66].

Serious AE.   A serious AE is one that occurs at any dose that results in any of the following outcomes: death, a life-threatening AE, in-patient hospitalization or prolongation of existing hospitalization, a persistent or significant disability/incapacity, or a congenital anomaly/birth defect. Important medical events that may not result in death, be life-threatening, or require hospitalization may be considered serious AEs when, based upon appropriate medical judgment, they may jeopardize the subjects and may require medical or surgical interventions to prevent one of the outcomes listed in this definition. Examples of such medical events include allergic bronchospasm requiring intensive treatment in an emergency room or at home, blood dyscrasias or convulsions that do not result in in-patient hospitalization, or the development of drug dependency or drug abuse.

Life-Threatening AE. This is defined as any AE that places the subject, in the view of the investigator, at immediate risk of death from the reaction as it occurred (i.e., it does not include a reaction that, had it occurred in a more severe form, might have caused death).

Disability. This is defined as a substantial disruption of a person's ability to carry out normal life functions.

Associated with the Use of the Drug. There is a reasonable possibility that the experience may have been caused by the drug.

Unexpected AE. An unexpected AE is any reaction, the specificity or severity of which is not consistent with the current Investigator's Brochure, or, if an Investigator's Brochure is not required or available, the specificity or severity of which is not consistent with the risk information described in the general investigational plan or elsewhere in the current application, as amended. For example, under this definition, hepatic necrosis would be unexpected (by virtue of greater severity) if the Investigator's Brochure referred only to elevated hepatic enzymes or hepatitis. "Unexpected," as used in this definition, refers to an adverse drug experience that has not been previously observed (e.g., included in the Investigator's Brochure) rather than one that has not been anticipated from the pharmacological properties of the pharmaceutical product.

When a serious adverse drug experience occurs, the investigator will provide the following information:

Subject identification number, age, and sex.
Duration of drug administration (includes dates of drug administration).
Dose administered (whether or not the code was broken in the case of a double-blind trial) and route of administration.

Indication of drug (diagnosis for use).

Description of adverse experience, including date and time of onset, as well as the date and time the event subsided. The outcome (recovered, alive with sequelae, dead) should also be stated. Any laboratory evaluations, ECGs, autopsy reports, etc., that are needed for understanding the adverse experience should be submitted.

Concomitant medication, including the dose and dates of administration.

Current disease state, diagnosis, and medical history.

Dechallenge and rechallenge information.

Whether the subject was in imminent danger of death at the time of the adverse experience.

Relationship to trial drug. The investigator should state whether there was a reasonable possibility that the adverse experience was caused by the drug/device.

Whether the adverse experience was unexpected.

The investigator should complete and sign the appropriate form as required by the FDA. The FDA Medical Products Reporting Program (MedWatch) issued FDA Form 3500A for use by user facilities, distributors, and manufacturers for "mandatory" reporting of adverse experiences and product problems during the use of drugs, biologicals, and devices. Form 3500 is for use by health care professionals and consumers for voluntary reporting. Adverse experiences associated with vaccines are reported to the FDA and the CDC using the VAERS.

If the AE was not resolved at the time of the initial contact with the investigator, the investigational site will be contacted on a regular basis to determine the status of the subject until the AE has resolved.

If the serious adverse experience is unexpected, fatal, or life-threatening and associated with the use of the drug, then the division of the FDA that has the responsibility for review of the IND will be informed by telephone or facsimile transmission as soon as possible, and no later than 7 calendar days after, of the first knowledge of the event. The initial notification must be followed by a complete written IND Safety Report within 15 calendar days. All investigators involved in a multicenter trial must be notified in writing within 15 calendar days. In addition, they, in turn, must apprise the individual governing IRBs of the report.

The FDA and all participating investigators will be notified in a written IND Safety Report of any adverse experience associated with use of the drug that is both serious and unexpected. Each notification must be made no later than 15 calendar days after receipt of the information.

2. Postmarketing Stage

Marketing authorization holders are required to develop written procedures for the surveillance, receipt, evaluation, and reporting of postmarketing AEs to the FDA. The definitions of postmarketing adverse experiences and unexpected adverse experiences are as follows [66]:

Adverse Experience. An AE is any experience associated with the use of a biological product in humans, whether or not considered product related, including the following: an AE occurring in the course of the use of a biological product in professional practice; an adverse experience occurring from an overdose of the product, whether accidental or intentional; an adverse experience occurring from abuse of the product; an adverse experience occurring from withdrawal of the product; and any failure of expected pharmacological action.

Unexpected AE. An unexpected AE is any that is not listed in the current labeling for the biological product. This includes events that may be symptomatically and pathophysiologically related to an event listed in the labeling, but differ from the event because of greater severity or specificity. "Unexpected," as used in this definition, refers to an adverse experience that has not been previously observed (i.e., included in the labeling), rather than one that has not been anticipated from the pharmacological properties of the pharmaceutical product.

The definitions of a serious and life-threatening AE are the same definitions as used for investigational drugs.

Adverse drug experiences that are both serious and unexpected, whether foreign or domestic, must be reported to the FDA as soon as possible, but no later than 15 calendar days after the initial receipt of the information (15-day Alert Reports). Form 3500A or the C10MS 1 form must be used for reporting. Additional information must be forwarded to the FDA in a follow-up report.

In addition, the frequency of reports of serious and unexpected AEs and reports of therapeutic failure must be reviewed periodically, and an increase in frequency must be reported to the FDA within 15 working days of determining the significant increase. Postmarketing periodic AE reports are required at quarterly intervals for 3 years from the date of approval of the NDA and then at annual intervals.

E. Assessment of Adverse Reactions

The most difficult part of ADR reporting is the accurate assessment of the causal relationship of a drug to an alleged reaction. The likelihood that a drug contributes to, or is responsible for, an adverse reaction with any degree of certainty can be established only if adequate information is available.

The degrees of causal relationship between a drug and a suspected adverse reaction are defined as follows:

1. A remote causal relationship between a drug and an event exists when the temporal association is such that the drug would not have had any reasonable association with the observed event.

2. A possible causal relationship between a drug and an event exists when the reaction (1) follows a reasonable temporal sequence from administration of the drug; (2) follows a known response pattern to the suspected drug; or (3) could have been produced by the subject's clinical state or other modes of therapy administered to the subject.

3. A probable causal relationship between a drug and an event exists when the reaction (1) follows a known response pattern to the drug; (2) is confirmed by withdrawal of the drug; or (3) cannot be reasonably explained by the known characteristics of the subject's clinical state.

4. A definite causal relationship between a drug and an event exists when the reaction (1) follows a reasonable temporal sequence from the time of drug administration or from the time the drug level has been established in body fluids or tissues; (2) follows a known response pattern to the suspected drug; or (3) is confirmed by improvement upon withdrawal of the drug (dechallenge) and reappearance of the ADR upon reintroduction of the suspect drug (rechallenge).

Accurate assessment of a causal relationship of a drug to an adverse reaction is beset with many difficulties. Most prominent among these are (1) incomplete time-related drug-related information; (2) multiplicity of drugs administered in most cases; (3) lack of an objective means of demonstrating a direct relationship between a drug and an adverse reaction; and (4) the limited number of reaction patterns of the body to the entire range of physical, chemical, and biological causes of disease. Because of these and other potential problems, the majority of drug-induced diseases fall into the "possible" category. Very few can unequivocally be labeled as definite.

V. SUMMARY

The main objective of all AE and ADR reporting programs continues to be the collection of data sufficient to evaluate, in a meaningful way, the benefit-to-risk ratio of new drugs. In this way, significant drug hazards may be detected and corrective measures implemented at an early stage. In extreme cases, this may even involve total withdrawal of the drug from further clinical investigation or, in the case of approved drugs, from general clinical use. Whereas a number of official regulations governing clinical research may seem to be overly restrictive at times, the overall concern for proven safety and established efficacy of new drugs cannot be questioned. All new drug development efforts must be supported by scientific presentation of accurate data and the continuing recognition of the rights of all subjects participating in clinical drug trials.

REFERENCES

1. Federal Register. May 9, 1997; Vol. 62. No. 90.
2. Lazarou J, Pomeranz BH, Corey PN. Incidence of adverse drug reactions in hospitalized patients: a meta-analysis of prospective trials. JAMA 1998; 279: 1200.
3. Turner P, Richens A. In: Clinical Pharmacology. Edinburgh: Churchill Livingstone, 1973.
4. Nicholson HO. Cytotoxic drugs in pregnancy. J Obstet Gynecol Br Cwlth 1968; 75:307.
5. Shaw EB, Steinbach HL. Aminopterin induced fetal malformation. Am J Dis Child 1968; 115:477.
6. Brandner Nussle M. Foetopathie due a l'aminopterine avec stenose congenitale de l'espace medallaire des os tubulaires longs. Ann Radiol 1969; 12:703.
7. Warrell DW, Taylor R. Outcome for the foetus of mothers receiving prednisolone during pregnancy. Lancet 1968; 1:117.
8. Elmes PC. Antibacterial drugs used in miscellaneous infections. In: Meyler L, Herxheimer A, eds. Side Effects of Drugs. Amsterdam: Excerpta Medica, 1972.
9. Kouvalainen K, Unnirus V, Wasz-Hockert O. Side effects of chloramphenicol in prematurely born infants. Ann Paediatr Fenn 1967; 13:23.
10. Hirsh J, Cade JF, Gallus AS. Fetal effects of coumarin administered during pregnancy. Blood 1965; 26:623.
11. Mahairas GH, Weingold AB. Fetal hazard with anti-coagulant therapy. Am J Obstet Gynecol 1963; 85:237.
12. Crooks J. Thyroid and antithyroid drugs. In: Meyler L, Herxheimer A, eds. Side Effects of Drugs. Amsterdam: Exerpta Medica, 1972.
13. Zucker P, Simon G. Prolonged symptomatic neonatal hypoglycemia associated with maternal chlorpropamide therapy. Pediatrics 1968; 42:824.
14. Hussar A. The hypoglycemic agents—their interactions. J Am Pharm Assoc 1970; 100:169.
15. ICM Harmonized Tripartate Guideline (S5B). Detection of Toxicity to Reproduction for Medicinal Products.
16. ICM Harmonized Tripartate Guideline (S5B). Toxicity to Male Fertility.

17. ICM Topic S_2B Document. Standard Battery of Genotoxicity Tests.
18. Kramer M. Delirium as a complication of imipramine therapy in the aged. Am J Psychiatry 1963; 120:502.
19. Bender AD. Pharmacodynamic consequences of aging and their implications in the treatment of the elderly patient. Med Ann 1967; 36:267.
20. Gibson JM II. Barbiturate delirium. Practitioner 1966; 197:345.
21. Hamilton LD. Aged brain and the phenothiazines. Geriatrics 1966; 21:131.
22. Ayd FJ Jr. Tranquilizers and the ambulatory geriatric patient. J Am Geriatr Soc 1960; 8:909.
23. Hollister LE. Nervous system reaction to drugs. Ann NY Acad Sci 1965; 123:342.
24. Ritama V, Vapaatalo HI, Neuvoner PJ. Phenothiazines and intestinal dilatation. Lancet 1969; 1:470.
25. Jick H, Slone D, Borda T. Efficacy and toxicity of heparin in relation to age and sex. N Engl J Med 1968; 279:284.
26. Pina LM. Drugs widely used off label in pediatrics, report of the pediatric use survey working group of the pediatric subcommittee. Draft (Federal Register), August 15, 1997; Vol. 62. No. 158.
27. Powell DA. Chloramphenicol: new perspectives on an old drug. Drug Intelligences Clinical Pharmacy 1982; 16:295.
28. Oski FA. Principles and Practice of Pediatrics. 2d ed. Philadelphia: J. B. Lippincott, 1994:864.
29. Nathan DG. Hematology of Infancy and Childhood. 4th ed. Philadelphia: W. B. Saunders, 1993:92.
30. Kauffman RE. Fentanyl, fads, and folly: who will adopt the therapeutic orphans. J Pediatr 1991; 119:588.
31. McCloskey JJ. Bupivacaine toxicity secondary to continuous caudal epidural infusion in pediatric patients. Anesth Analg 1992; 75:287.
32. Fisher DM. Neuromuscular effects of vecuronium (ORG NC45) in infants and pediatric patients during N_2O halothane anesthesia. Anesthesiology 1983; 58:519.
33. Agarwal R. Seizures occurring in pediatric patients receiving continuous infusion of bupivacaine. Anesth Analg 1992; 75:284.
34. Mevorach DL. Bupivacaine toxicity secondary to continuous caudal epidural infusion in pediatric patients. Anesth Analg 1993; 77:1305.
35. Cystic fibrosis and colonic strictures. Editorial. J Clin Gastroenterol 1995; 21:2.
36. Olkkola KT. A potentially hazardous interaction between erythromycin and midazolam. Clin Pharmacol Ther 1993; 53:298.
37. Hiller A. Unconsciousness associated with midazolam and erythromycin. Br J Anaesth 1994; 65:826.
38. Theodore J, Millen JE, Murdaugh HV. Prolonged postoperative apnea with pseudo-cholinesterase deficiency. Am Rev Respir Dis 1967; 96:508.
39. Evans DAP, Manley KA, McKusick VA. Genetic control of isoniazid metabolism in man. BMJ 1960; 2:485.
40. Goldberg A, Remington C. Diseases of porphyrin metabolism. Springfield, Illinois: Thomas, 1962.

41. O'Reilly RA, Aggler PM. trials in coumarin anti-coagulant drugs: hereditary resistance in man. Fed Proc 1965; 24:1266.
42. Trey C, Lipworth L, Davidson CS. Clinical syndrome of halothane hepatitis. Anesth Analg Curr Res 1969; 48:1033.
43. Siegal M, Lee SL, Peress NS. The epidemiology of drug-induced systemic lupus erythematosus. Arthritis Rheum 1967; 10:407.
44. Dewar HA, Peaston MJT. Three cases resembling polyarteritis nodosa arising during treatment with guanethidine. BMJ 1964; 2:609.
45. Baldwin DS, Levine BB, McCluskey T. Renal failure and interstitial nephritis due to penicillin and methicillin. N Engl J Med 1968; 279:1245.
46. Popper H. Cholestasis. Ann Rev Med 1968; 19:39.
47. Zupko AG. Drug interactions—a new professional responsibility. Pharm Times, 1969; 33(Sep), 38(Oct).
48. Autian J. Interaction between medicaments and plastics. J Mondial Pharm 1966; 316.
49. Cooper J. Interaction between medicaments and containers. J Mondial Pharm 1966; 259.
50. Kunin CM, Finland M. Clinical pharmacology of the tetracycline antibiotics. Clin Pharmacol Ther 1961; 2:51.
51. Brodie BB. Clinical effects of interaction between drugs. Displacement of one drug by another from carrier or receptor sites. Proc R Soc Med 1965; 58:946.
52. Eisen MJ. Combined effect of sodium warfarin and phenylbutazone. JAMA 1964; 189:64.
53. Goodman LS, Gilman A. The pharmacological basis of therapeutics. New York: MacMillan, 1980.
54. Burns JJ, Conney AH. Clinical effects of interaction between drugs. Enzyme stimulation and inhibition in the metabolism of drugs. Proc R Soc Med 1965; 58:955.
55. Vessle ES, Pasananti GT, Greene FE. Impairment of drug metabolism in man by allopurinol and nortriptyline. N Engl J Med 1970; 283:354.
56. Jackson JE, Powell RJ, Wandell M. Cimetidine-theophylline interaction. Pharmacologist 1980; 22:231.
57. Donovan MA, Heagerty M, Patel L. Cimetidine and the bioavailability of propranolol. Lancet 1981; 1:164.
58. Serlin MJ, Moisman S, Sibeon RG. Cimetidine: interactions with oral anticoagulants in man. Lancet 1979; 2:317.
59. Klotz U, Reiman I. Delayed clearance of diazepam due to cimetidine. N Engl J Med 1980; 320:1012.
60. Doering W. Quinidine-digoxin interaction. N Engl J Med 1979; 301:400.
61. Hartshorn EA. In: Francke DE, Handbook of Drug Interactions. Cincinnati, Ohio, 1970.
62. Cadwallader DE. Biopharmaceutics and drug interactions. Nutley, New Jersey: Roche Laboratories, 1971.
63. Hollister LE, The beneficial effects of drug interactions: sweet uses of adversity. New York, Symposium of Drug Interactions; Drug Information Association, January 1972.

64. Federal Register. March 1, 1994; Vol. 59. No. 40:9746–9748. International Conference on Harmonisation; Draft Guideline on the Extent of Population Exposure Required to Assess Clinical Safety for Drugs Intended for Long-Term Treatment of Non-Life Threatening Conditions.
65. Food Drug Cosmetic Law. Report No. 1626. November 29, 1993.
66. Federal Register, Vol. 62, No. 194. October 7, 1997 (21 CFR Parts 20, 310, 312, 314 and 600). Expedited Safety Reporting Requirements for Human Drug and Biological Products.

12

Biostatistics in Pharmaceutical Product Development—Facts, Recommendations, and Solutions

Mark Bradshaw
Covance, Inc., Princeton, New Jersey, U.S.A.

I. INTRODUCTION: THE ROLE OF BIOSTATISTICS IN LATE-STAGE PHARMACEUTICAL DEVELOPMENT

The premise of this chapter is that many of today's standard pharmaceutical development practices in experimental design, trial conduct, and statistical analysis are in need of review and revision if the goals of assuring the development and approval of safe, effective pharmaceuticals are to be maintained. The last four decades have confirmed the value of prospective, controlled, blinded, randomized clinical trials in pharmaceutical development. Refinements of experimental designs and statistical analyses, along with global harmonization of regulatory dossiers, have led to our present state, in which the basic tenets of Phase I–III clinical trials are ubiquitous. The current chapter will not cover a great deal of this old ground, but a sense of complacency with our status quo could lead us to ignore some serious problems with many of the current practices.

The role of the biostatistician in this process is more important than ever, but the statistical community must be challenged to develop better approaches to solving some old limitations and some new problems. Some of these problems will be explored in this chapter along with recommendations for solutions. The areas selected for review are those that in the author's opinion require the attention of statisticians in both pharmaceutical sponsor organizations and regulatory agencies. Some provocative examples will be highlighted in this introduction, and some will be covered in greater depth.

Alpha = 0.05. Biostatistical analysis of the human clinical trials that are required during the last stages of the pharmaceutical development process has effectively become a hurdle over which every drug, device, and biological must jump on its way to market. The all-important p-value is often used as a surrogate for comprehensive statistical and medical judgment by scientists and regulators whose job it is to take into account a wide variety of information, weigh it all against risks and benefits, and make the difficult decision either to provide a new medical miracle to awaiting subjects or to prevent a dangerous product from causing harm.

A cursory review of most introductory statistics texts will usually reveal a section on inferential analysis that explains how one can make a qualified leap from a sample to a population; then it will dutifully caution that a p-value should only be viewed as one type of evidence in evaluating that leap of faith. It is designed to be one of many ingredients leading to a rich, deep understanding of the phenomenon under study, when that phenomenon is surrounded by unexplained variability. Inferential statistics and the p-value are particularly useful when it is not possible to understand or control some of the sources of variability, and this clearly applies to human biological data.

Many texts caution that confidence intervals are more appropriate decision-making tools than an arbitrary gold-standard p-value (alpha) in this context. If a particular alpha level is to be used in decision making, its value should always reflect the circumstances of each different situation, taking into account both the risks of a false positive decision as well as the costs of a false negative. Nonetheless, the pharmaceutical approval process has effectively ignored these elementary cautions. It has instead established a single alpha value of 0.05 as the Procrustean bed into which every potential new product must somehow fit before it can be approved for the market.

The Price of Power. With regard to the demonstration of efficacy of a new product, achievement of a p-value ≤ 0.05 comparing the new therapy to the control group is critical as discussed above. However it is often not well understood that most products with even a modest potential therapeutic benefit can clear this hurdle if the company sponsoring the product is willing to spend enough money and/or time to perform a very large trial. Sample size can overcome the limitations of modest benefits. Hence the true decision criteria regarding effectiveness can sometimes be more financial than medical or scientific.

Is this the best model for the evaluation and approval of new therapies? Should a product's approval be based in large part on the financial strength of the sponsor, and the value of the product's future revenue potential?

These are the very real questions that the next generation of statisticians, medical scientists, and regulators must face.

Safety by Design. Safety concerns are the other half of the approval process. Surely sound statistical criteria should be used to quantify this critical process and ensure that public health concerns are addressed appropriately, both before and after approval. Safety is of concern for both the clinical trial participants and the future subjects if the product is approved. Yet the simple questions "How much safety data is enough?" and "Where do the greatest risks lie?" are usually answered based on regulatory precedent rather than any statistical modeling of risk or variability.

Precedent may be an adequate societal basis for common law and a good way to price real estate; but the unprecedented types of pharmaceutical products under development today must be evaluated against standards relevant to their unique risks. Historic precedents will be of little help in judging risk in the brave new world of tightly targeted therapies developed through genomics and proteomics.

Signal Detection and EDA (Exploratory Data Analysis). As clinical trials progress we are increasingly awash in a continuous flow of raw data, but the early detection of signals amidst the ocean of noise receives very little attention until a signal is made obvious by unfortunate and potentially avoidable human costs. Statistical principles can indeed be applied to build new models to estimate risk and create reasonable monitoring processes and criteria, but to date there is very little activity in this direction. Efficacy targets are required to be identified in advance along with analysis methodologies. Based on the results of both preclinical and Phase I clinical trials it is possible to identify for new drugs those areas of "reasonably foreseeable risk" for safety concerns.

Once identified biologically, targets for proactive surveillance during the clinical trials can be used by statisticians to develop highly sensitive monitoring schemes, trend analyses, and cross-variable signal and syndrome detection. Exploratory Data Analysis (EDA) techniques abound in other industries. However in pharmaceutical development we are far more advanced in real-time data collection technologies than in the use of statistical techniques for the ongoing analysis of trends and the detection of safety signals that may be present in the real-time flood of bits and bytes. This deficiency may be responsible in part for the postapproval withdrawal of a number of products from the market in recent years. The question for the biostatistician is whether a different paradigm for signal detection coupled with a priori targeting of reasonably foreseeable risks might identify safety issues much earlier in the clinical trial process, and well before approval and broad marketing exposure.

Sources of Bias. Finally, the very data on which safety and effectiveness decisions are made, while voluminous and scrupulously cleaned, may be of questionable value owing to the very process by which investigators and subjects are selected (not randomly sampled) and the data are revised (not simply cleaned) to fit our preconceived data models. Regulatory oversight has focused not on the scientific validity of the sampling frame or the meaningfulness of the data, but rather on adherence to a set of technical procedures that may assure neither. These three points deserve clarification.

Sampling. Statistical analysis relies on a clear distinction between random variability and variation in results due to deliberate manipulation of known factors in an experiment. Treatments are assigned systematically to subjects; while individual subject characteristics contribute to random variability. It is important to understand that studies are not performed to learn what happened to the participants—they are conducted to provide a basis for predicting what will likely happen to an entire future subject population if a product is approved and broadly marketed. Inferences from a sample to a larger population are only possible when certain statistical principles are followed in the selection of that sample. Those principles are rarely followed in clinical research today, and inferences to future subject populations are therefore not generally supported from a statistical standpoint.

Data Refinement. Data begins as clinical information collected from subjects in a trial. Initially it reflects some component of "truth" about treatment effects, and some component of variability or "error." Statistical analysis techniques can estimate the magnitude of the error component, and in turn use that as a metric to estimate the size and reliability of the truth component. But statisticians generally require consistent and relatively simple clinical assessments to create data tabulations and perform analyses. Raw data often does not meet this expectation. When we engage in data cleaning, the resulting altered data consists of three components: truth, error, and systematic bias. The impact of systematic bias introduced during the cleaning process is not normally assessed statistically, or even widely recognized as a factor. Yet as with the Heisenberg uncertainty principle, the act of making the data conform to our preferred measurement systems may obscure the very phenomena we seek to understand.

Regulatory Oversight. As discussed above, the pharmaceutical industry has drifted into a number of subject recruitment and data refinement practices that, though no doubt well-intentioned, may at times undermine the very basis for statistical analysis and decision-making. Regulators' scrutiny of the processes and the electronic systems for authorizing and tracking data changes, along with the industry's rigorous interpretation and adherence to the letter of those regulations, has effectively pointed the spotlight at the individual trees, missing the forest. Through extensive audit trails and authentication procedures we know who changed what to what, when they did it, and what reason they gave. But understanding the implications of the process by which investigators are influenced to "refine" data to fit preconceived data collection models is different from simply assuring that investigators have, at the end of the day, formally authorized each of these changes. Our industry appears focused on the latter, not the former.

In summary, the intention of clinical trials is to forecast accurately the benefits and risks of new therapies to the broad population of subjects seeking better therapies, while protecting the safety of those subjects who volunteer to provide the data needed to make that forecast. The design and conduct of the forecasting process in clinical trials is the role of the professional biostatistician. If we view the landscape from the perspective of the theoretical statistician, we would have to conclude that most of the studies performed today reveal little more than the outcomes for the subjects who participated in the trial, and even those outcomes can be clouded or biased by data refinement and categorization practices that are entirely compliant with current regulations and accepted practices. Strictly speaking, inference (forecasting) from such trial results to larger populations is not possible due to the violation of some critical principles of inferential statistics. Subject safety data, while voluminous, precise, and timely, is not monitored in the aggregate with adequate frequency or the best available exploratory analysis tools to assure the early detection of critical safety warning signals that could foreshadow unexpected risks.

It should be clear that the purpose of this chapter is not to review the normal role of the statistician in the pharmaceutical industry today. Instead, this chapter is intended to challenge the status quo and to highlight some critical problems and largely unmet needs that logically intersect both the expertise and the sphere of influence of professional statistician in the pharmaceutical industry. In some ways the intention is to revisit the basic tenets of experimental design and analysis to see where we have drifted away from sound scientific principles, and where we may have unexplored opportunities for the future—a future certain to be different from the past.

The topics are intended to be provocative, but there is no intent to criticize the profession or those individuals who diligently play a critical role in the industry today. As statisticians take up the challenges we face today, an expanded role for statisticians can evolve. This should lead to the ability to take full advantage of the statistical perspective, one that has already helped lead to important advancements in public health and can address the challenges of the future.

II. EXPERIMENTAL DESIGN IN CLINICAL TRIALS: THEORY AND PRACTICE

Clinical trials for a new drug, device, or biological typically are organized in three sequential phases prior to submission of the data to a regulatory agency for approval. To varying degrees the biostatistician is involved in the design and analysis of clinical trials in each of these phases.

A. Phase I trials normally involve a small number of volunteers who are not suffering from the medical condition the new entity is intended to treat. (Note that in some disease areas such as oncology, even Phase I trials are often conducted using patients as subjects, due to the adverse experiences caused by some new therapies.) One intention of these studies is to determine the nature and speed with which the new drug is distributed within the body, and then in what way and how quickly it is eliminated. This is the discipline of pharmacokinetics. Another is to determine the highest dose in man that is consistent with an acceptable level of adverse experiences.

B. Phase II comparative trials are usually the first to be conducted in subjects with the medical condition for which the new drug is targeted. The numbers of subjects are greater than in Phase I, but still well below the numbers required in Phase III. These studies usually provide the first opportunity in man to estimate the degree to which the drug may be effective in its intended therapeutic area, and the type of adverse experiences subjects may experience. Multiple dose regimens are often studied, and a large number of experimental tests and parameters are evaluated to assess both the effectiveness (efficacy) of the drug and its safety. At the conclusion of Phase II, sufficient evidence should be available to choose a specific dosing regimen, a detailed experimental design for proof of efficacy, a small set of pivotal efficacy variables to measure, and a target for the expected magnitude of clinical effect. In other words, a successful Phase II program provides encouragement that the drug will be safe and effective and at the same time sets the stage for the Phase III pivotal proof-of-efficacy trials.

C. Phase III comparative trials are usually large in numbers of clinical investigators and subjects, determined both by regulatory agency requirements and by statistical forecasts based on Phase II and other relevant data. The trials are often international in scope and cover multiple years in duration. A few predefined efficacy parameters are measured in a large number of subjects treated in a fashion similar to the intended treatment regimen for the drug, should it be approved for general use. Safety data are also collected in the form of adverse experience reports and (typically) a panel of laboratory analyses of blood samples collected from subjects at various time points during the trial. If the results of these trials demonstrate adequate safety, clinically meaningful efficacy results, and importantly a statistically significant benefit of the new drug over a control group, a marketing approval may be granted by the regulatory agency.

Sample Size and Experimental Design. An important role of the biostatistician is to collaborate with medical, regulatory, and data management experts in the design of these studies. Trial design includes the definition of what to measure, how often to measure it, how to select subjects and randomly assign treatments to them, and how to analyze the results. Everything must be prespecified in the clinical protocol, including the expected results, all analysis strategies, and the rationale for the number of subjects to be studied. The latter is called the sample size.

Although a statistician should be consulted on all the factors above, in practice the most common reason why a statistician is consulted at the beginning of a trial is to establish the sample size. Fortunately, to answer this single question, all the factors above must be considered, so that one way or another the statistician usually winds up in a collaboration on experimental design. Because the discussion often starts with sample size, we will also start there.

A clear understanding of the required sample size is particularly critical for Phase III trials, due to the requirement for the establishment of statistical significance in the final analyses of Phase III trials to support a submission for marketing approval. Even if a new drug seems to show evidence of clinical efficacy, without a statistically significant result the trial will normally not be accepted as pivotal evidence in support of an approval. Insufficient sample size is one of the leading causes of Phase III trial failures for drugs that otherwise appear to have adequate safety and efficacy for approval.

In principle, the results of Phase II should provide enough evidence to establish the required sample size for Phase III trials. Factors include the expected size of the clinical benefit of the new drug relative to the control group, the nature of the primary efficacy parameter (continuous, discrete, time-to-event, etc.), the variability one can expect to see in the data from the subjects in the trial, the p-value required to establish statistical significance (called the alpha level and normally set equal to or less than 0.050 by the regulatory agency), and the degree of risk the drug's sponsor is willing to take that the trial will fail to achieve the required alpha level even though the drug may in fact have the magnitude of efficacy predicted by the protocol. The last item, when described in a positive way as assurance instead of risk, is called statistical power. It is generally defined as the probability that a statistically significant outcome of a single trial will occur when the drug performs as expected.

This at first sounds quite odd. If a drug performs as expected, why shouldn't the trial always show a statistically significant benefit if the trial was designed correctly? The answer lies in the concept of a sample, and in a biological fact of life called unexplained variability.

We are actually not interested in the treatment results for the subjects in a clinical trial. We are instead very interested in the forecast that a trial allows us to make about the future results of treating an entire population.

Individual biological characteristics of humans along with the many differences in their daily lives plus the limitations of our understanding of biology and pharmacology make it impossible to predict with complete certainty how an individual subject will respond to a drug. This also means that the response of one individual cannot with certainty predict the response of another individual to the same drug. Yet the goal of clinical research is to predict the responses for both efficacy and safety of the entire population of subjects who may receive prescriptions for the drug if it is approved and marketed around the world.

Unpredictable variability in individual responses, coupled with the need to forecast the aggregate responses of an entire population of future subjects, provide the reasons why biostatisticians are involved in clinical trial design and analysis. Inferential statistics is the discipline of making inferences about populations by analyzing data from samples that were drawn from those populations in a prescribed way. If we could somehow look into a crystal ball and measure the actual future responses to a new drug from the entire population, there would be no need for clinical trials or inferential statistics. The best we can do, however, is to analyze a sample, and understand that the results from that sample are unlikely to match exactly what our crystal ball would show us about the population, owing to unexplained individual variability.

If we make an important assumption that the sample was drawn at random from the population, then the larger the sample, the closer the aggregate sample results will come to matching the future response of the overall population. Now we can answer the paradox raised earlier. A clinical trial may fail to show a significant result even if the drug being studied actually does meet its design criteria. The reason is that the trial is based on a sample. The aggregate results from the sample reflect both the overall population response and some degree of random variability. The larger the sample, the smaller the effect of the variability on the overall results. Inferential statistics allows us to quantify our uncertainty in this regard. Statistical power measures the degree to which the intended sample size can overcome unpredictable variability in subject response, and the degree to which we can be confident that the results of the sample will approximate the future response of the population.

Sensitivity and Cost. To put it simply, increasing the sample size in a trial increases the level of assurance that an effective drug will reach statistical significance when the results of the trial are analyzed using the normal statistical techniques. Because every sponsor of a new drug has some financial and time limitations, sample sizes are always a compromise between what is ideal and what is affordable. The biostatistician must be involved in defining the parameters around this compromise.

One consequence of these facts is that the sensitivity of a trial to detect a statistically significant efficacy effect for a new drug depends in part on sample size. All other things being equal, the larger the sample size, the less effective a drug must be to show a significant, and potentially approvable, result. Financial investment in the clinical trial process can be an important determinant of ultimate marketing approval. It is often not clearly understood that this statistical fact has important societal implications.

Recommendations. Although a major paradigm shift would be required in our thinking about statistical gold standards for approvals of new drugs, it would be consistent with sound statistical principles to abandon the rigid and ubiquitous alpha $= 0.05$ hurdle for regulatory approval. In its place could be an a priori process for establishing the treatment effect size consistent with clinically meaningful benefit, coupled with an agreement as to both the acceptable width of a confidence interval around that benefit and the degree of assurance required for that confidence interval. The latter could be specified for several confidence intervals, designed to show how differences in required precision affect the width of the interval. These parameters would be established based on known or expected risks, as well as the severity of the disease and the availability of alternative, effective, and safe therapies.

For example, a novel oncology therapy with a good (expected) safety profile relative to currently available therapies might be required to show a 20% improvement in median survival in subjects who have shown progression of disease after treatment with the best currently approved therapies. Because of the lack of effective alternatives for these subjects and assuming that a clean safety profile is established, an 80% confidence interval may be deemed adequate providing the lower bound does not include 0% improvement.

On the other hand, consider a trial vs. placebo on a new product with no claimed advantage over existing drugs in a therapeutic area already crowded with safe, effective products that use the same mechanism of action and have well-known safety profiles. Here the minimum therapeutic benefit could be based on known competitors, even if the clinical trial compared the study drug against placebo, owing to public health concerns of exposing subjects to unknown risks when a variety of safe and effective therapies already exist. The required confidence interval width may be quite narrow, and the assurance as to the width may need to be very high. Implications for sample size would clearly be very different as well. The challenge of course would be establishing a more flexible set of boundaries while maintaining objective decision parameters and repeatable decision processes. While these challenges are daunting in the face of the need to provide a regulatory atmosphere that encourages new drug development and predictable standards over the large number of years between compound discovery and marketing, the need for a more rich and thoughtful approach to the evaluation of efficacy and safety is clear, and the simplistic reliance on a single industry-wide standard p-value must be challenged.

Random Sampling. Underlying all of inferential statistics and the ability to forecast population benefits from clinical trials are two requirements with regard to random processes. First, it is necessary that the subjects in clinical trials represent a randomly chosen and representative sample of the population of future subjects in the total population eligible for the use of the drug, should it be approved. Second, it is essential for comparative trials that treatments be randomly assigned to clinical trial subjects. While most major trials carefully adhere to the second requirement, few if any follow the first.

In practice, medical professionals are selected to participate as investigators in clinical trials based on a number of factors, none of which reflect any element of random selection. Many self-select once they learn of a trial in their area of specialization. Others are selected because of the sponsor's past experiences with them in similar trials. Others are recruited for reasons ranging from their willingness to assure the recruitment of large numbers of subjects to their prominence as opinion leaders in a therapeutic area. Investigators and/or their institutions often receive financial grants for their participation. Subjects may be informed of the trial by a physician who is participating as an investigator, or they may be recruited through targeted advertisement or other means. Again, there is no random component to this process. Unlike statistical survey research, where careful, stratified random sampling is used to assure that the sample both represents the population of interest and is drawn within each stratum using a random process, the subjects in a typical clinical trial cannot be said to be representative of the target population for the drug in any statistical sense.

While this may seem to be an esoteric concern, it has an important consequence. As discussed earlier, the purpose of a clinical trial is to forecast outcomes for the population, not to focus on the results of the sample itself. Inferential statistics is the discipline used to make this forecast. Virtually all the commonly used statistical inferential analysis techniques for clinical trials require that the sample be drawn from the population using a random process. The p-value itself only has meaning in this framework, where it reflects the probability that two samples (subjects treated with the new drug vs. those treated with control) could have achieved the results seen in the trial if the two treatments in fact had the same effectiveness. This is often rephrased as the probability that the apparent benefit of the new drug over the comparator, as seen in the sample results of the trial, could have happened by chance alone. If this probability is very low (i.e., $p \leq 0.05$), we are willing to conclude that chance alone cannot account for the difference, and the drug must therefore have greater efficacy than the comparator. This is what is meant by "statistical significance."

When subjects are not drawn from the population using a random process and therefore cannot be said to represent a population, inferential statistics lose their meaning. Although it may be impractical to select either investigators or subjects for clinical trials at random, it is not generally understood that the p-value of 0.05, mandated by regulatory authorities as the standard alpha level and hurdle for approval, does not measure the relationship between the subjects in a clinical trial and the target population for the new drug.

There is a critical need for statisticians to develop inferential analysis models that are valid in the face of the realities of nonrandom subject recruitment. In addition, there is a need to consider whether the current trend toward highly selective inclusion and exclusion criteria for clinical trial subjects should be reversed to allow a more representative sampling frame.

Sponsors of new drugs are tending toward increasing restrictions to reduce variability in subjects' baseline characteristics, to minimize and standardize their use of concurrent medications, and to ensure, therefore, their likelihood to demonstrate consistently the benefits of the new therapy. However a less restrictive trial design would not only lead to more rapid recruitment but also result in a sample more closely matching the intended-population.

The pattern of nonrandom subject selection will likely become even more prominent for a number of reasons. Trials in many therapeutic areas are designed with inclusion criteria that require subjects never to have received any of an increasing number of standard therapies. Because of health care practices in the industrialized countries, this often means a search for subjects in less-developed countries, and a resulting sample that does not resemble the majority of the population for whom the drug is targeted. This trend seems to be increasing, limiting the generalizability of trial results to target populations.

Another factor that will soon create more pressure toward highly selected samples of subjects for clinical trials is the future development of therapeutics that are narrowly targeted to benefit subjects with certain genetic characteristics. Advances in genomics and proteomics promise a new world of pharmaceutical products, but products requiring even tighter selection of subjects to show benefits. This will likely provide breakthrough therapies in certain areas. However the implications for clinical trials are yet to be understood. Many new therapies will be particularly effective when used in combination with other therapies, yet our current practice is generally to study them in isolation even when future use will likely be in combination. Experimental designs and statistical analysis models will both need to be reconsidered in light of these new developments. Certainly the requirements of random sampling of subjects will not be easily met.

Recommendations. In a prospective randomized comparative clinical trial, the biostatistician should be primarily concerned with the ability to generalize from the results of the trial to the future population of subjects who may receive the new therapeutic product. To do so, the sampling frame must be constructed to represent the characteristics of that future population, and some element of random selection must be present when investigators and subjects are identified for the trial. If this is not possible in a strict sense owing to limitations on available subjects, then techniques such as advanced approaches to stratified sampling may be used. Note that if relative sizes of strata do not match those of the population to which inferences will be made, adjustments will be required at the time of the analysis to achieve the correct balance. This type of analysis is not commonly accepted, however, for pivotal trials; hence a good deal of work must be done by the statistical community to improve the relevance of trials to the population of subjects for whom drugs are intended. Trials targeting subjects who are not representative of the target population, such as some types of treatment-naïve subjects or subjects with an unusual set of inclusion criteria, should be avoided during Phase III as they are more applicable to establishing proof of concept in earlier phases.

III. DATA REFINEMENT

Pivotal trial designs in general, and the design of the data collection instruments in particular (usually called Case Report Forms or CRFs), have been developed to maximize the likelihood that the final clinical database will meet the needs of the statistician for analysis and reporting, and of the sponsor to establish sufficient evidence for approval. While a clinician treating a subject thinks in terms of that individual's detailed and unique medical history and prognosis, the statistician must look at groups of subjects in the aggregate. Paradoxically, the very uniqueness of each individual that the clinician is trained to observe and analyze gets in the way of aggregate analysis. Individual variation, to a statistician, is often called "error variance;" using the metaphor above, it is the "noise" that may mask a "signal." To the clinician, it is the signal.

It is therefore understandable that statisticians and the data managers who prepare databases for statistical analysis prefer to collect data in a way that minimizes individual variation. The question, "What percentage of subjects dropped out of the trial because of an adverse experience?" can only be answered if there is an explicit question on the CRF that requires a yes or no answer. Even though a paragraph written by a clinician describing the circumstances leading to a subject's withdrawal from the trial would be far more revealing from a medical perspective, the statistician cannot tabulate a paragraph of text and must instead have a clear binary answer to tabulate.

This simple logic leads to a forced categorization and structuring of efficacy and safety data in many of the more medically interesting and complex areas of information about how a subject fares under an experimental therapeutic regimen during a clinical trial. Questions on the CRF that lead to statistical analysis range from objective (blood pressure) to subjective (physician's global assessment); from immediate (pulse) to delayed (severity of pain last week); from office-based (erythema score) to home-based (urinary incontinence diary) to laboratory-based (hematocrit count).

The nature of the data is related to the degree to which "data refinement" or "data cleaning" activities may in fact change the intended message. If on the vital signs CRF page the subject's weight is recorded as 1.90 pounds, a query may be raised suggesting this is an error, and that based on the subject's previous visit CRF pages the value should perhaps be 190 pounds. The clinician agrees and signs the correction. This seems unlikely to create a biased result in the database. However here is a more worrisome hypothetical example. The physician is asked to categorize the subject's response on a five-point scale, from "much worse" to "much better;" but the physician responds "much better in terms of overall symptoms but prognosis is actually worse." This response does not fit into the analysis scheme, and through a process of structured interrogation called data cleaning, the physician does eventually agree (after some protest) to select a single category on the prescribed five-point scale. That category will however obscure the message that was intended. What if many subjects actually show improvement in symptoms, but something else about their condition raises concerns by their physicians regarding prognosis? Will the "filters" through which statisticians "refine" the data block this critical finding from our view?

Categorization of free-text data fields provides another important source of bias, particularly critical in the area of adverse experiences. In some areas where verbatim text is accepted in the CRF, there is a post hoc process called "coding" that maps a very wide variety of verbatim text strings into a much smaller number of categorized responses. So-called coding dictionaries such as MedDRA, ICD-10, and WHO-DRUG provide the basis for mapping experiences, diseases, conditions, and medications to a standard set of codes. These codes are then further mapped to broader categories, such as body systems for adverse experiences. Codes and categories can be tabulated, summarized and analyzed by statisticians; whereas thousands of unique verbatim text strings are only used when reading an individual subject's case history. However, the act of coding and categorizing inevitably discards a great deal of information. Depending on the way they are created and used, coding schemes can create order out of chaos and reveal important patterns in the data, or obscure critical findings. The relevance of data tabulations and analyses is limited by the nature of the coding schemes and activities.

Entire syndromes can be broken into multiple codes, and after such disassembly they may disappear entirely. Here is a hypothetical example that shows what can happen if an important verbatim term is either missing from a coding system or judged to be too vague for accurate coding.

A subject in a clinical trial visits the clinic and describes a complex adverse experience that occurred two months ago to a physician who records it simply as flu-like symptoms and added a sentence of further details. These include the subject's report of general weakness, light-headedness, headache, nausea, vomiting, and possible fever. During the subject visit the physician asked the types of questions consistent with years of training and experience. The physician took all this into account, along with the timing and relationship to other events such as study drug dosing and the use of concurrent medications. Three months later, after the data have been submitted and entered into a database, this visit is reviewed and handed over to coding experts who capture the primary term "flu-like symptoms." The physician then is asked in a written communication to please be more specific and concise. After a few iterations, and more than six months past the occurrence of the event itself, it is agreed to be resubmitted as two experiences – "nausea" and "vomiting" – each with its own indication of start date, stop date, severity, and outcome categorization. Yet the description the subject gave the physician at the visit plus the physician's own questions to the subject for clarification revealed much more information. Much of this has now been lost entirely from the perspective of the statistician, who will now focus only on the coded values for purposes of analysis and summarization.

What if this very syndrome, though not available in the coding system, is an important clue as to how the drug under study affects a small but important subgroup of subjects?

The following recommendations arise from examples such as these and are intended as directions toward possible solutions to a broad set of problems that can lead to bias through data refinement and categorization activities.

1. Categorize data captured during a clinical trial in terms of its objectivity/subjectivity, immediacy or delay of collection, and source (clinician, subject, or machine). Categorize it further as to whether it is hypothesis testing, hypothesis generating, or neither. For example, a predefined efficacy criterion such as reduction in serum cholesterol is hypothesis testing and has a predefined success criterion and known variance. In the same trial, body weight may be hypothesis generating if, whether suspected previously or not, the test drug is responsible for slight losses in body weight. Vegetarian diet (diet preference in general) may also be hypothesis generating. The question, "Which meal would you choose on an airplane given the following 5 choices?" may help understand variability in response to the drug. Safety data will usually be hypothesis generating and will be hypothesis testing for those areas targeted a priori based on reasonably foreseeable risk as discussed elsewhere in this chapter.

2. For objective data, especially when collected in an automated fashion, apply objective data cleaning criteria such as range checks and consistency comparisons. If apparent errors are found that are not simply transcription errors, delve deeply into the reasons and look for systematic errors such as incorrect units, miscalibrated devices, carelessness, or data fraud.

3. For subjective data, especially when a good deal of time has elapsed since its collection, exercise extreme caution when questioning values. (For diary data provided directly by subjects, do not make any changes no matter how unlikely the values may appear – the integrity of this type of data hinges on a reliance on the unaltered values provided directly by subjects.) When such data are either critical hypothesis testing or hypothesis generating, use the required audit trail to perform two types of analyses. The first is based on the final values after data cleaning. The second is a sensitivity analysis, based on the initial values before data cleaning. If there are differences in direction or trend or significance between the two analyses, look harder at the biases that may have been introduced. Report both sets of results.

4. Formalized coding schemes such as MedDRA should be augmented by a second classification based on syndromes, groupings, concurrent drug categories, types of medical conditions, etc. that are identified a priori as being particularly relevant to the drug or class of drug under study. Creation of this trial-specific classification scheme should be led by a medical expert intimately familiar with the drug under study, the preclinical and early human data available on it, and the disease or condition in question. In addition to adverse experiences, concurrent medications, and concurrent conditions, laboratory data should also be considered in the identification of relevant

syndromes, etc. In some cases other types of safety data such as ECGs and specialized laboratory data are relevant. The use of this information for safety surveillance and signal detection throughout the trial will be discussed below. At the end of the trial, analyses based on formalized coding systems should be compared with analyses based on the trial-specific system above. Differences must be explored and thoroughly understood before conclusions are drawn regarding the outcomes of the trial. This is far from a simple exercise and will require a great deal of thought by members of several disciplines. Yet without an adjunct to conventional coding, some of the most important information from the trial can be lost from the final analysis.

5. Data cleaning efforts for variables that are not identified as critical hypothesis generating, testing, safety, or subject identification and classification variables should be minimized. Further, the detailed audit trails mentioned earlier should be used to create a new type of quality assurance benchmark – perhaps it should be called the Data Refinement Index (DRI). The proportion of data fields that were changed from their original values at least once should be tabulated for each category of data above. Categories of fields with an unusually high degree of data refinement would have a high DRI, would be highlighted, and could then be investigated in detail for the possibility of bias. Just as a high error rate between CRF and database is cause for concern regarding the integrity of the data, an unusually high amount of refinement should cause an even greater concern. The overall average DRI for each category of data, and for the data as a whole, would become an important indicator of the reliability of the database. The goal would be to minimize DRI, while still delivering analyzable data. Bear in mind that every data "correction" carries with it some probability that the new value will introduce bias into the results of the trial. We should therefore rely more on the randomization process, the sampling frame, and the control group, than on individual data point refinement to lead to aggregate results that reflect the truth about the drug under study. Note that this philosophy will also require analytic approaches that are more tolerant of the types of data irregularities that characterize medical information but are not particularly compatible with current analysis techniques.

IV. SAFETY SIGNAL DETECTION AND EXPLORATORY DATA ANALYSIS

Ongoing individual subject safety monitoring is routinely managed in a clinical trial by the investigator, the medical monitor, drug safety specialists, the CRAs, Institutional Review Boards (IRBs) or other human safety committees, and often by trial-specific Data Safety Monitoring Boards (DSMBs) that meet according to a predefined schedule (typically anywhere from quarterly to annually). With the exception of DSMBs, however, the daily ongoing review of safety data is normally done on a subject-by-subject basis. This practice is consistent with the needs of each subject in conjunction with the management of the disease, but it does not provide a sensitive method for detecting subtle trends or emerging safety warning signals that are only seen when the data are viewed across subjects.

DSMBs are well-suited to see both the forest and the trees with regard to safety, but they meet infrequently, and they are far from a standard feature of the average clinical trial. In addition, they are often focused on predefined decision rules and hypotheses of interest, whereas the critical underrecognized need is for a more standard approach to looking for that which is not standard—the unexpected safety problem.

Fortunately, today's clinical trial technology can make available a wealth of detailed and timely safety data. These near-real-time globally available data feeds include highly precise central laboratory evaluations of blood and urine samples that can be available electronically from 24 to 48 hours after each subject visit; digitized ECGs that are remotely captured but centrally analyzed and available within 24 hours of the visit; serious adverse experience reports prepared within a few days of the event; electronic subject diary information that is often transmitted daily to a central repository; and e-CRF data available from a few days to a few minutes after a subject visit. With this wide array of near-real-time safety data, there is no longer any reason why the health of a trial cannot be monitored just as closely and frequently as the health of a subject who is in intensive care. Indeed, the health of hundreds or thousands of subjects is affected by the quality and intensity of this ongoing aggregate safety data monitoring.

There are several good reasons normally given to explain why aggregate subject safety data review is not done with the frequency or approach suggested above. During the typical trial the assignment of treatments to subjects is blinded and must remain so to protect the integrity of the trial. Conventional final unblinded analysis of safety data requires comparison between the groups which is not possible during the trial unless a DSMB has been formed and has in its charter the ability to become unblinded without impacting the trial's scientific validity. Yet a DSMB adds cost and meets infrequently. Second, in the event a possible safety concern is raised during the trial, it could impact the conduct of the rest of the trial in such a way as to bias the results. Investigators may change their behavior and their evaluation of subjects' responses based on the suggestion of a safety issue. This change in behavior could lead to a self-fulfilling prophecy effect on the data. Third, the appearance of subtle trends or signals may be illusory or transient, and may not reflect a real problem. An early termination may preclude the collection of enough solid data to draw any clear conclusions from the trial.

Recommendations. Solutions do exist that avoid the problems above yet provide more sensitivity to detect safety signals throughout the trial. There are three categories that will be covered here: (1) ongoing review of all pooled data irrespective of treatment group assignment, but with an understanding of what would be expected from similar subjects not participating in the clinical trial as a comparison; (2) the use of data displays borrowed from the discipline of exploratory data analysis (EDA); and (3) reasonably foreseeable risk projections to highlight in advance the hypotheses of interest.

1. Pooled Data Review: When we do not know which subjects are in which group, we can still look at the subjects in a trial as a single group without breaking the blind. There are always sources to reference to establish reasonable expectations for typical ranges of laboratory parameters, ECGs, experiences, etc. for subjects like those in the trial. Further, the tracking of changes from baseline, or changes visit by visit, is a powerful indicator of effects over time which are often caused by the study drug or the comparator. Ongoing review of the data based on preestablished thresholds of concern that take into account the dilution effect of looking at pooled data from all combined treatment groups can lead to the identification of potential safety signals. These can then be followed up in more detail, and even taken to an ad hoc safety monitoring committee with the authority to perform unblinded analyses when required. This multitier process can be both efficient and sensitive, yet avoid false alarms that would impact the trial needlessly.

If for example the trial has two equal-sized groups and we expect subjects with the disease under trial to show liver enzyme values 20% higher than normal individuals, we would expect the overall pooled average laboratory data to have this characteristic, if the study drug itself did not further increase liver enzyme abnormalities. An average value of $+20\%$ would not be seen as a safety signal. However if we learned that the study drug further increased liver enzyme abnormalities by an additional 10 percentage points, that would presumably show up in the final analysis as a difference between groups of 10% (20% in placebo subjects vs. 30% in the study drug group). Under this circumstance, the pooled result while we are still blinded would be expected to be 25% (average of 20% and 30% given equal subject numbers per group). Therefore we would know that a deviation from the expected "normal" results from subjects with this disease might show up in the aggregate pooled review as a deviation only half as large as experienced by the study drug-treated subjects. This knowledge can be used to set a threshold for concern, even though we have not broken the blind. The same process can be used for quantitative and categorical data, whether from a laboratory, an ECG, an incidence of endpoints, a survival analysis of median time to a specified event, or an incidence of adverse experiences.

2. Exploratory Data Analysis: While much of the work of the biostatistician in late-stage clinical development revolves around inference, testing of established hypotheses, and interpretation of p-values, some of the most interesting exploratory statistical methodology is designed to help understand experimental results, detect unexpected patterns, and develop new hypotheses to be tested and confirmed in future studies. One of the first lessons to be learned in this area is that the shape of the distribution of individual data points is more important to observe than the mean, or average, of the distribution. The latter is called a measure of central tendency and is a convenient one-number summary of a large amount of data. However it hides much of the critical information about the pattern of results. The mean is also influenced heavily by even a few outliers in the distribution, and distributions with widely disparate shapes can share exactly the same mean.

Graphical displays have become a standard, simple yet powerful way to show the shape of the actual distribution of the results, as well as several important summary values that round out the information carried in the mean value. The use of graphical displays of scatterplots of the actual individual subject visit values vs. baseline values is a quick way to spot overall trends as well as groups of subjects or areas on the scatterplot that differ from other groups or areas. Looking at the distribution will show at a glance whether it looks quite "normal," following the well-known symmetrical bell-shaped curve, or whether the distribution is skewed with a long tail containing extreme outliers, or even bimodal with evidence of two distinct groups of subjects, each with its own distribution. Each type of distribution can be an important clue to a clinical scientist or a statistician as to the effect of the study drug on various types of subjects at different time points in the trial. As the data accumulate, the ability to see trends and patterns increases in a way that is visually obvious even to the nonstatistician.

Variables plotted may be continuous or discrete, but plots of continuous variables generally contain more information. Sometimes it makes sense to plot one variable against time, for example, change in cholesterol vs. trial day. Or the plot of one variable against another may be more important, such as WBC vs. dose. Scatterplots are the first graphical display to consider. A useful addition to the scatterplot is often the regression line, showing the statistical relationship between one variable and another. The addition of confidence bounds on either side of the regression line can help distinguish between random fluctuation and true outliers. Dividing a scatterplot into quadrants may also add to the ability to see at a glance the concentration of subjects who are high on one parameter and low on the other, vice versa, high on both, or low on both. Next there are various summary displays that do not show any individual data points, but still show evidence of the shape of the distribution of results. These include so-called box-and-whisker plots that reflect mean, median, upper and lower quartile points, confidence limits, and outliers, all at a glance.

The list of available graphical displays goes beyond the scope of this chapter. The clear recommendation is to establish at the beginning of a trial the safety parameters of possible interest (see next point below), set the thresholds of expectation based on subjects not receiving the trial drug, create thresholds of concern by adjusting those thresholds of expectation to take into account the pooled sample, select graphical displays that will be sensitive to the clinical safety issues of interest and display the threshold data, and make updated displays available on a continuous basis to clinical, medical, and/or statistical experts. These individuals should be given the explicit ongoing responsibility not only to look for the expected issues but also to scan for the unexpected. Finally, some mechanism must be established to review any suspected signals in a blinded fashion at first, and then, if the information warrants, there must be an unblinded team available to pursue what appear to be stable patterns of concern. Technology is no longer a limitation, and the issues normally raised during a discussion of ongoing data-driven safety surveillance can be managed as outlined above.

3.   Reasonably Foreseeable Risk: Finally, it is important to point out that safety surveillance for the unexpected should always be an adjunct to a diligent and disciplined attempt to forecast areas of risk based on what we already know prior to the beginning of a trial. Phase II/III clinical trials are usually preceded by earlier human clinical trials, the results of which should be studied closely for indications of possible safety issues. Even Phase I first-in-man clinical research is done after thorough laboratory research which forms the basis for the determination that the drug is safe enough for initial testing in normal adults. The point is that there is always a great deal of data available before the start of a clinical trial that points to safety concerns, organ systems at risk, the potential for drug–drug interactions, etc. This information should be used to identify key variables for safety surveillance and circumstances that lead to heightened risk to subjects in a trial.

The a priori identification of specific risk hypotheses leads to the ability to take some of the methodology normally applied to hypothesis testing of efficacy results and apply it to safety assessment. The most important difference between these two analysis domains is that in the case of efficacy, outcomes of interest are identified a priori with great specificity, and clear statistical hypotheses are laid out in advance with complete analysis and decision rules documented in the clinical protocol. In practice, only a few efficacy variables are identified as primary, and only a few others as secondary. Sensitivity, statistical power, and sample size are all carefully analyzed in advance to assure the trial will have a high probability of detecting differences of interest in these few critical variables.

Safety analyses live at the other end of the spectrum, with very little if any prespecified hypotheses to test, no a priori specification of sensitivity or statistical power, and few if any clear decision rules. At a recent industry conference, the head of Biostatistics at the FDA suggested that this disparity may be one of the major reasons why a number of drugs were recently withdrawn from the market owing to safety issues not detected during Phase III clinical trials. It is time to apply the focused spotlight of efficacy analysis to the broad but critical area of safety assessment, both at the end of the trial and in safety surveillance throughout the trial. Statisticians must address this challenge, using both old and new tools and concepts to protect subjects in the trials as well as those who would receive the new therapy upon approval.

V. SUMMARY

The primary focus of late-stage clinical trials is to forecast accurately the benefits and risks of new therapies for the broad population of subjects seeking better therapies, while protecting the safety of those subjects who volunteer to participate in the process. Our present approach has steadily evolved and, for the most part, improved over time. But a number of challenges must be addressed and changes implemented for clinical trials to continue to deliver on their promise.

The current approach to clinical trials does not properly address the basic need to forecast the outcomes of the use of a new therapy for the intended population. Rigid and simplistic standards with regard to p-values and the assessment of inferential analyses do not allow the needed flexibility to address the enormous variety of therapeutic products and the circumstances of their intended use. Data cleaning, and the more general practice of categorizing raw trial information, can lead to systematic bias and a loss of critical outcome information. Safety assessments do not yet take advantage of the flood of near-real-time data coupled with exploratory aggregate data analysis tools. Pretargeted safety hypotheses based on reasonably foreseeable risk assessments of existing information are not normally established, but could assure that aggregate safety issues and trends are detected as early as possible in a trial and addressed appropriately.

Biostatistics as a discipline is at the heart of the issues discussed in this chapter. The development of the tools, techniques, and practices to address these issues is well within the scope and capabilities of the discipline. Some of these issues are already visible and important topics for pharmaceutical sponsors and regulators. Others will become more visible as new types of therapeutics approach the stage of development requiring human clinical trials. Applicability for many of the new therapeutics will be much narrower than in the past, stretching our current practices well beyond their limits. The challenge for biostatistics is to take the lead in forging the future of clinical trial design and analysis so that society's need for better, safer therapies will continue to be met while protecting the safety of those subjects who volunteer to make this process possible.

ACKNOWLEDGMENT

I would like to thank Dr. Lawrence A. Meinert, M.D., M.P.H., Sr. Vice President, Clinical Operations, Covance, Inc., for his ideas and inspirations, some of which are reflected in this chapter.

13

Industry and FDA Liaison

William M. Troetel
Regulatory Affairs Consultant, Mount Vernon, New York, U.S.A.

Richard A. Guarino
Oxford Pharmaceutical Resources, Inc., Totowa, New Jersey, U.S.A.

I. INTRODUCTION

One of the most important groups in a pharmaceutical company is the department of Drug Regulatory Affairs (DRA). Its personnel are largely responsible for establishing a liaison with their counterparts at the U.S. FDA. This chapter will describe the activities of the FDA, emphasizing the center responsible for the review and approval of INDs and NDAs, namely the Center for Drug Evaluation and Research (CDER).

The FDA is an agency within the PHS, which in turn is a part of the DHHS. The FDA regulates over $1 trillion worth of products, which account for 25 cents of every consumer dollar spent annually by American consumers. The FDA touches the lives of virtually every American, every day, for it is FDA's job to see that the food we eat is safe and wholesome, the cosmetics we use will not harm us, the medicines and medical devices we use are safe and effective, and radiation-emitting products such as microwave ovens will not cause harm. Feed and drugs for pets and farm animals also come under FDA scrutiny. The FDA also ensures that all of these products are labeled truthfully with the information people need to use them properly.

The FDA is one of our nation's oldest consumer protection agencies. Its approximately 9,000 employees monitor the manufacture, import, transport, storage, and sale of about $1 trillion worth of products each year. It does so at a cost to the taxpayer of about $3 per person. First and foremost, FDA is a public health agency, charged with protecting American consumers by enforcing the Federal Food, Drug, and Cosmetic Act and several related public health laws. To carry out this mandate of consumer protection, the FDA has some 1,100 investigators and inspectors who cover the country's almost 95,000 FDA-regulated businesses. These employees are located in district and local offices in 157 cities across the country.

A. Inspections and Legal Sanctions

These investigators and inspectors visit more than 16,000 facilities a year, seeing that products are made correctly and labeled truthfully. As part of their inspections, they collect about 80,000 domestic and imported product samples for examination by FDA scientists or for label checks. If a company is found violating any of the laws that the FDA enforces, the FDA can encourage the firm to correct the problem voluntarily or to recall a faulty product from the market. A recall is generally the fastest and most effective way to protect the public from an unsafe product.

When a company cannot or will not voluntarily correct a public health problem with one of its products, the FDA has legal sanctions it can bring to bear. The agency can go to court to force a company to stop selling a product and to have items already produced seized and destroyed. When warranted, criminal penalties, including prison sentences, are sought against manufacturers and distributors. About 3,000 products a year are found to be unfit for consumers and are withdrawn from the marketplace, either by voluntary recall or by court-ordered seizure. In addition, about 30,000 import shipments a year are detained at the port of entry because the goods appear to be unacceptable.

B. Scientific Expertise

The scientific evidence needed to back up the FDA's legal cases is prepared by the agency's 2,100 scientists, including 900 chemists and 300 microbiologists, who work in 40 laboratories in the Washington, D.C., area and around the country. Some of these scientists analyze samples to see, for example, if products are contaminated with illegal substances. Other scientists review test results submitted by companies seeking agency approval for drugs, vaccines, food additives, coloring agents, and medical devices. The FDA operates the National Center for Toxicological Research at Jefferson, Arkansas, which investigates the biological effects of widely used chemicals. The agency also runs the Engineering and Analytical Center at Winchester, Massachusetts, which tests medical devices, radiation-emitting products, and radioactive drugs.

Assessing risks—and, for drugs and medical devices, weighing risks against benefits—is at the core of the FDA's public health protection duties. By ensuring that products and producers meet certain standards, the FDA protects consumers and enables them to know what they are buying. For example, the agency requires that drugs—both prescription and over-the-counter—be proven safe and effective. The agency must determine that the new drug produces the benefits it is supposed to without causing side effects that would outweigh those benefits.

C. Product Safety

Another major FDA mission is to protect the safety and wholesomeness of food. The agency's scientists test samples to see if any substances, such as pesticide residues, are present in unacceptable amounts. If contaminants are identified, the FDA takes corrective action. They also set labeling standards to help consumers know what is in the foods they buy. The nation's food supply is protected in yet another way, as the FDA sees that medicated feeds and other drugs given to animals raised for food are not threatening to the consumer's health.

The safety of the nation's blood supply is another FDA responsibility. The agency's investigators routinely examine blood bank operations, from record-keeping to testing for contaminants. The FDA also ensures the purity and effectiveness of agents such as insulin and vaccines.

Medical devices are classified and regulated according to their degree of risk to the public. Devices that are life-supporting, life-sustaining, or implanted, such as pacemakers, must receive agency approval before they can be marketed.

The FDA's scrutiny does not end when a drug or device is approved for marketing; the agency collects and analyzes tens of thousands of reports each year on drugs and devices after they have been put on the market to monitor for any unexpected adverse reactions.

Cosmetic safety also comes under the FDA's jurisdiction. The agency can have unsafe cosmetics removed from the market. The dyes and other additives used in drugs, foods, and cosmetics are subject to FDA scrutiny. The agency must review and approve these chemicals before they can be used.

The FDA is headed by Commissioner Mark McClellan, M.D., Ph.D. The commissioner is appointed by the president of the United States, confirmed by the U.S. Senate, and serves at the president's discretion. The Office of the Commissioner oversees all of the agency's activities. Prior to his position with FDA, Dr. McClellan was confirmed as a member of the Council of Economic Advisers (CEA) appointed by the Senate. Before joining the CEA, he was Associate Professor of Economics at Stanford University,

Associate Professor of Medicine at Stanford Medical School, a practicing internist, and Director of the Program on Health Outcomes Research at Stanford University. He was also a Research Associate of the National Bureau of Economic Research and a Visiting Scholar at the American Enterprise Institute. Additionally, he was a member of the National Cancer Policy Board of the National Academy of Sciences, Associate Editor of the Journal of Health Economics, and co-Principal Investigator of the Health and Retirement Study (HRS), a longitudinal study of the health and economic well being of older Americans. From 1998 to 1999, he was Deputy Assistant Secretary of the Treasury for Economic Policy, where he supervised economic analysis and policy development on a wide range of domestic policy issues. He has twice received the Arrow Award for Outstanding Research in Health Economics. He earned his M.D. degree from the Harvard–MIT Division of Health Sciences and Technology and his Ph.D. in economics from MIT. He completed his residency training in internal medicine at Brigham and Women's Hospital, and he is board-certified in Internal Medicine.

II. FDA DIVISIONS

The Food and Drug Administration is divided into many centers, each center comprising a division with specific regulatory responsibilities. The following are the main centers:

CDER—Center for Drug Evaluation and Research
CBER—Center for Biologics Evaluation and Research
CDRH—Center for Devices and Radiologic Health
CFSAN—Center of Food Safety and Applied Nutrition
CVM—Center for Veterinary Medicine
NCTR—National Center for Toxicological Research

A. The Center for Drug Evaluation and Research (CDER)

The responsibility for reviewing new pharmaceutical products, including monoclonal antibodies and other well-characterized biotechnologically-derived products is now the responsibility of CDER. This work was, in the past, performed in part by the FDA's CBER and in part by CDER. This consolidation will allow CBER to concentrate its scientific expertise and effort in the crucial areas of vaccines and blood safety. In addition, CBER will be able to concentrate further its expertise on such other biological scientific areas as gene therapy and tissue transplantation. Therefore understanding how CDER is organized is important in the strategic planning of how best to interact with the various divisions and offices responsible for the new drug approval process. As of August 2003, there are 15 review divisions within CDER (including the Division of Over-the-Counter drug products) that are responsible for reviewing all INDs, NDAs, and chemistry and efficacy supplemental applications. Deciding which division will be assigned to a particular IND or NDA depends solely on the indication for the new drug. Divisions are organized on the basis of therapeutic uses for new products, and the divisions are staffed with experts in a particular pharmacotherapeutic area. The current divisions include Cardio-Renal; Neuropharmacological; Oncology; Pulmonary; Metabolic and Endocrine; Reproductive and Urologic; Gastrointestinal and Coagulation; Anesthetic, Critical Care, and Addiction; Medical Imaging and Radio-Pharmaceutical; Anti-Viral; Anti-Infective; Special Pathogen and Immunologic; Anti-Inflammatory, Analgesic and Ophthalmologic; Dermatologic and Dental, Drug Products.

The 15 divisions are grouped among one of five Offices of Drug Evaluation (ODEs). The ODE I, for example, has administrative control for the divisions of Cardiorenal, Neuropharmacological, and Oncologic Drug Products. The DDMAC also is a part of this Office. The organizational chart for CDER and its component parts is usually updated quarterly, and these updates may be found on the internet at http://www.fda.gov/cder/ cderorg.htm. The Center for Drug Evaluation and Research is organized into five main offices including: the Office of the Center Director (OCD); the Office of (Information) Management (OIM); the Office of Pharmaceutical Sciences (OPS); the Office of Pharmacoepidemioology and Statistical Science (OPaSS); and the Office of New Drugs.

The OCD encompasses the executive operations staff, the regulatory policy staff, the ombudsman, and the equal employment opportunity and diversity management staff. The executive operations staff provides support to the OCD, including coordinating executive and legislative activities, managing the preparation and coordination of center-level meetings, and responding to written correspondence from constituents. The regulatory policy staff initiates, develops, and reviews regulations, policies, procedures, and guidances that affect the drug review process. This includes creating and publishing CDER's Manual of Policies and Procedures, preparing *Federal Register* notices for publications, and responding to citizen petitions. The primary mission of the ombudsman is to receive complaints, investigate and act on them, mediate disputes, and, in general, attend to problems involving interpersonal working relationships.

The Office of Pharmaceutical Science (OPS) is an integral part of CDER's new and generic drug product application review process. The goal of OPS is to help establish common approaches to the manufacture and formulation of drugs among pharmaceutical manufacturers. OPS contributes to assuring the quality of drug products by providing uniform policies and review processes for the entire pharmaceutical industry. OPS coordinates its activities with its sister office, the Office of New Drugs (OND). The Office of Pharmaceutical Science has about 500 of CDER's 1,700 employees. OPS has four main offices:

- Office of Generic Drugs
- Office of New Drug Chemistry
- Office of Clinical Pharmacology and Biopharmaceutics
- Office of Testing and Research

Staff working in these offices have backgrounds in chemistry, biopharmaceutics, clinical pharmacology, pharmaceutical science, microbiology, pharmacology/toxicology and labeling.

Activities of OPS include:

- Supporting the review function within the Center for Drug Evaluation and Research (CDER).
- Promoting the adherence to and development of sound regulatory policy and decision-making.
- Managing discipline-related Coordinating Committees.
- Managing the Advisory Committee for Pharmaceutical Science.
- Managing the information technology infrastructure and initiatives that support the review process.

OPS provides scientific and regulatory support by:

- Developing and implementing review management and scientific policies pertaining to the new drug review process for chemistry, manufacturing controls, clinical pharmacology and biopharmaceutics.
- Evaluating and approving abbreviated new drug application (ANDAs) and their amendments.
- Developing and implementing policies and programs through applied regulatory research working with groups inside and outside FDA.
- Performing drug testing and scientific evaluation of drug products in support of the regulatory components of FDA.
- Developing and implementing standards and policies for both generic drugs and new drugs that enhance the drug development and regulatory review process.
- Providing scientific oversight, through the Center's Office of New Drug Chemistry, of chemistry and manufacturing controls (CMC) and the sterility sections of Investigational New Drugs, New Drug Applications and supplements.

- Validating the comparability of clinical safety and efficacy studies conducted during the IND phase of drug development, and evaluating the impact of drug-to-drug interactions and population characteristics on the safety and efficacy of drug products.

The Office of Pharmacoepidemiology and Statistical Science (OPaSS). OPaSS plays a significant role in the Center's mission of assuring the availability of safe and effective drugs for the American people by:

- Providing leadership, direction, planning, and policy formulation for CDER's risk assessment, risk management and risk communication programs;
- Working closely with the staff of CDER's other "super" offices, the Office of New Drugs and the OPS, to provide the statistical and computational aspects of drug review evaluation and research.

OPaSS, which includes the Office of Biostatistics and the Office of Drug Safety, was created as part of a 2002 CDER reorganization and has about 180 of CDER's 1,700 employees. Staff working in the Office of Biostatistics and the Office of Drug Safety have backgrounds in a variety of disciplines including medicine, epidemiology, pharmacology, pharmacy, statistics, regulatory science, health science, information technology, and administration and support services.

The Office of Information Management has been established to provide a more effective and efficient approach to information management within the Center. The Office provides a focal point for:

- Establishing standards for regulatory and health data standards; standards for paper and electronic submissions
- Training for use of review tools
- Coordination of systems development projects with the Office of Information Technology
- Reports and analysis of drug review information
- Oversight of CDER databases

The CDER drug review team members apply their individual, special technical expertise to review INDs or new drug applications.

Each review division uses *chemists* from the Office of New Drug Chemistry in the OPS who are responsible for reviewing the chemistry, manufacturing and controls sections of drug applications. In general terms, chemistry reviewers address issues related to drug identity, manufacturing control, and analysis. The reviewing chemist evaluates the manufacturing and processing procedures for a drug to ensure that the compound is adequately reproducible and stable. If the drug is either unstable or not reproducible, then the validity of any clinical testing would be undermined, because one would not know what was really being used in patients, and, more importantly, studies could pose significant risks to participants.

At the beginning of the chemistry and manufacturing section, the drug sponsor should state whether it believes the chemistry of either the drug substance or the drug product—or the manufacturing of either the drug substance or the drug product—present any potential human risk. If so, these risks should be discussed, with steps proposed to monitor them.

In addition, sponsors should describe any chemistry and manufacturing differences between the drug product proposed for clinical use and that used in the animal toxicology trials that formed the basis for the sponsor's conclusion that it was safe to proceed with the proposed clinical study. How these differences might affect the safety profile of the drug product should be discussed. If there are no differences in the products, that should be stated.

The *pharmacology/toxicology* review team is staffed by pharmacologists and toxicologists who evaluate the results of animal testing and attempt to relate animal drug effects to potential effects in humans. In the area of pharmacology and drug disposition, an application should generally contain (a) a description of the pharmacological effects and mechanism(s) of action of the drug in animals, and (b) information on the absorption, distribution, metabolism, and excretion of the drug. For toxicology studies, the types of studies needed depend on the nature of the drug but will typically include short- and long-term studies, including the potential for drugs to induce birth defects or cancer in humans.

Medical/clinical reviewers, often called medical officers, are almost exclusively physicians. In rare instances, nonphysicians are used as medical officers to evaluate drug data. Medical reviewers are responsible for evaluating the clinical sections of submissions, such as the safety of the clinical protocols in an IND or the results of this testing as submitted in the NDA. Within most divisions, clinical reviewers take the lead role in the IND or NDA review and are responsible for synthesizing the results of the animal toxicology, human pharmacology, and clinical reviews to formulate the overall basis for a recommended agency action on the application.

During the IND review process, the medical reviewer evaluates the clinical trial protocol to determine (a) if the participants will be protected from unnecessary risks, and (b) if the study design will provide data relevant to the safety and effectiveness of the drug. Under federal regulations, proposed phase 1 studies are evaluated almost exclusively for safety reasons. Since the late 1980s, FDA reviewers have been instructed to provide drug sponsors with greater freedom during phase 1, as long as the investigations do not expose participants to undue risks. In evaluating phase 2 and 3 investigations, however, FDA reviewers also must ensure that these studies are of sufficient scientific quality to be capable of yielding data that can support marketing approval.

Other reviewers include *statisticians, microbiologists,* and *biopharmaceutical experts.* Statisticians evaluate the statistical relevance of the data in the NDA, the main tasks being to evaluate the methods used to conduct the studies and those used to analyze the data. The purpose of these evaluations is to give the medical officers a better idea of the power of the findings to be extrapolated to the larger patient population in the country.

Clinical microbiology information is required only in NDAs for anti-infective and antiviral drugs. Because these drugs affect microbial rather than human physiology, reports on the drugs' in vivo and in vitro effects on the target microorganisms are critical for establishing product effectiveness. An NDA's microbiology section usually includes data describing

The biochemical basis of the drug's action on microbial physiology

The drug's antimicrobial spectra, including results of in vitro preclinical studies demonstrating concentrations of the drug required for effective use

Any known mechanisms of resistance to the drug, including results of any known epidemiological studies demonstrating prevalence of resistance factors

Clinical microbiology laboratory methods needed to evaluate the effective use of the drug.

Finally, a microbiological technical data section is necessary for any NDA for which a sterile claim is being made—this would include such products as large and small volume parenterals and sterile ophthalmic solutions.

Pharmacokineticists/biopharmaceuticists evaluate the rate and extent to which the drug's active ingredient is made available to the body and the way it is distributed in, metabolized by, and eliminated from the human body.

All team members work together to assure that the label and the labeling are accurate and provide clear instructions to health care practitioners or to consumers of OTC products.

A key member of the review team is the project manager, formerly called the consumer safety officer or CSO. The project manager evaluates regulatory information to determine compliance with current policies and regulations. In addition, project managers orchestrate and coordinate the drug review team(s') interactions, efforts, and reviews, and they serve as the CDER review team's primary contact with the drug industry. They may be considered as the liaison between the FDA and industry.

The total full-time equivalent staff working in CDER is just under 2000. The number of FDA staff has increased in recent years as a result of the PDUFA of 1992 and the renewal of the PDUFA in the FDA Modernization

Act of 1997. On average, each of the five ODEs has about 125 to 135 employees. Because there are essentially three divisions per office, the average staff in a particular division is about 40 to 45, including clerical, secretarial, and project management support. Updates of these organizational charts can be found on the internet at http://www.fda.gov/cder/cderorg.htm.

III. CONTACTS WITH THE FDA

One of CDER's primary goals is to work collaboratively and cooperatively with industry, academia, and others to improve the drug development and review process. It also strives to provide consumers and health care providers with drug information that is vital to improving the public health. The topics listed below provide an overview of the various means of communicating with CDER.

A.   Consumer/Industry Inquiries

The FDA's CDER is dedicated to ensuring that all persons involved in, or who depend upon, drug regulation excellence have the information needed to develop, review, market, dispense, prescribe, or use drugs safely and effectively.

To enhance the communications aspect of this process, the Center created the OTCOM's Division of Communications Management (DCM). This division enhances information exchange, strategic communications planning, and the development of communications products and initiatives. The Division of Communications Management works to ensure that pharmaceutical industry representatives, health care professionals, government officials, and consumers have easy and open access to information and are educated about the drug regulation process and the benefits and risks of drugs.

Any of these individuals or groups may request information on specific drugs, guidance documents, publications, or general information such as a description of the drug approval process.

There are a number of ways consumers and industry representatives can communicate with the Center or get reliable, current, and up-to-date information from it.

1. The newest and easiest method for getting information is the Center's world wide web homepage at http://www.fad.gov/cder.
2. For more specific or complex drug inquiries, individuals may telephone the Drug Information Branch at (301) 827-4573 or send an electronic mail message at dib@cder.fda.gov.

3. For specific inquiries from industry, CDER's Compendia Operations can be called at (301) 594-0104.

Other sources of information include

1. The FDA Office of Consumer Affairs at 1-800-532-4440, or locally at (301) 827-4420
2. The FDA's OPA at (301) 443-1130

In addition, consumers and industry representatives can contact

1. Acting CDER Ombudsman, Warren Rumble, at (301) 594-5443
2. FDA Freedom of Information Staff, at (301) 827-6567
3. FDA MedWatch Office, at 1-800-FDA-1088

B. Industry/FDA Inquiries

All meetings with the FDA are held at the pleasure of the agency and should be requested judiciously. Project managers (CSOs), a large percentage of whom are former FDA field investigators, are responsible for coordinating FDA/industry meetings. Their other duties include acting as the contact point between the division and the regulated industry, preparing minutes of FDA/industry meetings, and assisting the division with the FDA advisory committee meetings.

If a meeting with the FDA is deemed necessary, the first step is to telephone the project manager assigned to the firm's IND or NDA. The need for a meeting should be explained, a statement about the general topic of the meeting should be described, and an idea of when the meeting is needed should be offered. The project manager will likely return the call and indicate if a meeting will be granted. If the answer is positive, a confirmatory letter from the firm should be sent to the appropriate division. The document should include the fact that the meeting has been granted and what the date for the meeting will be. The names and titles of those representatives of the sponsor who will be attending the meeting, and the proposed agenda with the topics to be discussed spelled out in some detail, are provided. Typically it will be four, and more likely six, weeks after the initial telephone contact with the FDA before the meeting will be held. If the meeting requires an FDA review of the material, as a large percentage of meetings do, the premeeting document should be submitted with the letter. If the information to be discussed is already on file with FDA, the letter should detail by submission number what documents in an IND or NDA should be referred to. It is always appropriate to contact the project manager within the division by telephone to reconfirm the meeting about two weeks before the established meeting date. In February 2000, FDA issued a comprehensive guidance document entitled "Formal Meetings with Sponsors and Applicants for PDUFA Products". This guidance offers great detail on how to arrange meetings, the timing for such meetings and the scope and scheduling for submission of the pre-meeting documents that must be provided to FDA prior to the meeting.

C. FDA/Industry Meetings

There are three types or categories of meeting that industry can request of the agency. They are typically known as Type A, B, or C meetings.

Type A meetings are considered the most important. These are meetings immediately necessary for a delayed development program sometimes called a critical path meeting. Type A meetings are usually to dispute issues that arise during new drug development, or to resolve clinical holds that the FDA has deemed necessary, or at times they may pertain to protocol assessments after the FDA has critiqued the submitted protocols. These meetings are usually scheduled 30 days from FDAs receipt of a written request for a meeting. If the sponsors request a date beyond the 30 days, the meeting should occur no later than 14 days after the date requested.

Type B meetings are those that usually occur for a pre-IND, an End of Phase 1 (EOP1), an End of Phase 2 (EOP2), a Pre Phase 3, or a Pre-NDA or BLA. All of these meetings will be honored by the FDA. These meetings are usually scheduled 60 days from the time the agency received the written request. If the sponsor requests a date beyond 60 days, the meeting should occur no later than 14 days after the date requested.

Type C meetings are any other meeting not falling into Type A or B meetings. These are meetings that pertain to the review of human drug applications. These meetings are usually scheduled within 75 days of the agency's of the written request. If a sponsor requests a date beyond 75 days the meeting should be scheduled to occur no later than 14 days after the date requested.

1. Pre-IND/Preclinical Meetings

Prior to clinical studies, the sponsor needs to demonstrate evidence that the compound is biologically active, and both the sponsor and the FDA need data showing that the drug is reasonably safe for initial administration to humans; hence the filing of an IND. Preclinical meetings are occasionally conducted with the appropriate division that would review the IND or the drug marketing application, and these meetings are typically requested by the sponsor of a drug. Meetings at such an early stage in the process are sometimes useful opportunities for open discussion about testing phases, data requirements, and any scientific issues that may need to be resolved prior to IND submission. At these meetings, the sponsor and the FDA discuss and agree upon the design of the animal studies needed to initiate human testing, and perhaps discuss the types of clinical testing that would best demonstrate the safety and efficacy of the drug in humans.

It is sometimes difficult to know when it is necessary or prudent to request a pre-IND conference with the FDA prior to the filing of an IND. This decision frequently depends on the history of the new compound. If one is dealing with a new chemical entity that has been synthesized in the United States and on which minimal preclinical and clinical investigations have been conducted, there is seldom a need to review data with the FDA prior to submitting the IND. There are, however, exceptions to this statement. They reflect the nature of the proposed indication, the use of new technology (e.g., recombinant DNA techniques), the expected human toxicity based on animal data, the design of the initial clinical trials, or appropriate efficacy criteria to be monitored.

On the other hand, an IND may be submitted for a compound that hasbeen developed overseas and may even be marketed in one or more offshore countries. In this case, the data comprising the IND will be more voluminous. Many preclinical reports will need to be evaluated and summarized, and a large number of clinical reports and perhaps a significant amount of published literature may need to be reviewed, summarized, and presented to regulatory personnel. It is also possible that the sponsor has accumulated sufficient data on the compound from these sources to support both calculations regarding its safety and initiation of an IND with a phase 2 clinical investigation. Any or all of the above circumstances point to a discussion with appropriate division staff prior to IND filing—a staff that may help the FDA as well as the drug's sponsor. In the course of such a meeting, some agreement should be reached on a phase of clinical investigation that will be acceptable to the FDA for the initial study protocols to be included in the original IND submission. The FDA will then be alerted to the filing and can plan to review the IND armed with the prior information received during the meeting.

In preparing for a pre-IND meeting, the DRA representative should provide the FDA with summary documents of the subjects to be discussed. The question of confidentiality must be carefully considered. With no IND filing reference number, the information submitted should be general in nature. Complete details of the synthesis and chemical structure should not be provided. It is usually sufficient to describe vaguely the compound and identify it by code number.

The only division in CDER with an established policy regarding pre-IND consultation meetings is the Division of Anti-Viral Drug Products (DAVDP). Established in 1988, the DAVDP pre-IND Consultation Program is a proactive strategy designed to facilitate informal early communications between DAVDP and potential sponsors of new therapeutics for the treatment of AIDS and life-threatening opportunistic infections, other viral infections, and soft tissue transplantation. Pre-IND advice may be requested for issues related to drug development plans; data needed to support the rationale for testing a drug in humans; the design of nonclinical pharmacology, toxicology, and drug activity studies; data requirements for an IND application; and regulatory requirements for demonstrating safety and efficacy. All potential drug sponsors/developers working in the antiviral area are encouraged to initiate contact with the division as early in the drug development process as possible so that they will have the opportunity to consider the recommendations of DAVDP in planning their preclinical and clinical development programs. The individual to contact is the Pre-IND project manager within the DDAVP.

2. End-of-Phase 2 Meeting (EOP2)

The primary focus of "end-of-phase 2" meetings is to determine whether it is safe to begin phase 3 testing. This is also the time to plan protocols for phase 3 human studies and to discuss and identify any additional information that may be required to support the submission of an NDA. It is also intended to establish an agreement between the agency and the sponsor of the overall plan for phase 3 and the objectives and design of particular studies. These meetings avoid unnecessary expenditures of time and money because data requirements have been clarified.

One month before the end-of-phase 2 meeting, the sponsor should submit the background information and summary protocols for phase 3 studies. This information should include data supporting the claim of the new drug product, chemistry data, animal data and proposed additional animal data, results of phase 1 and 2 studies, statistical methods being used, specific protocols for phase 3 studies, as well as a copy of the proposed labeling for the drug, if available. This summary provides the review team with information needed to prepare for a productive meeting.

In the past, only selected NDA candidate drug sponsors were encouraged to request an end-of-phase 2 conference. Today, all holders of an IND for new chemical entities are entitled to this important conference. Depending on the workload of the division responsible for review of the IND, however, requests for a meeting for an end-of-phase 2 conference may be easier to arrange if the conference requested is for one of the following:

1. New molecular entities for a high priority review drug
2. Drugs with important toxicity problems
3. A compound representing a moderate therapeutic gain but not assigned as a high-priority drug
4. A marketed drug with an important new indication under study

3. Preparing for an End-of-Phase 2 Meeting

There are a number of checkpoints worth observing in preparing for the end-of-phase 2 conference. Key elements are listed here.

1. Ascertain that there have not been pauses in clinical studies between phase 1 and phase 2. The FDA's policies regarding no pauses apply to the usual situation in which research on a drug progresses without serious adverse incidents. This statement does not, however, take precedence over the FDA's responsibility, when necessary, to stop or limit clinical trials for reasons of safety. (Summary phase 1 data along with the necessary chronic toxicity reports should be submitted to support the safety of phase 2 studies when they are initiated.)

2. There also should be no pause between phases 2 and 3 clinical studies. For maximum benefit, the end-of-phase 2 conference should be timed as close as possible to the start of multiple phase 3 studies.

3. There is no clearcut dividing line between phase 2 and 3. (The latter usually includes well-controlled clinical trials of the type performed during phase 2, but in larger populations, under less-controlled conditions.) The sponsor of an IND should carefully determine the time when late phase 2 has been clearly passed (efficacy has been essentially demonstrated statistically to a sufficient degree of confidence) and the drug is ready for phase 3 development. At this point, with phase 3 plans defined, a meeting with the FDA is appropriate.

4. To aid in the review of phase 2 data, the sponsor must prepare a summary separately presenting the results and conclusions for each investigation or multi-investigator study; conclusions should be supported by appropriate statistical analyses. When results from more than one institution or investigator are presented under a single protocol, the information should be summarized so that data from each investigator or institution can be readily identified.

5. Be prepared to provide the following items for the end-of-phase 2 conference, representing each protocol under which the clinical studies have been performed:

a. Tables showing the number of patients (1) randomly assigned for each treatment category according to the protocol, (2) actually entered into each treatment category, (3) lost or prematurely withdrawn from the study, and (4) summarized by pertinent selection criteria.

b. A list explaining why patients were lost or prematurely withdrawn from the study and the number of subjects lost or withdrawn for each investigator. The number of days that each of the patients spent in the study also should be submitted.

c. A summary of the pertinent procedures used to obtain baseline information, measurements of effectiveness, and safety tests performed according to each applicable test or measure. Also prepare a table showing the frequency of testing, the unit of measurement, and the number of patients actually checked as of the reported date. Be sure to include normal values for each investigator's laboratory.

d. For each investigator, summarize baseline and final results of the study in terms of the appropriate variables used to measure safety and effectiveness of the drug under investigation.

e. A statement describing whether statistical analysis has been applied in evaluating the data, and justification of the adequacy of such analysis.

f. If requested, submit the "hard copy" of raw data used in the construction of the summary report. Clinical records or case report forms should be organized and identified for convenient reference and review. If large amounts of data are involved, automatic, processible formats such as easily accessible computer files on disk or computer tape may also be requested by the FDA.

The end-of-phase 2 conference should examine and appraise the adequacy of the phase 2 studies with respect to answering essential questions about the safety and effectiveness in humans for the claimed indications, the safety of proceeding to phase 3, the suitability of the phase 3 protocols, the completeness of the animal toxicity and pharmacology studies, and the manufacturing and controls data.

To address these and related matters, appropriate personnel from the company and the FDA should be present. The FDA will have medical reviewers and a statistician attend all meetings. Whether a pharmacologist, chemist, or microbiologist need attend these sessions will depend on the circumstances. An FDA consultant may be invited, or a review of the consultant's data may be presented in his or her absence. The sponsor also may bring to the meeting one or more consultants. Minutes of the conference will be prepared by the FDA, and allowances are made for the sponsor to prepare and submit the minutes to the file.

Finally, the draft meeting guidance discussed in Sec. III.B should be reviewed.

End-of-Phase 2 Conference—Summary. When a firm has reached the end of phase 2, it should contact the appropriate division at the FDA to arrange for a conference. All clinical data should be summarized, tabulated, and statistically analyzed, as described. These data, together with any additional preclinical and manufacturing and controls data, and plans and protocols for phase 3 should be submitted at least 1 month in advance of the scheduled meeting. A copy containing only clinical data, as a rule, plus the proposed protocols for phase 3, should be provided for the FDA statistician. The submission also should include any specific questions the firm wishes to discuss.

Discussions should be limited to those indications of the drug that the sponsor intends to claim. Agreements should be reached at the conference on the adequacy of, or deficiencies in, the submitted data, or the proposed protocols for phase 3 studies. Specific proposals for correcting deficiencies, for performing additional studies, or not performing what might be considered an excess of studies, should be reviewed and agreed to. The minutes of the conference and the follow-up letter from the firm will serve as a permanent record of these agreements. Barring new and significant scientific developments, a major improvement in the state of the art, unforeseen circumstances occurring during further investigation of the drug, or major inaccuracies in the summarized data noted after full review of the NDA, these agreements shall have the same status as advisory opinions in that they are binding on the FDA. The execution of the agreed upon studies, nevertheless, does not guarantee approval of the subsequent NDA. Any NDAs submitted after end-of-phase 2 conferences that are deficient in satisfying the recorded or subsequently modified agreements still may require additional studies to be considered approvable. Food and Drug Administration commitments will not necessarily be considered binding if the sponsor fails to comply with agreed-upon commitments.

4. Pre-NDA Meetings

The purpose of a pre-NDA meeting is to discuss the presentation of data (both paper and electronic) in support of the application. The information provided at the meeting by the sponsor includes

A summary of clinical studies to be submitted in the NDA.
The proposed format for organizing the submission, including methods for presenting the data
Other information that needs to be discussed

The meeting is conducted to uncover any major unresolved problems or issues; to identify studies the sponsor is relying on as adequate and well controlled in establishing the effectiveness of the drug; to help the reviewers to become acquainted with the general information to be submitted; and to discuss the presentation of the data in the NDA to facilitate its review. Once the NDA is filed, a meeting may also occur 90 days after the initial submission of the application to discuss issues that are uncovered in the initial review.

5. Advisory Committee Meetings

All of the FDA's current advisory committees are scientific and technical committees. Advisory committees have been established to advise and make recommendations on issues related to the agency's regulatory responsibilities.

The primary role of FDA advisory committees is to provide independent expert scientific advice to the agency in its evaluation of regulated products, and to help make sound decisions based on the reasonable application of good science. The committees are advisory in nature, and final decisions are made by the FDA. They consist of individuals with recognized expertise and judgment in a specific field who have the training and experience necessary to evaluate information objectively and to interpret its significance under various, often controversial, circumstances. Advisory committees weigh available evidence and provide scientific and medical advice on the safety, effectiveness, and appropriate use of products under FDA jurisdiction. Another role is to advise the agency on general criteria for evaluation and on broad regulatory and scientific issues that are not related to a specific product. Although advisory committees have a prominent role in the product approval stage, they are sometimes used earlier in the product development cycle and may be invited to consider postmarketing issues.

The charter of each of the advisory committees provides for at least one member to represent the consumer perspective. Consumer representatives make a valuable contribution by raising concerns that might not be otherwise addressed before products come to the marketplace. As they participate in the advisory committee process, consumer members become more knowledgeable about FDA issues and products that are often on the cutting edge of new research and technology. They gain the experience of working with nationally recognized scientific experts.

The current CDER advisory committees include the following:

Anesthetic and Life Support Drugs Advisory Committee
Anti-Infective Drugs Advisory Committee
Antiviral Drugs Advisory Committee
Arthritis Advisory Committee
Cardiovascular and Renal Drugs Advisory Committee
Dermatologic Drugs Advisory Committee
Drug Abuse Advisory Committee
Endocrinology and Metabolic Drugs Advisory Committee
Gastrointestinal Drugs Advisory Committee
Generic Drugs Advisory Committee
Medical Imaging Drugs Advisory Committee
Nonprescription Drugs Advisory Committee
Oncologic Drugs Advisory Committee
Peripheral and Central Nervous System Drugs Advisory Committee
Pharmaceutical Science Drugs Advisory Committee
Psychopharmacologic Drugs Advisory Committee
Pulmonary Allergy Drugs Advisory Committee
Reproductive Health Drugs Advisory Committee

At times, CDER may especially want a committee's opinion about a new drug, a major indication for an already approved drug, or a special regulatory requirement being considered, such as a boxed warning in a drug's labeling. Committees may also advise CDER on necessary labeling information or help with guidelines for developing particular kinds of drugs. They may also consider questions such as whether a proposed study for an experimental drug should be conducted or whether the safety and effectiveness information submitted for a new drug is adequate for marketing approval.

In October 1998, FDA published a guidance for industry entitled *Advisory Committees: Implementing Section 120 of the Food and Drug Administration Modernization Act of 1997*. This document provided guidance for industry on changes to the policies and procedures being used by CDER regarding advisory committees in response to section 120 of the FDA Modernization Act of 1997 (FDAMA). This section of the FDAMA directed the FDA to establish panels of experts, or to use already established panels of experts, to provide scientific advice and recommendations to the agency regarding the clinical investigation of drugs or the approval for marketing of drugs. The FDA has defined the term "panel of experts" to mean "advisory committees."

Section 120 of the FDAMA amended section 505 of the FD&C Act by adding section 505(n). This new section includes provision for the following: (a) additional members to be included in new advisory committees, (b) new conflict of interest considerations, (c) education and training for new committee members, (d) timely committee consideration of matters, and (e) timely agency notification to affected persons of decisions on matters considered by advisory committees.

Advisory committee meetings can be very advantageous to sponsors who are filing an NDA for similar drug categories. It would behoove these sponsors to attend advisory committee meetings. The sponsor should get to know the advisory committee members and what the advisory committee is looking for. Assess carefully the issues that are important to the advisory committee and make careful notes as to their concerns. Heed their recommendations and consider them seriously when you are developing your products.

IV. FDA INITIATIVES TO SPEED DRUG APPROVAL

The FDA has instituted several programs designed to hasten the drug approval process for effective drugs. Pharmaceutical regulatory professionals should be aware of any and all ways that can be recommended to their research and management staff for more rapid drug approval. These FDA pathways to expeditious new drug approval are described below.

Subpart E in Section 312 of the Code of Federal Regulations establishes procedures to expedite the development, evaluation, and marketing of new therapies intended to treat people with life-threatening and severely debilitating illnesses, especially where no satisfactory alternatives exist.

A.   Accelerated Development/Review Program

The first is the accelerated development/review program. Accelerated development/review (see Federal Register, April 15, 1992) is a highly specialized mechanism for speeding the development of drugs that promise significant benefit over existing therapy for serious or life-threatening illnesses. This process incorporates several novel elements aimed at making sure that rapid development and review are balanced by safeguards to protect both the patient and the integrity of the regulatory process.

Accelerated development/review can be used under two special circumstances: (1) when approval is based on evidence of the product's effect on a "surrogate end point," and (2) when the FDA determines that safe use of a product depends on restricting its distribution or use. A surrogate end point is a laboratory finding or physical sign that may not be a direct measurement of how a patient feels, functions, or survives, but it is still considered likely to predict therapeutic benefit for the patient. The fundamental element of this process is that the manufacturers must continue testing after approval to demonstrate that the drug indeed provides therapeutic benefit to the patient. If not, the FDA can withdraw the product from the market more easily than usual.

B.   Treatment IND

Treatment INDs (see Federal Register, May 22, 1987) are used to make promising new drugs available to desperately ill patients as early in the drug development process as possible. The FDA will permit an investigational drug to be used under a treatment IND if there is preliminary evidence of drug efficacy and the drug is intended to treat a serious or life-threatening disease, or if there is no comparable alternative drug or therapy available to treat that stage of the disease in the intended patient population. In addition, these patients are not eligible to be in the definitive clinical trials, which must be well under way, if not almost finished.

An immediately life-threatening disease means a stage of a disease in which there is a reasonable likelihood that death will occur within a matter of months, or in which premature death is likely without early treatment. For example, advanced cases of AIDS, herpes simplex encephalitis, and subarachnoid hemorrhage are all considered immediately life-threatening diseases. Treatment INDs are made available to patients before general marketing begins, typically during phase 3 studies. Treatment INDs also allow the FDA to obtain additional data on the drug's safety and effectiveness.

C. FDA Guidance Documents/Guidelines

A regulatory professional must be aware of the guidance documents that the FDA has made available to assist industry to understand expectations regarding drug development and the approval process. The website providing the complete list of FDA guidances is updated almost daily. It may be accessed at http://www.fda.gov/cder/guidance/index.htm.

The FDA comprehensive list of all guidances available is found on the internet at http://www.fda.gov/cder/guidance/guidlist.pdf.

The FDA guidance page is subdivided into the following sections for ease of use: advertising; biopharmaceutics (final and draft); chemistry (final and draft); clinical/antimicrobial (draft); clinical/medical (final and draft); compliance (final and draft); generics (final and draft); industry letters; information technology; international congress on harmonization (final and draft); IND; labeling; microbiology; modernization act; OTC; pharm/tox; and procedural.

V. FREEDOM OF INFORMATION ACT (FOIA)

Freedom of information is another important way in which regulatory personnel may readily obtain information from the FDA. The FDA has published a guidance handbook intended to facilitate requests for both public information and records not originally prepared for distribution by the FDA. This handbook has been updated in response to the Electronic Freedom of Information Act (FOIA) amendments of 1996.

A. Obtaining Public Information

Certain documents that are prepared for public distribution—press releases, consumer publications, speeches, and congressional testimony—are available from the FDA without having to file an FOI request. Many of these documents are available on the FDA's internet site (http://www.fda.gov/). Consumers with questions about FDA-related matters also may write to the Office of Consumer Affairs, HFE-88, Food and Drug Administration, 5600 Fishers

Lane, Rockville, MD 20857, or call toll free, 1-888-FDA-INFO (1-888-322-4636).

B. Obtaining Information Through the FOI

The Freedom of Information Act allows anyone to request copies of records not normally prepared for public distribution. It pertains to existing records only and does not require agencies to create new records to comply with a request. It also does not require agencies to collect information they do not have or to do research or analyze data for a requestor. In addition, FOI requests must be specific enough to permit an FDA employee who is familiar with the subject matter to locate records in a reasonable period. Under the FOIA, certain records may be withheld in whole or in part from the requestor if they fall within one of nine FOIA exemptions. Six of these exemptions most often form the basis for the withholding of information by the FDA:

Exemption 2 protects certain records related solely to the FDA's internal rules and practices.

Exemption 3 protects information that is prohibited from disclosure by other laws.

Exemption 4 protects trade secrets and confidential commercial or financial information.

Exemption 5 protects certain interagency and intraagency communications.

Exemption 6 protects information about individuals in personnel, medical, and similar files when disclosure would constitute a clearly unwarranted invasion of privacy.

Exemption 7 protects records or information compiled for law enforcement purposes when disclosure (a) could reasonably be expected to interfere with enforcement proceedings, (b) would deprive a person of a right to a fair trial or an impartial adjudication, (c) could reasonably be expected to constitute an unwarranted invasion of personal privacy, (d) could reasonably be expected to disclose the identity of a confidential source, (e) would disclose techniques and procedures for law enforcement investigations or prosecutions, or would disclose guidelines for law enforcement investigations or prosecutions, if such disclosure could reasonably be expected to risk circumvention of the law, or (f) could reasonably be expected to endanger the life or physical safety of an individual.

In the event the FDA relies on one or more FOIA exemptions to deny a requestor access to records, a letter stating the reasons for denying the records will be sent to the requestor. The letter will also notify the requestor of the right to appeal the agency's denial determination. More specific information on these exemptions and on other aspects of the FOIA programs are contained in the FDA's FOIA implementation regulations codified in 21 CFR Part 20.

C. How to Make an FOI Request

All FOI requests must be in writing and should include the following information:

1. Requestor's name, address, and telephone number.
2. A description of the records being sought. The records should be identified as specifically as possible. A request for specific records that are releasable to the public can be processed much more quickly than a request for "all information" on a particular subject. Also fees for a more specific and limited request will generally be less. Information on major information systems maintained by the FDA can be obtained by using the Department of Health and Human Services Government Information Locator Service (GILS) site. This information may be useful in narrowing a request.
3. Separate requests should be submitted for each firm or product involved.
4. A statement concerning willingness to pay fees, including any limitations.

All FOI requests must be in writing. The FDA does not accept FOI requests sent by e-mail. Requests should be mailed to Food and Drug Administration, Freedom of Information Staff (HFI-35), 5600 Fishers Lane, Rockville, MD 20857. Or requests may be sent by fax to (301) 443-1726. If there are problems sending a fax, call (301) 443-2414.

D. Fees

Requestors under FOIA may have to pay fees covering some or all of the costs of processing their request. Requestors may want to include the maximum dollar amount they are willing to pay. If the fees exceed the maximum amount stated, FDA will contact the requestor before filling the request. Requestors are generally billed for fees after their requests have been processed; however, if total fees are expected to exceed $250.00, the FDA may require payment in advance of processing.

1. Commercial Use Requestors

Search and review time: $14, $29, or $52 per hour, depending upon the grade level of the FDA employee filling the request

Duplication: $0.10 per page for standard in size paper or actual cost per page for odd-size paper; $0.50 per fiche for microfiche
Certifications: $10 each
Computer charges: actual cost for time involved
Electronic forms/formats: actual cost for form/format requested

2. Noncommercial Use Requestors, Such as Representatives of the News Media, Public Interest Groups, and Educational and Noncommercial Scientific Institutions

Duplication charges are issued at the same rates listed above, with no charge for first 100 pages of duplication.

3. Other Requestors, Including Consumers

Search and duplication charges are issued at the rates listed above, with no charge for the first 2 hours of search and the first 100 pages of duplication.

Requestors should not send payment with their requests. They will be billed if the total processing charges are $15 or more. The FDA does not accept credit cards. Payment must be made by check or money order.

VI. SUMMARY

The true value of a pharmaceutical firm's regulatory specialist is largely measured by his or her success in dealing with an FDA counterpart. In the course of routine dealings with the FDA, the regulatory expert should occasionally address the following questions:

1. How expeditiously are the firm's submissions reviewed by the FDA compared with other pharmaceutical manufacturers?
2. How many filings require follow-up submissions with additional data? Would adequate review prior to the initial filing have disclosed the deficiencies cited by FDA reviewers?
3. What additional steps can be implemented to speed the drug review or support process?
4. Is there an accord between the DRA department representatives and FDA personnel?
5. How difficult is it to arrange meetings with FDA staff members? Can the relationship be improved?

A knowledge of how the FDA operates is essential to the success of a DRA department. All dealings with the FDA—or other regulatory agencies for that matter—must be well conceived and adequately planned. Without knowledge, conception, planning, and an understanding of how the other half works, significant delays in drug approval frequently and painfully occur. Whether the regulatory goal is to speed the approval process for a new product or to keep a product on the market, the firm must know how best to work with the FDA. Will patience work? Should there be a legal confrontation? Should the commissioner be involved? These and other questions must be addressed and constructively resolved by the regulatory professional. Perhaps it pays to heed the words of Tolstoy in *War and Peace*: "The strongest of all warriors are... Time and Patience."

14

Chemistry, Manufacturing, and Control Requirements of the NDA and ANDA

Evan B. Siegel
Ground Zero Pharmaceuticals, Inc., Irvine, California, U.S.A.

I. INTRODUCTION

With the enactment of the FDA Modernization Act of 1997 (FDAMA) and multiple reauthorizations of the Prescription Drug User Fee Act of 1992 (PDUFA), the drug approval process by the FDA is expected to be streamlined further. The agency has aggressively generated guidance documents to implement the provisions of the statute, and it continues the process to this date. Therefore it is up to the drug sponsor to prepare drug submissions that are complete and in a format that will facilitate the review and lead to a rapid approval.

One of the most critical portions of an NDA or ANDA is item 4 of the Form FDA 356h, the chemistry section. This section, more commonly referred to as CMC (for chemistry, manufacturing, and controls), is actually subdivided into three subsections: the chemistry, manufacturing, and controls information; samples; and methods validation package. Although the chemistry section of a typical application comprises only 5% of a submission, 25% of FDA guidance documents generated refer to CMC issues, making the chemistry section the most highly regulated part of the application.

Nonclinical and clinical studies are usually completed during the investigational phases of drug development. The final formulation(s) for the product, however, along with the associated analytical methodologies and manufacturing procedures, may not be finalized until the latter part of phase 3 clinical trials. Even with no change in the safety, efficacy, and manufacturing process of a drug in the market, the CMC information on a drug filed with the FDA is always updated as long as the company manufactures the drug, whereas clinical and preclinical information are not, except where postmarketing experience dictates labeling changes to provide updated guidance to healthcare professionals, patients, and consumers regarding safe and effective use of the product. Chemistry, manufacturing, and controls issues exist throughout the life cycle of a product.

It is clear that the FDA considers that appropriate construction and submission of the CMC section has the potential to decrease significantly the NDA review and approval times. In addition to the issuance of guidance documents and CMC initiatives, the regulations permit the submission of item 4 material 90 to 120 days in advance of other sections of the NDA (21 CFR 314.50(d)(iv)) as a further means of expediting the regulatory review process. The changes in regulatory procedure stimulated and mandated by the FDAMA and the PDUFA have included a more consistent series of approaches to the setting of levels of change in manufacturing processes that require either more or less advance notification to the FDA prior to their incorporation in drug manufacture; prior review; and intensity of concern for agency reviewers. The newer guidelines provide detailed information for sponsors on these issues. In addition, the ICH has generated a series of additional guidelines since 1997 on product quality that also provide critical information for sponsors.

Sponsors can help both themselves and the FDA chemistry reviewer by providing sufficient documentation in NDA submissions, particularly regarding the following: (1) methods of synthesis, (2) validation of analytical assay methods for both the drug substance and the finished dosage form(s), (3) container/closure systems, and (4) stability testing. Deficiencies in these key areas also are common causes for the delayed approval of ANDAs. It is important to ensure that the CMC section of an application accurately reflects the actual manufacturing and control processes for the batches to be marketed. This will have great impact on the way the FDA conducts a preapproval inspection for the application. In the pages to follow, recommendations as to what information should be provided in both NDAs and ANDAs will be discussed. Appropriate reference(s) to the applicable guideline(s) will be presented throughout, and Table 1 lists them all for convenience. These guidelines and other pertinent publications issued by the FDA can be obtained by mail or through the FDA website (htpp/www/FDA.gov). Differences in the information provided for original and abbreviated new drug filings will also be highlighted.

The FDA has provided a guidance intended to provide recommendations to sponsors of INDs on the CMC documentation that should be sub-

Table 1 FDA Manufacturing and Controls Guidelines

1. Guideline for the Format and Content of an Application Summary
2. Guideline for the Format and Content of the Chemistry, Manufacturing, and Controls Section of an Application
3. Guideline for Impurities in Drug Substances
4. Guideline for Stability Studies for Human Drugs and Biologics
5. Guideline for Packaging of Human Drugs and Biologics
6. Guideline for Submitting Supporting Documentation in Drug Applications for the Manufacture of Drug Substances
7. Guideline for Submitting Supporting Documentation for the Manufacture of Finished Dosage Forms
8. Guidelines for Drug Master Files
9. Guidance for Industry: Changes to an Approved Application for Specified Biotechnology and Specified Synthetic Biological Products
10. Guidance for Industry: INDs for Phase 2 and Phase Studies: Chemistry, Manufacturing, and Controls Content and Format
11. Guidance for Industry: Nonsterile Semisolid Dosage Forms Scale-Up and Postapproval Changes: Chemistry, Manufacturing, and Controls; In Vitro Release Testing and In Vivo Bioequivalence Documentation
12. Guidance for Industry: Container Closure Systems for Packaging Human Drugs and Biologics: Chemistry, Manufacturing, and Controls Documentation
13. Guidance for Industry SUPAC-SS: Nonsterile Semisolid Dosage Forms Manufacturing Equipment Addendum
14. Liposome Drug Products: Chemistry, Manufacturing, and Controls; Human Pharmacokinetics and Bioavailability; and Labeling Documentation
15. Guidance for Industry: Drug Master Files for Bulk Antibiotic Drug Substances
16. Guidance for Industry: Monoclonal Antibodies Used as Reagents in Drug Manufacturing
17. Guidance for Industry: Nasal Spray and Inhalation Solution, Suspension, and Spray Drug Products—Chemistry, Manufacturing, and Controls Documentation
18. Guidance for Industry AC-ATLS: Postapproval Changes—Analytical Testing Laboratory Sites
19. Guidance for Industry: Analytical Procedures and Methods Validation: Chemistry, Manufacturing, and Controls Documentation
20. Guidance for Industry SUPAC-MR: Modified Release Solid Oral Dosage Forms Scale-Up and Postapproval Changes: Chemistry, Manufacturing, and Controls; In Vitro Dissolution Testing and In Vivo Bioequivalence Documentation
21. Guidance for Industry: Botanical Drug Products
22. Guidance for Industry: Stability Testing of Drug Substances and Drug Products
23. Guidance for Industry: SUPAC-IR/MR: Immediate Release and Modified Release Solid Oral Dosage Forms; Manufacturing Equipment Addendum
24. Guidance for Industry: Environmental Assessment of Human Drug and Biologics Applications
25. Guidance for Industry: Changes to an Approved NDA or ANDA
27. Guidance for Industry: Changes to an Approved NDA or ANDA. Questions and Answers
28. Guidance for Industry: Container Closure Systems for Packaging Human Drugs and Biologics. Questions and Answers
29. Submitting Applications According to the ICH/CTD Format—General Considerations
30. Guidance for Industry: Drug Product: Chemistry, Manufacturing, and Controls Information
31. Guidance for Industry: Current Good Manufacturing Practice for Medical Cases
32. Guidance for Industry: Integration of Dose-Counting Mechanisms into MDI Drug Products

mitted for phase 2 and phase 3 studies conducted under INDs. The recommendations in the guidance provide regulatory relief for IND sponsors in three specific areas. First, the phase 3 supplementary data and information corroborating the quality and safety criteria established in earlier investigational phases need not be submitted before the initiation of phase 3 studies and can be generated during phase 3 drug development. Second, a sponsor may elect to delay submitting data elements obtained in earlier investigations until phase 3 if they do not affect safety. This allows sponsors to postpone the submission of data and information, even if generated before and during earlier investigational phases. Third, a sponsor may submit summary reports annually and does not need to resubmit data and information already submitted.

The importance of the updating of the regulatory process through these changes cannot be overemphasized, since successful NDAs, for which appropriate documentation has been submitted during the IND phases, provide relevant correlations established between data generated during early and late drug development. The movement toward a continuum of drug development from the early phases through NDA review and approval is accelerating at the FDA. In addition, the transfer of most therapeutic biological product INDs from CBER to CDER should allow for a harmonization of marketing application requirements across therapeutic areas.

A pre–new drug application (pre-NDA) meeting may be requested by the sponsor to address outstanding questions and scientific issues and aid in the resolution of problems. The CMC portion of the pre-NDA meeting is a critical interaction between the CMC review team and the sponsor to ensure the submission of a well-organized and complete NDA. Examples of CMC issues that could be addressed in pre-NDA meetings include, but are not limited to

> Discussion of the NDA format, including provision of an electronic submission
> Confirmation that all outstanding issues discussed in earlier meetings will be adequately addressed in the proposed NDA
> Assurance that all activities for the proposed NDA have been coordinated, including the full and timely cooperation of DMF holders or other contractors and suppliers
> Discussion of the relationship between manufacturing, formulation, and packaging of the product used in phase 3 studies and the product intended for marketing
> Assurance that the submission will contain adequate stability data in accordance with stability protocols agreed upon earlier
> Confirmation that all facilities (e.g., manufacturing, testing, packaging) will be ready for inspection by the time of the NDA submission

Identification of any other issues, potential problems, or regulatory issues that should be brought to the attention of the agency or sponsor

II. THE NDA SUMMARY

The FDA regulations published February 22, 1995, provide for the preparation of a summary of the NDA, including a condensation of the CMC section. (The Guideline for the Format and Content of an Application Summary is available to aid in the preparation of this document.) Properly presented, the summary will provide all of the NDA reviewers a general overview of CMC information for both the drug substance and the drug product. It should be written in sufficient detail and in a style that can meet the editorial standards required for publication in refereed scientific journals. The following subsections detail what should be included in the NDA summary regarding CMC information.

A. The Drug Substance

1. Names

Include the generic name(s), synonyms, and code designation(s) that have appeared in the published literature or in nonclinical or clinical reports being submitted with the application, the proprietary names (brand name or trademark) if known, identification number (e.g., Chemical Abstracts Service [CAS] registry number), and chemical name(s). List the preferred chemical name first, if available. This information can be found in a reference book called the *U.S. Adopted Names Council* (USAN) *Handbook*, if a generic name for the drug substance has been accepted by the council.

2. Physical and Chemical Properties

Describe the physical and chemical properties of the drug substance. Include, as applicable, appearance, odor, taste, physical form, solubility profile, melting point, boiling range, molecular weight, structural and molecular formulae (Wisswesser line notation), isomers, polymorphs, pKa, pKb, and pH. A description of the data obtained to elucidate the structure (e.g., spectroscopic characteristics) should also be included.

3. Stability

The results of studies conducted on the drug substance should be summarized and related to the anticipated storage conditions and container/closure system, as well as the retest plan to be used by the sponsor. Statements on whether additional studies are ongoing or planned for the future should be included. Also provide a statement regarding the suitability of the methods used (see the section below on specifications and analytical methods).

4. Manufacturer

The name(s) and address(es) of the manufacturer(s), i.e., entity(ies) performing the manufacturing, processing, packaging, labeling, and control operations of the drug substance, must be listed. Include a description of the responsibilities of each manufacturer listed, if more than one is used.

5. Method of Manufacture

Information concerning the method of manufacture may be presented in the form of a flow chart. Supply a brief description of the methods of isolation (e.g., synthetic process, fermentation, extraction, recombinant deoxyribonucleic acid [DNA] procedure) and purification (solvent recrystallization, column chromatography, distillation). Include all synthetic pathways that have been adequately characterized during the investigational stages of drug development.

6. Process Controls

Provide a brief description of the control checks performed at each stage of manufacturing and packaging of the drug substance.

7. Specifications and Analytical Methods

Describe the acceptance criteria and the test methods used to assure the identity, strength, quality, particle size and polymorphic integrity, and purity of the drug substance. The guidelines also indicate that applicable information should be provided regarding actual or potential impurities in the drug substance (by-products, degradation products, antigenic substances, viral contaminants, isomeric components, heavy metal contaminants, extraction solvents, and so forth). As the summary may also be used by the FDA as a reference document in the preparation of the Summary Basis of Approval (SBA) for the product, releasable to the public under the FOI regulations, the information included in the summary regarding impurities should be well considered.

8. Container/Closure System

Describe the characteristics of, and test methods used for, the container, the closure, and other component parts. In addition, highlight stability data and any other information that support their suitability for packaging the drug substance.

B. The Drug Product

1. Composition of the Dosage Form

A quantitative composition, including the name and amount of each active and inactive ingredient contained in the drug product, should be provided. In addition, an overall description of the dosage form should be included. This should be in sufficient detail to characterize it fully with regard to its type, release properties (i.e., immediate versus sustained or controlled release), and physical characteristics such as shape, color, type of coating, hardness, scoring, and identification marks.

2. Manufacturer

The information provided for the manufacturer is analogous to that provided for the drug substance. In this case, however, there are likely to be more facilities listed. Contract packagers, for example, are used frequently for preparing samples or unit dose presentations such as blister packages.

3. Method of Manufacture

Briefly describe the manufacturing and packaging process for the finished dosage form(s) of the product (e.g., wet granulation, direct compression, and lyophilization).

4. Specifications and Analytical Methods

Detail the regulatory specifications and test methods used to assure the identity, strength, quality, purity, and bioavailability of the drug product. The emphasis lies in the assay methodology(ies) used to quantitate the presence of degradation products and to assure stability of the drug product.

5. Container/Closure System

A description of all the container/closure system configurations for the drug to be marketed should be presented. In addition, stability data and any other information that support the suitability of the container/closure components, including specifications and test methods, should be indicated.

6. Stability

The proposed expiration dating period and storage conditions for the product, along with justifications for them based on data obtained from stability studies, should be stated.

7. Test Formulations

Provide quantitative compositions and lot numbers of each finished dosage form used in nonclinical safety studies, clinical studies, and stability during the investigational phases of development for the drug product. In addition, formulation differences should be explained, and each formulation should be cross-referenced to the study or studies in which it was used.

If these points are clearly and concisely presented, FDA reviewers should have a general understanding of the data and information submitted in the CMC section.

III. CHEMISTRY, MANUFACTURING, AND CONTROLS INFORMATION

This part of an application contains a precise description of the composition, methods of manufacture, specifications, and control procedures for the drug substance and the drug product. It also includes an environmental impact analysis statement for the manufacturing process and for the ultimate use of the drug. (Refer to the Guideline for the Format and Content of the Chemistry, Manufacturing, and Controls Section of an Application and 21 CFR 314.50(d)(1), which set forth specific data requirements for this section.)

In preparation of the documents for the CMC section, one of the first items to consider is the selection of a representative batch of the drug substance and the drug product for the NDA. Ideally, the representative drug substance batch selected was used to manufacture the representative drug product batch. This will provide a good and consistent data flow in the CMC section.

A. The Drug Substance

1. Names

Include the established (generic) and proprietary (trade) name(s), synonyms (e.g., different names being used for the same drug in other countries), CAS registry number, and code number(s). Most drugs early in their investigation are referred to by some alphanumeric code number until a generic name has been officially approved by the USAN and/or by the WHO as an INN.

2. Structural Formulae and Chemical Name(s)

The chemical structure(s), molecular formula(e), molecular weight(s), and chemical name(s) should be shown. List all chemical names by which the drug was referred to during its development, and highlight the preferred names assigned by USAN or WHO at the time a generic name was approved.

3. Physical and Chemical Properties

The description provided in this section should include, as applicable, information on the following: (1) organoleptic properties (e.g., appearance, odor, taste); (2) solid-state form (i.e., the preferred crystalline polymorph); (3) solubility profile (limit data to aqueous solubility, pH effect, and at most one or two organic solvents); (4) pH, pKa, or pKb; (5) melting and boiling range; (6) specific gravity or bulk density; (7) spectroscopic characteristics such as a specific rotation, refractive index, and fluorescence; and (8) isomeric composition.

The FDA has issued a guidance that provides recommendations to applicants on the chemistry, manufacturing, and controls (CMC) documentation for liposome drug products submitted in NDAs. A liposomal formulation of an active moiety that has already been approved or marketed in the United States is not classified as a new molecular entity (Type 1 NDA). When submitted in an NDA, the drug is classified as a Type 3 NDA unless it is a new ester, new salt, or other noncovalent derivative of the approved drug substance. In that case, the NDA would be classified as a Type 2,3. Special attention should be paid in the NDA for a liposomal drug product to describe fully the physicochemical properties of the membrane layer, control of lipid component excipients, and analytical testing methodologies supporting the specifications.

4. Proof of Structure

A reference standard batch of the drug substance is used to conduct structure elucidation and confirmation studies. The elucidation and confirmation of structure should include physical and chemical information derived from applicable analyses, such as (1) elemental analysis; (2) functional group analysis using spectroscopic methods (i.e., mass spectrometry, nuclear magnetic resonance); (3) molecular weight determinations; (4) degradation studies; (5) complex formation determinations; (6) chromatographic study methods using HPLC, GC, TLC, GLC; (7) infrared spectroscopy; (8) ultraviolet spectroscopy; (9) stereochemistry; and (10) others, such as optical rotatory dispersion (ORD) or x-ray diffraction.

5. Stability

Information on the stability of a drug substance under defined storage conditions is an integral part of the systematic approach to stability evaluation.

Stress testing helps to determine the intrinsic stability characteristics of a molecule by establishing degradation pathways to identify the likely degradation products and to validate the stability indicating power of the analytical procedures used. Stress testing is conducted to provide data on forced decomposition products and decomposition mechanisms for the drug substance. The severe conditions that may be encountered during distribution can be covered by stress testing of definitive batches of the drug substance. These studies should establish the inherent stability characteristics of the molecule, such as the degradation pathways, and lead to identification of degradation products and hence support the suitability of the proposed analytical procedures. The detailed nature of the studies will depend on the individual drug substance and type of drug product. This testing is likely to be carried out on a single batch of a drug substance. Testing should include the effects of temperatures in 10°C increments above the accelerated temperature test condition (e.g., 50°C, 60°C) and humidity, where appropriate (e.g., 75 percent or greater). In addition, oxidation and photolysis on the drug substance plus its susceptibility to hydrolysis across a wide range of pH values when in solution or suspension should be evaluated. Results from these studies will form an integral part of the information provided to regulatory authorities. Light testing should be an integral part of stress testing.

The results from studies conducted to evaluate the stability of the new drug substance should be described fully in the NDA. In addition, on the basis of these results, recommendations for the storage conditions and retesting period should be discussed. Data should be submitted from studies of the product stored in open and closed containers analogous to the container in which the drug substance is to be stored. Generally, manufacturers do these studies in 1 to 5 kg containers fabricated from the same materials used for bulk manufacturing storage.

Other studies, conducted at accelerated storage conditions, such as freezing or 5°C, 40–50°C, or higher temperatures, humidity of 75% or greater, and exposure to light, should be submitted. These studies generally help define what handling precautions are necessary for bulk storage and during manufacture of the dosage form. The FDA also recommends that studies be conducted on solutions or suspensions of the drug substance to evaluate the effects of acid and alkaline pH, high oxygen and nitrogen atmospheres, and the presence of added substances, including chelating agents and antioxidants. Indicate the stability indicating method(s) used to quantitate the drug substance, its impurities, and its degradation products. Define the possible degradation profile of the drug substance. The availability of samples of these impurities or degradation products permits the validation of assay method(s) used to quantitate their levels in the drug substance. Also, either the same method (preferably) or another method of sufficient sensitivity—at least to

0.1% of active drug—must be used to quantitate levels of degradation products.

To avoid or limit problems in this area after submission of the NDA, the validation of analytical methods and the conduct of stability studies should be planned from the initial phases of clinical research. This will provide the type of data approvable by the FDA. The reader is directed to the Guideline for Stability Studies for Human Drugs and Biologics and updates, and the final ICH Guideline for the Stability of Drug Substance and Drug Product for assistance in fulfilling this essential requirement.

6. Manufacturer

Under this section, the name and address of each facility (including contract testing laboratories) used in the manufacture and control of the drug substance should be provided. Each building involved in the manufacture of the drug substance should be properly identified by street address and, if appropriate, building number. If more than one building is used, state the part of the operation being carried out in each building. The operations that should be covered include manufacturing, processing, packaging, labeling, and control of the drug substance.

For foreign facilities, manufacturing site facilities, operating procedures, and personnel information must be included in this section. This information can also be available as a DMF, in which case a letter from the DMF holder to the FDA that authorizes the use of applicable data in conjunction with the review of the sponsor's application is sufficient for this section.

7. Method of Manufacture

a. Starting Materials—Specifications and Tests. The starting material(s) used to synthesize the drug substance should comply with the FDA's definition of a starting material. For a material to be considered a starting material, it should be (1) commercially available; (2) a compound whose name, chemical structure, and chemical and physical properties are generally known; (3) described in the literature; and (4) obtained by commonly known procedures (including starting materials extracted from plant or animal sources, and precursors to semisynthetic antibiotics obtained by fermentation procedures). Most of the time, a material will meet several of these criteria. If it does not meet any of them, it probably is not the starting material.

Describe the analytical controls used to ensure the identity, quality, and purity of each batch of starting material. The source of the starting material need not be specified, but it may be requested.

   b. Solvents, Reagents, and Auxiliary Materials. List all reagents, solvents, and auxiliary materials and a statement of the quality of each material (i.e., USP, NF, ACS, or Technical). Describe the specifications and tests used to accept each batch of material. A specific identity test should be included. The need for additional testing depends on the role of the material used in the preparation or isolation of the drug substance.

   c. Drug Substance Synthesis. Provide a full description of the method used in the isolation (e.g., synthesis, extraction, fermentation, recombinant DNA procedures) and purification of the drug substance. The description of the isolation of the drug substance should include a diagrammatic flow chart. Such charts should contain (1) chemical structures of reactants, molecular weights, and names or code designations, (2) stereochemical configurations, if applicable, (3) structures of intermediates, both in situ and isolated, (4) solvents, (5) catalysts, (6) reagents, and (7) significant side products that may interfere with the analytical procedure or that are toxic.

   Describe the processes involved in the synthesis of the drug substance. The synthesis description should include information on the following: (1) pieces of equipment used; (2) quantities of starting material(s), reagents, solvents, catalysts; (3) workup and isolation procedures; (4) reaction conditions such as temperature, pH, and time; (5) purification procedures; (6) manipulative details including addition rate, stirring speed, pressure, and order of addition; and (7) yields (crude and/or purified weight and percent).

   The FDA has given approval in the past to the concept of a "pivotal intermediate." This is an analyzed and well-characterized synthetic intermediate that is usually isolated one to two steps before synthesis of the crude final product, but may be obtainable by more than one synthetic route. To obtain approval, material produced by the several routes must be characterized, especially with regard to the identity and level(s) of impurities and the relative qualities of the finished bulk drug substance produced. In addition, a fairly rigorous set of specifications for the intermediate has to be established to assure its ultimate quality by whichever approved route is used in its production (see section on process controls below). The benefit to the sponsor is that the level of detail describing the various routes used to make the pivotal intermediate does not have to be as great as normally required. This permits some latitude for implementing modifications to those steps occurring up to the synthesis of the pivotal intermediate without the necessity of receiving prior FDA approval, as long as the quality and impurity profiles of the pivotal intermediate are unaltered from those on file at the FDA.

   It also should be noted that the FDA may request additional preclinical toxicology studies. This will depend on the degree(s) of difference(s) in the profiles, identities, and levels of impurities in bulk drug substances produced from the pivotal intermediate made by the various routes of synthesis, and whether the finished drug is intended for short-term or chronic use.

The final steps in the workup, isolation, and purification of the bulk or microencapsulated drug substance should be written in detailed fashion. The description should address the following issues: (1) crude product yield (a range should be given); (2) tests performed on the crude product, preferably including at least one purity test appearing in the finished drug substance specifications; (3) the isolation and purification procedures; (4) alternate purification procedures (polymorphic changes should be considered); (5) yield of purified product (again it is recommended that a range be provided); and (6) evidence that the purification procedure actually improves the purity of the crude product (e.g., chromatographic illustrations).

Any alternate method or permissible variation, such as different starting material, reagent, solvent, or conditions, should be reported with an indication of the circumstances under which it will be used, and comparative analytical data should be provided.

d. Antibiotics and Other Products Obtained by Fermentation Processes. Similar information is needed for the preparation, isolation, and purification of antibiotics and other drug substances isolated from microbial or cell culture sources. The components of the fermentation media should be defined and specifications established, including, if applicable, a defined degree of purity. The role of each ingredient, if known, should be stated.

Because the specific microorganism cultured is the most critical factor in any antibiotic process, strain identification, including morphological, cultural, and biochemical characteristics, should be performed. The source of the microbial isolate (e.g., soil, air, water), as well as any genetic engineering or mutation procedures, should be documented. Microbial deposition should be reported (e.g., American Type Culture Collection or Type Culture Collection of the U.S. Department of Agriculture).

The stability of the cell culture to repeated transfer should be defined, because numerous transfers lead to strain degradation (attenuation). The factors that should be defined are the number of transfers from individual colonies that do not result in a significant decrease of antibiotic production, and the proper method(s) and conditions for maintaining an active culture.

The monitoring and control of the fermentation process should be reported in detail. Parameters to be addressed include the media preparation and sterilization, inoculation procedures, and the fermentation process. Provide a detailed description of the media composition, the method for its sterilization (temperature and duration), and the pH after sterilization. The inoculation stage description should include quantity (by volume percent) and age of the inoculum to be used, as well as information on the morphological stage of the mycelium, if this parameter is controlled. The fermentation stages should be characterized by duration, temperature, pH, aeration rate (volume of air per volume of medium), concentration of dissolved oxygen, the critical elements regarding agitation, and the pressure in the fermenting vessel. Also cite the name and concentration of any antifoaming agents and precursors or inducers of biosynthesis used. The monitoring of antibiotic concentration in the fermentation broth is one of the most critical parameters in the production process, so the concentration and the method(s) used for its determination should be reported. If a microbiological method is used, the assay microorganism should be indicated, and information should be provided on the sensitivity and reproducibility of the method along with pertinent literature references. In addition, the microbiological and biochemical methods used to control the fermentation process should be described as well as an indication regarding their frequency of use.

Some antibiotic-related considerations concerning extraction and isolation that should be addressed include (1) the presence of impurities and side products, along with their quantitation and the results of tests assessing their immunological and toxicological properties, (2) the development of specific analytical techniques capable of differentiating the product from related antibiotics, and (3) identification of minor active components as well as their levels and respective antimicrobial activities.

Approved applications for bulk antibiotic drug substances were converted to Type II DMFs when section 507 of the Federal Food, Drug, and Cosmetic Act was repealed as part of the enactment of the Food and Drug Administration Modernization Act. The FDA gave each affected holder the newly assigned DMF number. Holders are expected to reference the new DMF number on all letters of authorization or other correspondence relating to the DMF for the bulk antibiotic drug substance and maintain the DMF in accordance with the NDA regulations.

An FDA guidance provides recommendations on the use of monoclonal antibodies as reagents in the manufacture of drug substances that are regulated by CDER or CBER. The guidance focuses on the chemistry, manufacturing, and control (CMC) issues that should be addressed in NDAs, ANDAs, and supplements to these applications. The sponsor or applicant should submit information (e.g., production process, specification) to support the use of the monoclonal reagent or a letter of authorization to a DMF that contains this information. A description of the manufacturing process should be provided. The description is used to assess the potential impact on the biological safety, quality, and purity of the drug substance and/or drug product. The monoclonal reagent should be adequately characterized, and its identity, purity, and structural integrity should be assessed. A description of the purification process for the monoclonal antibody should be provided in the CMC documentation, along with complete stability information. Changes in the monoclonal supplier or in the manufacturing process of the antibody or solid support are considered to be drug substance manufacturing process changes that can have an effect on the safety and effectiveness of the drug substance and final product.

e. Drug Substances Isolated from Plant or Animal Sources. Botanical drug products have certain unique characteristics that should be taken into account when CMC documentation is provided for NDAs covering them. Botanical drugs will be different from synthetic or highly purified drugs, whose active constituents can be more readily chemically identified and quantified. Active constituents in a botanical drug might not need to be identified in an NDA submission if this is shown to be infeasible. In such circumstances, the FDA will rely instead on a combination of other tests (e.g., spectroscopic or chromatographic fingerprints, chemical assay of characteristic markers, and biological assay), controls (e.g., strict quality controls of the botanical raw materials and adequate in-process controls), and process validation (especially for the drug substance) support for the NDA for the botanical drug.

For drug substances obtained from plants, the description of their collection and preparation should include the following: (1) botanical species and plant section(s); (2) geographical location(s) where plants with acceptable levels of drug substances are found (the same species can have different levels, when harvested from different locales, because of differences in climate and soil constituents); (3) storage and transportation conditions; (4) drying conditions; (5) grinding procedures; (6) testing procedures to identify and assay crude material, as well as a listing of typical results; and (7) extraction and isolation procedures, where applicable.

The description of drug substances isolated from animal (including human) sources should contain (1) species and organ(s) or tissue(s) used, (2) statement(s) demonstrating compliance with USDA or other applicable requirements, and (3) information corresponding to items c–g for plant-derived drug substances described above.

f. Process Controls. A brief description of the control checks performed at each stage of the manufacturing process, and of the packaging of the drug substance, should be provided. The controls applied to the intermediates should be adequate to assure the correct operation of synthetic and purification procedures, as well as the production of the desired products with the necessary purity. The tests should include identifying the material using at least one physical property (e.g., melting or boiling range, refractive index, and optical rotation), detecting impurity/contaminant levels, and monitoring yield. Testing for pivotal and key/critical intermediates should address all of these criteria.

For a pivotal intermediate (one that can be prepared by several different routes), specifications should be rigid and methodologies used should minimize the possibility of the presence of previously undetected or vagrant impurities. The number of steps between the pivotal intermediate and the penultimate intermediate determines the extent of detail and degree of purity required (i.e., the closer they are, the greater the detail and degree of purity required). It should be noted that the pivotal intermediate and the penultimate intermediate can be one and the same.

For a key/critical intermediate (defined as one in which an essential molecular characteristic[s] is first introduced), specifications and test methodologies should be used that assure that the molecular architecture intended to be conferred (e.g., chirality, stereospecificity) has occurred in the expected yield and required purity. At least one test methodology should be used that can quantitate levels of undesired impurities, such as isomers, reaction by-products, or starting materials. For other intermediates, controls may not have to be as extensive. One or more tests monitoring the progress of the synthesis may be all that is necessary.

g. Reprocessing. It is expected that operating conditions during the manufacture of the drug substance may occasionally deviate from the synthesis description. If a standard reprocessing procedure has been developed and validated and is expected to be used routinely in the synthesis of the drug substance, include this information in this section.

h. Reference Standard Preparation. Describe how the reference standard used to perform the proof-of-structure studies was prepared and how new lots of reference standards will be qualified. If the method of synthesis is the same as that of the drug substance, a statement referencing this fact is sufficient, along with a detailed description of any additional purification procedures performed. These procedures (e.g., recrystallization) should be repeated until important parameters, including assay and levels of impurities, remain unchanged after two successive purification procedures as demonstrated by appropriate tests (e.g., chromatography).

The primary reference standard is normally prepared on a laboratory scale using pure starting materials, reagents, and solvents and should be of the highest purity that reasonably can be obtained. The synthetic procedure used to make it, and the method(s) used for its purification, also should be provided. (If applicable, the method of manufacture section can be referenced.) The purification procedure is normally performed until little or no change is observed through two consecutive cycles in assay purity and levels of impurities.

An analytical reference standard or working standard usually derived from a production batch is normally established as the comparative standard for routine analyses of the bulk drug substance for release purposes. It should be characterized against the primary standard.

i. Specifications and Analytical Methods. The regulatory specifications and analytical methods used to assure the identity, potency, quality, and purity of the drug substance should be submitted. The following are examples of attributes that should be monitored:

APPEARANCE/DESCRIPTION. Color, taste, odor, crystalline form(s), and feel.

PHYSICAL PROPERTIES. Melting or boiling range, pH, specific rotation, refractive index, dissolution characteristics in various solvents (including water), and crystallinity (type, such as orthorhombic, cubic, amorphous).

SPECIFIC IDENTITY TESTS. At least one specific identity test that is capable of distinguishing the drug substance from related compounds must be included. Spectrometric tests are usually used, such as ultraviolet, infrared, nuclear magnetic resonance, and mass spectroscopy. Retention times or factors derived from thin-layer, gas-liquid, and HPLC are also used as identification tests to verify a more specific spectral identity test.

IMPURITY PROFILE. Because it requires many hours of work by synthetic and analytical chemists, deficiencies in this area are rather frequent. Impurities should be identified, and at least the major ones should be characterized. Other impurities, when possible, should also be elucidated structurally. Specifications should include limits for each major impurity, as well as a limit for the total level of all impurities. These limits should be based on the known or anticipated toxicological properties of each impurity, referencing, if necessary, the toxicological profiles of similar compounds. They also should be based on a review of levels in batches used in longer term toxicology and clinical studies and demonstrated in these studies to be safe. The reader is referred to the Guideline for Industry on Impurities in New Drug Substances and the Guidance for Industry NDAs: Impurities in Drug Substances. The agency strongly recommends that ICH guidances on identification, qualification, and reporting of impurities should also be considered when evaluating impurities in drug substances produced by chemical syntheses that are not considered new drug substances. This recommendation applies to applicants planning to submit NDAs and supplements for changes in drug substance synthesis or process. Examples of NDAs affected by the recommendation include those submitted for new dosage forms of already approved drug products, or drug products containing two or more active moieties that are individually used in already approved drug products but have not previously been approved or marketed together in a drug product.

ASSAY. The methods for the drug substance and the impurities should be stability indicating. If the identity test is specific and impurities are adequately controlled by other methods, a less specific method to assay the drug substance may be used. If possible, the same procedure should be used to measure both the overall purity of the drug substance and the levels of impurities or degradation products. The limits for purity should be established on the basis of scientific review of the impurity profile of the drug substance and review of results obtained from individual batches.

OTHER. Most drug substances used to manufacture dosage forms are solids. It is therefore necessary to consider other properties that may affect the bioavailability with the possibility of eliciting adverse reactions. These parameters, which should be adequately addressed both in the specifications and in the characterization/structure elucidation section, include the nature and extent of solvation, the possibility of different polymorphs, and particle size.

The extent of solvation is routinely monitored by LOD testing conducted at a temperature previously defined by TGA. Either the basis for concluding the existence of only one solvated form or information comparing the respective solubilities, dissolution rates, and physical/chemical stability of the different solvates should be provided.

Polymorphism is customarily monitored by melting point or infrared spectral analysis. However, other methods, such as x-ray diffraction, thermal analytical, and solid-state Raman spectroscopy, also can be used. It is expected that the sponsor will conduct a diligent search by evaluating the drug substance recrystallized from various solvents with different properties. Either the basis for concluding that only one crystalline form exists or comparative information regarding the respective solubilities, dissolution rates, and physical/chemical stability of each crystalline form should be provided.

Particle size determination may not be important if (1) the drug substance demonstrates good water solubility, (2) particle size reduction or compaction is performed as part of the dosage form manufacture, or (3) the drug substance is intended to be administered in solution (not suspended). However, the sponsor should be prepared to address with the FDA reviewer why it is not important. The appropriate part of the dosage form manufacturing section, where the data are to be found, should be cross-referenced.

REFERENCE STANDARD. Characterization and structure elucidation data are typically derived from tests conducted on the primary reference standard. Its suitability must be documented by information much more extensive than prescribed in the specifications. In addition to the prescribed analyses—especially levels of impurities—other tests normally conducted include elemental analysis and ultraviolet, infrared, nuclear magnetic resonance, and mass spectrometry, along with reviews of each, providing assignments of the important features supporting the structure(s) of the drug substance. Other tests, such as optical rotation, refractive index, x-ray crystallography, phase solubility analysis, and differential scanning calorimetry, may be provided as well to support its purity and elucidate its structure. Finally, some compounds may require bioassays for full characterization.

j. Container/Closure System. Provide explicit information regarding the characteristics of, and quality control test methods used by both the manufacturer and the sponsor for, the container, closure, and any other component parts (e.g., desiccant bags) to assure suitability for their intended use. If this information is on file at FDA in the form of a DMF, provide a copy of the letter from the holder of the DMF to the FDA authorizing the use of applicable data in conjunction with the review of the sponsor's application. Whenever possible, a similar letter from the fabricator(s) should be obtained and included. In addition, stability data supporting the use of the components should be cross-referenced. Detailed information concerning this subject can be found in the Guideline for Packaging of Human Drugs and Biologics.

If most of the CMC information drug substance is covered by a DMF, the sponsor needs a letter of authorization to this DMF. The sponsor has to indicate in this section how the drug substance is accepted, maintained, and qualified in its facilities prior to use in the production of the drug product.

Further guidance regarding the required information to be included in support of the manufacture and control sections of the new drug substance can be found in the Guideline for Submitting Supporting Documentation in Drug Applications for the Manufacture of Drug Substance.

IV. DRUG PRODUCT

A. Components

Provide a list of all substances used in producing the finished dosage form intended for commercial distribution, regardless of whether they are ultimately contained in the product. This includes excipients as well as in-process materials, such as water or other solvents used in the granulation process and later removed by drying. The quality specifications or grade (ACS, USP, or NF) should be indicated for each substance.

If proprietary mixtures (colorants, coating mixtures, flavors, controlled release matrices, imprinting inks) are used as components, information on their compositions should be provided. Any alternates that have been evaluated and determined to be interchangeable also may be included. The sponsor should be prepared either to delete the alternative from the application or to generate further information, including effects on the bioequivalency, in support of retaining the alternative if the FDA initially does not accept it.

B. Composition

The statement of composition identifying each active or inactive ingredient per unit of dosage form (e.g., tablet, capsule, or mL) should be provided. In addition, include a batch formula that is representative of the scale of manufacture to be used. Besides the name, strength, and type of dosage form, the name and weight of each active ingredient and the identification of all components should be given. This should include their grades in the same manner as defined under Components. Information to be included will usually consist of the weights and measures of each component using the same weight system, any calculated excesses, and the theoretical weight and number of doses to be obtained. Reasonable variations in the amounts of inactive components (e.g., ±10%) are usually permitted and are generally indicated on the quantitative composition. Dosage forms, however, must be formulated to contain 100% of the desired potency. Whereas the allowable range for the potency of a drug might be 90% to 110% of its labeled potency during its labeled shelf-life period, a sponsor cannot change the formulation to achieve 95% of the labeled potency in an effort to reduce the cost of manufacturing.

C. Specifications and Analytical Methods for Inactive Components

Inactive components are sometimes referred to as inactive ingredients, ingredients, or excipients. These are all the items in the listing of components used to manufacture the drug product except the drug substance(s). If an inactive component is USP/NF grade, it is acceptable just to reference the current monograph for that component. If the inactive ingredient is non-USP/NF but belongs to a foreign compendium, provide a copy of the actual monograph for this inactive component. The FDA will at times accept the specifications and test methods indicated in the foreign compendium but can ask for validation data for the assay method. The FDA has placed its approved inactive ingredients list on the CDER web site in a searchable format (previously it was available in a series of .pdf files). A simple search by name will provide the range of concentrations and quantities of each inactive ingredient found in the formulations of approved NDAs. An ingredient intended for use in an NDA or ANDA that is found in this list, and that is intended for use within the approved limits across marketing applications, will be acceptable in the new drug. Acceptable food or color additives are indicated in the 21 CFR, and batch certifications are needed for some of the color additives before they can be released for production. A batch certificate for the NDA batch should be included.

Indicate which tests will be performed routinely by the sponsor on each lot received. Most sponsors will perform all tests specified in the monograph for the first few batches until comparative data are achieved with the manufacturer's Certificate of Analysis; then they rely on Certificates of Analysis and perform an identity test for each batch.

In the case of noncompendial materials, specifications and complete descriptions of the test methodologies to be used for quality control release purposes by the sponsor should be included. In addition, it may be necessary for the sponsor to obtain a letter authorizing reference to a DMF from the supplier concerning the manufacturing and controls procedures used to make these materials, such as mixtures of colorants or flavors. It may be necessary to obtain toxicity data if the mixture or component has little or no history of human use (e.g., new polymers). If it is anticipated that an "untried" component will be used, it is recommended that discussions be initiated with the FDA's reviewing chemist and pharmacologist. These sessions should be scheduled as soon as possible to minimize the possibility of delays in NDA approval caused by inadequate information to support the use of the material.

D. Manufacturer

The names(s) and address(es) of all manufacturers, contract packagers, and contract analytical laboratories used for testing raw materials or the drug product should be given. If the manufacturing site is in the United States, a general description of site facilities and operations should be incorporated, because information on these facilities is available in the FDA District Offices. If the manufacturing site is in a foreign country, letters authorizing FDA reference to site DMFs (type I) on behalf of the sponsor should be included. If a DMF is not available, then information that is needed to prepare a type I DMF should be obtained by the sponsor from the manufacturer. This information is then placed in this section. Refer to the Guideline for Drug Master Files.

E. Method of Manufacture, Packaging Procedure, and In-Process Control

In this section, include a general description of the manufacturing procedure, including all processing alternatives previously validated as producing acceptable product. The FDA also wants copies of the proposed or actual master production and control record, as well as a copy of a completed production and control record for a typical batch. It is also helpful to provide a schematic diagram for the flow of materials, the production process, and an indication of the equipment to be used.

For other than manual operations (e.g., computerized automated plants), the schematics are more critical to assure that the FDA reviewer understands the process. The description should also indicate the various points of sampling.

The piece(s) of equipment that renders the batch homogeneous before packaging should be identified, with both the useful working and total capacities noted.

Regarding reprocessing operations, adequate information should be submitted to permit approval of such procedures for bulk, in-process, or finished drug products that do not conform to established specifications. The original application may include proposals for such steps to cover foreseeable deviations, such as unacceptable weight variation, content uniformity, and tablet coating. Deviations not covered in the original application should be covered by a supplemental application and must receive approval before commercial distribution of such reprocessed product. All proposals should include a description of the material that includes a statement of the deviations(s), a detailed description of the reprocessing procedure, including additional controls to be used over and above those established for routine production, and information on the maximum allowable time between initial manufacture and initiation of reprocessing operations, along with the applicable storage conditions to be used during this interval.

A sample packaging record(s) that describes the packaging and label operations also should be included with the manufacturing and control record and the completed production and control record for a typical batch.

1. Regulatory Specifications and Analytical Methods for Drug Product

Consistency in the quality of the drug product batches is controlled by the specifications and analytical methods set for that product. This means that when the drug is taken by a patient, the expected clinical response will occur. Specifications and analytical methods evolve throughout the investigational phases of drug development. By NDA time, a sponsor has learned much about the nature of the drug product and the critical parameters that have to be monitored to provide maximum assurance of its safety and efficacy. It is at this point that the regulatory specifications and analytical methods are determined for the drug product. These are established to assure the safety and efficacy of every batch of drug product up to the date of its expiration. The NDA also should include appropriate information on in-process controls and a listing of the number or amount of drug product needed to perform each of the regulatory analytical methods.

Regulatory specifications may differ from product release specifications. Regulatory specifications assure acceptable product potency until the labeled expiration date or shelf life. In general, in-house release specifications are tighter than regulatory specifications. Refer to the Guideline for Submission of Supportive Analytical Data for Methods Validation in the New Drug Application.

The following items should also be considered.

a. Tablets, Capsules, and Other Dosage Forms

1. Weight variation.

2. Content uniformity for tablets, capsules, sterile solids, and sterile suspensions. A common deficiency is the use of different analytical methodologies for uniformity and for assay purposes without supporting their equivalency or adequately defining correction factors.

3. Dissolution rate tests for tablets, capsules, suspensions, suppositories, or other dosage forms. Controlled-release dosage forms or drug delivery systems also should be monitored by appropriate testing methodology. The FDA has provided a Guidance to Industry: In Vitro Dissolution Testing for Modified Release Solid Oral Dosage Forms.

4. Moisture content. In some formulations of relatively water-insoluble drug substances containing anhydrous lactose, storage under high humidity (75% or higher) has been shown to affect dissolution rates adversely.

5. Loss on drying, where applicable.

6. Physical characteristics such as color, appearance, odor, shape, hardness, thickness, friability, and coating. Fading and brittleness (powdering) are common problems.

7. Softening or melting points and particle size distribution of suspended drug (suppositories).

8. Assay(s) for the active drug substance in the drug product, for impurities, and for degradation products.

For sponsors who intend to change (1) the components or composition, (2) the manufacturing (process and equipment), (3) the scale-up/scale-down of manufacture, and/or (4) the site of manufacture of immediate release and modified release solid oral dosage forms during the postapproval period, the FDA has provided aid on assessing (1) the levels of change, (2) the recommended CMC tests to support each level of change, (3) recommended in vitro release tests and/or in vivo bioequivalence tests to support each level of change, and (4) documentation to support the change.

b. Solutions and Suspensions

1. Clarity, limit for the presence of particulate matter, preservative effectiveness and assay, isotonicity (ophthalmics and injectables), and pH

2. Sterility of ophthalmics

3. Sterility, apyrogenicity, and container fill of injectables

4. Leakage test for presentations such as ampules, vials, sachets, aerosols, strips, and tubes

5. Spray pattern and container pressure for aerosol products; for a metered dose product, reproducibility of actuated dose and defined limits for dose administered per actuation

6. Particle size specifications for the active component; resuspendability, viscosity, sedimentation rates, caking, and syringeability of suspensions

7. Completeness and clarity of constituted solutions

For sponsors who intend to change (1) the components or composition, (2) the manufacturing (process and equipment), (3) the scale-up/scale-down of manufacture, and/or (4) the site of manufacture of nonsterile semisolid preparations (e.g., creams, gels, lotions, and ointments) intended for topical routes of administration during the postapproval period, the FDA has provided aid on assessing (1) the levels of change, (2) recommended CMC tests to support each level of change, (3) recommended in vitro release tests and/or in vivo bioequivalence tests to support each level of change, and (4) documentation to support the change.

For nasal spray and inhalation solution, suspension, and spray drug products intended for local and/or systemic effect, CMC recommendations may vary depending on the specific drug product and stage of development. Changes in components of the drug product or changes in the manufacturer or manufacturing process can affect key parameters and should be carefully evaluated for their effect on the safety, clinical effectiveness, and stability of the product.

c. Plastic Devices Containing Active Drugs

1. In vitro rates and identity testing of all plastic components. If applicable, determine sterility and measure levels of residual ethylene oxide and its decomposition products.

2. Additional physical tests, such as frame memory, resiliency, tensile strength, and seal integrity.

d. Diluent Solution. Full specifications and analytical methods, including preservative levels.

2. Container/Closure System(s)

CDER approves a container/closure system to be used in the packaging of a human drug or biological as part of the NDA or BLA for the drug. A packaging system found acceptable for one drug product is not automatically assumed to be appropriate for another. Each application should contain enough information to show that each proposed container closure system and its components are suitable for its intended use.

The type and extent of information that should be provided in an application will depend on the dosage form and the route of administration.

The responsibility for providing information about packaging components rests foremost with the applicant of an NDA or ANDA, or the sponsor of an IND. This information may be provided to the applicant by the manufacturer of a packaging component or material of construction and may be included directly in the application.

Any information that a manufacturer does not wish to share with the applicant or sponsor (i.e., because it is considered proprietary) may be placed in a DMF and incorporated into the application by a letter from the manufacturer to the applicant that authorizes reference to the DMF. The letter of authorization should specify the firm to whom authorization is granted, the component or material of construction being described, and where the information and/or data is located in the file by page number and/or date of submission.

a. General Requirements. Describe all the packaging configurations to be used for the drug product. List the components that comprise each container/closure system to be used. Specific information to be submitted is described in Table 2.

The Guideline for Packaging of Human Drugs and Biologics includes specific recommendations for the format and content of this section. Some points need to be emphasized, however, to help the sponsor avoid delays in NDA approval because of deficiencies in container/closure information. The FDA issued a guidance in 1999 that supersedes the FDA Guideline for Submitting Documentation for Packaging for Human Drugs and Biologics, issued in February 1987. Section 505(b)(1)(D) of the act states that an application shall include a full description of the methods used in the manufacturing, processing, and packing of such drug. This includes facilities and controls used in the packaging of a drug product. Information on container closure systems used for storage of bulk drug products need not be included in the application. However, these container closure systems should be shown to be suitable for their intended use. The suitability of the storage containers should be supported by data retained by the applicant and/or manufacturer and should be made available during FDA inspection upon demand.

The information regarding the container closure system used by a contract packager that should be submitted in the CMC section of an NDA, ANDA, or DMF, and which is referenced in the application, is no different

Table 2   Container/Closure Information for an Application for Any Drug Product

General description of the container closure system.
For each packaging component,
    Name, product code, manufacturer, physical description
    Materials of construction (name, manufacturer, product code)
    Description of any additional treatments or preparations
    Protection (by each component and/or the container closure system, as appropriate):
       light exposure, reactive gases (e.g., oxygen), moisture permeation, solvent loss or
       leakage, microbial contamination (sterility/container integrity, increased bioburden,
       microbial limits), filth, other
    Safety (for each material of construction, as appropriate): chemical composition of all
       plastics, elastomers, adhesives, etc.; extractables (as appropriate extraction/toxico-
       logical evaluation studies, USP testing, reference to the indirect food additive
       regulations, other studies as appropriate)
    Compatibility (for each component and/or the packaging system): component/dosage
       form interaction (USP methods are typically accepted), may also be addressed in
       postapproval stability studies
    Performance (for the assembled packaging system): functionality and/or drug delivery,
       as appropriate
    Quality control for each packaging component received by the applicant: applicant's
       tests and acceptance criteria, dimensional (drawing) and performance criteria.
       Method to monitor consistency in composition, as appropriate
For each packaging component provided by the supplier,
    Manufacturer's acceptance criteria for release, as appropriate, and brief description of
       the manufacturing process

from that which would be submitted if the applicant performed its own packaging operations.

When more than one plastic resin is used to fabricate bottles, it is necessary to demonstrate the equivalency of the container produced using the different resins. In addition, comparative data derived from light transmission, chemical resistance, extractables, and moisture permeation/vapor transmission tests described in the USP should be provided as applicable to the type of product. (For example, moisture permeation for an aqueous dosage form would not be necessary.) Whereas the compendia discuss these tests only in the context of polyethylene, the guideline makes no distinction as to the resin used. It also should be verified that copies of letters authorizing FDA reference to appropriate DMFs from manufacturers of the resins used to fabricate bottles and from the bottle fabricator(s), if available, are included. Although most resin suppliers include information on extractables data in their DMFs, it should be pointed out that fabricators may have to add release agents or other additives not covered by extractables data in the DMF of the resin supplier.

Manufacturers of glass components, in most cases, do not have DMFs. It is recommended that letters be obtained from fabricators certifying that the glass used will meet appropriate compendial requirements (i.e., US type I or type II glass).

For closures, compatibility of the drug product with the inner liner/ contact surface should be evaluated. This is usually done as part of stability studies conducted on a product stored inverted. If available, appropriate DMF authorization letters should be obtained to support suitability of the closure and liner.

Provide information on any adhesives used for blistered packages. Defect classification data should be considered. Permeation and leaching/ migration testing should be conducted and reported. (Information in a DMF or data from studies conducted by the fabricator may be sufficient.)

For elastomers (e.g., stoppers), leaching of components is a concern, as is the possibility that components, especially active drug substance from the formulation, will migrate into the closure. Therefore test data should be provided that demonstrate drug product/closure compatibility. A letter from the closure manufacturer authorizing FDA reference to their DMF should be obtained and included.

Finally, for any unusual or uncommon containers and closures, sufficient information about the materials of fabrication, design performance, and other information that conclusively demonstrates their suitability for use with the dosage form should be provided.

b. Inhalation, Injectable, and Ophthalmic Drug Products. There are special considerations for certain types of products, such as inhalation, injectable, and ophthalmic drug products.

Inhalation drug products include inhalation aerosols (metered dose inhalers); inhalation solutions, suspensions, and sprays (administered via nebulizers); inhalation powders (dry powder inhalers); and nasal sprays. The CMC and preclinical considerations for inhalation drug products are unique in that these drug products are intended for respiratory-tract compromised patients. This is reflected in the level of concern given to the nature of the packaging components that may come in contact with the dosage form or the patient.

Any contaminants present (as a result of contact with a packaging component or due to the packaging system's failure to provide adequate protection) can be rapidly and completely introduced into the patient's general circulation. Although the risk factors associated with ophthalmic drug products are generally considered to be lower than for injectable drug products, any potential for causing harm to the eyes demands caution.

Injections are classified as small-volume parenterals (SVPs) if the solution volume is 100 mL or less and as large-volume parenterals (LVPs) if the solution volume exceeds 100 mL. The potential effects of packaging component/dosage form interactions are numerous. Hemolytic effects may result from a decrease in tonicity, and pyrogenic effects may result from the presence of impurities. The potency of the drug product or concentration of the antimicrobial preservatives may decrease due to adsorption or absorption. Injectable drug products require protection from microbial contamination (loss of sterility or added bioburden) and may also need to be protected from light or exposure to gases (e.g., oxygen).

The American Academy of Ophthalmology (AAO) recommended to the agency that a uniform color coding system be established for the caps and labels of all topical ocular medications. An applicant should either follow this system or provide an adequate justification for any deviations from the system. Although ophthalmic drug products can be considered topical products, they have been grouped with injectables because they are required to be sterile [21 CFR 200.50(a)(2)], and the descriptive, suitability, and quality control information is typically the same as that for an injectable drug product.

F. Stability

This section, as previously discussed, frequently poses problems leading to delays in NDA approval. Particular attention should be paid to the development of adequate data from studies conducted with commercial formulations packaged in container/closure system(s) to be marketed. It is critical that adequately validated analytical methods be used as early as possible in the investigational phases of drug development—no later than the initiation of phase 3 studies. Common defects in stability studies submitted to the FDA reflect the lack of acceptable long-term or short-term accelerated stability data to support the approval of an expiration date for the product. Another common problem occurs when studies are conducted using only one container size, yet the sponsor is applying to market two or more sizes. As a general rule, the FDA wishes to see data from studies conducted on at least the smallest and largest sizes to be marketed (e.g., 100- and 500-tablet bottles or 2- and 32-ounce bottles). Blister packs are generally exceptions to the rule because each dosage unit is individually packaged.

With drug products containing preservatives, the stability protocol should include preservative efficacy testing. Microbial challenge testing should be conducted at appropriate intervals—at least once a year unless significant losses are observed earlier as a result of assay procedures.

Other items worth considering in the design of a stability protocol are the effects of heat, humidity, freezing (for solutions, emulsions, and semisolids), and light. These data are needed to support the recommended storage conditions required to be on the product labeling. The information also helps answer the inevitable questions from the field (e.g., the product has been stored in a warehouse whose air conditioning unit broke, and the customer wants to know if the product is still good after storage for a month at 110°F). Simulated use tests are also recommended, in which the same bottles are opened and closed a number of times and the data are compared with the stability of drugs stored in unopened containers.

For products intended to be reconstituted, it is necessary to conduct stability studies on the final product form to determine the maximum allowable storage time after reconstitution. Data from these studies, usually conducted over a period of a week or less, support recommendations required to be on the labeling for storage time and conditions after reconstitution (e.g., "Administer within 3 hours after reconstitution. Store until use under refrigeration [2° to 8°C or 35° to 45°F]"). If previous studies have demonstrated light or heat sensitivity, these conditions should be considered in designing studies of the reconstituted product.

In addition to potency, other design considerations that may need to be incorporated in the stability protocol for various dosage forms include the following:

TABLETS. Appearance, friability, hardness, color, odor, moisture, and special emphasis on dissolution rates.

CAPSULES. Moisture, color, appearance, shape, brittleness, and especially dissolution rates.

EMULSIONS. Appearance (particularly with regard to phase separation and color), odor, pH, viscosity, and the effects of heating and cooling.

ORAL SOLUTIONS AND SUSPENSIONS. Appearance (clarity, the presence of a precipitate, cloudiness), pH, color, odor, redispersibility (suspensions), and storage both in upright and inverted positions to determine if the closure or liner adversely affects stability.

ORAL POWDERS. Appearance, color, odor, moisture content of powder, and, if intended for reconstitution, appearance, pH, and dispersibility/dissolution properties.

METERED-DOSE INHALATION AEROSOLS. Quantity of delivered dose, total number of acceptable doses delivered, color, solvate formation with propellant, particle size distribution, weight loss of canister (i.e., loss of propellant), pressure, valve corrosion, and storage in both upright and inverted positions.

TOPICAL AND OPHTHALMIC PREPARATIONS. Appearance (clarity, color, and especially homogeneity), odor, pH, resuspendability, consistency, particle size, weight loss (of more importance if plastic containers are used). Sterility and preservative levels also must be considered if the product is intended for ophthalmic administration.

SMALL VOLUME PARENTERALS (SVP). Appearance, color, clarity (particulates), pH, and sterility checks at reasonable intervals are minimum standards. Powders for reconstitution should also include residual moisture and stability checks after reconstitution. Except for ampules, upright and inverted storage of final product should also be evaluated.

LARGE VOLUME PARENTERALS (LVP). Similar evaluations as described for SVPs should be conducted. In addition, if plastic containers are used, volume and extractables data should be evaluated. Another important parameter to consider, if applicable, is the maintenance of adequate preservative levels over the expiration dating period.

SUPPOSITORIES. Appearance, melting range, dissolution at 37°C (body temperature) and aging with respect to hardening and polymorphic transformation.

DRUG ADDITIVE. Compatibility of admixture, appearance over 24 hours including evaluations of both drug and additive for assay, pH, color and clarity, and interaction with the container at the time of mixing (time 0) and 2–3, 6–8, 12, 24, and 48 hours after mixing. Some intervals may be deleted or the time intervals adjusted as considered appropriate or cost effective.

STATISTICAL ANALYSES. The statistical analyses of data submitted to support a proposed expiration date should be described fully. In addition, as part of the stability protocol, provide detailed plans for such analyses of future batches.

STABILITY REPORTS. These reports are frequently deemed incomplete because adequate information for each lot of product is missing. Data must be provided describing formulation; batch number; scale of manufacture, including designation as to whether a laboratory, pilot, or production lot; site(s) of manufacture; and the analytical methodology(ies) used, reflecting changes, if any, made during the course of the investigation. Notations regarding the status of each lot (whether it is terminated or continuing on stability) should also appear on each table of data.

STABILITY PROTOCOL. A postapproval stability protocol should be submitted documenting future plans. It should include information on time points and storage conditions to be evaluated, and indicate whether extensions of expiration dating are intended based on sponsor evaluation of data obtained following the protocol. These data will still have to be submitted, as well as the details of the extensions of expiration dating being implemented, in the annual reports filed with the FDA. Also indicate how many batches of drug product will be placed on stability in a year.

BIOTECHNOLOGICAL/BIOLOGICAL PRODUCTS. These products have distinguishing characteristics to which consideration should be given in any well-defined testing program designed to confirm their stability during the intended storage period. For such products in which the active components are typically proteins and/or polypeptides, maintenance of molecular conformation, and hence of biological activity, is dependent on noncovalent as well as covalent forces. The products are particularly sensitive to environmental factors such as temperature changes, oxidation, light, ionic content, and shear. To ensure maintenance of biological activity and to avoid degradation, stringent conditions for their storage are usually necessary. The evaluation of stability may necessitate complex analytical methodologies. Assays for biological activity, where applicable, should be part of the pivotal stability studies. Appropriate physicochemical, biochemical, and immunochemical methods for the analysis of the molecular entity and the quantitative detection of degradation products should also be part of the stability program whenever purity and molecular characteristics of the product permit use of these methodologies.

With these concerns in mind, the applicant should develop the proper supporting stability data for a biotechnological/biological product and consider many external conditions that can affect the product's potency, purity, and quality. Primary data to support a requested storage period for either drug substance or drug product should be based on long-term, real-time, real-condition stability studies. Thus the development of a proper long-term stability program becomes critical to the successful development of a commercial product.

G. Environmental Assessment

The format and content of this section for NDAs and ANDAs can be found under 21 CFR 25 Subpart C. In addition, the FDA has generated a guidance document that provides a more in-depth description and clarification of items to include in this section. This document is entitled "Guidance for Industry on the Environmental Assessment in Human Drug and Biologics Applications, July, 1998." The FDA guidance provides information on when an EA should be submitted; it also makes recommendations on how to prepare EAs for submission of drug or biological applications to CDER and CBER. Topics covered include (1) when categorical exclusions apply, (2) when to submit an EA, (3) the content and format of EAs, (4) specific guidance for the environmental issues that are most likely to be associated with human drugs and biologics, (5) test methods, (6) an applicant's treatment of confidential information submitted in support of an EA, and (7) master files for drugs and biologics.

V. SAMPLES

Identify all samples being set aside for FDA validation. The samples should include drug substance, drug product, major impurities, and degradation products being controlled for, reference standard, and internal standard (the latter is not required if commercially available but is recommended to facilitate FDA laboratory work). If appropriate, blanks and any other materials not commercially available but specified in the analytical procedures should be provided. The samples are to be maintained by the sponsor until the FDA's reviewing chemist provides instructions as to where they should be forwarded. The total quantities and the manner of their subdivision (e.g., 400 tablets, 4 100 tablets/ bottle) should be indicated. The amounts provided should be adequate to permit at least three separate determinations, excluding sterility, by two different laboratories.

VI. METHODS VALIDATION PACKAGE

A recent FDA guidance provides recommendations to applicants on submitting analytical procedures, validation data, and samples to support the documentation of the identity, strength, quality, purity, and potency of drug substances and drug products. The recommendations include drug substances and drug products covered in NDAs, ANDAs, and supplements to these applications. The principles also apply to drug substances and drug products covered in drug master files (DMFs). Each NDA and ANDA must include the analytical procedures necessary to ensure the identity, strength, quality, purity, and potency of the drug substance and drug product, including bioavailability of the drug product. Data must be available to establish that the analytical procedures used in testing meet proper standards of accuracy and reliability.

Unlike the full NDA, which is submitted in duplicate, the methods validation section must be provided in triplicate because copies are forwarded to two FDA laboratories. These laboratories will assess the validation data and test the drug substance and drug product to verify the validity of the regulatory specifications and test methods indicated in the NDA. Documents in this package that were taken from the CMC section should retain the original pagination in the CMC section. Intended to expedite the NDA review and FDA laboratory validation of proposed regulatory methods, it is recommended that the submission include the following items.

A. Test Methods and Specifications

Copies of regulatory specifications and analytical methods for the drug substance and drug product should be provided. These documents should retain the original pagination they had in the CMC section.

B. Supporting Data

Validation information to support the suitability of the regulatory analytical method(s) is shown by providing data on accuracy, specificity, sensitivity, precision, ruggedness, and linearity over the range of interest. The emphasis for analyzing drug substances is the control of the presence of impurities. With drug products, it is more important to quantify the active drug substance and level of degradation products throughout the expected shelf life of the product. (Levels of impurities that are not degradation products are adequately controlled in the bulk drug substance-release testing.)

Documentation (or lack thereof) provided in support of specificity, sensitivity, and ruggedness is a frequent source of FDA comment and delays in NDA approval.

SPECIFICITY. It is not advisable to rely on drug substance assay results (and assay specificity demonstrated only with respect to impurities) on the assumption that degradation products behave similarly. Specific studies to determine degradation pathways must be conducted. These should include exposing the drug substance to acid(s), base(s), heat, light, oxidizers, reductants, and combinations of the above, as appropriate. In the absence of suitably designed degradation studies, it is not possible to know the intrinsic stability of the drug substance or to determine in future studies whether any given peak on a chromatogram is an artifact or a real degradation product. It also may be difficult to establish whether the chromatogram is run long enough to permit the observation of peaks from degradation products. In addition, excipients in the dosage form may interfere with one or more peaks of interest. The specificity of the method(s) should be evaluated by treating the formulation minus the active ingredient(s) in similar fashion to the dosage form before injecting or spotting. It is strongly recommended that the methods include retention information for all degradation products known or still in the process of being identified to facilitate their monitoring by different analytical chemists during the course of the stability studies.

SENSITIVITY. This can be a source of FDA comment, when information is not included in the validation documentation on the sensitivity(ies) of the method(s) to detect and quantitate the drug substance and the degradation products. In addition, the methodology description should include the appropriate mathematical formula(e) to be used for calculating their respective levels. Even if the sponsor uses a computerized system that provides the number directly, these formulae should still be provided to facilitate manual calculations.

RUGGEDNESS. This is also an important consideration, because it is directly linked with the probability of success for the FDA laboratories validating the methods internally (i.e., analyst-to-analyst, lab-to-lab reproducibility results). It is recommended that the sponsor have a second laboratory perform the method using a different instrument and column, if possible. By following this recommendation, potential misunderstandings regarding the performance of the various operations and manipulations can be identified and rewritten for clarity to facilitate the use of the selected method. In addition, in the case of chromatographic systems (HPLC or GC), the appropriate peaks and their minimum resolution (separation) factor can be determined and noted in the method of description as the parameters to be monitored by the analyst to assess the suitability and effectiveness of the operating system before conducting the assay. This assessment should be performed routinely and is commonly referred to as "system suitability testing."

OTHER AREAS.   Those that can lead to approval delays include (1) use of instrumentation not commercially available and the absence of a detailed description of the components and assembly, (2) use of single source specifications to permit duplication, (3) use of specialized tools or equipment not available to the FDA chemists for sample preparation, (4) use of an in-house standard or other noncommercial reagent, and (5) failure to provide a system suitability test on chromatographic procedures.

Data from these and similar sources should not be submitted unless it can be demonstrated that no acceptable alternatives are available.

Include documentation supporting the integrity of the reference standard.

For additional information, the reader is directed to the Guideline for Stability Studies for Human Drugs and Biologics and the Guideline for Submission of Supportive Analytical Data for Method Validation in New Drug Applications.

C. Test Results

Provide the certificates of analysis for drug substance, drug product, and reference standard for the lots where the samples were obtained.

In support of samples of impurities, degradation products, and internal standards, it is recommended that copies of relevant spectra and other supportive analyses used to elucidate or verify their structures be included.

VII. THE COMMON TECHNICAL DOCUMENT

The ICH has created a new format for the marketing applications, the Common Technical Document (CTD), which is acceptable to all signatories, including the EU, Japan, and the U.S. CMC information is presented in detail in Module 3 ("Quality") and is summarized in Module 2, the CTD summaries. This format is described in ICH and FDA guidances (M4: The Common Technical Document for the Registration of Pharmaceuticals for Human Use, M4: CTD–Quality and Submitting Applications According to the ICH/CTD Format–General Considerations). The CTD is intended to be a precise, detailed, universal and uniform approach to the organization of all technical data to support a marketing application. It does not materially add to, or subtract from, the required information for an NDA, as delineated in this chapter. However, the organization of the CTD allows for a uniform approach to marketing applications across ICH regions and regulatory review agencies, thus allowing a single CTD to serve as the basis for approval of a new product in all applicable jurisdictions. The CTD format will be mandatory for new marketing submissions in the various ICH regions in the years 2003–2004.

VIII. ABBREVIATED NEW DRUG APPLICATION

There are distinct differences and some unique problems likely to be encountered in the preparation of manufacturing and controls sections for ANDA submissions. Some of them are highlighted below.

A. Summary

A summary is not required by the FDA. Its preparation, however, might help the sponsor pinpoint potential deficiencies. If the application is among the first being submitted for a drug whose patent is about to expire, the summary may help the FDA's reviewing chemist become familiar with the drug.

In lieu of a summary, information should be provided that shows the proposed product is the same as a listed product (eligible products are listed in the FDA publication, "Approved Drug Products with Therapeutic Equivalence Evaluations") with respect to its indications for use, active ingredients, route of administration, dosage form, strength, bioavailability, and labeling. Patent certification information and any indications for which the ANDA sponsor is not eligible because they were exclusively approved for a previous NDA sponsor should also be provided.

B. Drug Substance Sources

Drug substances that are used in the manufacture of drug products that are the subject of ANDAs are usually obtained from one or more external manufacturers, frequently located overseas, and imported into the United

States. Under the FOI it is important to obtain a copy of a potential supplier's most recent EIR describing the FDA's findings. This document should be reviewed by the sponsor to assess the likelihood of the supplier's acceptability to the FDA as a manufacturer. In addition, the supplier should have a DMF available at the FDA for reference purposes. This will describe the facilities, personnel, equipment, and manufacturing and controls procedures used at the site(s) where the bulk drug substance is made. The ANDA sponsor can then submit a much simplified drug substance section because the letter of reference to the DMF serves in place of providing specific details regarding the manufacturing procedures, controls, stability data, and identification of impurities. These and other relevant issues should be assessed by direct discussion with the manufacturer and, if necessary, one should arrange to have the manufacturer update the DMF.

C. Specifications

This subject is usually not a problem if compendial (USP) monographs exist. Analytical methodology, however, can be a troublesome item. This is especially true with older drugs when the assay methodology specified in the monograph is not sufficiently specific, and in the case of drugs for which there are no published compendial monographs. An FOI request to the FDA for a copy of the pertinent regulatory assay method will prove helpful in minimizing the amount of analytical development work to be carried out.

It is prudent to evaluate impurity peaks observed in a supplier's bulk substance and compare them with those observed in the drug product. The extent that the peaks differ may determine the need to obtain further information, including toxicity. Samples of impurities/degradation products methods should be appropriately validated by the ANDA sponsor for their sensitivities and specificities. It also is recommended that the sponsor of an ANDA set up and maintain a stability program for the bulk drug substance.

D. Drug Product Requirements

Drug product requirements are similar to those described previously for the NDA. The extent of stability data submitted, however, is much less than that usually available for an NDA. Specifications are usually defined by a published compendial monograph. It must be emphasized that analytical methodologies for many older drugs, as set forth in their monographs, may not be sufficiently specific to be accepted by FDA as "stability indicating." It is also possible that the drug product may not have a published monograph. A request should be made under the FOI to obtain a copy of the regulatory assay method. Adequate validation studies should be carried out to verify the accuracy, precision, specificity, recovery, and sensitivity of the method(s) conducted by the sponsor's own laboratory or contract facility. It is also important to compare the release characteristics of the sponsor's product with those obtained with the original brand name product using the same methodology. For example, data comparing the dissolution characteristics and performance of the sponsor's and the brand name tablet or capsule products at several different time points (as applicable to obtain 95% or more of drug in solution)—otherwise referred to as a comparative dissolution profiling— should be obtained.

The FDA issued a guidance in 1999 which supersedes the packaging policy statement issued in a letter to industry dated June 30, 1995, from the Office of Generic Drugs. Section 505(b)(1)(D) of the act states that an application shall include a full description of the methods used in the manufacturing, processing and packing of such drug. This includes facilities and controls used in the packaging of a drug product. The information regarding the container closure system used by a contract packager that should be submitted in the CMC section of an ANDA or in a DMF, which is referenced in the application, is no different from that which would be submitted if the applicant performed its own packaging operations.

All significant phases of the manufacturing and processing of a drug product (including packaging) should be described as part of the CMC section of an ANDA or in a DMF referenced in the application. The only exception is the repackaging of solid oral drug products for which an approved application already exists.

E. ANDA Expiration Dates

Generally, the FDA will tentatively approve a 2-year expiration date for a product if satisfactory data reflecting at least 3 months' storage under accelerated conditions is submitted. The sponsor is also expected to provide a commitment to continue to monitor the stability of the product, periodically to report the results to the FDA, and to remove from the market any batches failing to meet specifications prior to the product's labeled expiration period. Final approval for the expiration date is obtained when acceptable shelf life data for 2 years or more for one production lot are made available to the FDA. In contrast to NDAs, for which the extended term data are frequently available prior to approval, the importance of the stability protocol describing future plans, including the basis that the sponsor deems appropriate to support an extension of a product's expiration dating, is magnified for an ANDA. In fact, an ANDA will most likely not be approved without the inclusion of a suitable stability protocol.

The FDA generated a guidance document regarding the content and format of an ANDA entitled Guidance for Industry: Organization of an Abbreviated New Drug Application and an Abbreviated Antibiotic Application (February, 1999). Depending upon the availability of significant information on, and the complexity of, these drug products/dosage forms, the amount of information necessary to support these applications may vary from that proposed for NDAs.

IX. CHANGES TO AN APPROVED NDA OR ANDA

Section 506A of FDAMA provides requirements for making and reporting manufacturing changes to an approved application and for distributing a drug product made with such changes. The FDA has issued a guidance to provide recommendations to holders of NDAs and ANDAs who intend to make postapproval changes in accordance with Section 506A. The guidance covers recommended reporting categories for postapproval changes for drugs, other than specified biotechnology and specified synthetic biological products. Recommendations are provided for postapproval changes in (1) components and composition, (2) manufacturing sites, (3) manufacturing process, (4) specifications, (5) package, (6) labeling, (7) miscellaneous changes, and (8) multiple related changes.

The FDA's guidances on postapproval changes have provided a great deal of detail on the preferred approach to CMC submissions. These guidances, for example, provide recommendations to pharmaceutical sponsors of NDAs and ANDAs who intend to change an analytical testing laboratory site for components, drug product containers, closures, packaging materials, in-process materials, or drug products during the postapproval period. The documents provide guidance on a less burdensome approach to providing notice (i.e., Changes Being Effected [CBE] supplements) of certain postapproval changes. A guidance document has been released by the FDA providing suggestions on changes to an approved application for specified biotechnology and specified synthetic biological products, recombinant DNA–derived protein/polypeptide products, and complexes or conjugates of a drug with a monoclonal antibody.

Section 506A of the Act provides for four reporting categories that are distinguished as follows:

1. A major change is a change that has a substantial potential to have an adverse effect on the identity, strength, quality, purity, or potency of a product as they may relate to the safety or effectiveness of the product (506A(c)(2)). A major change requires the submission of a supplement and

approval by the FDA prior to distribution of the product made using the change (506A(c)(1)). This type of supplement is called, and should be clearly labeled, a Prior Approval Supplement.

2. A moderate change is a change that has a moderate potential to have an adverse effect on the identity, strength, quality, purity, or potency of the product as they may relate to the safety or effectiveness of the product. There are two types of moderate change. One type of moderate change requires the submission of a supplement to the FDA at least 30 days before the distribution of the product made using the change. This type of supplement is called, and should be clearly labeled, a Supplement—Changes Being Effected in 30 Days. The product made using a moderate change cannot be distributed if the FDA informs the applicant within 30 days of receipt of the supplement that a prior approval supplement is required. For each change, the supplement must contain information determined by the agency to be appropriate and must include the information developed by the applicant in assessing the effects of the change. If the FDA informs the applicant within 30 days of receipt of the supplement that information is missing, distribution must be delayed until the supplement has been amended with the missing information. The FDA may identify certain moderate changes for which distribution can occur when it receives the supplement. This type of supplement is called, and should be clearly labeled, a Supplement—Changes Being Effected. If, after review, the FDA disapproves a changes-being-effected-in-30-days supplement or a changes-being-effected supplement, the FDA may order the manufacturer to cease distribution of the drugs that have been made using the disapproved change.

3. A minor change is a change that has minimal potential to have an adverse effect on the identity, strength, quality, purity, or potency of the product as they may relate to the safety or effectiveness of the product. The applicant must describe minor changes in its next Annual Report. An applicant can submit one or more protocols (i.e., comparability protocols) describing tests, validation studies, and acceptable limits to be achieved to demonstrate the absence of an adverse effect from specified types of changes. A comparability protocol can be used to reduce the reporting category for specified changes. A proposed comparability protocol should be submitted as a prior approval supplement, if not approved as part of the original application.

X. CONCLUSION

In the context of the guidance documents issued by the FDA, this chapter has explored the various issues, and described a number of recommendations, concerning the documentation requirements for NDA and ANDA submissions. It is anticipated that as industry representatives become more familiar with these guidance documents, the quality of CMC documentation will be improved, and it is hoped that the frequency and extent of deficiencies will diminish. One of the most positive contributions will be the economical one, because reproducible manufacture of new drugs in well-designed dosage forms can be prescribed by physicians with confidence. The careful preparation of the manufacturing and controls section in an NDA or ANDA can facilitate the FDA processing, review, and approval procedures. The result is potentially faster commercialization of new products benefiting both pharmaceutical manufacturers and the patients they ultimately serve.

BIBLIOGRAPHY

Buday PV. Manufacturing controls sections of new drug applications. Drug Cosmet Ind 1976; 119:62; 126–127; 129–131; 133–135. Reports 1981; 43:T&G\4, December 14. Washington D.C.: F-D-C Reports.

Code of Federal Regulations, Title 21, Part 314. Applications for FDA Approval to Market a New Drug or Antibiotic Drug.

Cook J, Prunella P, Stringer S, Yacura M. Approvals and non-approvals of new drug applications during the 1970s. OPE Study 57, PB 81-14865. Rockville, MD: U.S. Food and Drug Administration, 1980.

FDA Letter to Industry. FDA letter describing efforts by CDER and ORA to clarify responsibilities of CDER chemistry review scientists and ORA field investigators in the new and abbreviated drug approval process in order to reduce duplication and redundancy. October 14, 1994.

Federal Food, Drug and Cosmetic Act, as Amended. Superintendent of Documents. Washington, DC: U.S. Government Printing Office, November, 2002.

Federal Register February 22, 1985; 50(36):7452–7519.

Food and Drug Administration. Guidelines: Manufacturing and Controls for INDs and NDAs. FDA Papers 1971; 5:4–14.

Food and Drug Administration. Requirements of Laws and Regulations Enforced by the U.S. Food and Drug Administration. U.S. Department of Health, Education, and Welfare, Public Health Service, HEW Publication (FDA) 1979: 79–1042.

Food and Drug Administration Modernization and Accountability Act of 1997.

Fry EM. The role of the inspection in pre-market approval for drug products. Paper presented at the Pharm Tech Conference, Sheraton Centre Hotel, New York, NY, September 1981, 22–24.

Karlton P. Meeting the challenge of FDA's CMC initiatives. J Pharm Tech, October, 1996.

Kumkumian CS. Manufacturing and controls guidelines for INDs and NDAs—1978. Paper presented at the 25th National Meeting of the Academy of Pharmaceutical Sciences, Hollywood, FL, November 14, 1978.

Kumkumian CS. New drugs: filing the manufacturing and controls sections of INDs and NDAs. Paper presented at the Pharm Tech Conference, Sheraton Centre Hotel, New York, NY, September 22–24, 1981.

Kumkumian C. New Drug Application Chemistry Review. Format and Content Guide. June, 1992.

McDermaid R. FDA's foreign inspection program. Paper presented at the Pharm Tech Conference, Sheraton Centre Hotel, New York, NY, September 22–24, 1981.

Personeus GR, Ascione P. Preparation and use of drug master files in the pharmaceutical industry. J Parenter Sci Technol 1981; 35:63–69.

Phelps Hyman, PC McNamara. The Food and Drug Modernization Act of 1997: A Summary 1997.

Schultz RC. New drug stability guidelines. Paper presented at the 11th Annual Industrial Pharmacy Management Conference, Concourse Hotel, Madison, WI, November 1, 1978.

The United States Pharmacopeia/National Formulary. United States Pharmacopeial Convention, Rockville, MD. Edition updated every 5 years; supplements published approximately yearly.

15
Data Presentation for FDA Submissions: Text and Tabular Exposition

Patricia Blaine
Blaine Pharmaceutical Services, Inc., Matawan, New Jersey, U.S.A.

I. INTRODUCTION

Over the years, representatives of both the FDA and the pharmaceutical industry have published in pharmaceutical journals or presented at workshops many helpful suggestions to facilitate NDA review of submissions and to avoid elements that impede the review. Several authors and presenters have expressed the FDA reviewers' frustration at having to review a submission that is incoherently assembled or confusing in its presentation.

It is to the advantage of an NDA sponsor to make the FDA review process as effortless for the reviewer as possible. The difference in time to approval between a difficult-to-review submission and a clear, well-presented submission may be many months, as the reviewer might require the sponsor to correct the deficiencies before the review can proceed. The marketing personnel of the sponsoring company can all too readily compute the thousands and millions of sales dollars lost for every month of delay in approval or, conversely, the revenue gained from a quick review and approval. In the worst case, a submission that might be marginally acceptable (fileable) on the merits of a therapeutic agent's effectiveness and safety data alone may generate an RTF action if errors in indexing, presentation, and assembly make a meaningful review tedious or even impossible.

The ideas in this chapter for improving the text and the tables in NDA submissions (or other regulatory submissions) will be representative rather than comprehensive and will focus more on general methods for improving the quality of the text and the tables than on specific styling conventions. Many pharmaceutical and biotech companies have their own style guides to promote uniformity and quality of documents throughout a submission. Other companies use a standard style guide, such as the *Manual of Style* published by the American Medical Association [1]. Although the examples given in this chapter will be derived from the clinical area, the ideas transcend the different disciplines. Finally, it is beyond the scope of this chapter to discuss graphic presentations, which can greatly enhance the interpretation of data.

II. TEXT EXPOSITION

A. Content

Most NDA submissions contain an enormous amount of data, which cannot be presented entirely within the body of a document. Although all the data collected for an individual subject or patient (or groups of subjects or patients) may be important, critical judgment must be exercised in the selection of key data for presentation and discussion within a given document. Data necessary for the development of a specific thesis should be presented within the body of the document rather than placed into a remote appendix, which will impede the review. Less important data can be summarized briefly, clearly referenced in text, and placed in appendices. Additionally, data that have been collected over the years of a drug's development but add nothing to the evaluation of the effectiveness or safety of a therapeutic agent need not be presented at all. Any data submitted will have to be evaluated, so the inclusion of extraneous data will slow the review of the application. The submission should note the existence of such data and have it available upon request of the FDA.

B. Tone

The tone of the text should be formal without being stilted. Avoid legal language on the one hand and colloquial or informal language on the other.

C. Conciseness

Be mindful that FDA reviewers must read through many volumes of an NDA to make a report on their conclusions. Having to pour through dense, inflated, entangled text to ascertain the point being made will slow the review process. Whereas scientific data are more complex and require more effort to comprehend than most general reading material, a skillful writer will ensure that the complexity derives only from the material and not from the presentation.

Wordiness and needless elaborations impede the progress of the review. Also, much of the textual data should be presented in tables to make the comparison of data easier. The following points address ways of making NDA documents more concise.

1. Keep the language simple and straightforward. Simple language is not unscientific; rather it promotes clear, fast understanding. Edit out inflated language. For example, "prior to the initiation of the study" can be changed to the much simpler "before the study began"; and "subsequent to the initial administration of study drug" can be changed to "after the first dose of study drug." Why say "The patient experienced a fall and suffered a fracture of her right hip" when "The patient fell and fractured her right hip" will convey the meaning just as well?

2. Use acronyms and initialisms to speed up the flow of text if they are easily recognized and have been spelled out at first mention. Those that may be confused with another used in the same document should be spelled out.

3. Eliminate redundancies. A careful review of the text will find many words, phrases, and even sentences that can be omitted. Sentences can often be combined by the deletion of redundant phrases, thus improving the flow of the text. Be prepared to come up against style mavens when implementing this task. For example, many "house styles" insist on units after each number in a range (e.g., 10 mg/kg–20 mg/kg). Whereas some units are brief and may not interfere with the flow of the sentence, a range such as "10 mg of iodine/mL to 20 mg of iodine/mL" would interrupt the sentence flow. This redundancy adds considerably to the length of the sentence, and the burden on the reviewer is further compounded if multiple ranges are compared within one sentence. Consider dispensing with this nicety to improve flow and comprehension.

D. Correctness

The textual presentation should agree with the tabular data in the document; in turn, the tabular data should agree with the data source (which agrees with the case report form and other clinical documentation). This is critical to the scientific merit of the submission. When lack of agreement between in-text data and source documents is found, the entire submission may be suspect, and the reviewer will be inclined to spend much more time evaluating the raw data to be sure of the conclusions.

E. Consistency

Consistent punctuation, capitalization, abbreviations, and other styling conventions are much desired in any document, but use judgment before applying the consistency rule unquestioningly. Does the adherence to consistency improve the document or confound it? For example, should all section headers at the same level have the same grammatical structure or would another structure better describe the content of the section? Be critical before insisting on consistency at any cost. A pundit once said, "Foolish consistency is the hobgoblin of little minds."

F. Clarity

The FDA reviewer should be able to read through an application expeditiously and not have to stop to try to discern the meaning of a textual presentation. The sponsor of the application should have someone who is familiar with the material in general, but not with the specific document, read it for clarity before submission. If a particular presentation is not clear to this reader, then most likely an FDA reviewer will have the same problem understanding it. Clarity is facilitated by careful attention to the following:

1. Punctuation. *In The Art of Plain Talk*, author Rudolf Flesch said that punctuation "is the most important single device for making things easier to read" [2]. Omission of punctuation marks, especially commas, can force the reviewer to reread a sentence to ascertain the meaning.

2. Sentence structure and length. If long sentences are needed to report equivalent statistics that will be evaluated together, it is helpful to keep the structure of the sentence straightforward and simple. In this kind of sentence, put the thrust of the sentence at the beginning so reviewers have a reference point for the subsequent statistics as they read them. Series items should be in order, not random, and be free of interrupting material. Vary sentence lengths to avoid boredom. If possible and feasible, use active rather than passive voice.

3. Misplaced modifiers. Every style book covers this topic, but the rule on avoiding misplaced modifiers is often violated. A careful reading of the text by a good editor will eliminate this error.

4. Parallelism. Because much of the data in an NDA involves comparisons of one group to another, parallel structure is important in presenting the data. Style books for scientific writing will supply good examples of this concept.

G. Outline of Sections and Subsections

The clear relationship of one section to another is critical to the review of a document. If no definite structure is apparent, the reviewer will become lost.

The decimal system is a very popular outlining system; it is easy to use and can be set up automatically in most current word processing software applications. This author strongly advises against going beyond three or four levels in the decimal system, because it is difficult to figure out by then which level you are reading. For example, is section 3.1.2.1.2.1.1.1 on the same level as section 3.1.2.1.2.1.1 or is it a subsection of the former? If no other formatting characteristics identify the subordination of one section to another or are not recognizable as clear distinctions (e.g., all caps, bold versus initial caps, bold), the reviewer has difficulty figuring out the relationship of one section to another. This is also true of another popular outlining system, the alphanumeric system, where letters and numbers alternate as section headers. After a few levels, the distinctions become obscured, and reviewers will become lost.

H. Indenting

Avoid indenting large sections of text. Most text should be flush to the left margin with appropriate headers to identify the section. Multiple and sequential indenting wastes space and is confusing. Short lists are appropriately indented, and conventions like indenting with bullets are useful to break up long sections of text.

I. Global to Specific

For any section, begin with global statements or data and then discuss the specifics. For example, in the discussion of adverse events, the overall presentation of the events should precede the presentation by severity, by relationship, by subgroup, etc. It is particularly important in the discussion of the populations evaluated in a particular document. Begin with the all-inclusive population first, then define the subpopulations. One NDA this author worked on had about 10 different populations, many of which were close in numbers of patients (e.g., all patients entered, all patients treated in controlled studies, all patients treated in uncontrolled studies, patients treated with test drug in controlled studies, patients treated with active comparative agents or with placebo in controlled studies). This caused great confusion until a table was constructed to identify each population, beginning with the largest population.

III. TABULAR PRESENTATION

In-text tables should be used whenever they simplify the presentation and allow for substantial reduction in text. Comprehensive multipage tables that interrupt text should be avoided, if possible, unless they are critical to the development of the thesis of the section. However, if the tables are very important, they can be placed in the same volume in an appendix. Usually, data can be collapsed to be included in the in-text table, with reference to the full table in an easy-to-locate appendix. It should be mentioned here that any tables, figures, or graphs in the appendices must have in-text references.

Information from the tables should not be repeated in the text except as part of a concluding statement about the tabular data or trends seen in the data. The commentary on data from the tables should precede the table, beginning with an introduction to the table by number and a statement identifying what type of data it contains. Additional commentary related to the table but not derived from the tabular data may follow the table.

A. Title

All tables require concise but descriptive titles. Sequences of tables that are similar should identify their differences very conspicuously in the title, such as at the end of the title after a colon (e.g., Treatment-Related Adverse Events: by Age; ... by Sex ... by Race).

B. Data Source

Every table should identify the source of the data contained in it. This is usually done in a footnote to the table (e.g., Data source: Statistical Table 23, Volume XX, p. xx). The volume and page numbers will be inserted at the end of the project. Exact referencing of in-text tables will facilitate the review process.

C. Footnotes

Footnotes should be assigned letters (superscripted), not symbols or numbers, which can be confused with the data. Asterisks (*, **, ***) are generally reserved for levels of statistical significance. In multipage tables, footnotes should be assigned letters in the order in which they appear on the specific page of the table. Always begin such tables on a new page to avoid changing the footnotes as the tables shift with the addition of preceding text.

D. Orientation

Portrait tables are always preferable to landscape tables. Remember that the volumes in a submission will be about 2 inches thick. It is cumbersome, annoying, and disruptive for an FDA reviewer to have to move the volume around repeatedly to coordinate the text presentation with the tabular data. If data appear not to fit in the portrait orientation, try changing the axes of the table, so that the axis with more individual descriptors is vertical, whereas the axis with fewer items is horizontal (column headings). Also consider revising the table into separate sections under the same column headers, with descriptive headings for each section spanning the width of the table.

E. Order of Data Presentation

In multiple tables with similar data, present the data in the same order as much as possible. If the first column always has the active drug and the second column the placebo or comparative agent, then keep this order throughout the tables. In the analysis of data by demographic or disease subgroup, it is helpful to keep the subgroup of concern (i.e., women, the elderly, racial subgroups, impaired renal function) in the same column in each table.

F. Present Meaningful Data Together

Try to present the data that will be evaluated and compared as close together as possible rather than scattered around the table. For example, if the tabular data represent both evaluable and nonevaluable patients who have been either previously treated or previously untreated, place the evaluable patients together rather than present them by previous treatment.

IV. CONCLUSION

The suggestions presented in this chapter for improving text and tables are meant to be neither complete nor sacrosanct, but simply considered. Indeed, the suggestions may be countermanded by particular constrictions and style conventions of the company sponsoring an NDA or other submission. However, the ability of the writer to look at a document through the eyes of an NDA reviewer will reinforce the suggestions in this chapter. The goal is to speed up the review process and obtain fast approval for a new drug entity. Any suggestions that facilitate this endeavor should be welcome.

REFERENCES

1. American Medical Association. Manual of Style. 8th ed. Philadelphia, PA: Williams and Wilkins, 1989.
2. Flesch R. The art of plain talk, 1962. In: Trimble JR, ed. Writing with Style: Conversation on the Art of Writing. Englewood Cliffs, NJ: Prentice-Hall, 1975: 101.

16
Preparing for FDA Inspections: Manufacturing Sites

Timothy Urschel
EpiGenesis Pharmaceuticals, Inc., Cranbury, New Jersey, U.S.A.

I. INTRODUCTION

A. Purpose of a PAI

The FDA PAI program was intended to have two purposes:

1. To provide an opportunity to perform a full GMP inspection of the applicant's facilities to determine the applicant's capability to manufacture the new drug in the submitted application *and to verify that the data submitted are authentic.*
2. To provide an opportunity to review the applicant's GMP compliance profile *and systems.*

B. When Does a PAI Occur?

Under the current policy, the FDA may inspect an applicant's facilities under any of the following scenarios:

1. Drug products that are difficult to manufacture and replicate
2. Drug products with a narrow therapeutic range, such as drugs used to treat epilepsy, asthma, high blood pressure, and heart disease
3. Drugs that are new chemical entities
4. Drugs that represent a new dosage form for the applicant

5. Drugs to be manufactured by a firm with a history of noncompliance with cGMPs
6. Drugs to be manufactured by an applicant who has not previously submitted an NDA or ANDA
7. Drugs to be manufactured by an applicant who has been manufacturing over-the-counter products and who is seeking approval of its first prescription drug product
8. Other reasons as determined by the local district office

In addition to the above, a firm may receive a PAI for the filing of a supplement for NDA/ANDA changes:

1. Changes in the manufacturer or manufacturing site(s)
2. Changes in the supplier of the active ingredient
3. The introduction of a new dosage form
4. The use of new facilities or equipment or significant changes in manufacturing facilities or equipment

For the suppliers listed in the application, a PAI is valid for 2 years for a domestic supplier and 3 to 4 years for a foreign supplier.

Regarding the manufacturing of clinical supplies, one should not be as concerned with meeting minimum cGMP requirements, but rather documentation and controls beyond cGMPs that would be required to satisfy a future PAI. The PAI actually serves as a second review of the CMC section of an application. The FDA's time frame is to conduct the PAI within 45 days after FDA headquarters's acceptance of the application for filing. If a firm is not ready for inspection (the FDA expects the firm to be ready for a PAI upon submission of the application), it is advised that they notify the local district office and provide a date when they will be ready.

The Center for Drug Evaluation and Research during 2001 evaluated 822 plants in support of new drug applications. Also, the FDA evaluated 1,268 domestic firms in support of generic drug applications.

II. FOCUS OF THE PAI

The PAI inspection team must determine if there is valid and scientific justification for the failure to report data that demonstrate that the product failed to meet its predetermined specifications. Inspections should compare the results of analyses submitted with results of analyses of other batches that may have been produced. The PAI will determine if data submitted in the application are authentic and accurate and if procedures listed in the application were actually used to produce the data contained in the application.

These procedures must be specific and well documented. The PAI, in addition, focuses on the following:

1. An evaluation of the firm's compliance with cGMP requirements, including coverage of the specific batches used to demonstrate bioequivalence
2. An evaluation as to whether the firm has adequate facilities, equipment, procedures, and controls to manufacture the product in conformance with the NDA application
3. Collection samples of the biobatch from the bioequivalence laboratory

Extensive emphasis is also placed on the development of research batches to clinical and production batches and the validation of the transfer and scale-up.

III. GENERAL INSPECTION COVERAGE

A. Points of General Inspection Coverage

1. In-depth evaluation of data to support manufacturing process and controls
2. Data review for clinical and biobatches
3. Comparison between submitted and actual procedures
4. Production controls

    a. Supported with scientific evidence
    b. Qualified and verified to include installation and operational qualification of equipment

5. Technology transfer difficulties
6. Batch production in full-scale equipment
7. Facilities and controls review of bio/clinical batch manufacturing

    a. Qualified facilities; validation of equipment
    b. Accurate documentation
    c. Compliance with cGMPs
    d. Validated processes
    e. Training of staff

8. Review NDA filing

    a. Compare against manufacturing procedures for bio/clinical batches
    b. Check R&D notebooks for development support

    c. Check inventory and receiving records for drug substance (accountability, evidence of falsification)

9. Review validation report to support filed data (to include scale-up equivalency from biobatch to proposed production batch)
10. Review chemical and bioequivalency changes (justification of)
11. Review process, change system, and logs (compliance with SOPs and documentation)

IV. REASONS FOR RECOMMENDATION TO WITHHOLD APPROVAL RESULTING FROM A PAI

The FDA cites the following as the most frequently occurring reasons for disapproval of an application after a PAI:

1. The sponsor's lack of facilities or equipment to manufacture the product
2. Raw material specifications that are not documented in the development report
3. Biobatch and scale-up production lots that differ in formulation and manufacturing procedure
4. A biobatch that is too small or misrepresented
5. Discrepancies in bioavailability studies
6. A scale-up that is not documented or supported with adequate data
7. Manufacturing procedures that are not specific as to manufacturing equipment and instructions
8. Lack of data supporting the processes and controls of the manufacturing process
9. Inadequate development data
10. Insufficient record keeping and controls
11. Discrepancies suggesting fraud or deception
12. The lack of sound validation protocols
13. The lack of validated analytical methods, or the failure of test methods to perform reliably
14. Failure to follow stability protocol or to include stability failures with the filing

V. PAI AUDIT STRATEGY AND GOAL

The goal of a PAI audit is to confirm that the process and controls proposed for the production of the commercial batch will produce a product that is bioequivalent to the clinical batch. The strategy of a PAI audit is to confirm cGMP compliance for all batches produced and to confirm that the biobatch provides an adequate bioequivalence linkage between the clinical batch and the proposed commercial product.

VI. "HOW TO" OF A MOCK PAI AUDIT

The best way to prepare for an FDA PAI is to perform a mock PAI. The mock inspection is usually best performed by an independent auditor who has reviewed the appropriate sections of the submission and has gained some familiarity with the product and the production process used in manufacturing the drug product. The main difference between a routine GMP audit and a PAI audit is that a GMP audit usually follows product flow (materials receipt through distribution of finished product), whereas a PAI focuses on the review of the manufacturing process and controls, and begins with a review of records and the actual submission to the FDA. It is recommended that a flow chart be generated during the cursory review of the production process identifying the processing sequence, components, equipment, parameters, and specifications at each stage.

After a cursory review, the NDA/ANDA submission should be fully received, checking for contradicting information in the various sections of the submission. The FDA correspondence file should be reviewed and assessed as to whether all FDA questions have been adequately addressed. The summary section should be examined for inclusion of all batches used in developmental scale-up and stability studies.

A. Clinical Batch Record

The clinical batch record should be reviewed for GMP compliance and documentation requirements. The biobatch and stability batch records should be reviewed for equivalence to the information included in the NDA/ANDA submission. Process controls, specifications, bioequivalence data, and other information supported with foreign data should be submitted with a certified translation of those data.

B. Batch Size and Scale-Up

Regarding batch size and scale-up, a minimum batch size of 10% of the proposed commercial production batch should be used for producing test batches of solid, oral-dosage nonantibiotic products. All scale-up procedures should be validated. It is important to keep in mind that the scale-up process should not result in a change in the method of manufacture.

C. Drug Formulation and Development

Regarding drug formulation and development, the safety and efficacy studies should be evaluated to check if they were performed using the formulation for the proposed dosage form. Bioequivalency should be demonstrated if a different dosage form or formulation was used to conduct the study. Proposed changes should be critically evaluated for their impact on product quality, integrity, purity, safety, efficacy, bioactivity, uniformity, and stability. One should ensure that an adequate change control system is in place that complies with the systems and procedures established.

D. Product Components

Concerning product components, the name and address of each source of component used in the manufacturing and packaging of the drug product, as well as receiving and inventory (including reconciliation) records for the active ingredient, should be available. The name, address, and operation of each facility involved in the various steps to produce and test the final drug product also should be available. Approved specifications, test procedures, and results for components used should be given. Lots of components should not be accepted on the basis of the supplier's Certificate of Analysis results unless appropriate validation of the reliability of the test results is available.

E. Physical Specifications

Development of physical specifications for the active drug substance (particle size, density) should be specified. Absence of physical specifications must be justified with supporting documentation and should be part of the developmental report 21 CFR 211.84(d). Impurities should be detected, identified, quantified, and characterized. The USP has a limit of 2.0% for ordinary impurities. Data may be required to support the classification of an impurity as ordinary. The FDA expects complete identification of impurities at levels down to 0.1%. A review of active component specifications should be evaluated for changes during development. Changes or discrepancies should be explained. The impurities profile for the NDA drug substance should not differ from lots used in the toxicology and clinical studies. Specifications and microbiological test procedures should be established for pharmaceutical water. Validation of the water system may be required.

F. Bulk Drug Substances

Regarding production of bulk drug substances, specifications for contaminants should be established for all solvents used in the process. A comparison should be performed between the manufacturer's Certificate of Analysis and the submitted specifications, and any discrepancies should be justified. A full description for the route of synthesis should be given, as this is important for the testing and control of impurities and process solvent residues. The FDA expects that, at the time of submission, it will be determined if the drug substance exists in a multiple solid-state form (racemic mixture; stereoisomer) and whether this affects the dissolution and bioavailability of the drug product.

A check on the data should be performed to ensure that dosage forms produced from different manufacturers are equivalent. To demonstrate equivalence, at least one batch of the drug product should be manufactured for each source of the new drug substance to verify for bioequivalence against each clinical batch used in the pivotal studies.

In vivo bioequivalence studies may be necessary for each additional source of new drug substance if the drug product is known to produce bioequivalency problems resulting from the new drug substance.

The FDA requests that, for NDA/ANDA products, one batch of each strength be manufactured from each listed source of active ingredient. Three months of accelerated stability data, including comparative dissolution, should be available for inspection.

Regarding the components of bulk fermentation processes, the strain of the organism used to manufacture the drug substance for the clinical study should be compared with the strain to be used in commercial production. Strain identification includes microbiological, cultural, and biochemical characteristics. A comparison of the media composition and method of sterilization, sterilization parameters, and the pH of the medium after sterilization should be done. All fermentation stages, parameters, and conditions should be described in detail (i.e., temperature, pH) and documented. With regard to bulk drug substances derived from animals, the following should be specified in the submission:

1. Species and organ or tissue used
2. Conditions for storage and transport
3. Processing conditions (i.e., drying)
4. Impurities

G. Equipment

Concerning equipment, comparability is needed when different pieces of equipment are to be used for production batches. Validation of equivalency may be required.

Mixing equipment should be evaluated for the presence of dead spots, which may affect blend uniformity (i.e., valves and discharge ports). All production equipment should be assessed for suitability of use in the manufacturing process; this should include ease of cleaning and ability to maintain control parameters (including sterilization, if applicable). Test results consistently at or near the upper or lower limits indicate problems with the process or incompatibility with the equipment. All equipment should be adequately identified in each batch record. A detailed description of all equipment should be given in the submission as well. The suitability of the equipment for the process can be determined by a review of the installation and operational qualification reports to ensure that equipment can operate at the ranges specified in the manufacturing procedure.

H. Production Controls and Process

In the review production controls, the proposed production process, which must be manufactured in full compliance with GMPs, should be identical to the process used for the manufacture of the biobatch and the stability batch. Any changes in SOPs, controls, or formulation between test batches and proposed production batches should be justified (i.e., addition of ingredients by automated equipment). For bulk drug substances, a change in solvents may require prior FDA approval if these can be considered a significant change. A review of product annuals will indicate if there are problems with manufacturing or controls (for example, where there have been frequent reworks or failures, and at what percentage). In establishing operating parameters, supporting data are required (retest batches, equipment rating, or characteristics). Time limits should be specified for each phase of processing, including a clear explanation of the starting and end times, where necessary. A detailed sampling plan (showing source and location of each sample) for development batches should be included. In addition, a flow chart of the manufacturing process should be provided.

Batch records for the packaging and labeling of clinical batches should be available and similar in content to those to be used for marketed products.

I. Laboratory Records and Controls

Regarding laboratory controls, a review of laboratory notebooks and chromatograms should be done to check the reliability and authenticity of the supporting data in the methods development and testing of the clinical, bio, and stability batches. Reference standards used should be certified as standards. The FDA expects that, for bulk substances, the suitability of reference standards should be more extensive than that of bulk drug substance specifications. A comparison of analytical methods and specifications for lots of drug substance used in clinical batches and biobatches should be performed to see if any deletions or revisions to any specifications occurred.

One should verify that the method of recordkeeping in the development laboratory follows what is stipulated in the FDA's "Laboratory Inspection Guide," from June 1992. The system should also be evaluated for the transfer of validated analytical methods. "On-site" validation of the method is required for analytical methods validated at another laboratory. A written procedure should be available covering both the transfer of methods and on-site validation and revalidation. When contract laboratories are being used, verification that the laboratory is using the correct analytical methods and specifications should be performed.

J. Validation of Analytical Methods

Concerning validation of analytical methods, all methods must be validated prior to the PAI. The validation should include an approved validation protocol and report. The validation protocol should include

1. Method of evaluating validation results
2. Acceptance criteria for all analytical parameters

Compendial methods for drug substances generally do not require any additional validation; however, drug products may require some limited validation to demonstrate that the drug matrix does not interfere with the compendial method.

Acceptance by FDA headquarters of specifications in the submission does not necessarily mean the FDA field office will accept them. The FDA field office during the PAI will check for appropriate development data to support filed specifications and ensure that these specifications are realistic. The submitted specifications should be supported with reliable and reproducible data and be sensitive and discriminating, so that changes in raw materials or products can be detected.

K. Equipment Cleaning

Regarding the cleaning of equipment, a review of the cleaning procedures for the new drug product and assurance that the cleaning procedures have been validated should be undertaken. One should check for possible cross-contamination with highly insoluble or sensitive drugs. Inspection of pipes and hoses and other areas difficult to clean should be considered. A check for validated cleaning procedures in the development area is recommended to determine whether cleaning procedures have been validated against the products manufactured. Cleaning validation includes residue limits and methods of sampling that the FDA expects as achievable and verifiable at the ppm level. The swabbing method is expected to be used with other sampling methods.

L. Process Validation

Equipment qualification and process validation are expected for clinical and biobatches to show batch uniformity and process control. A master validation plan should be available and include the company's philosophy of the matter (what will be validated, who will validate, when and under what conditions will revalidation be undertaken). Full validation of the manufacturing process is not required before a facility receives a PAI. Validation of bulk drugs for each batch size is not required prior to the PAI; however, at minimum a validation protocol should be available. Problems found with a process validation done prior to a PAI does not constitute disapproval; the firm would have the opportunity to correct deficiencies before shipping the new approved drug product. Process validation should include data generated at various operating conditions to bracket the manufacturing parameters and limits. The key to validation of bulk drug substances is proving that the actual production process can consistently operate within the defined critical parameters according to the FDA. Validation studies for bulk substances should include the following:

A flow chart of the process

A discussion concerning the scientific basis for the process, including its limitations and efficiency

A narrative discussion of each step of the synthesis, including what each step accomplishes, its limitations, the quality level of the intermediate produced at each step, and the impurities (if any) generated from each step

The identification of critical steps in the process and how they are monitored and controlled

A discussion of the established parameters for the critical steps and what happens if actual conditions are outside these established parameters

A discussion of any recovery procedures, how they work, and their limitations (for example, to demonstrate that recovered solvent is suitable for its intended use or comparable to virgin solvent)

A discussion of the process refinements to lower impurities

A discussion of the quality and equivalence of product recovered from the mother liquor to the first crop

For reworks, a description of the cause for the process failures that would result in a rework and the contaminants or impurities the rework is intended to remove

M. Master Batch Record

Documentation and recordkeeping of a separate master record with original signatures from the QA or QC departments to indicate their approval should be maintained. A master batch record should not be used as a batch record even if only one batch is to be produced from the master batch record. All manufacturing conditions and equipment usage should be recorded. This information is considered critical to support the proposed scale-up manufacturing process. Investigation reports should be available to address all production problems or difficulties. The batch record for clinical supplies should be a stand-alone document; any references made in the batch record and all supporting documentation should be included as part of the batch record.

For aseptically produced products, a justification for using aseptic processing instead of terminal sterilization should be provided. A batch record for clinical batches should include a specimen label as required by 21 CFR 211.186. Any development batch that failed specifications should include an explanation and a full investigation in accordance with 21 CFR 211.192. Reasoning as to why these batches were not included in the submission should be documented and justified. In review of stability studies, a formal stability program should be available specifying container closure system, storage conditions, test intervals, and parameters. The processing and control parameters used for stability batches should cover limits specified for the proposed production batches. Test batches on stability should be manufactured at the proposed manufacturing site.

Strict accountability for all clinical supplies is important to avoid any suspicion of drug diversion or fraud. Records covering drug returns, distribution, and destruction should be available.

N. Quality Assurance

Quality assurance procedures and controls should be similar to those used for marketed products. Complete and comprehensive follow-up investigations, including a written report, are required for any failures or discrepancies. Any investigation report should at minimum include

The reason for the investigation

A summation of the process sequences that may have caused the problem

An outline of corrective actions necessary to save the batch and prevent a similar recurrence

A list of other batches and products possibly affected, the results of investigation of these batches and products, and any corrective action.

Specifications or processing parameters should not be changed to accommodate or correct the failure unless there is conclusive evidence that a specific parameter or specification is responsible for the failure.

Where reprocessing is considered, supporting data must be available to show that reprocessing will result in a product equivalent to the original.

O. Development Report

The development report of the drug product is crucial for a PAI. In narrative form, it should summarize the development process, thereby linking all information and data to demonstrate equivalency of the proposed manufacturing formulation, process, and controls to the clinical trials. A good development report indicates that the applicant has the appropriate level of knowledge and control over the product and manufacturing process. The FDA often uses the development report to identify potential process-related problems or difficulties in technology transfer, which then would be subject to in-depth coverage during the actual PAI. At present, there are no standard industry practice or FDA guidelines regarding development reports. Recent FDA recommendations of the contents for a development report should include the product formulation, manufacturing instructions, laboratory reports, and the rationale and validation for manufacturing processes, raw material specifications, and release parameters. Specifically, the development report should include or be supported by the following available data:

1. The physical and chemical properties necessary to characterize fully the drug substance, which include, but are not limited to, identification of impurities, particle size, solubility, bulk density, polymorphism, and hygroscopicity
2. The manufacturing procedures used to manufacture development batches, biobatches, and batches used for pivotal clinical studies, which must be specific and well documented
3. Granulation studies (if applicable) to include sieve analysis, bulk density, moisture, blend uniformity
4. Finished product test results to include content uniformity, assay, hardness, friability, etc.
5. Dissolution profile (at minimum for the biobatch and pivotal clinical batches)
6. Stability

During the PAI, the investigator will review underlying raw data and analytical worksheets to assure the accuracy and reliability of the data reported.

Regarding sterile dosage forms, the additional developmental data needed to support the filed process would include physical factors (extrusion force, particulate levels), metal/light sensitivity, filter compatibility and integrity, oxygen sensitivity, container requirements, preservative effectiveness, heat sensitivity (autoclavability), drug substance (source, chemical, microbial purity), manufacturing procedures and equipment, in-process test data, and final dosage form test results.

The development report should identify critical variables for the process and how to monitor and control these variables during scale-up, as well as show correlation of the production batches with the biobatch and clinical batches. A system for the technology transfer from research and development to production should also be provided, and at minimum an SOP describing such a procedure should be available. The rationale for the formulation should include a discussion of the chosen raw materials. (Raw material inventory records should be available during the PAI, because the investigator will review them to evaluate the quantities of materials used, the testing performed, and the source of the raw material). A discussion of the equipment used during development, including a comparison of any different pieces of equipment used to manufacture the developmental batches, should be part of the report. It is also important to include the justification and documentation of any deviation from the established manufacturing procedure, as the investigator will look to see what changes were made or what conclusions were drawn, if any, as a result of the deviation. The conclusion of the development report should be a discussion of the consistency of the process, failures (if any), scale-up problems (if any), bioequivalency among batches, and rationale of decisions made as a result of failures and problems.

VII. POST PAI

A PAI, of course, is not statutorily required for approval of an application to market a drug product. A PAI may be requested by FDA headquarters's staff or conducted at the district office's discretion. Generally, if deficiencies are noted, at the conclusion of the PAI, the investigator will provide a letter to the company explaining its decision to recommend that approval be withheld until the center reviews the field's data. There are several layers of review within the agency after a PAI. The supervisory inspector, branch director, compliance officer, and district director may review any resulting deficiencies in the FDA district office. The FDA headquarters's review will be performed by the Office of Compliance in the Center of Drugs when the district recommends withholding approval of the application. Upon receipt of written certification from the company stating that the noted deficiencies have been corrected, the FDA field office is obligated to clear the application within 45 days if the correction is adequate. In providing responses to deficiencies, a company may have to conduct some additional or repeat tests where the records were lost. On the basis of the data and records that do exist, one may need to obtain a professional's opinion about the data to demonstrate that the lost records will not have a material impact on the product or process. Careful thought and analysis and discussion of the lost records with the agency are generally the best approach under these situations.

REFERENCES

1. Code of Federal Regulations, Title 21, Part 314. Applications for FDA Approval to Market a New Drug or Antibiotic Drug.
2. Code of Federal Regulations, Title 21, Part 211. Current Good Manufacturing Practice for Finished Pharmaceuticals.
3. Davis R. A guide to inspection of pharmaceutical quality control laboratories. Pharmaceutical Engineering, Sept./Oct. 1992.
4. D'Eramo P. Preparing acceptable development reports. Paper presented at DIA Annual Conference, 1993.
5. Federal Register Sept. 8, 1993; 58(172):47340–47352.
6. The Gold Sheet. FDA Pre-Approval Inspection Management Nov. 1991; 25(11).
7. Lee J. GMP compliance: clinical supplies to pre-approval inspections. Presentation in Fort Lauderdale, FL, Feb. 1993.
8. Lee JY. Documentation requirements for preapproval inspections. Pharm Technol 1993; 154–164.
9. Lynch M. Current drug GMP compliance issues. Paper presented at the RAPS annual conference, Washington, DC, September 1997.
10. Morningstan K. Preparing for and passing an FDA inspection. Paper presented at the RAPS annual conference, Washington, DC, September 1997.
11. Perry V. FDA facility inspection. Paper presented at the RAPS annual conference, Washington, DC, September 1997.
12. Points to consider: Commissioner's industry exchange meetings pre-approval inspection program. Regulatory Affairs 1993; 5:281–316.
13. Valazza M. GMP issues and documentation for bulk pharmaceutical contract manufacturers. Pharm Technol Nov. 1992; 48–51.

17

Technology Change: Advantages in the Pharmaceutical Industries

Brian J. Chadwick
LookLeft Group, New York, New York, U.S.A.

I. INTRODUCTION

The life sciences industry faces a number of challenges on the road ahead. Significant market events are converging to create unprecedented opportunities for those organizations that can respond:

   The deciphering of the human genome and the rapid maturation of the disciplines of genomics and proteomics

   Technology innovation such as high throughput screening (HTS) and combinatorial chemistry creating a tsunami of potential new drug candidates coming over the wall from discovery

   Significant consolidation across pharmaceutical and related market segments in pursuit of scale economies of operation and production across a global reach

   The emergence of the Internet as a pervasive operating environment enabling execution of eBusiness strategies that embrace all mission critical, company critical, and back officer functions

   Favorable market conditions for rapid emergence of focused biotech organizations with the agility to leverage the deepening understanding of the nature of disease and the potential for technology to enhance and accelerate traditional rates of development

Overall increase in market velocity due to enabling technologies and
market expansion

Simultaneously, there is economic and social pressure from all sides:

Healthcare reform
Increases in discovery
Increasing number of clinical trials (for NDA)
Escalating costs
New competition
Increasing organizational complexity
Shortages in key skills and overall resources
Explosion of available data and information
Changing political and regulatory environments
Expanding market opportunity

These events of change are pressuring life sciences companies to move
toward the promise that technology will positively impact decision support,
improve the velocity of the new product development process and the capacity
of the new product development enterprise, and enhance relationships inside
and outside the enterprise.

Indeed, it seems that by leveraging technology to allow individuals and
groups working together to be more productive, one can reduce the time it
takes to reach conclusions about products in the development cycle. Clearly,
time is the most significant factor in the calculation of cost—and the cost of
bringing a new product to market is staggering. Just as clearly, less time spent
bringing a new product to market should translate into greater revenue potential. But there is a grander goal still, and that is the promise and value of
knowledge management.

> Knowledge Management caters to the critical issues of organizational
> adaptation, survival and competence in face of increasingly discontin-
> uous environmental change ... Essentially, it embodies organizational
> processes that seek synergistic combination of data and information
> processing capacity of information technologies, and the creative and
> innovative capacity of human beings [1].

This chapter will describe a variety of emerging technology solutions
that can positively change the new product development process for life
sciences companies as well as the implications of such change. The life sciences
industry is conservative and risk adverse by its nature, and change therefore
comes slowly. Yet there are sufficient events in the life sciences marketplace
that suggest that *technology change is upon us*.

II. PEOPLE, PROCESS—AND THEN TECHNOLOGY

The major life sciences companies tend to have a brick-and-mortar perspective. New product development processes have been labor intensive and paper based for more than a century in some cases. In order for any new technology solution to work within such an environment there are a number of considerations that should be addressed.

First and foremost, the needs of the stakeholders must be assessed, including but not limited to

Needs analysis
Business requirements
Stakeholder requirements
Financial parameters and available resources
Process change analysis
Technology integration objectives
Technology direction (other technologies that will be implemented)
Strategy for technology deployment
Strategy for driving user adoption

Once a corporate perspective has been established, a technology and vendor assessment process should be defined, encouraged, and supported, including but not limited to

Business profile
Regulatory compliance
Domain knowledge
Experience
References
Support, help desk
Scalability
Pricing
Customization and optimization
Future development plans
Ancillary tools
User interface/ease of use
Integration profile/configuration requirements
Pilot program

While any such effort must be flexible, a vendor qualification process should be established. And if life sciences organizations are proceeding down this path without appropriate executive support, financial commitment, and necessary resources—with substantial attention to people and process—there will be significantly less chance for success.

Equal attention must be paid to the processes for change management and the technology and the vendor. Typically, technologies have been implemented with insufficient design considerations for integration with other manual and technology solutions or business processes. While the technology clearly needs to work within the constraints of the highly regulated, multinational, and absolutely secure requirements of the life sciences Industry, technology itself may represent only 25% of the overall change requirements. There is a long list of business processes—in both the internal and external environments—that must be proactively addressed, including but not limited to

Creating/modifying

Standard operating procedures (SOPs)
Business continuity practices (BCPs)
Work practices (WPs)

Regulatory compliance
HIPAA implications
CDISC and other standards
Pilot program/metrics analysis
"Best test not just stress test" process
Avoidance of "perpetual piloting syndrome"
"Next steps plan" in place

Implementation planning should address

User adoption tactics
Training—for the various stakeholders
User documentation requirements
User process-readiness evaluation
Help desk solution—internal, subcontractor, vendor
Technology administration
Hardware qualification and procurement
Asset management/hardware maintenance

If *technology change is upon us*—and for that change to bring value—life sciences companies' decision makers must identify key criteria for decision making with attention to *people, process—and then technology.*

III. TECHNOLOGY ADOPTION LIFE CYCLE

In his *Crossing the Chasm,* author Geoffrey A. Moore describes the process by which a new technology is absorbed into a community.

"Through his technology adoption life cycle, Moore offers a vision of how technology is absorbed into a community in phases that correspond to psychological and social profiles of population segments within the community. The most critical point in developing a high-tech market, he states, lies at the transition from an early market dominated by a few visionary customers on the technological cutting edge to a mainstream market of a larger number of customers with more pragmatic views. The latter are willing to make substantial investments in a new technology only after well-established paths to success begin to emerge".

"Moore assigns the term "early market innovators" to those visionary enthusiasts in the first phase who aggressively seek out the latest technological advancements and possess the skill to assess the technology's value. Innovators influence the early adopters to buy into the product concepts early in their life cycles. Early adopters, in turn, influence the next group, the early majority, to embrace the technology. This early majority combined with a late majority comprises two thirds of the market and holds the key to the success of the technology in a community" [2].

The life sciences industry is currently in the early majority phase. Technologies such as combinatorial chemistry and high throughput screening (HTS) have significantly increased the numbers of compounds coming out of discovery. Preclinical (or nonclinical) development groups are evaluating computer simulation and the creation of more specific animal models to decrease the numbers of animals necessary to fulfill preclinical regulatory requirements. They are looking at animal research management systems and applications that can be integrated with a variety of digital measurement tools. In clinical development, most life sciences companies are experimenting with a variety of solutions collectively being referred to as eClinical applications. And in the marketing environment, interactive voice response systems and handheld computers supported by web sites and portals for direct to consumer (DTC) interactions are emerging. Life sciences companies are using web-based eProcurement tools for supply chain management and offering ePrescribing solutions to expedite prescription fulfillment and billing processes.

So *change is upon us*. Slower than other industry verticals (like capital markets and financial services)—reflecting the very conservative and risk adverse nature of the life sciences industry. But there are still insufficient standards in place with a number of relatively new regulatory implications such as 21 CFR Part 11 and HIPAA—further complicated by varying interpretations of these regulations. And change itself is costly and resource intensive and must deal with behavioral modification and human nature's resistance to change.

Technology solutions are starting to cross the chasm—but many have fallen into the chasm on the way across. Patience and persistence rule the day.

IV. THE INTERNET

The Internet has changed the way we do just about everything. It is a wonderful vehicle for rapid access to and exchange of information. And while it has not (yet) achieved the level of ubiquity, according to Global Reach www.glreach.com), an Internet statistics provider, there are currently more than six hundred million web users in the world today.

The 2002 AMA Study on Physicians' Use of the World Wide Web examined Internet behaviors among 977 physicians (limited to the United States). "Sixty-seven percent use the Internet on a daily basis for an average of 7.1 hours per week." This number is expected to increase to 96% by the end of 2003, and every life sciences company, large or small, uses the Internet as a part of the activities of daily business.

A. Intranets and Extranets

The Internet provides individuals and businesses a way of transferring information of every type, *quickly*, *easily*, and *inexpensively*. Corporate intranets provide an internal network for transferring information. While Internet security has gotten extremely good, and the application service provider (ASP) business model is growing (see below), an Intranet still provides more control over access and content management.

Because the enterprise has become the extended enterprise, involving internal and external participants, it has become vital to extend the work group to the world. Many companies have built extranets to facilitate a more secure route for the exchange of confidential information. Firewalls, 128 bit encryption, public key interface (PKI), biometric signatures, and identity management are all components of the advancing state of security for information traveling around the intranet and across Internet and extranets alike.

Over the last decade, computer users have extended their environment from the desktop to the network. The network has been extended by work group applications. Over the past several years, the work group has been extended to include all the other computers in the world through the Internet! The key to success in deploying technology is leveraging the resources of secure global networking to help knowledge workers accomplish their jobs *quickly*, *easily*, and *inexpensively*.

B. The Application Service Provider (ASP) Business Model

The ASP model is a service that provides access to applications through a secure extranet. The Application Service Provider assumes all responsibility for software maintenance and upgrades, regulatory compliance, and data and document storage. Servers and databases are colocated in two and sometimes three geographically disparate areas with regular redundancy and backup procedures. Such data storage facilities have substantial physical security. This model can provide more robust security, business continuity practices, and disaster recovery processes than many corporations—especially mid-tier and smaller companies. Companies availing themselves of this service, by definition, no longer need to purchase software applications. And this can be for a single application or for the entire IT infrastructure. Users merely need a browser. Businesses require less internal IT organization. Each company's and/or user's data are protected and accessible only by the individuals that are given permission to access that data (by the owner of that data). The ASP model has been referred to as "the app. on tap."

While adoption for this model has been slow and will probably continue to be slow, since corporations and individuals alike prefer to keep their data in their own location, the ASP can level the technology playing field. Smaller companies can have access to technologies that they previously could not afford. It is also a way to experiment with applications. There is little commitment, and the risk is shifted to the application service provider. This model has real potential, and the future may find users in front of dumb terminals (again) connected through a secure extranet (or security applied to the Internet).

C. Security

The protection of information, both corporate intellectual property and personal data, is on the top of everyone's list in a world that depends more and more on knowledge sharing (in real time). While those who want to steal information can be clever, since 21 CFR Part 11 (Title 21 Code of Federal Regulations: Electronic Records; Electronic Signatures) was issued by the FDA in March 1997 and electronic signatures were approved as legal authorization by federal law in October, 2000, what is referred to as identity management has become a key part of the IT strategy for the logical and physical security of hardware, software, databases, and networks. The Health Insurance Portability and Accountability Act (HIPAA), which is enforceable as of April 2003, has heightened even more the level of legislation around the privacy of individuals' personal health information (PHI).

Electronic or digital signatures are therefore an important link in the security chain. The objectives of the digital signature, through an advanced process referred to as public key interface (PKI), are three:

> *Authentication* is the verification of the identity of an individual or organization sending information.

Providing verification that a message or document is genuine and has not been manipulated or changed since its original creation (or signing) is called *integrity*.

Nonrepudiation ensures that the originator of a message or transaction cannot subsequently disown it.

Access to data can be managed at the *atomic level*. This means that an individual with the proper administrative permission could allow a user access to a single data point in a huge database. This is very powerful and further facilitates internal and external collaboration.

V. HARDWARE

There are dozens of choices of popular hardware platforms, depending on the size of your business or your personal preference. Software runs your business. The hardware requirements of the software define the hardware needed. Activities of daily business or lifestyle further define hardware requirements. Personal digital assistants or "handheld computers" have significantly improved user mobility. As wireless technology emerges, users will enjoy even greater flexibility. But at the end of the day, most hardware, even stand-alone home computers (with Internet connectivity), are networked.

For networked computers, two basic types of machines exist—servers and workstations. Servers should be as powerful and upgraded as frequently as software requirements and the budget permit. In today's very competitive new product development marketplace, speed and processing power impact the efficiency of the knowledge worker. Management must find the balance on that delicate line between cost and productivity.

VI. SOFTWARE

A. General Software Applications

Applications software that is not targeted to a particular industry is termed horizontal, because it fits into a wide range of industries. The basic group of software is the office suite of applications, consisting of word processing and spreadsheet software as well as e-mail. This suite of applications is generally extended to include presentation, database, collaboration, and Internet software.

Applications that are sold as a package provide a seamless data flow between them. For example, raw data in a database can be called into a spreadsheet and analyzed. The resulting analysis can be merged into a word-processed document. The resulting document can then be sent by e-mail to its intended audience, or posted on the Internet, intranet, or extranet for review. The key to choosing applications software is that it provides the feature sets needed by the enterprise (or for personal use). It is also important to ensure interoperability with all the users in the enterprise. It becomes a bit trickier when it is necessary to extend that interoperability to users in the extended enterprise—and trickier still as interoperability or integration becomes a requirement across disparate applications and systems.

B. eDiscovery Software

Recent scientific and technological advances have introduced new paradigms for drug discovery research. The drugs developed over the last four decades have been aimed at about 500 different biological targets. With the sequencing of the human genome, over 100,000 new biological targets will be recognized. It has been estimated that at least 10% of these could be potential targets for drugs. This creates additional decision support issues for the already thinly-spread resources of the life sciences industry.

High throughput screening (HTS) is a system for analyzing compound libraries and natural products in order to identify new therapeutic hits and leads on potential targets. "HTS arose in the 1990s as 96 microtitre plates were selected over test tubes as the receptacle of choice for biological assays" [4]. In combination with combinatorial chemistry, it resulted in a paradigm shift from knowledge-based sequential synthesis and testing to parallel processing of multiple compounds. For improving success rates and cycle times for discovering new hits, HTS has become one of the cornerstones of drug discovery. With the advent of high-throughput approaches in genomics, combinatorial chemistry, and screening, the life sciences industry should face no shortage of novel targets or promising lead compounds. Once again, choosing the right compounds to enter the clinical development process still requires a bit of luck and has been referred to by some as "planned serendipity."

C. ePreclinical Software

In the preclinical (nonclinical) stage of new product development, an investigational drug must be tested extensively in living organisms (in vivo) and in cells in the test tube (in vitro) to provide information about the pharmaceutical composition of the drug, its safety, how the drug will be formulated and manufactured, and how it will be administered to the first human subjects. Regulatory agencies require testing that documents the characteristics—chemical composition, purity, quality, and potency—of the drug's active ingredient and of the formulated drug. Pharmacological testing determines the effects of the candidate drug on the body. General toxicology and reproductive toxicology studies are conducted to ensure that any risks to humans are identified.

There are numerous opportunities to infuse software into the preclinical phase of new product development such as

Animal facility software management systems that include on-line IACUC, protocols, census, animal orders, and an e-mail notification system

Breeding colony management software that tracks projects, lines, matings and litters, injections, implantations, pedigrees, phenotypes, and genotypes

An important requirement in selecting preclinical software solutions is the ability to interface with peripherals such as scales, automatic vital signs (i.e., arterial line), bar code readers, animal ID scanners, and others.

But the primary limitation to automating the preclinical testing environment is budget. Financial support for preclinical software solutions pale significantly relative to budgets to improve the clinical phases of new product development. This has resulted in a very slow transition to software automation—significantly slower than in the clinical phases of new product development—which, as mentioned earlier, is pretty slow.

D. eClinical Software

So, while technology solutions are indeed being introduced across the new product development life cycle, the clinical development phase is the most critical and most expensive phase of new product development. It is, therefore, the area that is receiving the most attention in attempts to increase the velocity of the new product development process and improve the capacity of the new product development enterprise. To date, this marketplace has been dominated by numerous "point solutions" providers that are challenged by the requirements of scale, and have not been able to convince life sciences companies that they have the bandwidth and/or clout worthiness for those life sciences companies to place sufficient trust in such offerings. Further, the issue of systems integration—that is, the integration of disparate software applications—has proven a great challenge. Thus the new product development enterprise still awaits the technology shift that will truly change the way new products are developed. While large software companies have dabbled in this marketplace, the effort required to "verticalize" their horizontal solutions has not proven valuable enough (as yet) to align such solutions with the very idiosyncratic nature of the functional requirements of new product development software solutions.

1. Electronic Data Capture (EDC) and Patient Diaries

The terms electronic data capture (EDC) and remote data collection (RDC) are generally used as synonymous in describing the technology-based collection of clinical trial data from physicians participating as investigators in a clinical trial. These are web-based (on-line), client server (off-line), or hybrid (combined on-line/off-line) software applications. And there are implications to be considered when choosing an on-line, off-line and/or hybrid solution. However, ING Barrings differentiates RDC from EDC.

> RDC is about capturing information at the clinical site rather than at some centralized location. RDC may occur over the fax, via the phone or through a computer connection—but the case report form (CRF) remains the primary data source. EDC, which involves the Internet or other data network, relies on an electronic CRF (eCRF) as the primary data source [5].

Regardless of specific interpretation, the shift away from paper CFRs has been slower than many expected. In fact, although it has been "fifteen years since the introduction of the concept, it is unclear whether more than 5–10% of the industry's clinical trials use EDC technologies" [6].

While using software that can facilitate cleaner data faster *just seems to make sense*, the following list has some of the reasons why EDC has yet to replace the paper-based clinical trial data collection process:

The technology is still perceived to be in the maturation phase.
Cost in dollars/cost in time.
Lack of confidence of the value proposition and ROI.
Process reengineering requirements.
Work flow.
Resistance to change.
Lack of economic pressure due to pharmaceutical companies' pattern of sustained prosperity and total shareholder return.
Lack of economic ability due to hospitals', HMOs', and private practice patterns of unwillingness or inability to make the types of investments necessary to implement technology solutions.

Another variety of electronic data capture is in the area of direct-to-patient solutions such as patient diaries and quality of life questionnaires. While as an industry, we have been collecting this type of information for years, paper-based collections of direct patient input was never given much credibility. It was not because that data is perceived to be unimportant but rather that the paper-based approach to such data collection made that data, which usually must be collected at an appointed time (i.e., two hours after a dose of a medication), unreliable. There was no guarantee that the information requested was indeed completed at that appointed time. There are many anecdotes of patients in the waiting room scrambling to complete weeks worth of "daily diary" data before their appointment with the physician. Nonetheless, the use of electronic tools such as the PDA (personal digital assistant) have resuscitated the huge value that direct input from the patient can bring to clinical trial data. Data entry sessions can now be date and time stamped. There can be alarms that go off to remind patients of a data entry session. That data can be sent in real time across the Internet. There are still issues with usability. The PDA is small and requires a certain manual dexterity that many elderly patients find challenging. There are viable alternatives such as IVRS (interactive voice response systems), which uses the good old telephone for the transmission of direct patient information. All in all, advances in technology have brought a new value to data that was always seen to be worthy of collection, though until now there were insufficient vehicles to enable this.

PDAs have found another area of value in the community of physicians involved in drug and device development as well as in practice management. PDAs are small and powerful tools. ePrescriptions, patient's notes, schedules, and even eDetailing have moved the PDA into the daily work flow of more and more physicians. As this technology evolves, we can expect to see an increasing role of the PDA in the world of drug and device development and in healthcare in general.

2. Clinical Trials Management Systems (CTMS)

Clinical trials management systems (CTMS) are currently receiving significant attention as the life sciences industry orients itself to the value of relationship management. And, as competition for the relatively limited pool of qualified investigators continues to grow, building a database with investigator/site capabilities and objectives rather than self-reported investigator performance metrics is perceived to be more valuable than ever before. Further, the number of codevelopment and comarketing partnerships is growing exponentially, and the requirement to share and/or merge information about the status of ongoing clinical trials has become critically important. Most CTMS offer and/or can be integrated with off-the-shelf project management and resource management tools.

3. Collaboration Software

Collaboration software could include any application that has groupware functionality. But this section is focused on on-line meetings, eLearning, and document exchange applications.

a. On-line meetings or virtual meetings solutions are becoming increasingly popular as an alternative to and/or adjunct of the traditional (in person) meeting. Unfortunately, part of that popularity is the result of the tragic events of 11 September, 2001. But life sciences companies were in the process of reevaluating the huge costs associated with investigators' meetings, and on-line meetings offer a significantly less expensive option. This new market opportunity is evolving in two forms: self-administered web-based meetings and service-based on-line meetings. On-line meetings seem to provide a rare win–win solution. Life sciences companies spend less money, and since, in addition to safety concerns, the burden of travel has become an issue of "time away from the office" and/or "time away from the family" (quality of life) for many investigators and coordinators, especially the group of investigators that perform a number of clinical trials each year, on-line meeting technology and services providers should prosper.

b. eLearning applications are often integrated with and a key part of on-line meetings. There are regulatory, quality, and maybe even liability issues that have raised interest in eLearning. Like on-line meetings, eLearning has proven to be a less expensive alternative to classroom-based learning and broadens significantly the reach of knowledge transfer. It is easier to certify that participants in clinical trials have learned. And the return on investment (ROI)—through an increased understanding of protocol requirements—should be better quality data and improved regulatory compliance.

c. Document exchange applications are also referred to as digital workspaces. Again, this technology is most powerful when integrated with eLearning and on-line meetings offerings—truly collaborative solutions. A digital workspace (secure web site) is created where structured and unstructured data—documents of all kinds, but mostly study start-up documents—are posted for secure access by investigators and their staffs. Content access—security—is at the document level. This means that individuals only see the documents that they have been given permission to see. Using digital signature technology, those documents can be signed and returned to create on-line regulatory files. To be in compliance with 21 CFR Part 11 requirements, there must be complete audit trails of every transaction and each access.

4. Database Management Systems (DBMS)

In many life sciences companies the database management system is the center of their clinical trials data universe. Most other eClinical solutions (noted above) are expected to integrate with the corporate database management system. This is easier said than done in 2003, since DBMS are complex systems, and although there are only a few significant providers of DBMS, each life sciences company tends to create its own data standards. And this makes integration by the other (disparate) eClincal systems a complex process. (And indeed, integration issues have been one of the primary limiting factors to the success of eClinical technology in general.) These systems are the clinical data repositories from which statistical analysis is done, reports are created, and electronic regulatory submissions (ERS) evolve.

5. Document Management Systems

Developing a new drug leads to a great deal of documentation, compounded by doing an FDA application. Managing the documents can become a significant task. Just finding documents can be difficult if a user does not know the location of the file on disk. In most cases, documents also need to track revisions through an audit trail of user modifications. The systems work by using a library approach to documents. New documents are created and checked into a library under an appropriate heading or study name. These documents are then checked out as users need to modify them, and this transaction is logged. This approach ensures that only one user can modify a document at a time and that an audit trail exists. Security can be set up to define which users are allowed to change documents. Upon completion, a document can be locked to disallow further changes. The document system also generally provides an index of documents in the library. Through the index, a user can quickly search for documents with specific contents. Any part of any document can also be cross-referenced to other sections. These features are especially useful in an Electronic Regulatory Submission (ERS)— the electronic version of a New Drug Application—where volumes of paper documents can be stored electronically and readily cross-referenced. Integrated with clinical development data from a DBMS, a regulatory reviewer could have an entire NDA accessible on the desktop.

6. Portals

Using the metaphor of a web site as a store makes a portal a shopping mall— enabling access to multiple stores (applications). Portal technology may be the first solution to help sort the integration problem of connecting otherwise not integrated disparate eClinical applications. Future integration solutions will incorporate data standards. Using tools sometimes called gadgets, portal technology allows users with proper security clearance to reach into multiple eClinical applications to surface specific data of interest to that specific user. The user can integrate that data (from multiple disparate applications) into a single report. In an age when too much data is as bad as too little data, the ability to personalize access to multiple applications and generate integrated reports has huge potential. The "digital dashboard" is the portal interface that facilitates the opportunity to control and report on individualized information on a regular basis. Portal solutions can be very expensive, and therefore to date only major life sciences companies have been truly able to take advantage of this technology.

VII. CONCLUSION

Over the past few years technology has started to play a major role in most life sciences companies' attempts to make faster and less expensive the new product development process. But the investment has been, and will continue to be, significant. And while, intuitively, most life sciences companies' executives believe the future of new product development will be based on technology decisions being made today, the return on investment (ROI) has yet to prove dramatic.

To succeed with technology in new product development is clearly dependent upon *people and process—then techhnology.* For technology solutions in the life sciences industry to *cross the chasm*, applications must allow users to do what they need to do *quickly, easily, and inexpensively.* And as standards evolve and integration becomes easier, as personalization, work flow, and artificial intelligence improve application functionality and further enable knowledge workers—helping to drive user adoption, as the more computer savvy generations of knowledge workers assume more leadership roles and responsibilities, and as the Internet becomes pervasive, indeed, technology will realize its role as a core piece of the new product development puzzle. Nonetheless, *change is upon us.*

REFERENCES

1. Tool@work. Deciphering the knowledge management hype. Journal for Quality and Participation Jul/Aug 1998; 21(4):58–60.
2. Bien M. Pioneers, perceptions, promises: it's time for a second look at remote data entry. July 1999; white paper.
3. The 2002 AMA Study on Physicians' Use of the World Wide Web. AMA Website www.ama-assn.org.
4. Gordon EM. Combinatorial Chemistry and Molecular Diversity in Drug Discovery. Wiley-Liss, 1998:17–38.
5. Mathieu MP. Parexel's Pharmaceutical R&D Statistical Sourcebook. Parexel 2001:91.
6. Fitzmartin R. The synergistic relationship of computers and medical sciences in the twenty-first century: impact on biopharmaceutical drug development. Drug Information Journal 34.

18

The Common Technical Document for the Registration of Pharmaceuticals for Human Use

Duane B. Lakings
Drug Safety Evaluation Consulting, Inc., Elgin, Texas, U.S.A.

I. INTRODUCTION

The year is 1999. You, a pharmaceutical or biotechnology company sponsor or a sponsor's agent or a CRO under contract by the sponsor, have all the drug discovery reports and/or publications, nonclinical study reports, clinical study reports, and the chemistry, manufacturing, and control (CMC) information and documentation on a drug candidate necessary for the preparation of a regulatory agency submission for a marketing application. Your charge is to prepare the necessary summaries to "tell the story" of the discovery and development of the drug candidate and to integrate the information in the appropriate formats for submissions to each of the countries where marketing approval is being sought. To complete this endeavor, you need to know the marketing application submission requirements for each of these countries. These requirements vary substantially from country to country and often require the preparation of different summaries to be presented in a different order for each country. In addition, each country has some differences in formatting (e.g., binding and binder size and color, paper and page size, font and font size, heading and subheading type and style) stipulations. Thus you end up preparing multiple submissions, probably one for each country. The process takes substantial time and resources, sometimes 6 months (if everything goes smoothly and according to plan) to a year (or longer if unexpected surprises are encountered). After the submissions are made, you start to receive questions and queries from the regulatory agencies in various countries. Each question has to be carefully considered, in light of the information in the submission to that country, and appropriately answered. The time necessary to prepare the submissions and to respond to queries from the various regulatory agencies shortens the time of marketing exclusivity after approvals are received, causing a reduction in revenue, which may be substantial if the delays in approval are long and the drug candidate has a projected fifth year sales of $365,000,000 or one million dollars a day.

Fast forward to late 2002. The International Conference on Harmonisation (ICH) prepared a guideline on the Organization of a Common Technical Document for the Registration of Pharmaceuticals for Human Use of a CTD. This ICH guideline, designated M4, is recommended for adoption at Step 4 of the ICH process and is published, and thus available for use, by the three ICH regions (the European Agency for the Evaluation of Medicinal Products for the European Union, the Pharmaceutical and Medical Safety Bureau for Japan, and the Federal Drug Administration for the United States). Since most nonsignatory countries also follow ICH guidelines, the ICH CTD guideline provides a format for the preparation of a marketing application submission that is acceptable to most, if not all, countries in which a sponsor wishes to obtain marketing approval. Thus the scenario described above for 1999 and before is no longer applicable and sponsors submitting a marketing application prepared according to the ICH CTD guideline recommendations should be able to obtain quicker marketing approvals with fewer questions and queries from regulatory agencies.

This chapter provides summary information on the recommendations listed in the ICH CTD guideline. Readers who desire more details on the information in this ICH M4 guideline should obtain a copy of the document, which is available electronically at various Internet sites, including the ICH web site at http://www.ich.org.

II. CTD OVERVIEW

The ICH M4 guideline provides the agreed-upon common format for the preparation of a well-constructed Common Technical Document (CTD) for applications that will be submitted to regulatory authorities for marketing approval. The goals of using a common format for the technical documentation are

1. To reduce significantly the time and resources needed to compile applications for registration of human pharmaceuticals.
2. To ease the preparation of electronic submissions.

3. To facilitate regulatory agency reviews and communications with the sponsor.
4. To simplify the exchange of regulatory information between regulatory agencies.

Important points for sponsors to know (and to remember) include

1. The ICH CTD guideline addresses the organization of the information to be presented in registration applications for new pharmaceuticals, including biotechnology-derived products.

2. The ICH CTD guideline does NOT indicate which research studies are required to support an application or how research studies are to be designed and conducted.

3. The overall organization of a CTD, as outlined in the guideline, should not be modified by the sponsor.

4. The display of information in a CTD is to be unambiguous and transparent in order to facilitate review of the basic data and to assist reviewers in becoming quickly oriented to the application's contents.

5. Text, tables, and figures should be prepared using margins that allow the document to be printed using paper employed by the various ICH regions.

6. Example templates for various tables recommended for inclusion in a marketing application are given in the ICH CTD guideline and these templates, or appropriate modifications of the templates, should be employed for summary presentations of results. A designation of ETA, for "example template available," will be used throughout this chapter to alert sponsors that recommended table formats are available for their consideration.

7. The left-hand margin should be sufficiently large so that information is not obscured by the method of binding.

8. Font sizes (Times New Roman, 12-point font or equivalent) for text and tables should be large enough to be easily legible, even after photocopying.

9. Every page should be numbered, with the first page of each module designated as page 1.

10. Acronyms and abbreviations should be defined the first time they are used in each module and in the opinion of this author should be uniform among the various modules.

11. References should be cited in accordance with the 1979 Vancouver Declaration on Uniform Requirements for Manuscripts Submitted to Biomedical Journals or equivalent.

The most important point above, in this author's opinion, is the second. The sponsor is responsible for determining which research studies are necessary for characterizing and developing a drug candidate, when these studies should be conducted in relation to other experiments, how these studies are designed, where the studies are conducted, and how the results are interpreted. The sponsor is also responsible for preparing, or having prepared, the study reports that document the studies and the generated results. The ICH CTD guideline only provides a common template for the order of presentation of the summaries describing completed research studies and the individual study reports. A CTD is to be organized in five modules. Module 1 is region specific and should contain documents, such as application forms or proposed label for use, specific to the region. Modules 2, 3, 4, and 5 are intended to be common for all regions and each of these modules will be discussed in more detail in the following sections. Much of the discussion in this chapter was paraphrased from the text in the ICH CTD guideline and thus should provide the reader with an overview of the material provided in more detail in ICH M4. Since Module 1 is region specific, no further information will be provided for this module. Module 2 provides summary information on the detailed data and results presented in Module 3 for Quality or CMC information, Module 4 for Nonclinical Study Reports, and Module 5 for Clinical Study Reports.

III. MODULE 2: COMMON TECHNICAL DOCUMENT SUMMARIES

From the standpoint of telling the story of the discovery and development of a drug candidate and integrating the results from the various research studies conducted to define manufacturing processes and to characterize the physiochemical properties, pharmacology or efficacy, pharmacokinetics, and toxicology or safety of the drug candidate in animal models and in humans, Module 2 is by far the most important module of a CTD. This module provides summary information on all aspects of the discovery and development processes, including CMC information and nonclinical and clinical evaluations. The writers of each of these summaries need to have a good understanding of the overall story so that each author can compare, contrast, and integrate the results in his/her summaries with the information in the summaries prepared by other authors.

Most large pharmaceutical corporations have trained and experienced scientific and medical writing groups who have as one of their primary functions the drafting of these quality, nonclinical, and clinical summaries for regulatory agency submissions. Smaller pharmaceutical firms and some larger biotechnology companies may have a few science writers on the staff and when the time comes to prepare a marketing application, these writers may be asked to draft summaries both inside and outside their areas of expertise. Most small biotechnology firms do not have the resources to have an independent scientific writing staff; they frequently rely on partners (i.e., large pharmaceutical companies who have licensed or are codeveloping a drug candidate with the discoverer) to perform these important aspects of the drug development process. Whatever the size of the sponsor, resources may not, at times, be available to complete the task within the desired time frame. When that is the case, sponsors may contract with a CRO, a medical writing service organization, or independent science writers to draft the summaries. Many independent science writers belong to the American Medical Writers Association (AMWA) and information on their background and qualifications can be found on the AMWA web site at http://www.amwa.org. The sponsor should carefully assign or select the scientific and medical writers, whether in-house or contract, to ensure that the summaries are appropriately prepared and reviewed. For example, having an expert in clinical or CMC aspects of drug development prepare the nonclinical summaries may result in incomplete or inaccurate descriptions of preclinical and nonclinical study results. However, having the clinical or CMC experts review the nonclinical summaries is highly desirable so that the information shared is effectively integrated with the summaries from the other areas.

Whoever prepares the summaries to be included in Module 2 of a CTD, the information should be presented using the order of presentation described in the ICH CTD guideline. Module 2 is to begin with a short (not to exceed one page) general introduction on a drug candidate and is to include the pharmacological class, the mode of action, and the proposed clinical use. The Introduction is to be followed by the Quality Overall Summary or QOS, then the Nonclinical Overview and the Clinical Overview. Following the QOS and overviews are the Nonclinical Written Summaries and the Nonclinical Tabulated Summaries and the Clinical Summary.

A. Quality Overall Summary (QOS)

The QOS is a summary that follows the scope and outline of Module 3 and should not include information, data, and/or justifications that are not included in Module 3 or in another part of a CTD. The primary purpose of a QOS is to provide sufficient information so that a reviewer is given an overview of the data in Module 3. A QOS should emphasize key parameters of a drug substance (or a drug candidate, as a compound under development is commonly referred to in nonclinical and clinical research efforts; both designations are utilized throughout this chapter) and a drug product and should include discussions of issues that integrate information from sections in Module 3 with supporting information from Modules 4 and 5. The length of a QOS (excluding tables and figures) should generally not exceed 40 pages of text. However, for most biotechnology drug candidates and for candidates manufactured using more complex processes, a QOS may be longer but should not exceed 80 pages of text.

The recommended order of presentation for a QOS in Module 2 and the more detailed quality information in Module 3 is described in Table 1, where S designates drug substance and P denotes drug product. A QOS is to start with an Introduction that includes the proprietary name, nonproprietary name, and/or common name of a drug substance; company or sponsor name; dosage form(s), strength(s), and route(s) of administration; and proposed indication(s). After the introduction, summary information on a drug substance and then a proposed drug product are provided. Following the summaries and primarily for biotechnology-derived drug candidates, appendices on facilities and equipment and on safety evaluations for adventitious agents are provided. Finally, regional information is documented.

In a General Information on a Drug Substance section, the nomenclature, structure, and general properties of a drug substance are to be provided. Nomenclature could include the recommended international nonproprietary name, compendial name, chemical name(s), sponsor code, other nonproprietary name(s), and/or Chemical Abstracts Service (CAS) registry number. For small organic molecules or NCEs, the structural formula, including relative and absolute stereochemistry (if relevant), the molecular formula, and the relative molecular mass are to be provided. If a drug substance is chiral, information is to be provided on the specific stereoisomer or mixture of stereoisomers (i.e., a racemic mixture) used in nonclinical and clinical studies and on the stereoisomer(s) that is (are) to be used in the final drug product intended for marketing. For protein or polypeptide macromolecules, the schematic amino acid sequence with glycosylation sites and/or other post-translational modifications identified and the relative molecular mass are to be given. For other macromolecules, such as nucleic acids or carbohydrates, sufficient structural information should be provided to describe the chemical structural and the interactions between the various moieties or subgroups. Information on general properties is to include summaries of the physiochemical and other relevant characteristics of a drug substance, including biological activity for macromolecules.

The Manufacture section is to include the name, address, and responsibility (e.g., production or testing facility) of each manufacturer, including contractors. A brief description of a drug substance's manufacturing process is to describe adequately the synthesis and process control. The use of a flow diagram for NCEs and macromolecules prepared by synthetic procedures is recommended. The diagram should include molecular formulas; weights; yield ranges; and chemical structures of starting materials, intermediates, and drug substance (reflecting stereochemistry, if relevant) and should identify operating conditions and solvents. The diagram is to be explained using a sequential procedural narrative that includes information on the quantities of raw materials, solvents, catalysts, and reagents and that identifies critical

Table 1 Order of Presentation for Quality Overall Summary (Module 2) and Quality (Module 3)

Material			Module	
S	P	Sequence of presentation	2	3
		Table of Contents		X
		Body of Data		X
		Introduction	X	
X		General Information on Drug Substance	X	X
X		Nomenclature		X
X		Structure		X
X		General properties		X
X		Manufacture of Drug Substance	X	X
X		Manufacturer(s)		X
X		Description of manufacturing process and controls		X
X		Control of materials		X
X		Control of critical steps and intermediates		X
X		Process validation and/or evaluation		X
X		Characterization of Drug Substance	X	X
X		Elucidation of structure and other characteristics		X
X		Impurities		X
X		Control of Drug Substance	X	X
X		Specification		X
X		Analytical procedures		X
X		Validation of analytical procedures		X
X		Batch analyses		X
X		Justification of specification		X
X		Reference Standards or Materials	X	X
X		Container Closure System	X	X
X		Stability of Drug Substance	X	X
X		Stability summary and conclusions		X
X		Postapproval stability protocol and commitment		X
X		Stability data		X
	X	Description and Composition of Drug Product	X	X
	X	Pharmaceutical Development	X	X
	X	Components of the drug product (drug substance and excipients)		X
	X	Drug product (formulation development, overages, physicochemical and biological properties)		X
	X	Manufacturing process development		X
	X	Container closure system		X
	X	Microbiological attributes		X
	X	Compatibility		X
	X	Manufacture of Drug Product	X	X

Table 1 Continued

Material			Module	
S	P	Sequence of presentation	2	3
	X	Manufacturer(s)		X
	X	Batch formula		X
	X	Description of manufacturing process and controls		X
	X	Control of critical steps and intermediates		X
	X	Process validation and/or evaluation		X
	X	Control of Excipients	X	X
	X	Specifications		X
	X	Analytical procedures		X
	X	Validation of analytical procedures		X
	X	Justification of specifications		X
	X	Excipients of human or animal origin		X
	X	Novel excipients		X
	X	Control of Drug Product	X	X
	X	Specification(s)		X
	X	Analytical procedures		X
	X	Validation of analytical procedures		X
	X	Batch analyses		X
	X	Characterization of impurities		X
	X	Justification of specification(s)		X
	X	Reference Standards or Materials	X	X
	X	Container Closure System	X	X
	X	Stability of Drug Product	X	X
	X	Stability summary and conclusion		X
	X	Postapproval stability protocol and commitment		X
	X	Stability data		X
		Appendix on Facilities and Equipment	X	X
		Appendix on Adventitious Agents Safety Evaluation	X	X
		Regional Information	X	X
		Key Literature References		X

S = drug substance, and P = drug product.

steps, process controls, equipment, and operating conditions (e.g., temperature, pressure, pH, time).

For protein macromolecules, a manufacturing process usually starts with vial(s) of the cell bank and includes cell culture, harvest(s), purification and modification reactions, and storage and shipping conditions. Again a flow diagram is recommended to illustrate the manufacturing route from the original inoculum to the last harvesting operation. Relevant information (e.g., population doubling levels, cell concentration, volumes, pH, cultivation times, holding times, and temperature) is to be included and critical steps and intermediates are to be identified. A brief text description of each process step in the flow diagram is to be provided and should include summary information on scale, culture media and other additives, major equipment, and process controls (e.g., in-process tests and operational parameters, process steps, equipment, and intermediates with acceptance criteria).

Another flow diagram along with a brief text description is to be provided to illustrate the purification steps and is to include all steps, intermediates, and relevant information for each stage with critical steps for which specifications are established identified. Reprocessing procedures with criteria for the reprocessing of any intermediate or drug substance is to be summarized. Procedures used to transfer material between steps, equipment, areas, and buildings are to be listed. A description of the filling procedure for a drug substance, process controls, and acceptance criteria is to be provided. The container closure system for storage of a drug substance and storage and shipping conditions for a drug substance are to be delineated. Where appropriate, tabulated summaries and graphs should be employed.

All materials (e.g., raw materials, starting materials, solvents, reagents, catalysts) used in the manufacture of a drug substance need to be controlled and a list identifying where each material is used in the process should be provided. Information demonstrating that materials meet standards appropriate for their intended use is to be included.

Test and acceptance criteria performed at critical steps of the manufacturing process are to be summarized to ensure that the process is controlled. For intermediates isolated during the process, information on their quality and control is to be listed. For protein macromolecules, stability data to support storage conditions is recommended.

Process validation and/or evaluation studies for aseptic processing and sterilization are to be briefly described and should contain sufficient information to demonstrate that the manufacturing process is suitable for its intended purpose and to substantiate selection of critical process controls and their limits.

A brief description and discussion of the manufacturing process development history is recommended and should provide summary information on significant changes made to the process or site used in the production of nonclinical, clinical, scale-up, pilot, and production scale (if available) batches. Where appropriate, the significance of the change(s) should be addressed to describe the potential impact of the change(s) on the quality of a drug substance.

Characterization of a drug substance is to include elucidation of structure. For NCEs, confirmation of structure can be provided by spectral analysis techniques and should include summary information on the potential for isomerism, the identification of stereochemistry, and/or the potential for forming polymorphs. For protein macromolecules, structural details should include information on primary, secondary, and higher-order structure, post-translational forms, biological activity, purity, and immunochemical properties (when relevant).

Information on impurities, including their structure, acceptance limits, and control, is to be briefly described.

For control of a drug substance, specifications (including justifications) and analytical procedures (including validation information) used for testing are to be summarized. Data on reference standards or reference materials used for drug substance testing are to be provided. Information on batches and the results of batch analyses are to be described.

A brief description and discussion of the container closure system for a drug substance is to include the identity of and specification for materials of construction of each primary packaging component. The suitability of each component should be summarized.

A summary, including tabular and graphic presentations of results, of the stability studies undertaken on a drug substance is to include information on testing conditions, batches, and analytical procedures and a discussion of the results and conclusions. Also to be included are the proposed storage conditions, retest dates, or shelf life (where relevant) and a summary of the postapproval stability protocol.

The description and composition of a proposed drug product is to be summarized and is to include a description of the dosage form, a list of all components and their amounts on a per-unit basis, the function of the components, and a reference to their quality standards. If appropriate, a brief description of accompanying reconstitution diluent(s) is to be provided. Information on the type of container and closure used for a drug product and accompanying diluent(s) is to be summarized. Using tables and graphs as appropriate, the pharmaceutical development of a proposed drug product is to be summarized. Information to be shared should include development studies conducted to establish that the dosage form, the formulation, the manufacturing process, the container closure system, microbiological attributes, and usage instructions are appropriate for the intended purpose. In addition, a summary should be provided to identify and describe critical formulation and process parameters that might influence batch reproducibility, drug product performance, and drug product quality.

The name, address, and responsibility of each manufacturer, including contractors, and each proposed production site or facility involved in manufacturing a drug product are to be provided. A flow diagram is recommended to present the steps of a drug product manufacturing process and should indicate where materials enter the process. The critical steps where process controls, intermediate tests, and final drug product controls are conducted are to be identified. Also to be included is a brief description of the manufacturing process and the controls, including process validation and/or evaluations, that are intended to result in the routine and consistent production of drug product of appropriate quality.

A brief summary on the quality of excipients is to include information on specifications and their justification, analytical procedures and their validation, excipients of human or animal origin, and novel excipients.

Using tables and graphs as appropriate, control of a drug product is to be briefly described and is to include information on specifications and their justification, analytical procedures and their validation, and characterization of impurities. Also, information on reference standards or materials used for control of a drug product should be provided.

A brief description of a drug product container closure system is to include the identity of materials of construction for each primary packaging component and their specifications. Where appropriate, noncompendial methods and their validation should be summarized.

Summary information on the stability studies conducted on a drug product are to include conditions tested, batches analyzed, and analytical procedures used. A brief discussion of the results and conclusions, with respect to storage conditions and shelf life, from drug product stability studies and an analysis of the data is to be provided. Tables and graphs should be used where appropriate to describe stability data. A brief description of the postapproval stability protocol for a drug product is to be included.

For a macromolecule drug candidate, appendices to QOS are to include a summary of facility information for the production of a drug substance and a drug product and a discussion of measures implemented to control endogenous and adventitious agents during production. A diagram is recommended to illustrate the manufacturing flow, including movement of raw materials, personnel, waste, and intermediate(s) into and out of the manufacturing areas. A tabulated summary of the reduction factors for viral clearance is desirable.

The last section of a QOS is to be a brief discussion, when appropriate, of the information specific for the region for which marketing approval is being sought.

B. Nonclinical Overview

A Nonclinical Overview is to present an integrated and critical assessment of the pharmacological, pharmacokinetic, and toxicological evaluations of a drug candidate in in vitro systems and animal models and should not exceed about 30 pages of text. Where relevant guidelines (e.g., ICH safety guidelines) on the conduct of nonclinical studies exist, these guidelines are to be taken into consideration and any deviations are to be discussed and justified. In addition, the nonclinical testing strategy (i.e., the nonclinical drug development plan) should be discussed and justified and comments included on the status of compliance with GLP Regulations for the research studies being submitted. Where appropriate, any association between nonclinical findings and the quality characteristics of a drug candidate, the results from clinical trials, and/or the effects seen with related drug products is to be described.

Except for macromolecules, an assessment of the pharmacological and toxicological effects of the impurities and degradants present in a drug substance and a drug product is to be included. This assessment should form part of the justification for proposed impurity limits and be appropriately cross-referenced to the quality documentation in the QOS and Module 3. The implications of any differences in the chirality, chemical form, and/or impurity profile between the compound evaluated in nonclinical studies and a drug substance in a drug product to be marketed is to be discussed. For a macromolecule, comparability of material used in nonclinical studies, clinical trials, and proposed for marketing is to be addressed. If a drug product contains a novel excipient, an assessment of the information on this material's safety is to be included.

If references to published scientific literature are to be used in place of nonclinical studies conducted by a sponsor, the information in these citations are to be supported by a detailed justification that reviews the design of the studies, including the quality of the drug substance, and that documents any deviations from available guidelines.

The recommended sequence for the nonclinical overview is

1. Overview of the nonclinical testing strategy or nonclinical drug development logic plan.
2. Pharmacology.
3. Pharmacokinetics.
4. Toxicology.
5. Integrated overview and conclusions.
6. List of literature citations.

The material summarized in each section of a nonclinical overview should contain appropriate references (i.e., Table X.X, Study/Report Number) to the Tabulated Nonclinical Summaries.

In vitro and animal studies conducted to evaluate and establish the pharmacodynamic effects, the mode of action, and potential adverse effects are to be evaluated with consideration given to the significance of any issues that are noted. In addition, in this author's opinion, any animal model developed or utilized to evaluate the pharmacological activity of a drug candidate should be fully summarized and, when available, information on the relevance and predictability of the animal model to the human disease or disorder for which a marketing approval is being sought should be provided. Assessments of nonclinical pharmacokinetic (PK), toxicokinetic (TK), and drug metabolism (DM) results should address the relevance of the bioanalytical chemistry methods and the pharmacokinetic models and derived PK or TK parameters. Where appropriate, cross-referencing may be necessary to the more detailed information on certain issues (e.g., impact of disease state, changes in physiology, anti-drug candidate antibodies, cross-species considerations) within the pharmacology and toxicology studies and any inconsistencies in the data should be discussed. Interspecies, including with humans, comparisons of metabolism (both extent and metabolite profile) and systemic exposure comparisons in animals and humans are to be described and the limitations and utility of the nonclinical results for prediction of potential adverse effects in humans delineated.

For animal species evaluated in toxicology studies, the toxic effects (onset, severity, and duration) and their dose-dependency and degree of reversibility or irreversibility and species- and/or gender-related differences are to be evaluated. Important aspects are to be discussed with regard to (a) pharmacodynamics, (b) toxic signs, (c) causes of death, (d) pathological findings, (e) genotoxic activity, (f) carcinogenic potential and risk to humans, (g) fertility, embryo-fetal development, pre- and postnatal toxicity, (h) studies in juvenile animals, (i) the potential consequences of use before and during pregnancy, during lactation, and during pediatric development, (j) local tolerance, and (k) studies conducted to clarify special problems.

An overview evaluation of toxicology studies is to be arranged in a logical order to allow all relevant data for describing a given adverse effect to be discussed together. Extrapolations of toxicity data from animals to humans are to be considered with relation to (a) animal species evaluated, (b) number of animals studied, (c) routes of administration employed, (d) dosages evaluated, (e) duration of treatment, (f) systemic exposure in the toxicology animal species at the no-observed-adverse-effect levels (NOAEL) and at doses that produce a toxic effect in relation to the human systemic exposure at the maximum recommended human dose, and (g) the toxic effects of a drug candidate observed in animal models to that expected or observed in humans. Tables and figures are recommended for summarizing these extrapolations.

If alternatives to whole-animal experimentation are employed to evaluate the pharmacology, pharmacokinetics, and/or toxicology of a drug candidate, the scientific validity of the alternatives is to be discussed.

An integrated overview and conclusions of nonclinical results are to define clearly the characteristics of a drug candidate as demonstrated by the results of the nonclinical research studies and are to arrive at logical, well-argued conclusions supporting the safety of a drug candidate for the intended clinical use. Using the pharmacology, pharmacokinetic, and toxicology results, the implications of the nonclinical findings for the safe human use of a drug candidate are to be discussed.

C. Clinical Overview

A Clinical Overview provides a critical analysis of the clinical data generated during the development of a drug candidate and is to reference appropriately the information in the more detailed Clinical Summary and in the individual clinical study reports in Module 5 and other relevant study reports. A primary purpose of this overview is to present the conclusions and implications of the clinical results and to provide a succinct discussion and interpretation of these findings in conjunction with other relevant information, such as nonclinical data or quality issues that may have clinical implications. While primarily intended for use by regulatory agencies for the review of the clinical section of a drug candidate's marketing application, the Clinical Overview can also be a useful summary to the overall clinical findings for reviewers of other sections of a CTD. This overview should

1. Describe and explain the overall clinical development plan for a drug candidate and include critical clinical study design decisions.

2. Assess the quality of the design and performance of the clinical studies and include a statement regarding compliance with GCP regulations.

3. Provide a brief summary of the clinical findings, including important limitations (e.g., absence of data on some patient populations, on pertinent endpoints, or on use in combination therapy; lack of comparisons with relevant active comparators).

4. Discuss and evaluate risks and benefits based on the conclusions of pivotal clinical trials and include interpretations of how safety and efficacy results support the proposed dose(s) and target indication(s); include also an evaluation of how prescribing information will optimize benefits and manage potential risks.

5. Address particular safety and efficacy issues encountered during clinical development and how these issues were evaluated and resolved.

6. Explore unresolved issues, discuss why these issues are not considered as barriers to approval, and present plans to resolve the issues.

7. Discuss the basis for important or unusual aspects of the prescribing information.

A Clinical Overview will generally be a relatively short document of approximately 30 pages but the length will depend on the complexity of the clinical development program. The use of in-text tables and figures to facilitate understanding of key clinical information is encouraged. Also encouraged is cross-referencing to the more detailed information provided in the Clinical Summary or in the clinical study reports located in Module 5.

The recommended organization and order of presentation for a Clinical Overview is

1. Product development rationale
2. Overview of biopharmaceutics
3. Overview of clinical pharmacology
4. Overview of efficacy
5. Overview of safety
6. Risks and benefits conclusions
7. References

A discussion of the clinical development rationale for a drug candidate is to (a) identify the pharmacological class of the candidate, (b) describe the target indication (i.e., the particular clinical or pathophysiological condition that a drug candidate is intended to treat, prevent, or diagnose), (c) summarize the scientific background that supported the investigation of a drug candidate for the indication(s) that was (were) studied, (d) briefly describe the clinical development program for a drug candidate and include information on ongoing and planned clinical studies and the basis for submitting the marketing application at this point in the program, and (e) briefly describe plans for the use of foreign clinical data to support the application. In addition, this rationale should note and explain concordance or lack of concordance with current standard research approaches (i.e., GCP regulations) regarding the design, conduct, and analysis of the clinical studies. Pertinent published literature is to be referenced. Regulatory guidance and advice are to be identified and formal advice documents (e.g., official meeting minutes, official guidance, letters from regulatory authorities) are to be referenced with complete copies included in the reference section of Module 5.

The purpose of an Overview of Biopharmaceutics subsection is to present an analysis of any important issues related to the bioavailability of a drug candidate that might affect the safety and/or efficacy of a proposed drug product for marketing. These issues could include dosage form and strength proportionality, differences between a proposed drug product and the formulation(s) of a drug candidate evaluated in clinical trials, and the influence of food and the time of eating on the extent and duration of exposure.

An Overview of Clinical Pharmacology subsection is to present an analysis of PK, pharmacodynamic (PD), and related in vitro data. This analysis is to consider all relevant data, discuss how and why the data support the conclusions drawn, and emphasize unusual results and known or potential problems. Items to be addressed in this sub-section include

1. Pharmacokinetics including, but not limited to, comparative PK in healthy subjects, patients, and special populations; PK related to intrinsic factors (e.g., age, gender, race) and to extrinsic factors (e.g., environmental

factors, diet); rate and extent of absorption; distribution; metabolism and the pharmacological and/or toxicological activity of formed metabolites; rate(s) and route(s) of excretion; stereochemistry issues; clinically relevant drug–drug and drug–food interactions.

2. Pharmacodynamics including, but not limited to, information on the mechanism of action; favorable or unfavorable PD effect to plasma concentration of a drug candidate and/or active metabolite(s) (i.e., PK/PD relationships); PD support for proposed dose, dosing interval, and dosing duration; possible genetic differences in PD response.

3. Interpretation and implication of immunogenicity and clinical microbiology studies.

A critical analysis and evaluation of the clinical data pertinent to the efficacy of a drug candidate in the intended patient population is to be presented in an Overview of Efficacy subsection. All relevant data, both positive and negative, are to be considered with discussions on why and how these data support the proposed indication and prescribing information. The studies considered relevant for the evaluation of efficacy are to be identified and the reasons that any adequate and well-controlled studies are not being considered should be discussed. Issues that should be considered in this overview include, but are not limited to

1. Relevant features of the patient population (e.g., demographics, disease stage, important but excluded patient populations, and participation of children and elderly).

2. Implications of the study design(s) and justification of any surrogate endpoints employed.

3. Statistical methods and any issues that might affect the interpretation of study results.

4. Similarities and/or differences in results among studies and in different patient subgroups within studies.

5. Observed relationships between efficacy, dose, and dosage regimen for each indication both in the overall patient population and in different patient subgroups or special populations.

6. For a drug product intended for long-term use, findings pertinent to the maintenance of long-term efficacy, the determination of long-term dosage regimen, and the potential for developing tolerance.

7. Data suggestive that treatment may be improved by drug candidate plasma concentration monitoring and the optimal plasma concentration range.

8. The clinical relevance of the magnitude of the observed efficacy.

An Overview of Safety is a critical analysis of the safety data and an indication of how the safety results support and justify the proposed prescribing information. Topics that should be considered in this analysis of safety include

1. Adverse experiences (AEs) considered characteristic of the pharmacological class.

2. Approaches employed for monitoring of particular AEs (e.g., QT interval prolongation, ophthalmic changes).

3. Findings in relevant animal toxicology and/or drug substance and drug product quality information that affect or could affect the evaluation of clinical safety.

4. The nature of the patient population and the extent of exposure for both a drug candidate and any control treatment(s) evaluated. Limitations of the safety database as related to inclusion and exclusion criteria and subject/patient demographics is to be considered and discussed.

5. Common and nonserious AEs with reference to the tabular presentations of AEs in the clinical summary.

6. Serious adverse experiences (SAEs) (with appropriate cross-reference to tabular presentations in the Clinical Summary) with a discussion on absolute numbers and frequency of SAEs, including deaths, and other significant AEs for a drug candidate and control treatments. Any conclusions regarding causal relationship, or the lack thereof, to a drug product should be provided. Laboratory findings that reflect actual or possible serious medical effects are to be discussed.

7. Similarities and/or differences in safety results among clinical studies and how these observations affect the interpretation of the safety data.

8. Any differences in the rates of AEs or SAEs in population subgroups or special populations.

9. Possible relation of AEs to dose, dosage regimen, and dose duration.

10. Methods to prevent or manage AEs.

11. Reactions due to overdose and the potential for dependence, rebound phenomena, and abuse or the lack of data on these issues.

12. Worldwide marketing experience and, where appropriate, support for the applicability to the new region of data generated in another region.

A Risks and Benefits Conclusions subsection is to integrate all the conclusions reached in the other subsections of the Clinical Overview and to provide an overall assessment of the risks and benefits of the use of a drug product in clinical practice. Also, the implications of any deviations from regulatory advice, regulations, or guidelines and any important limitations in the available data are to be discussed. An analysis of risks and benefits is expected to be quite brief but should identify the most important conclusions and issues concerning

1. The efficacy of a drug product for each proposed indication
2. Significant safety findings
3. Dose–response and dose–toxicity relationships and optimal dose ranges and dosage regimens
4. Efficacy and safety in subgroups and special populations
5. If applicable, results in children of different age groups
6. Risks to patients for known and/or potential drug–drug and drug–food interactions

A list of references cited in a Clinical Overview is to be included with copies of all relevant references provided in Module 5.

D. Nonclinical Written and Tabulated Summaries

The information presented in the Nonclinical Written and Tabulated Summaries section of the ICH CTD guideline is intended to assist sponsors and authors in the preparation of nonclinical pharmacology, pharmacokinetic, and toxicology summaries in a format acceptable to the various ICH regions and is not intended to indicate what nonclinical research studies are required or how these studies are to be designed or conducted. Since no guideline can cover all possibilities, a sponsor can modify, if needed, the format to provide the optimal presentation of the generated results in order to facilitate the understanding and evaluation of the information. General points to be considered by a sponsor and authors for inclusion in these summaries include that

1. Age- and gender-related effects in animal models are to be discussed.
2. Relevant findings on stereoisomers and/or drug candidate metabolites, as appropriate, are to be included.
3. Consistent use of units throughout the nonclinical summaries (and throughout the quality and clinical sections of a marketing application) will facilitate review and, if needed, a table for converting units may be useful.
4. During discussions, information is to be integrated across studies and across species and exposure in the animal models is to be related to exposure in humans given the maximum intended dose.
5. When available, results from in vitro studies should precede results from in vivo studies.
6. When multiple studies of the same type are to be summarized, the studies are to be ordered by species, by route, and then by duration with the shortest duration first.

7. Species and routes of administration are to be ordered as shown in Table 2.
8. When considered desirable to display results more effectively, tables and figures may be used within the text or grouped together at the end of each subsection.
9. References to citations in the tabulated summaries are to be included throughout the text and are to be in the following format: (Table X.X, Study/report number).

In general, the total length of the three nonclinical written summaries should not exceed 100 to 150 pages.

The order of presentation recommended for the Nonclinical Written and Tabulated Summaries in Module 2 and the nonclinical study reports in Module 4 is presented in Table 3.

The aim of an Introduction is to introduce a reviewer to a drug candidate and the proposed clinical use. This introduction should contain brief information on a drug candidate's structure and pharmacological properties and on the proposed clinical indication, dose, and duration of use. For a Pharmacology Written Summary, a brief summary of approximately 2 to 3 pages should describe the principal findings from the in vitro and animal pharmacology studies. This summary should include a short discussion of the pharmacological data package and should point out any notable aspects (such as the lack of a relevant animal model or the potential predictability of an animal model to a human disease or disorder).

A subsection on Primary Pharmacodynamics (i.e., studies on the mode of action and/or effects of a drug candidate in relation to the desired therapeutic target) should, when possible, relate the pharmacology of a drug candidate to available data (e.g., selectivity, safety, potency) on other drugs in

Table 2 Presentation Order for Species and Routes of Administration for Nonclinical Studies

Species order	Route of administration order
Mouse	Intended route for human use
Rat	Oral
Hamster	Intravenous
Other rodent	Intramuscular
Rabbit	Intraperitoneal
Dog	Subcutaneous
Nonhuman primate	Inhalation
Other nonrodent mammal	Topical
Nonmammals	Other

Table 3 Order of Presentation for Nonclinical Written and
Tabulated Summaries (Module 2) and Nonclinical Study Reports
(Module 4)

	Module	
Sequence of presentation	2	4
Table of Contents		X
Introduction	X	
Pharmacology	X	
Brief summary of pharmacology	X	
Primary pharmacodynamics	X	X
Secondary pharmacodynamics	X	X
Safety pharmacology	X	X
Pharmacodynamic drug interactions	X	X
Discussion and conclusions	X	
Tables and figures	X	
Tabulated summary of pharmacology	X	
Pharmacokinetics	X	
Brief summary of pharmacokinetics	X	
Methods of analysis	X	X
Absorption	X	X
Distribution	X	X
Metabolism	X	X
Excretion	X	X
Pharmacokinetic drug interactions	X	X
Other pharmacokinetic studies	X	X
Discussion and conclusions	X	
Tables and figures	X	
Tabulated summary of pharmacokinetics	X	
Toxicology	X	
Brief summary of toxicology	X	
Single-dose toxicity	X	X
Repeat-dose toxicity	X	X
Genotoxicity	X	X
Carcinogenicity	X	X
Reproductive and developmental toxicity	X	X
Studies in juvenile animals	X	X
Local tolerance	X	X
Other toxicity studies	X	X
Tables and figures	X	
Tabulated summary of toxicology	X	
Key Literature References		X

the pharmacological class. Where appropriate, secondary pharmacodynamic results (i.e., studies on the mode of action and/or effects of a drug candidate not related to the desired therapeutic target) should be summarized by organ system. The results from conducted safety pharmacology evaluations (i.e., studies conducted to investigate the potential undesirable pharmacodynamic effects of a drug candidate on physiological functions in relation to exposure within and above the therapeutic range) should be summarized and evaluated. Since the results of some secondary pharmacodynamics studies may predict or assess potential adverse effects in humans and thus may contribute to the safety evalutions on a drug candidate, these results should be considered along with the data from safety pharmacology studies. If performed, drug interaction studies on pharmacodynamic effects (i.e., synergy or antagonism of the pharmacological response when two or more compounds are concurrently administered) should be summarized.

A Discussion and Conclusion subsection allows a sponsor to explain the results from the nonclinical pharmacological evaluations and to consider the significance of any issue that was noted or uncovered. A Tabulated Summary of Pharmacology should provide, in the same order as the written text and by study with in vitro studies preceding in vivo studies, brief descriptions of (a) the type of study, (b) the testing facility, (c) an indication of GLP compliance, (d) the indication tested, (e) the study design, (f) the study numbers (i.e., animals/sex/group), (g) the dose levels and method of administration, (h) a synopsis of results, (i) reference to publication citation and/or study report number, and (j) any other information that might assist a reviewer in better understanding the results from a given study. Recommended pharmacology tables (ETA) include a pharmacology overview, primary and secondary pharmacodynamics, safety pharmacology, and pharmacodynamic drug interactions.

The recommend order of presentation for a Pharmacokinetic Written Summary is given in Table 3. A brief summary of approximately 2 to 3 pages should provide information on the scope of the nonclinical PK evaluations and should indicate whether the animal species and strains studied were the same as those employed in animal pharmacology and toxicology experiments and whether the formulations tested were similar to or different from the formulations employed in other animal studies. As with the nonclinical pharmacology section, in-text tables and figures can be used, as appropriate, throughout the pharmacokinetic section or they can be grouped at the end of the section.

An introductory summary is to be followed by a brief description of the bioanalytical chemistry methods employed for the quantification of a drug candidate and known metabolites in physiological matrices. Where appropriate, method validation results for each species and each matrix, including limits of quantification and stability in physiological specimens, should be summarized. While not listed in the ICH CTD guideline, this author recommends that this section also include information on the synthesis of any radiolabeled compound used to evaluate the pharmacokinetics and drug metabolism, including mass balance and tissue distribution, of a drug candidate. Information on the site of the radiolabel in the chemical structure of a drug candidate and on the chemical and metabolic stability of the radiolabeled material should be included. In addition, any developed metabolic profiling assay should be summarized.

A subsection on Absorption should discuss available data on the extent and rate of absorption as determined from in vivo and in situ studies and on the relative bioavailability and/or bioequivalence animal studies conducted to evaluate changes in formulation or to bridge studies using different routes of administration. A Distribution subsection is to summarize results from protein binding and distribution in blood cell experiments, single and repeat dose (if conducted) tissue distribution studies, and placental transfer studies conducted to support reproductive and developmental toxicology studies. A primary purpose of conducting metabolism studies is to determine if the metabolic profile (number and amount of metabolites) of a drug candidate is similar or dissimilar in the animal models used for pharmacology and toxicology studies when compared to humans. In a subsection on nonclinical metabolism, this interspecies comparison is to be presented and should include information on the chemical structures and quantities of metabolites in physiological specimens from each species evaluated. The possible metabolic pathways for a drug candidate in each species, including humans, should be described using figures, as appropriate. For a drug candidate to be administered orally, information on the extent of presystemic metabolism (i.e., metabolism in the GI tract or first-pass metabolism by the liver) should be included. Any in vitro metabolism studies conducted to identify the enzyme systems (i.e., CYP450 isozymes) or individual enzymes (i.e., glucuronidases, esterases) responsible for metabolism of a drug candidate should be discussed and any information on metabolizing enzyme induction and inhibition should be included. Research studies conducted to evaluate the rate and extent of excretion of a drug candidate and metabolites or mass balance studies in rodent and nonrodent animal models are to be summarized. In addition, if available, information on the extent of excretion in milk should be provided as supportive data for completed reproductive and developmental toxicology studies.

If performed, the results from nonclinical PK drug–drug interaction studies should be summarized. The results from any other conducted nonclinical PK studies (i.e., drug–food interaction studies, renally impaired animals, juvenile and/or aged animal evaluations) should be briefly discussed. Using a Discussion and Conclusion subsection, a sponsor-designated author, either in-house or contracted, should discuss any nonclinical PK issues and consider the significance of these findings to the overall development of a drug candidate.

A Pharmacokinetic Written Summary is to be followed by a Pharmacokinetic Tabulated Summary. This tabulated summary should be ordered the same as the written summary and include an overview of all PK studies conducted on a drug candidate with indication of which of these studies were conducted in compliance with GLP Regulations, the study or report number, and the location of the study report in Module 4 of a marketing application. This overview is to be followed by tabulated summaries (ETA) of each conducted individual study, such as (a) bioanalytical chemistry methods and validation reports, (b) absorption after single and repeat doses, (c) tissue distribution, (d) protein binding, (e) study in pregnant and/or nursing animals, (f) metabolism (in vitro and in vivo) and possible metabolic pathways, (g) induction and/or inhibition of drug metabolizing enzymes, (h) excretion (urinary, fecal, biliary, expired air), (i) drug–drug interactions, and (j) other pharmacokinetic studies).

The order of presentation recommended for a Toxicology written summary is shown in Table 3. A brief summary of the principal Toxicology findings should be described in a few pages, generally not more than six, and should include a discussion in relation to the proposed clinical use. If desired and without including toxicology results, a summary table describing the extent of the toxicological evaluations on a drug candidate and a comment on compliance with GLP Regulations for each study conducted can be provided.

Results from single-dose or acute toxicology studies should be briefly presented by species and by route. Repeat-dose toxicology studies, with supportive TK evaluations, should be summarized by species, by route, and by duration and should provide summary information on methodology and highlight important findings (e.g., target organs, dose or exposure relationship to toxicity, NOAEL, maximum tolerated dose or MTD). Nonpivotal toxicology studies can be summarized in less detail than pivotal studies, which are the definitive GLP-regulated toxicology studies specified in the ICH M3 guideline).

Genotoxicity studies are to be summarized with in vitro nonmammalian cell system evaluations followed by in vitro mammalian cell system studies and then in vivo mammalian system experiments, which may have supportive TK evaluations. For carcinogenicity studies, with supportive TK results, a brief rationale, including the selection of doses, should be used to explain the types of studies chosen. The results from individual carcinogenicity studies are to be summarized with long-term or lifetime studies first and then short- or medium-term studies. The studies are to be ordered by species and to include dose range-finding studies that cannot be appropriately included under repeat-dose toxicity or PK subheadings.

Reproductive and developmental toxicology studies, with information on range-finding studies and supportive TK evaluations, are to be ordered by nonpivotal studies and pivotal studies, which include fertility and early embryonic development to implantation, effects on embryo-fetal development, effects on pre- and postnatal development including maternal function. If conducted, studies in which juvenile animals are dosed and evaluated are to be included in this section.

If local tolerance studies were conducted (and are considered by this author to be necessary for a drug candidate administered by any of a number of routes including, but not limited to, intravenous, intramuscular, subcutaneous, dermal, buccal, nasal, pulmonary, rectal, and vaginal), the results should be summarized by species, by route, and by duration and one should provide brief details of methodology and highlight important findings.

If other toxicology studies have been performed to support the development of a drug candidate, the results should be summarized with a rationale for conducting the studies and a brief discussion of the methodology and significant findings. Other toxicology study types include antigenicity, immunotoxicity, mechanistic studies (if not summarized elsewhere in the marketing application), dependence, and metabolite(s) and/or impurity(ies) evaluations.

A Discussion and Conclusions subsection on the toxicology results allows a sponsor's author to discuss the toxicity findings with reference to the significant issues that were noted or observed. The use of in-text tables and figures for highlighting these findings is recommended.

A Toxicology Tabulated Summary is to follow a Toxicology Written Summary. A tabulated summary should be ordered the same as a written summary and start with an overview of all toxicology and toxicokinetic studies conducted on a drug candidate with indication of which studies were conducted in compliance with GLP Regulations, the study or report number, and the location of the study report in Module 4 of the marketing application. Following the overview are to be the tabulated summaries (ETA) of the individual studies (single-dose toxicity, repeat-dose toxicity, genotoxicity, carcinogenicity, reproductive and developmental toxicity, studies in juvenile animals, local tolerance, and other toxicity studies).

E. Clinical Summary

A Clinical Summary is to provide a detailed, factual summarization of all the clinical information in a marketing application, including results within clinical study reports, from meta-analyses and/or other cross-study analyses reports, and, if appropriate, postmarketing data. The length of a clinical summary (excluding tables and figures) will usually be in the range of 50 to 400 pages. The recommended order of presentation, which corresponds to the

Table of Contents, for the various items to be included in a Clinical Summary is provided in Table 4.

A Clinical Summary is to start with a subsection on Biopharmaceutical Studies, and Associated Analytical and Bioanalytical Chemistry Methods conducted during the clinical development of a drug candidate. The background of the formulation development process is to be briefly provided and is to include information on in vitro and in vivo dosage form performance and the general approach and rationale for developing the bioavailability (BA), comparative BA, bioequivalence (BE), and in vitro dissolution profile database. Also to be included is a summary of the analytical and bioanalytical chemistry methods and the validation characteristics of these methods.

A tabular listing (ETA) of all biopharmaceutical studies conducted is recommended. Brief narrative descriptions (e.g., similar to an abstract for a journal article) are to share relevant features and outcomes of each study that provided important in vitro or in vivo data and information relevant to the BA and/or BE of a drug candidate. These narratives can be abstracted from clinical study reports (i.e., the synopsis of reports prepared according to ICH guideline E3) and should include reference to the full report. A comparison of results across studies, using both text and tables, is to pay particular attention to differences in in vitro dissolution, BA, and comparative BA results. This comparison is to consider

1. The effects of formulation and manufacturing changes on in vitro dissolution and bioavailability.
2. Where appropriate, the effect of food (i.e., meal type and/or timing of the meal in relation to dose administration) on bioavailability.
3. Evidence of, or lack of, correlations between in vitro dissolution and bioavailability, including the effect of pH on dissolution, and conclusions on dissolution specifications.
4. Comparative BA of different dosage form strengths.
5. If appropriate, comparative BA of a drug candidate formulation(s) used in clinical trials and a proposed drug product to be marketed.
6. The source and magnitude of observed inter- and intrasubject variability for each formulation in a comparative BA study.

A Summary of Clinical Pharmacology Studies is to provide reviewers of a marketing application with an overall view of the clinical pharmacology of a drug candidate and is to include information on clinical studies conducted to evaluate human PK and PD and on in vitro studies performed with human cells, tissues, or related material (i.e., human biomaterials) and considered pertinent to PK processes. Types of in vitro studies include permeability assessment (e.g., intestinal absorption, blood–brain barrier transport, protein binding, hepatic metabolism). For a vaccine product, immune response data is to be provided to support the selection of dose, dosing schedule, and the

Table 4 Order of Presentation for Clinical Summary (Module 2)

Table of Contents
Summary of Biopharmaceutical Studies and Associated Analytical Methods
  Background and overview
  Summary of results of individual studies
  Comparison and analyses of results across studies
  Appendix (tables and figures not included in text)
Summary of Clinical Pharmacology Studies
  Background and overview
  Summary of results of individual studies
  Comparison and analyses of results across studies
  Special studies (e.g., immunogenicity, clincal microbiology)
  Appendix (tables and figures not included in text)
Summary of Clinical Efficacy
  Background and overview of clinical efficacy
  Summary of results of individual studies
  Comparison and analyses of results across studies
    Study population
    Comparison of efficacy results of all studies
    Comparison of results in subpopulations
  Analysis of clinical information relevant to dosing recommendations
  Persistence of efficacy and/or toxic effects
  Appendix (tables and figures not included in text)
Summary of Clinical Safety
  Exposure to drug candidate
    Overall safety evaluation plan and narratives of safety studies
    Overall extent of exposure
    Demographic and other characteristics of study population
  Adverse events of experiences (AEs)
    Analysis of AEs
      Common AEs
      Deaths
      Other serious AEs (SAEs)
      Other significant AEs
      Analysis of AEs by organ system or syndrome
    Narratives
  Clinical laboratory evaluations
  Vital signs, physical findings, and other observations related to safety
  Safety in special groups and situations
    Intrinsic factors
    Extrinsic factors
    Drug interactions
    Use in pregnancy and lactation
    Overdose
    Drug abuse
    Withdrawal and rebound
    Effects on ability to drive or operate machinery and impairment of mental ability
  Postmarketing data
References
Synopses of Individual Studies

formulation of a proposed final drug product. The summary is to start with a brief overview of conducted human biomaterial studies followed by the clinical studies conducted to characterize the PK and PD of a drug candidate, and any PK/PD relationships, in healthy subjects and patients. Critical aspects of study designs and data analysis are to be noted and may include rationale for the choice of singe or repeat doses, the study population, the choice of intrinsic and extrinsic factors studied, and the choice of PD endpoints.

A tabular listing (ETA) of all clinical pharmacology studies is recommended and is to be accompanied by brief narrative descriptions, with appropriate reference to the full reports, of the relevant features and outcomes for each of the critical individual studies. The summary information on individual clinical pharmacology studies is to be followed by a comparison and analyses of results across studies. Using, as appropriate, tables (ETA), figures, and text, the comparison is to provide a factual presentation of all data pertinent to

1. In vitro drug metabolism and in vitro drug–drug interaction studies and possible clinical implications of the results.
2. Human PK studies, including estimates of standard PK parameters, sources of variability, and evidence supporting dose and/or dose individualization in the target patient population and in special populations.
3. Comparison between single- and repeated-dose PK studies.
4. Population PK analyses.
5. Dose–response and/or concentration–response relationships.
6. Major inconsistencies in the human biomaterial, PK, and/or PD database.
7. PK studies conducted to determine if foreign clinical data might be extrapolated for supporting a marketing application in a new region.

In addition, a Clinical Pharmacology subsection should include information on research studies that provide special types of data that are relevant to a specific type of drug candidate. These study types may include immunogenicity studies for a protein drug candidate and in vitro assessments to characterize the spectrum of activity for an antimicrobial or antiviral drug candidate. For a vaccine or other type of drug product intended to induce specific immune reactions, immunogenicity data is to be described in the section on efficacy. Similarly, clinical studies that include characterization of the susceptibility of clinical isolates to a drug candidate as part of the efficacy determination are to be included in the section on efficacy.

A Summary of Clinical Efficacy subsection is to describe the program of controlled clinical studies and other pertinent clinical trials that evaluated efficacy specific to the indication(s) sought. If a marketing application is for more than one indication, separate clinical efficacy sections are to be provided for each indication unless the indications are closely related. The use of tables (ETA) and figures is recommended to enhance the readability of the document; if appropriate (i.e., owing to the length of tables or the size of figures), they can be provided in an appendix at the end of the subsection. A Clinical Efficacy subsection is to begin with an overview of the design of the controlled clinical trials (e.g., dose response, comparative efficacy, long term efficacy, efficacy in patient population subgroups) that were conducted to evaluate efficacy. Critical features like randomization, blinding, choice of control treatment, choice of patient population, study duration, endpoints, and statistical analysis plan are to be discussed.

A tabular listing of all clinical studies that provided (or were designed to provide) data relevant to the efficacy of a drug candidate is recommended and is to be accompanied with brief narrative descriptions, with references to the full clinical study reports, of important clinical trials. These narratives can be abstracted from the synopses of reports prepared according to the ICH E3 guideline.

Narratives for any bridging study using clinical endpoints (i.e., clinical trials for extrapolating certain types of foreign clinical data to a marketing application to a new region) are to be included. A comparison and analysis of efficacy results across clinical studies is to summarize all available data that characterizes the efficacy of a drug candidate. This summary is to include analyses of all data, irrespective of whether the data support the overall efficacy conclusion, and is to discuss the extent to which the results of the relevant clinical studies do or do not reinforce each other. Major inconsistencies regarding efficacy are to be addressed and any area needing further evaluation is to be identified. Important differences in study design (e.g., endpoints, control groups, study duration, statistical methods, patient population, dose or dose range, drug candidate formulation) should be identified. Analyses will generally be two types: (1) comparison of results of individual clinical studies and (2) analysis of data combined from various clinical studies. Comparisons of efficacy results across studies should primarily focus on prespecified primary endpoints. Also, important evidence that supports efficacy and were summarized in a clinical pharmacology section should be cross-referenced.

The demographic and other baseline characteristics of patients across all efficacy studies are to be described and should provide information on

1. The characteristics of the disease (e.g., severity and duration) prior treatment in study patients and inclusion and exclusion criteria.
2. Differences in baseline characteristics of the study population in different studies or groups of studies.

3. Any differences between populations included in critical efficacy analyses and the overall patient population who would receive a drug product after marketing approval has been obtained.
4. Assessment of the number of patients who dropped out of or were terminated from the studies, the times of withdrawal, and the reasons for discontinuation.

Overview analyses of efficacy in specific populations should be summarized to demonstrate whether the claimed treatment efforts are consistently observed across all relevant population subgroups. Owing to the limited sample size in many individual clinical trials, analyses across multiple studies may be necessary to evaluate efficacy effects for major demographic factors and for relevant intrinsic and extrinsic factors. Factors of special interest may arise from general concern (e.g., treatment of the elderly) or from specific issues related to the pharmacology of a drug candidate or identified during earlier drug development. Efficacy in the pediatric population should routinely be analyzed in marketing applications for a proposed indication that occurs in children.

An integrated summary and analysis is to be provided on all data that pertain to dose–response or drug candidate plasma concentration–response relationships of effectiveness and thus to contribute to dose selection, dosing interval, and dosage duration. Relevant data from nonclinical and clinical studies should be referenced and, where appropriate, summarized to illustrate further and describe these relationships. Any identified deviations (e.g., nonlinearity of pharmacokinetics, delayed effects, tolerance, enzyme induction) from relatively simple relationships should be discussed. Also, any evidence of differences in the relationships that result from the age, gender, race, disease status, or other factors of the patients should be described. How the potential for these deviations and differences were evaluated, even if no differences were found, should be described.

Available data on the persistence of efficacy over time should be summarized. The number of patients for whom long-term efficacy data are available and the length of exposure should be provided and any evidence of tolerance over time should be noted.

A summary of data relevant to safety in the intended patient population is to integrate the results of individual clinical study reports. Safety-related data are to be displayed at three levels:

1. The extent of exposure (e.g., dose, dosing duration, number of patients, type of patients) to determine the degree to which safety can be assessed from the database.
2. The identification and classification of the occurrence of the more common AEs and changes in laboratory test values.
3. The occurrence of SAEs and other significant AEs with the events examined for frequency over time.

With the appropriate use of tables and figures, the safety profile of a drug candidate is to be described on the basis of analysis of all clinical safety data and is to be outlined in a detailed, clear, and objective manner.

For the assessment of exposure to a drug candidate, the overall safety evaluation plan is to be briefly described and is to include considerations and observations concerning nonclinical data, any relevant pharmacological class effects, and the sources of the safety data. A tabular listing (ETA) of all clinical studies, grouped appropriately, that provided safety data is recommended. Narrative descriptions of these studies should be provided, or be appropriately cross-referenced, and should include sufficient detail to allow reviewers to understand the exposure of study subjects/patients to a drug candidate or control agent(s) and how the safety data were collected. A table (ETA) and appropriate text should be employed to summarize the overall extent of drug candidate exposure from all phases of the clinical development program. The table should indicate the number of subjects/patients exposed in clinical studies of different types and at various doses, routes of administration, and durations of dosing, which can, if necessary, be grouped in an appropriate manner. Dose level designations could be the maximum dose received by a subject/patient, the dose with the longest exposure, the mean daily dose, and/or the cumulative dose. Duration of exposure can be summarized by the number of subjects/patients exposed for specific periods of time (e.g., 1 day or less, 2 days to 1 week, 1 week to 1 month, 1 month to 6 months, 6 months to 1 year, more than 1 year). A summary table (ETA) should provide an overview of the demographic characteristics of the population that was exposed to a drug candidate during clinical development and the choice of age ranges studied should be taken into account. Additional tables should be used to describe relevant characteristics of the population and the number of subjects/patients with special characteristics, such as (a) severity of disease, (b) hospitalization, (c) impaired renal function, (d) concomitant illnesses or diseases, (e) concomitant or concurrent use of particular medications, and (f) geographical location. Any imbalance(s) between a drug candidate and placebo and/or comparator(s) regarding demographic characteristics should be discussed, particularly in relation to differences in safety outcomes. Separate demographic tables should be prepared for each indication evaluated, unless the indications are closely related and the risks to the study populations are considered to be the same. Tables (ETA) and text should be used to describe the frequency of AEs. All AEs occurring or worsening after the initiation of treatment are to be summarized in tables listing each AE, the number of subjects/patients in whom the AE occurred, and the frequency of occurrence in subjects/patients treated with a drug candidate, comparator drug(s), and placebo. These tables could also present AE results for each drug candidate dose level and could be modified to show AE rates by severity, by time from onset of therapy, or by assessment of causality.

When the safety data is not concentrated in a small number of clinical studies, grouping the studies and pooling the safety results to improve estimates and sensitivity to differences may be considered. However, while often useful, pooling of safety data across studies is to be approached with caution since in some cases, interpretations can be difficult and may obscure real differences. When pooling safety data, items that should be considered include

1. Combining safety data from clinical studies that are of similar design is often appropriate.

2. A safety estimate from pooled data is usually less informative if the incidence of a particular AE differs substantially across the clinical studies in the pool.

3. An unusual AE pattern for any clinical study is indicative that the safety data for that study should be presented separately.

4. The appropriate extent of analysis is depedent on the seriousness of the AE and the strength of evidence of drug candidate causation.

5. Examination of which subjects/patients experience extreme laboratory abnormalities may be useful in identifying subgroups who are at risk for certain AEs.

When a sponsor decides to pool safety data from several clinical studies, the rationale for selecting the method used for pooling should be described. AEs in pooled studies should use standardized terms to describe events and their frequencies and synonymous terms should be collected under a single preferred term. The use of MedDRA is recommended but other specified dictionaries can be used.

Tables of AE rates are recommended to compare rates in treatment and control groups. Combining the AE severity and causality categories may be helpful in providing a simpler side-by-side comparison of groups. While causality categories, if used, may be reported, the recommended presentation of the safety data is to include total AEs (whether considered related or unrelated to treatment with a drug candidate), since evaluations of causality are considered to be inherently subjective and may exclude unexpected AEs that are in fact treatment related. Another useful examination is to evaluate more closely the more common AEs that are considered to be drug candidate related (e.g., show an apparent dose–response relationship and/or a clear difference between drug candidate and placebo rates) for possible correlation with relevant factors such as (a) dosage, (b) dose level expressed in terms of mg/kg or mg/m^2, (c) dosing regimen, (d) dosing duration, (e) total dose administered, (f) demographic characteristics, (g) concomitant medication use, (h) other baseline features, (i) efficacy outcomes, and/or (j) drug candidate plasma concentrations (where available). Also possibly useful for the apparently drug-candidate-related events is a summary of AEs results based on time of onset and duration of the experience. Rigorous statistical evaluations of the possible relationships of specific AEs to each of the factors mentioned above are often not necessary, particularly when inspections of the safety data show no apparent evidence of a significant relationship between AE rate and a given factor.

A table, usually located in an appendix to a clinical safety subsection, is to list all deaths occurring while subjects/patients are on study, including deaths that occurred shortly following (e.g., within 30 days) treatment termination. Only deaths that are clearly disease-related as described in a clinical study protocol and are not related to the administration of a drug candidate can be excepted from this table. All deaths should be examined for any unexpected patterns between study treatment arms and further analyzed if unexplained differences are noted. Deaths are to be examined individually and analyzed on the basis of rates in individual clinical trials and appropriate pools of trials, considering both total mortality and cause-related deaths. Potential relationships of death to demographic, intrinsic, and extrinsic factors should also be considered.

Summaries of all SAEs, other than death but including SAEs associated with or preceding death, are to be displayed in a table and discussed in text. The display should include major laboratory abnormalities, abnormal vital signs, and abnormal physical observations that are considered to be SAEs. Results of analyses and/or assessments of SAEs across clinical studies should be presented and examined for frequency over time, particularly for a drug candidate projected for chronic clinical use. Potential relationships of SAEs to demographic, intrinsic, and extrinsic factors should also be considered.

Other than those reported as SAEs, marked hematologic and other laboratory abnormalities and any experience that led to a substantial intervention (e.g., premature discontinuation of drug candidate treatment, dose reduction, or substantial additional concomitant therapy) should be displayed. Experiences that led to premature discontinuation of drug candidate administration are considered to represent an important safety concern and deserve particular attention in the evaluation of safety data. AEs leading to treatment discontinuation should be considered as possibly drug-candidate related even if the event was thought to represent intercurrent illness. Reasons for discontinuation should be discussed and rates of discontinuation should be compared across clinical studies in relation to rates for placebo and/or active control treatment groups and for potential relationships to demographic, intrinsic, and extrinsic factors.

Assessments of causality of, and risk factor for, death, other SAEs, and other significant AEs is frequently complicated by the fact that these events are uncommon in most clinical development programs. Thus consideration of related events as a group may be of critical importance in understanding the safety profile of a drug candidate. In addition, summarizing AEs by organ system or syndrome is often useful so that AEs may be considered in the content of potentially related experiences, including laboratory abnormalities.

The locations in a marketing application of individual narratives of subject/patient deaths, other SAEs, and other significant AEs should be referenced. These narratives themselves will normally be a part of the applicable clinical study report. In cases where no clinical study report has been generated, narratives can be placed in an appropriate section of Module 5.

A subsection on Clinical Laboratory Evaluations is to describe changes in patterns of laboratory tests with drug candidate use. As mentioned earlier, marked laboratory abnormalities and those that led to a substantial intervention are to be reported in the subsection on SAEs. The appropriate evaluations of laboratory values will usually be determined by the results observed and should include comparison of the treatment and control groups. Normal laboratory ranges, given in standard international units, should be provided for each analyte measured. A brief overview of the major changes in laboratory data (e.g., hematology, clinical chemistry, urinalysis, and other data as appropriate) at each time (e.g., at each clinical visit) over the course of the studies should include information on

1. The central tendency as determined by the group mean and median values.

2. The range of values and the number of subjects/patients with abnormal values or with abnormal values of a predefined certain size.

3. Abnormalities, including those that led to discontinuation, considered important for an individual subject/patient.

The technique employed for presenting cross-study observations and comparisons of vital signs (e.g., heart rate, blood pressure, temperature, respiratory rate), weight, and other data (e.g., ECGs, x-rays) related to safety should be similar to that used for laboratory variables. If an effect is evident, any relationship to a drug candidate or to other variables (e.g., disease, demographics, concomitant therapy) should be identified and discussed for clinical relevance.

Separate subsections in a Clinical Summary are recommended to summarize safety in special groups and situations. These subsections may include brief overviews of safety data pertinent to individualizing therapy or patient management for

1. Intrinsic ethnic factors that may include age, gender, height, weight, lean body mass, genetic polymorphism, body composition, other illness, and organ dysfunction (e.g., renal or hepatic impairment).

2. Extrinsic ethnic factors that may include environment (e.g., geographic location), use of tobacco, use of alcohol, use of other drugs, and food habits.

3. The potential impact on safety (e.g., changes in pharmacological effect, AE profile, and/or drug candidate plasma concentrations) for drug–drug and drug–food interactions.

4. Use during pregnancy and lactation.

5. Overdose including signs and/or symptoms, laboratory findings, therapeutic measures and/or treatments, and antidotes, if available.

6. Drug abuse and dependence potential, including particularly susceptible patient populations.

7. Withdrawal and rebound effects, including events that may occur, or increase in severity, after discontinuation.

8. Effects (e.g., drowsiness) on ability to drive or operate machinery or impairment of mental ability.

If a drug candidate has already been or is being marketed, all relevant postmarketing data (e.g., published and unpublished, including, if available, periodic safety update reports) available to a sponsor of a marketing application should be summarized. Details to be provided include the number of subjects/patients estimated to have been exposed and categorized, as appropriate, by indication, dosage, treatment duration, and geographic location. A tabulation of SAEs reported after a drug is marketed is recommended and should include information on any potentially serious drug–drug interactions.

A list of references cited in a Clinical Summary should be included and copies of important references provided in Module 5. Any reference not included in Module 5 should be available upon request.

The last section of a Clinical Summary is recommended to contain a table entitled Listing of Clinical Studies (ETA). This table is also to be included in Module 5. Following the table are to be individual clinical study synopses organized in the same sequence as the clinical study reports in Module 5. The ICH E3 guideline on Structure and Content of Clinical Study Reports provides an example of a format for a clinical study report synopsis, which can be used for marketing applications in all ICH regions.

IV. MODULE 3: QUALITY

Information to be presented in Module 3 on quality is to be an expansion of the summary descriptions provided in a QOS. As shown in Table 1, the order of presentation is to be same as that utilized for QOSs with subsections under the main headings for each item for a drug substance and a drug product.

Detailed descriptions, using flow diagrams, figures, and narrative text, of the manufacturing processes for a drug substance and drug product are to be provided under the appropriate headings. Alternate processes, if available, should be explained and described with the same level of detail as the primary process. A detailed development history discussion is recommended and should provide information on the significant changes made in the manufacturing process and/or manufacturing site for a drug substance and drug product.

Validation protocols and reports, with acceptance and rejection criteria and specifications and experimental data, for all analytical chemistry methods developed and used for the characterization of a drug substance and drug product are to be included within the designated sections. These methods may include, but are not limited to, (a) identity assays for a drug substance, intermediates, and excipients; (b) content assays for a drug substance, intermediates, and excipients; (c) impurity profiling and quantification assays for a drug substance and drug product; (d) dissolution assays for a drug product; and (e) stability-indicating assays for a drug substance and drug product.

Descriptions of batches and the results of batch analyses for a drug substance and drug product are to be provided under the appropriate sections.

For both drug substance and drug product, the types of stability studies conducted, the protocols used, and the results are to be included in the designated sections. Study types may include forced degradation, stress conditions, and shelf life conditions. Results from stability studies are to be presented using an appropriate format that includes tables, figures, and narrative text. Conclusions with respect to storage conditions and shelf life are to be provided. A postapproval stability protocol and stability commitment for both drug substance and drug product are to be included.

For a macromolecule drug substance and drug product, appendices to Module 3 are to include detailed information on facilities and equipment and safety evaluations on adventitious agents. The flow diagram presented in a QOS for facilities and equipment should be included. In addition, information is to be presented with respect to adjacent areas that may be of concern for maintaining the integrity of a drug substance and drug product. Information on all developmental or approved products manufactured or manipulated in the same areas as a sponsor's drug substance or drug product are to be included. In addition and as appropriate, information on the preparation, cleaning, sterilization, and storage of specified equipment and materials is to be provided. Also to be included is information on procedures (e.g., cleaning and production scheduling) and design features of the facility to prevent contamination or cross-contamination of areas and equipment where operations for the preparation of cell banks and drug substance and drug product manufacturing are performed. For nonviral adventitious agents, detailed information is to be provided on the avoidance and control of these agents. Examples of information include certification and/or testing of raw materials and excipients and control of production processes for a given agent. For viral adventitious agents, detailed information is to be discussed from viral safety evaluation studies, which demonstrate that the materials used in production are considered safe and that the approaches used for testing, evaluating, and eliminating the potential risks during manufacturing are suitable. Information essential for the evaluation of the virological safety of materials of animal or human origin is to be provided. For cell lines, data on the selection, testing, and safety assessment for potential viral contamination of cells and viral qualification of cell banks should also be included. The selection of virological tests, including the sensitivity and specificity of the test and the frequency of testing, that are performed during manufacturing is to be justified. Test results to confirm that a drug substance and drug product are free from viral contamination at an appropriate stage of manufacture are to be provided. In addition, the rationale and action plan for assessing viral clearance and the results and evaluations of viral clearance studies are to be delineated.

A final section of Module 3 provides additional drug substance and drug product information that is region specific. Sponsors need to consult the appropriate regional guidelines and/or regulatory authorities for additional guidance. Examples of region-specific information include

1. Executed batch records (US only)
2. Method validation package (US only)
3. Comparability protocols (US only)
4. Process validation scheme for drug product (EU only)

At the end of Module 3, key quality literature references cited in the text are to be included.

V. MODULE 4: NONCLINICAL STUDY REPORTS

The organization and order of presentation for the Nonclinical Study Reports in a marketing application prepared in the recommended CTD format is given in Table 3 and is the same as described earlier (Sec. III.D) for a nonclinical Written Summary. Individual-animal results are to be located in the corresponding nonclinical study report or as an appendix to that report. Module 4 of an application should start with a Table of Contents that lists all the nonclinical study reports included and that gives the location of each study report in a submission. The last section in a Nonclinical Study Reports module is to provide copies of key nonclinical literature references that were cited support the pharmacological, pharmacokinetic, and toxicological characterization and development of a drug candidate.

For some nonclinical studies, primarily drug discovery efforts and pharmacology evaluations conducted in-house by a sponsor, technical reports may not have been prepared but reprints of published journal articles may be available. While this situation is not discussed in the ICH CTD guideline, this author recommends that these publications not be included in place of a technical report. If both a publication and report are available, the technical report should be included since a study report should contain all the data generated during the study while the publication may only summarize these results and might only contain those data that are supportive of the

Table 5 Order of Presentation for Clinical Study Reports and Related Information (Module 5)

Table of Contents of Clinical Study Reports
Tabular Listing of All Clinical Studies
Clinical Study Reports
    Reports of biopharmaceutical studies
        Bioavailability (BA) study reports
        Comparative BA and bioequivalence (BE) study reports
        In vitro and in vivo correlation study reports
        Reports on bioanalytical and analytical methods for human studies
    Reports of studies pertinent to pharmacokinetics using human biomaterials
        Plasma protein binding study reports
        Reports on hepatic metabolism and drug interaction studies
        Reports of studies using other human biomaterials
    Reports of human pharmacokinetic (PK) studies
        Healthy subject PK and initial tolerability study reports
        Patient PK and initial tolerability study reports
        Intrinsic factor PK study reports
        Extrinsic factor PK study reports
        Population PK study reports
    Reports of human pharmacodynamic (PD) studies
        Healthy subject PD and PK/PD study reports
        Patient PD and PK/PD study reports
    Reports of efficacy and safety studies
        Study reports of controled clinical studies pertinent to the claimed indication
        Study report of uncontrolled clinical studies
        Reports of analyses of data from more than one study, including any formal integrated analyses, meta-analyses, and bridging analyses
        Other clinical study reports
    Reports of postmarketing experience
    Case report forms and individual patient listings
Copies of References

conclusions being made by the publication's authors. A copy of the publication, along with copies of other key literature references, should be included in an appendix.

VI. MODULE 5: CLINICAL STUDY REPORTS

The recommended organization for the placement of clinical study reports and related information in a marketing application is described in Module 5 of the ICH CTD guideline. The placement of the individual clinical study reports is to be determined by the primary objective of a clinical trial and each report is to appear in only one section with appropriate cross-referencing to other sections when a trial has multiple objectives. An explanation, such as "not applicable" or "no study conducted" should be provided when no clinical study report or information is available for inclusion in a given section or subsection. This author recommends that sponsors use a similar practice when information is not available for inclusion in a quality (Module 3) or nonclinical (Module 4) section or subsection. Table 5 provides the recommended order of presentation for clinical study reports and related information. In general, this order of presentation is similar to the order of presentation in a Clinical Summary and is to start with a Table of Contents for Clinical Study Reports and then a tabular listing of all clinical studies. The tabular listing (ETA) is to be the same listing as is utilized at the end of a Clinical Summary.

VII. CONCLUSIONS

This chapter has described and discussed the various modules of a Common Technical Document (CTD) as presented in ICH M4. A sponsor preparing a marketing application for submission to any of the three ICH regions and to most other regulatory authorities around the world can, and probably should, utilize the recommend orders of presentation outlined in the ICH CTD guideline for quality, nonclinical, and clinical results generated to support the characterization and development of a drug candidate.

Using the recommended orders of presentation provides a sponsor of a marketing application submission with a number of benefits, which include, but are not limited to

1. The compilation of the generated data and results in an order that is acceptable to various regulatory agencies.

2. Easier and more timely evaluation of a marketing application by regulatory agency reviewers, since the data and results are presented in a defined order and under the same headings as in other submissions.

3. An indication of missing results (e.g., key research studies not conducted during the drug development process or insufficient information being available to complete a description of manufacturing procedures) that may be critical for obtaining marketing approval.

This author recommends that sponsors consider using the CTD-recommended order of presentation for quality, nonclinical, and clinical results as a generic template for the definition of a drug development logic plan (as described in Chap. 1). The results from drug discovery efforts, preclinical research experiments, and earlier CMC evaluations can be appropriately summarized and placed in the desired locations of the CTD-recommended format. This compilation of data can then be utilized to support a regulatory agency submission for a first-in-human clinical trial. As clinical studies are completed and additional nonclinical and manufacturing information becomes available, the results can be summarized and placed in the appropriate sections or subsections of a CTD. Using this approach, once a sponsor believes that sufficient clinical data on the safety and efficacy of a drug candidate in the proposed disease indication(s) have been generated, the time needed to prepare a marketing application should be greatly reduced (i.e., a few months versus a year or more).

19
Obligations of the Investigator, Sponsor, and Monitor

Richard A. Guarino
Oxford Pharmaceutical Resources, Inc., Totowa, New Jersey, U.S.A.

I. INTRODUCTION

The Good Clinical Practices (Gcps) regulations section (21 CFR 312) in the Code of Federal Regulations outlines the responsibilities of the clinical investigator, the drug sponsor, and the clinical trial monitor involved in investigational new product development. In addition to this regulated conduct of clinical investigations, each participant has a moral and ethical responsibility for the safety of subjects who participate in these trials. Good clinical practices have long been the norm for the investigator, as written in the 1572 Form, but the first proposed regulations pertaining to investigator, sponsor, and monitor were circulated in 1977 and 1978. In 1987, 10 years later, GCPs were published as final regulations in the Code of Federal Regulations. Today, investigators, sponsors, and monitors are obligated by law to follow these GCPs.

To conduct clinical research that meets the requirements of the FDA for new product approval, it is essential to understand these regulations and their subsequent impact on the clinical development process of drugs, devices, and biologics.

The 1987 IND regulations specified within the current Code of Federal Regulations identify (more clearly than in previously proposed GCP guidelines) the delegation of responsibilities in the conduct of clinical trials. Not only do investigators have a key responsibility in assessing subjects' efficacy and safety response to new drugs, devices, or biologics, but the sponsor and monitor also have equal responsibility for the subjects' safety and welfare.

To clarify who are the people obligated under GCP regulations, the following definitions will be applied throughout this chapter:

1.   Investigator: The individual who conducts a clinical investigation (i.e., under whose immediate direction the drug is administered or dispensed to the subject). If an investigation is conducted by a team of individuals, the investigator is the responsible leader of the team. The subinvestigator is any other individual member of that team. These individuals are usually licensed physicians or individuals working under the direction of a licensed physician.

2.   Sponsor/investigator: An individual who both initiates and conducts an investigation under whose immediate direction the investigational drug is administered or dispensed. This category refers mostly to physician investigators who are conducting clinical research under an investigator IND (see Chap. 3).

3.   Sponsor: An individual or organization that takes responsibility for and initiates a clinical investigation. This may be an individual, a pharmaceutical company, a governmental agency, an academic institution, or a private or other organization.

4.   Monitor: The person selected by the sponsor who is qualified by training experience to facilitate and oversee the progress of the investigation.

II.   INVESTIGATOR OBLIGATIONS

In 21 CFR 312.53, the regulations deal with the descriptive information provided on form FDA 1572, the Statement of Investigator form. Also included in 21 CFR 312.53 are the selection requirements for clinical investigators. Previously, to conduct trials designated as phase 1 and 2, investigators were required to complete a Statement of Investigator form FDA 1572; investigators conducting trials designated as phase 3 or phase 4 completed a different Statement of Investigator form, which was known as form FDA 1573. As a result of the IND rewrite regulations, form FDA 1573 is no longer used for any clinical trials. At present, for phases 1 through 4, only the Statement of Investigator form FDA 1572 is required. This describes the obligations of investigators conducting clinical research. The new information required on form FDA 1572 includes the name and address of any clinical laboratory facility and address of the Institutional Review Board that is responsible for the review and the approval of the individual investigators participating in the trial. This part also states that the sponsor is charged with the responsibility of selecting qualified investigators who are defined as those capable of conducting the trial by virtue of their training and experience. By using the phrase "training and experience," the FDA means that clinical investigators conducting a trial of a particular disease should have enough experience in the clinical specialty to observe correctly the signs, symptoms, and progress of that disease while experimenting with a new investigational drug. For example, if a new drug is designed for an OB-GYN practice, a pediatrician would not be expected to have the expertise to assess this drug, nor would a cardiologist have expertise in evaluating a gastrointestinal drug.

Investigators are defined as those who have signed and completed form FDA 1572, or sub-or coinvestigators listed on that form, and who are considered to have the academic and experiential qualifications for participating in the clinical program.

The fine print on the reverse side of form FDA 1572 is a written agreement whereby the investigator assures the sponsor that he will conduct the trial in accordance with the appropriate trial plan (i.e., the protocol) and will observe the GCP tenets. Implicit in this agreement is that the investigator will have obtained signed Informed Consent (IC) forms from patients or subjects participating in the clinical research under their jurisdiction. Form 1572 also charges the investigator with the reporting of adverse experiences that occur during the investigation and provides assurance that the investigator has read and understood the investigator's brochure. In addition, he or she assures that all individuals participating in the supervision of any clinical trial, under the direction of the investigator, are aware of their responsibilities. Once form 1572 has been signed by the investigator, he or she further assures compliance with the requirements of providing trial materials, protocols, and other pertinent information to an authorized Institutional Review Board (IRB) for review. Along with these documents, a CV should be provided along with assurance that the investigational plan set forth in the trial protocol will be followed.

To summarize, the primary responsibilities of investigators in clinical trials are the ethical and moral obligations to all the participating patients and subjects in the trial. Investigators must provide a measure of safety for each participant in the trial so that the subject is protected ethically and morally from any endangerment that might occur during a trial of an investigational drug. After the investigator's responsibilities are outlined and he or she has signed form FDA 1572, any additional information from the sponsor that might be necessary should be requested and any concerns regarding procedures should be raised. An investigator is responsible (a) for ensuring that an investigation is conducted according to the signed investigator statement, the investigational plan, and applicable regulations; and (b) for protecting the rights, safety, and welfare of subjects participating in a clinical investigation on any unapproved product. Also, the investigators must maintain complete control of drugs under investigation. An investigator shall obtain the informed consent of each human subject to whom the drug is administered and shall administer the drug only to subjects under the investigator's supervision or under the supervision of a subinvestigator responsible to the investigator. The investigator shall not supply the investigational drug to any person not participating in the clinical program.

The investigators are required to maintain adequate records of the disposition of the drug, including dates, quantity, and use by subjects. If the investigation is terminated, suspended, discontinued, or completed, the investigator shall account for and return the unused supplies of the drug to the sponsor, or otherwise provide written documentation for disposition of the unused supplies of the drug. An investigator is required to maintain accurate case histories designed to record all observations and other pertinent data on each individual treated with the investigational drug. (Usually this is accomplished by completing case report forms and maintaining medical records.)

All investigators shall retain records of all subjects enlisted in investigational trials for 2 years after a marketing application for the drug is approved for the indication being investigated. If no application is to be filed, or if the application is not approved for such indication, records must be maintained for 2 years after the investigation is discontinued and the FDA has notified the sponsor of the status of the application.

The investigator shall furnish all reports to the sponsor of the drug. The sponsor is responsible for collecting and evaluating the results obtained. The sponsor also is required to submit annual reports to the FDA on the progress of the clinical investigations. Investigators shall promptly report to the sponsor any adverse effect that may reasonably be regarded as caused by, or probably caused by, the investigational drug. If the adverse effect is alarming, the investigator shall report the adverse effect immediately (see ADR reporting, Chap. 11).

An investigator shall provide the sponsor with an adequate report shortly after completion of the investigator's participation in the trial.

III. OTHER INVESTIGATOR RESPONSIBILITIES

Prior to signing a 1572 the investigator must have a good understanding of the content in the Investigator Brochure (see Chap. 3). Based on this document, an investigator is usually assured that sufficient pharmacology and toxicology allows trial subjects to be prescribed an investigational drug.

The investigator must assure that an IRB who reviews the clinical investigational protocol complies with the regulations established in CFR (see Chap. 20) and that the IRB is responsible for the initial and continuing review and approval of the proposed clinical trial. The investigator must also assure that he or she will promptly report all changes in the research activity and all unanticipated problems involving risk to human subjects (AEs and ADRs) or others to the IRB. In addition, the investigator will not make any changes in the protocol without IRB approval, except where necessary to eliminate apparent immediate hazards to human subjects.

An investigator shall, upon request from any properly authorized officer or employee of the FDA, at reasonable times, permit such officer or employee to have access to, copy, and verify any records or reports made by the investigator. The investigator is not required to divulge subject names unless the records of particular individuals require a more detailed trial of the cases, or unless there is reason to believe that the records do not represent actual case trials, or do not represent actual results obtained.

A. Investigator Penalties

What are the results if an investigator has repeatedly or deliberately either failed to comply with these GCP requirements, or has submitted false information in any report to the sponsor? First, the Center for Drug Evaluation and Research (CDER) or the Center for Biologics Evaluation and Research (CBER) will furnish the investigator with written notice of the matter complained of and offer the investigator an opportunity to explain the matter in writing. On the other hand, at the option of the investigator, an informal conference could be requested. If the explanation offered by the investigator is not accepted by CDER or CBER, the investigator will be given an opportunity for a regulatory hearing. At this hearing, the issue of whether the investigator is entitled to receive investigational drugs will be addressed. After evaluating all available information, including any explanation presented by the investigator, the FDA commissioner determines whether the investigator has repeatedly or deliberately failed to comply with GCP requirements or has deliberately or repeatedly submitted false information to the sponsor in any required report. The commissioner will then notify the investigator and the sponsor of any investigation in which the investigator has been named as a participant not entitled to receive investigational drugs. If there is reasonable cause for this action, the investigator becomes subject to further investigation for each IND and each approved application submitted to the FDA containing data reported by this investigator. Therefore every investigational trial conducted by this investigator will be examined to determine whether the investigator has submitted unreliable data. Other investigations that are conducted under the same protocol will be temporarily put on hold.

Conversely the commissioner may determine, after eliminating the unreliable data by the investigator, that the remaining data justify continuing other of the same investigations at other sites. However, if a danger to the public health exists, the commissioner will terminate the IND immediately; the sponsor will be notified and will have an opportunity for a regulatory hearing before the FDA on the question of whether the IND should be reinstated. If the commissioner determines that the data submitted are unreliable and data submitted by the investigator cannot be justified, the commissioner will proceed to withdraw approval of the drug product in accordance with the provisions of the FD&C Act. As a result, an investigator who has been deemed to be ineligible to receive investigational drugs will be blacklisted and unable to participate in any experimental trials. The investigator may be reinstated when the commissioner determines that he or she has presented adequate assurances that the investigator will use investigational drugs in compliance with FDA regulations.

In conclusion, before an investigator accepts the responsibilities of conducting a clinical investigation with an IND drug, he or she must be aware of the legal obligations agreed to when form FDA 1572 is signed. Investigators must comply with the protocol and the rules, regulations, and guidelines of GCPs. The investigators must realize that they are subject to a federal offense and can jeopardize their reputation and ultimately their ability to conduct further clinical research. Investigators must know that precise collection of data is mandatory in the conduct of clinical research. Research must be designed to assess the efficacy of the product and, above all, to ensure that the safety of the subject remains the primary concern.

IV. SPONSOR OBLIGATIONS

The sponsor's primary responsibility is clearly delineated in 21 CFR 312.50, which ensures that clinical trials are conducted in compliance with FDA regulations. The sponsor is responsible for selecting qualified investigators and for providing them with the information they need to conduct an investigation in accordance with the published regulations. Usually the sponsor accomplishes this task by supplying the potential investigator with an investigator's brochure and a protocol of the clinical investigation on the agent to be investigated (see Chaps. 10 and 3). An investigator's brochure contains all information from nonclinical trials and reports, and any previous human efficacy and safety trials reports that reflect previous experiences of subjects on the investigational agent.

Of primary interest in the obligations is the option of a sponsor to transfer total or partial responsibility for the conduct of a clinical trial to a CRO. CROs play a significant role in new drug development (see Chap. 25). However, CROs who contract with sponsor companies are obligated under the same GCP regulations as defined in this chapter. A CRO may be the sponsor or the monitor with equal obligations as defined in 21 CFR 312. The current regulations noted in 21 CFR 312.52 are specific and require that any transfer, whether in total or in part, be described in writing and agreed to by both parties. The FDA states that any obligations not specifically described by the sponsor in the written transfer of responsibilities will be considered as not transferred to the CRO; the liability for these undefined responsibilities therefore remains with the sponsor. The FDA further requires the CRO (once any transfer of responsibilities has been made by the sponsor) to comply with all applicable regulations, and notes that the CRO is subject to the same regulatory actions as a sponsor if the CRO does not satisfy FDA regulations in the fulfillment of its contracted duties. As a result of these regulations, it is possible for a CRO to act on behalf of a sponsor once this legal transfer of obligations has been completed. Although the CRO must assure complete compliance with the responsibilities assigned (and described in writing), it remains the sponsor's responsibility to ensure the quality and integrity of data generated under the supervision of a CRO. In this situation, the sponsor would be expected to act as a quality assurance auditor of the data, even though assignment for the conduct of a trial has been delegated to the CRO. The regulations also charge the sponsor with responsibility for the inventory and control of the drug. Only investigators participating in a clinical trial may receive and have access to investigational drug and materials. It must be emphasized that the sponsor is always responsible for the conduct and reporting of all clinical research originating from their directive.

V. SPONSOR AND MONITOR OBLIGATIONS

One of the most important responsibilities of the sponsor is to monitor the progress of every clinical investigation conducted under its direction (21 CFR 312.56). A monitor's obligations, under the auspices of the sponsor, are to ensure that the deficiencies created during the conduct of clinical investigations are corrected or justified by the investigator and that the investigator adheres to the investigational plan (the protocol; see Chap. 10). The appointed monitors for any clinical investigation conducted under a sponsor's IND have an obligation to assure that an investigator is complying with the signed Form FDA 1572 and the general investigational plan, and that the clinical protocol is being followed. If an investigator does not correct his errors and mistakes and no improvement is noted in the progress of the trial, the monitor shall promptly secure compliance or discontinue shipment of the investigational drug to the investigator and end the investigator's participation in the clinical program. Another responsibility while monitoring the progress of a clinical investigation is evaluating the evidence relating to the drug's safety and effectiveness. At the same time, sponsors shall make such reports to the FDA regarding information relevant to the safety of the drug, as they are required to do under section 312.32 of the FDA regulations.

When a monitor reports an adverse experience (see Chap. 11) to a sponsor during an investigational trial, it is the sponsor's obligation to determine whether there is an unreasonable and significant risk to the subject or patient. At that time, the sponsor must determine if the investigational trial is to be discontinued. Important among the procedures of reporting adverse experiences is the sponsor's obligation to the FDA, and to all investigators who, at any time, participate in clinical trials and who are prescribing the experimental drug. It is up to the investigators to report any AEs or ADRs to the IRB. The monitor should assure that this has been done.

The sponsor should report to the FDA any AEs or ADRs that are unexpected, fatal, or life-threatening within 7 calendar days of receipt of information. ADRs that are both serious and unexpected and related to drug administration should be reported within 15 calendar days of receipt of information. Subsequent to this, the sponsor should furnish the FDA with a complete report no later than 8 days from filing the report. The decision to discontinue the investigation will be contingent on the severity of the drug related reports and the number of similar reports. (See ADR Reporting, Chap. 11).

It is important to understand that the obligations of monitors include the responsibility for assuring that all records and data recorded on case report forms reflect valid data gathered by the investigator, and that they coincide with corresponding medical and hospital records of the subject participating in the investigational trial. Detailed auditing and documentation assure the sponsor that the monitor is overseeing the clinical data collected by the investigator and that GCPs are being followed. One misconception of many monitors who audit clinical investigations is that their only task is to assure correct entry of data. In fact, one of the monitor's primary obligations is to note any adverse effects or deviations in laboratory values that could signify a safety problem in investigational trial subjects. This is especially true in large multiclinic trials, when many centers are conducting investigational trials following the same protocol, and many monitors are auditing data. If any abnormal reactions or laboratory deviations are noted from center to center, the monitors should compare observations and assess an accumulative percentage of occurrence of these deviations. At times, a sporadic, apparently minor deviation can turn out to be significant when calculated across all centers. If monitors are astute, they can often prevent recurrence of adverse experiences that might jeopardize the safety of the subjects participating in investigational drug trials.

Another responsibility of the monitor is to assure maintenance of accurate records showing the receipt, shipment, or other disposition of the investigational drug. These records are required to include, as appropriate, the name of the investigator to whom the drug is shipped, the date, the quantity, and the batch number of each shipment. A sponsor shall retain these records and reports for 2 years after a marketing application is approved for the drug, or, if an application is not approved, until 2 years after shipment and delivery of the drug for investigational use is discontinued and the FDA has been notified. The sponsor shall also assure the return of all unused supplies of the investigational drug from each investigator whose participation in the investigation is discontinued or terminated. The sponsor may authorize alternative disposition of unused supplies of the investigational drug, provided this alternative disposition does not expose humans to risks. Although the overall responsibilities of drug inventory is assigned to sponsors, it is the monitors' underlying responsibility for drug accountability as they represent the sponsor.

In turn, the investigators, during experimental research, are also responsible for record retention similar to that of the sponsor. They are required to maintain adequate records of the disposition of the drug, including dates, quantity, and use by the subjects or patients. The investigator is also obligated, if he is terminated, suspended, or discontinued, or if he has completed a trial, to return all unused supplies of the drug to the sponsor or otherwise provide documentation of how the unused supplies of the drug were disposed. (It is always recommended that the unused trial medication be returned to the sponsor to assure drug accountability.) An investigator is required to prepare and maintain accurate case histories (designed to record all observations and other data pertinent to the investigation) on each individual treated with the investigational drug. An investigator shall retain records from the trial for a period of 2 years after a marketing application is approved for the drug for the indication for which it was being investigated; again, if no application is to be filed or if the application is not approved for the indication, an investigator must retain records for 2 years after an investigation is discontinued and the FDA has been notified. Although these investigator obligations have been previously discussed, the monitor should assure that these procedures are adhered to and reported in a timely fashion.

One of the monitor's responsibilities is to assure that the investigator fulfills their obligations. An often neglected investigator responsibility is the requirement to submit periodic reports to the sponsor. Many investigators assume that the case report forms are sufficient in providing periodic reports. However, an investigator should be prepared to provide the sponsor with progress reports. These should include an update of the ongoing investigational trial. Annual reports to the FDA on the progress of the clinical investigations are required to be submitted by the sponsor. These reports contain information based or the investigators' progress reports. The monitor should make sure that the safety reports are promptly reported to the sponsor, including any adverse experiences that may reasonably be regarded as caused by or likely caused by the investigational drug. Alarming adverse experiences (i.e., severe adverse reactions that jeopardize a subject's safety in any way) must be reported immediately by the investigator to the sponsor. Lastly, when an investigator has completed or terminated an investigational trial, a final report should be submitted to the sponsor. This comprehensive report should be completed shortly after an investigator's participation in the investigation is over. The report summarizes the final observations of the trial and any adverse experiences that occurred during the course of the clinical investigation. Monitors should be responsible for encouraging investigators to complete and submit these reports. In this case, constant follow-up may be necessary. In most cases, the clinical monitor will provide the investigator with these reports. They are usually based on the summary of findings in the closeout visit (see Chap. 22).

Legal repercussions can occur from any neglect of the obligations by investigators, sponsors, or monitors. The Code of Federal Regulations stipulates in 21 CFR 312.58 that the FDA can inspect the sponsor's records or reports upon request from any properly authorized officer or employee of the FDA. These inspections normally occur at reasonable times and permit the FDA to have access to copy and verify any records or reports relating to a clinical investigation conducted under an IND. Upon written request by the FDA, the sponsor may be asked to submit the records, reports, or copies of them to the FDA. Under these regulations, the sponsor is also obligated to discontinue shipments of the drug to any investigator who has failed to maintain or make available records or reports of the investigation. Subsequently, an investigator shall, upon request from any properly authorized officer or employee of the FDA, at reasonable times, permit such an officer or employee to have access to or copy and verify any records or reports made by the investigator. The investigator is not required to divulge subject or patient names unless the records of particular individuals require a more detailed trial of the cases. The monitor must assure that all these investigator responsibilities are completed. (See Chap. 22).

The investigators', sponsors', and monitors' obligations must be fulfilled by complying with GCP rules and regulations. Sponsors' and monitors' consistent and persistent managing roles are vital in assuring that each person involved in conducting clinical trials meet the legal obligations. The success of any clinical program will depend on the cooperation, understanding, and compliance of this triad working together. With this agreement of responsibilities and a well-organized clinical plan the combination can only result in valid data to support a new drug application.

20

Institutional Review Board/ Independent Ethics Committee and Informed Consent: Protecting Subjects Throughout the Clinical Research Process

Rochelle L. Goodson
R. L. Goodson Consulting, Inc., New York, U.S.A.

I. INTRODUCTION

The US Food and Drug Administration (FDA) statutes that are published in Title 21 of the Code of Federal Regulations (21 CFR) identify and define the activities involved in the clinical research process. These codified regulations are designed to protect the rights, safety, and welfare of subjects of clinical investigations. An amendment to Title 21, dated July 27, 1981, specifically required that the conduct of clinical investigations would include (1) obtaining the informed consent of all subjects and (2) approval of all research proposals by Institutional Review Boards (IRBs).

More recently, the Department of Health and Human Services, Food and Drug Administration, published the guideline entitled "Good Clinical Practice: Consolidated Guideline," which underscored the importance of these and other regulated activities. Although the guideline is not perceived by the FDA as a substitute for the codified regulations, the FDA's recognition of this guideline is evidenced by a statement noting it as representative of the agency's current thinking on good clinical practices. The significance of the guideline "The International Conference (ICH) on Harmonisation of Technical Requirements for Registration of Pharmaceuticals for Human

Use" is that it supports the concept and implementation of a unified standard for designing, conducting, recording, and reporting trials that involve the participation of human subjects in clinical investigations in the US, Japan, and the European Union. Informed consent and IRB activities are discussed throughout the document to address how studies are conducted.

Despite federal regulations and established guidelines mandating good clinical practice procedures, the complexity of protecting research participants continues to challenge the research community. As recently as the late 1990s, several tragic and widely reported research-related events, including several deaths, prompted the DHHS to commission the Institute of Medicine (IOM) to assess the current national system of regulated research. An IOM committee formulated the concept of implementing a human research participant protection program (HRPPP) in all research environments. In its first report (issued in 2001) the committee outlined key elements and activities to ensure protection of every research participant. Most significant, however, was the recommendation of accreditation programs that assess protection activities in a uniform and independent manner, as indicated by the report's title "Preserving Public Trust: Accreditation and Human Research Participant Protection Programs." To date, two independent organizations have developed accreditation standards. The National Committee for Quality Assurance (NCQA) was contracted by the Veteran's Administration to develop an accreditation program specifically for VAs, and The Association for the Accreditation of Human Research Protection Programs under a grant from the IOM developed an interim accreditation program for broad-based research programs. At present, accreditation is voluntary, and the debate continues in the research community as to whether mandatory accreditation will be required in the future.

II. BACKGROUND

The National Research Act passed by Congress on July 12, 1974, mandated the establishment of IRBs, which for the first time formalized the review of federally funded research. Also, this act provided for a National Commission for the Protection of Human Subjects of Biomedical and Behavioral Research and resulted in the publication of the Belmont Report in 1979. Although the Belmont Report was never officially adopted by Congress, it provided a fundamental guideline for the protection of human subjects in research.

Historically, private practitioners conducting clinical research were exempt from the IRB and informed consent regulations required of institutional, i.e., university or hospital researchers. The amended regulations on July 27, 1981, requiring IRB review and approval of all research, increased the need to establish IRBs that would review and approve research proposals that might not be affiliated with a major research center, teaching hospital, or university. In the current regulatory environment, all New Drug Applications (NDAs) submitted to the FDA in support of all drugs, biologicals, or medical devices require proof that IRB approval was obtained before implementation of the research. Evidence of continuing review by the IRB throughout the trial must also be demonstrated. The only exemptions from IRB review are investigations that started before July 27, 1981, and that fit categorical descriptions defined in the regulations.

III. INSTITUTIONAL REVIEW BOARD DUTIES

The goal of the IRB (a.k.a. Independent Ethics Committee or IEC) is the protection of the rights, safety, and welfare of human subjects involved in clinical research investigations. The review board is, therefore, primarily responsible for the evaluation of the proposed research. All evaluations should have the following objectives: (1) to determine that the research is properly designed; (2) to determine that the benefit of the intended therapy will outweigh the potential risk; and (3) to determine that the patient will be provided with adequate information to enable him or her to make an informed decision regarding participation in the clinical trial.

If the benefits do not sufficiently outweigh the risks, the IRB may either refuse to award approval of the project/study protocol or require a modification to research that limits the risk/benefit ratio by approving it for a more defined or limited patient population.

Since IRB review/approval and continuing review processes are required for all clinical investigations performed in support of a research application or a marketing permit for FDA regulated products, it is important to ensure that projects are not initiated before these approvals are obtained.

It is also important to note that, although IRBs are subject to codified regulations stipulating their functions and responsibilities, other key players in the clinical research process are intrinsically involved in review processes to ensure the protection of subjects' rights. Specifically, clinical investigators are bound by 21 CFR 312.66 (Assurance of IRB review) to obtain initial and continuing approval reviews, to report changes in research activity, to report unanticipated problems relating to risks to subjects, and to provide study status. In addition, sponsors of clinical trials are bound by 21 CFR 312.53 (Selecting investigators and monitors) to inform the IRB, albeit through the investigator, of these obligations. The sponsor secures the investigator's agreement to fulfill these obligations by obtaining a signed and dated Investigator's Statement before initiating a trial.

IV. INSTITUTIONAL REVIEW BOARD MEMBERSHIP AND RESPONSIBILITIES

The composition of an IRB membership is specifically defined by the FDA in Title 21 CFR Part 56 and must include the following basic requirements, which must be adhered to:

- Members of both sexes at each meeting
- Scientific (e.g., physician, research scientist) and nonscientific (lawyers, clergy) members; a minimum of one nonscientific member at each meeting
- A minimum of one member who is unaffiliated with the institution at each meeting
- No member with a conflict of interest
- A minimum of five voting members at each meeting

Some IRBs have expanded their working policies or standard operating procedures to include the following additional requirements:

- One member representing cultural or ethnic diversity
- One member representing a special interest group, if applicable (e.g., handicapped)
- The considerations of socioeconomic factors and local attitudes
- Financial considerations

Because there are some IRBs with a large membership and all members may not attend every meeting, it is imperative that the basic requirements for constituting an IRB be met by all present and voting members. A standard roster or an IRB Membership List should be maintained, which lists the alternative members and indicates that they have equal professional status and meet the basic qualifications.

All IRBs are ultimately responsible for the unbiased determination of whether a proposal for clinical research is acceptable in terms of the standards of professional practice, the institution or individual undertaking the research, and the patient population. Therefore proposals considered for approval at convened meetings must receive approval of a majority of the members present at that meeting.

If a voting member has a conflicting interest in the review, e.g., a member who will be directly involved in the proposal being reviewed for approval, he/she may provide information but must abstain from voting. In addition, individuals with expertise in a specialized area may be invited to assist in reviews at a meeting; however, these individuals will not be permitted to vote.

V. IRB DOCUMENTATION AND OPERATIONS

IRBs must maintain written procedures of all operations. All activities associated with the following operations must be recorded:

- Conducting initial review and continuing review/approval of research
- Conducting expedited review/approval of research
- Ensuring that changes in research activity are reported
- Ensuring that changes in previously approved research are not implemented without review and approval
- Reporting of serious risks
- Reporting of significant findings

All IRBs are required to maintain records (minutes) of meetings and documents for at least 3 years after the completion of a study. In addition, IRBs are responsible for reporting investigator noncompliance to their institutions, sponsors of clinical research, and the FDA. It is important to note that IRBs have the regulatory authority to suspend or terminate research they previously approved if the research ceases to be conducted in accordance with the IRB's requirements. Research that has been associated with unexpected and/or serious harm to research subjects may be suspended or terminated.

VI. INFORMATION REQUIRED FOR IRB REVIEW

All information submitted to an IRB for review of a research protocol is provided by the clinical investigator seeking approval to conduct the research. The standard documents typically provided are the research protocol, a sample of the intended informed consent, and the Investigator's Brochure or Package Insert. It has become common practice recently also to provide patient information sheets or instruction guides, advertising that will be used to recruit subjects, and any scheduled reimbursements to compensate patients for their time or expenses incurred during participation in a trial. Although the regulations do not require these additional documents, FDA information sheets suggesting that they be provided have served as guidelines or references for common practices that facilitate regulated activities. The regulations require that the Investigator's Brochure be submitted for studies conducted under an investigational new drug application in the section defining IND content and format (21 CFR 312.23(a)(5) and in the section regarding informing investigators (21 CFR 312.55(a). In the ICH GCP Guideline, it is specifically stated that certain documents be obtained for review, as part of the responsibility of the IRB/IEC (Sec. 3.1. Responsibilities, 3.1.2).

The review of the protocol ensures that there are adequate selection criteria and procedures to protect vulnerable study populations. In addition, information within the protocol, the informed consent, and the Investigator's Brochure are reviewed to assess safety information that may affect subjects. IRBs are empowered with the authority to approve or disapprove research activities that are covered by regulations, as well as to require modifications to secure approval. Informed consents will be reviewed to assure that all the information provided is in accordance with 21 CFR 50.25; the IRB may also require that additional information be provided to study subjects in a separate format, such as a patient information sheet. If this requirement is waived, a written statement may be given to the subject. If a very short window of opportunity exists to dispense a research treatment to avoid a devastating or fatal outcome, a waiver for this requirement may be requested. It is important to note, however, that the sponsor must clearly describe or define the situations that would require testing without administering a written informed consent. Also, provisions that will be made to obtain the consent from family members must be in place. This issue will be discussed in more detail in the section on informed consent. In summary, the following criteria are used by IRBs to approve research:

- Minimal risk
- Risk/benefit ratio
- Equitable patient population
- Informed consent documentation
- Planned study management/monitoring
- Patient privacy and confidentiality
- Rights and welfare of a vulnerable population

The FDA does not prohibit the use of advertising. However, since it has become an increasingly popular tool for increasing the enrollment rate of subjects in clinical studies, the FDA has created an Information Sheet, *Advertising for Study Subjects*, to serve as a guideline. This guideline recognizes advertisements as an extension of the informed consent and subject selection process and defines them as a research activity and subject to review, primarily to protect subjects from misleading advertisements. Since advertisements are perceived as a research activity, they should be submitted for review and approval, although the regulations do not specifically require a review.

The Information Sheet notes what the contents of advertisements should be limited to as follows:

- The name and address of the clinical investigator
- The purpose of research and, in summary form, the eligibility criteria that will be used to admit subjects into the study

- A straightforward and truthful description of the benefits (e.g., payments for free treatment) to the subject from participation in the study
- The location of the research and the person to contact for further information

Sample advertising submitted to the IRB may be in various media formats. Whether the advertisement is in the form of newspaper advertisements, posters, brochures, leaflets, radio or television advertisements, and even notices posted on the Internet, they are all subject to the same requirements noted above. All copy, including audio or video scripts or videotape, should be submitted for review and approval before use. All of the requirements for written copy apply to all advertising modes.

The IRB must ensure that advertising does not include misleading information or statements implying that the drug or device is safe or effective for the indication being investigated or that the drug or device is equivalent or superior to any other drug or device. In addition to misleading potential subjects, statements that could be considered to be promotional claims would be in violation of statutes regulating the promotion of investigational drugs or devices.

The issue of subject reimbursement also has to be considered by the IRB to ensure that subjects are not induced to participate in a study because of excessive payments, but rather are remunerated adequately for the time and inconvenience that they experience in order to participate. If subjects participate in studies involving more than one study visit, the amount of reimbursement on a per visit basis should be stated. Visits that require additional time and/or cause inconvenience to the subject and have higher remunerations should be stated when applicable. Conversely, it should be stated if there are visits for which no reimbursement is scheduled. Finally, subjects should be informed when there is a caveat that, if the study is not completed, a prorated amount will be reimbursed rather than the total amount indicated for study completion. All of these items should be delineated in the informed consent.

Informed consents, which must be signed by subjects before they participate in a study, reflect payments that will made and, as mentioned, should include how they will be scheduled. The review of this information falls under the purview of IRB responsibility for two reasons. First, payment is perceived as a benefit, and it is the IRB's responsibility to determine that the benefit does not reflect an unduly coercive amount that may persuade a subject to participate in a study he or she ordinarily would not consider. Second, the IRB is also responsible for evaluating the investigator's responsibilities regarding the submission of this document.

VII. INITIAL APPROVAL AND CONTINUING REVIEW

The critical documents required for approval of research, i.e., protocol, informed consent, and Investigator's Brochure, are usually presented to an IRB chairperson by the principal investigator. Copies of the pertinent documents are supplied to the IRB members for thorough review before they vote on the proposed research project. Any and all elements of the project may be deliberated and may result in recommendations to modify any part of the research.

Clinical investigators will be notified, in writing, of all IRB decisions regarding the approval or disapproval of research or modifications to the research that will be required to obtain approval. Approvals will identify the study and include the date of approval and the IRB chairperson's signature. If a decision to disapprove a research proposal is rendered, the notification will include the reasons to provide the investigator with an opportunity to respond in person or in writing. All written documentation between the IRB and the clinical investigator should be accompanied by a transmittal letter to ensure verification after any action or decision. All correspondence should be date-stamped upon receipt, and all study documentation should be stamped with the date of IRB approval. In addition, documentation submitted to the clinical investigator (and the IRB) should be dated to distinguish between final documents and draft versions to avoid accidental approval of a draft document.

Regulations regarding the IRB review of research require the continuing review of protocols at least once per year; however, the intervals are based on the degree of risk to the subject and are usually specified by the IRB at the time of initial approval. Finally, IRBs have the authority to observe or designate a third party to observe the consent process and the research.

VIII. EXPEDITED REVIEWS

Expedited reviews are used by IRBs to review and approve minor changes in previously approved research, either because the change is administrative in nature or because the research (or change in the research) involves no more than minimal risk to the subject. This procedure requires only the IRB chairperson's review or review by one or more reviewers designated by the chairperson who are voting members of the IRB. In addition, when and if the expedited procedure is invoked, every member must be advised of all approvals made via this procedure. It is important to note that expedited review procedures are used only under the limited circumstances addressed above and do not replace a full IRB review of research proposals.

The original documentation of all IRB reviews and decisions should be maintained by the principal investigator; copies should be maintained by a trial's sponsor.

IX. THE INFORMED CONSENT FORM

Overall, the informed consent regulations (21 CFR, Part 50) apply to all clinical investigations regulated by the Food and Drug Administration, including clinical investigations that support applications for research or marketing permits for products the FDA regulates. The general requirements for informed consent are discussed below.

As mentioned earlier, the clinical investigator is ultimately responsible for assuring that a subject in a clinical investigation is not only fully informed of the project but also apprised of the procedures to be followed and the risks and benefits of the therapeutic regimen proposed in the research. The informed consent process requires that a written consent is obtained from each patient (or his legally authorized representative) to verify that the above-referenced obligations have been satisfied. On November 5, 1996, the FDA published a final rule, i.e., a change to an existing regulation, requiring that a consent form signed by the subject or the subject's legally authorized representative be dated by the subject (or legally authorized representative) at the same time it is signed. This ruling became effective on December 5, 1996, enforcing via regulation a good clinical practice procedure that has been routinely implemented by clinical researchers in recent years. In addition, the FDA amended the regulation regarding case histories (21 CFR 312.62) to specify that case histories must document that informed consent was obtained before a subject participated in a study and to clarify what should be included in a case history.

The IRB's oversight responsibility regarding informed consent is highlighted by this amendment, which was enacted to ensure that an informed consent is obtained before any clinical trial–related procedures are performed.

During the informed consent process, clinical investigators should plan to allot sufficient time for patients to review a consent and ask questions regarding the research. Patients must be permitted to take the form with them while they are considering participation; however, the form must be signed in front of a witness. In addition, the IRB may request that a witness sign the informed consent, as well. The principal investigator may not serve as a witness. A copy of the consent document must be provided to the patient.

Informed consents should be written so that they can be understood by a layperson. In general, the overall document should not contain words or explanations that could not ordinarily be understood by an individual who has completed an eighth-grade level of education. All technical, medical, or legal terminology should be explained to a prospective subject. Patients unable to read English should have the informed consent made available in their native language. The translation of the informed consent should be documented as being completed by a qualified individual. It is recommended that translation be used only in instances where a significant amount of the proposed study population would require a translation.

Finally, informed consents should not contan any coercive language that unfairly persuades or influences a subject's decision to participate. The consent should not contain exculpatory language that either requires or appears to require a subject to waive any legal rights or releases or appears to release an investigator, sponsor, institution, or any other agent of a clinical investigation from liability for negligence. The moral and legal ramifications of this type of language are obvious.

Aside from the general requirements for informed consent that have been discussed, there are basic elements that must be included in all informed consents. Additional elements are to be included only when they are deemed appropriate.

X. BASIC ELEMENTS OF THE INFORMED CONSENT (21 CFR 50.25)

1. A statement that the study involves research, an explanation of the purposes of the research, the expected duration of the subject's participation, a description of the schedule of events to be followed, and identification of any procedures that are experimental.

2. A description of any reasonable foreseeable risks or discomforts to the subject.

3. A description of any benefits to the subject that reasonably may be expected as a result of the research.

4. A disclosure of appropriate alternative procedures or courses of treatment, if any, that may be advantageous to the subject.

5. A statement describing the extent to which the confidentiality of records identifying the subject will be maintained, including mention of the possibility that the FDA may inspect the records.

6. Since all clinical research investigations entail more than minimal risk, a statement describing compensation (if any) that will be paid and an explanation as to whether any medical treatment is available if an adverse reaction occurs, what the treatment consists of, and/or where further information can be obtained.

7. A list of people to contact in the event of a study-related adverse experience and to answer pertinent questions about the research, including the subject's rights.

8. A statement that participation in the study is voluntary, that refusal to take part in the research will not result in penalty or loss of benefits to which the subject is otherwise entitled, and that that subject may withdraw from the study at any time without penalty or loss of benefits to which he or she is otherwise entitled.

XI. ADDITIONAL ELEMENTS OF THE INFORMED CONSENT (21 CFR 50.25(B))

1. A statement that the particular treatment or procedure may involve currently unforeseeable risks to the subject (or embryo or fetus, if the subject is or may become pregnant).

2. Circumstances under which the subject's involvement may be terminated by the investigator without regard to the subject's consent.

3. Additional costs to the subject, if any, that may result from participation in the research.

4. Consequences that may result from the subject's decision to withdraw from the research, and the procedures for an orderly termination of the subject's participation.

5. A statement that, during the course of the study, any significant new findings related to the subject's willingness to continue in the program will be presented and reviewed with him or her.

6. The approximate number of subjects involved in the study.

All consent documents and the entire informed consent process should be designed and implemented to be in compliance with the above-stated regulations, as well as consistent with the principles of the Declaration of Helsinki, World Medical Assembly, Revised 1996, 48th General Assembly, the accepted basis for clinical trial ethics incorporated into the ICH GCP Guideline.

The ICH GCP Guideline encompasses the procedures involved in the administration of the informed consent process that is included in the US CFR. However, it is worth noting that, in addition to expanded explanations for some of the basic and additional elements of informed consent in the regulation, other items are included.

The guideline's descriptions of the procedures also require that the probability for random assignment for each treatment be included in the discussion. Also, the guideline explicitly states that invasive procedures must be explained when they are part of the treatment. Furthermore, the guideline states that if there are anticipated prorated payments to the subject for participating in the trial, the subject should be informed via the consent form. This is somewhat of a departure from the US regulations, which do not require that this information be stated in the informed consent. However, the FDA Information Sheets state that payments should not be contingent on study completion, and that the proposed schedule should be evaluated by the IRB to determine that payments are reasonable and do not unduly influence a patient to remain in a trial. Since payments are perceived as a benefit, it is suggested that the outline of the payment schedule and the conditions determining the payments be outlined in the informed consent.

The guideline specifically states that an explanation of the subject's responsibilities must be discussed during the informed consent discussion and included in the consent form and any other written information.

Good clinical practice procedures dictate that the safety and welfare of clinical subjects is intrinsic to the clinical research process and is an integral responsibility of the clinical investigator, the IRB, and the sponsor; therefore the importance of a correctly documented informed consent and an adequately implemented consent procedure cannot be stressed enough. In addition to understanding these requirements, one should be equally mindful that there are situations that may deviate from the norm but require equal attention. This includes the necessity of resubmitting an informed consent and obtaining reapproval from an IRB when a consent has been significantly revised or altered, usually because of a protocol amendment. A full explanation of the revisions and any associated changes in the study procedures should be provided to each subject who signed the original consent form, and he or she must be required to resign a revised form before any changes in the research are performed. All revised forms must be submitted to the IRB for review and approval. If, during the course of a trial, an informed consent was signed by a legally authorized representative because a subject was incompetent or a minor, the consent should be readministered to obtain the signed and dated signature of the patient who regained competency or reached the age of majority, respectively.

Although the age of majority in most states is 18 years, approximately 10 states permit higher or lower consent ages. Also, some local and state laws permit consent at lower ages dependent on various circumstances, e.g., abortion, prevention, treatment, or diagnosis of a sexually transmitted disease (STD), pregnancy, and drug or alcohol abuse.

XII. ORAL CONSENT

A short form written consent document, stating that the elements of informed consent required by 21 CFR 50.25 have been presented orally to the subject or the subject's legally authorized representative, is included in the regulations. However, clinical investigators do not recognize oral consent as a practical or appropriate alternative to obtaining documented informed consent whenever possible. The following requirements are necessary when the use of a short form informed consent is implemented:

- A witness to the oral presentation must be present.
- The IRB must approve a written summary of what will be said to the subject or representative.
- The short form is to be signed by the subject or representative.
- The short form and summary will be signed by the witness.
- The person administering the consent will sign a copy of the summary.
- Copies of the short form and the summary will be given to the subject or representative.

Any research conducted in the United States must comply with the federal regulations regarding informed consent, despite the type of form or procedure used. It is important for those involved in patient safety and welfare issues to know that there are some state or local laws that may have additional requirements regarding informed consent procedures. The California Research Subjects Bill of Rights is an example of a state law that requires all research subjects to be provided with a document entitled "Experimental Subjects Bill of Rights" before they participate in a research trial.

XIII. EMERGENCY USE OF INVESTIGATIONAL DRUGS AND BIOLOGICS

The regulations include a provision for the emergency use of an investigational drug or biological when a human subject is (1) in a life-threatening situation in which no standard acceptable treatment is available and (2) there is not sufficient time to obtain IRB approval (21 CFR 56.102).

When a human subject does not meet the criteria stipulated in an existing study protocol or if an approved study protocol is not available, the manufacturer of the test article should be contacted to determine if the company will make the test article available for emergency use under the manufacturer's IND. If an emergency occurs before an IND submission and the manufacturer agrees to make the test article available, the FDA would have to authorize shipment.

The specific regulation (21 CFR 56.104) is actually an exemption from prior review and approval by the IRB; however, it can be used only when the specific conditions described in 21 CFR 56.102 are met, and it allows for only one emergency use of the investigational product. The investigator must file a report of its use within 5 days to comply with the exemption regulation. Also, some institutions require IRB notification before the emergency use. Finally, the manufacturer may require an emergency use approval letter or at least a written statement that the IRB has been informed of the emergency use and acknowledges that the requirements stipulated in the exemption regulation have been met. All subsequent uses of an unapproved test article are subject to usual IRB review and approval procedures.

XIV. INFORMED CONSENT DURING EMERGENCY USE

In an emergency use situation where an investigator has determined that there is not sufficient time to obtain informed consent from a subject or legally authorized representative, he or she is required to have the determination reviewed by a physician who is not participating in the clinical investigation and to obtain a written certification of the following informed consent requirements (21 CFR 50.23) before use:

- The subject is confronted by a life-threatening situation necessitating the use of the test article.
- Informed consent cannot be obtained because of an inability to communicate with the subject or obtain legally effective consent from the subject.
- Time is not sufficient to obtain consent from the subject's legal representative.
- No alternative method of approved or generally recognized therapy is available that provides an equal or greater likelihood of saving the subject's life.

Although it is optimal for both the investigator and a physician independent of the clinical trial to determine the necessity for emergency use of an investigational product prior to its use, if this is not possible, the investigator must have the determination of use reviewed, evaluated, and submitted to the IRB within 5 working days after use of the test article.

XV. HEALTH INSURANCE PORTABILITY
AND ACCOUNTABILITY ACT (HIPAA)

In 1996, the DHHS passed the Health Insurance Portability and Accountability Act (HIPAA) to facilitate the sharing of information while protecting patient confidentiality (medical records); subsequently, associated privacy regulations were issued in 2000 (Privacy Rule). Amendments to the Privacy

Rule were proposed on March 27, 2002, to address research-related situations, and become effective on April 14, 2003. In essence, the Privacy Rule is the governing law for the use and disclosure of individually identifiable protected health information (PHI) by "covered entities," defined as health care providers, health plans, or health clearing houses. HIPAA-compliant consents that include elements specified in federal regulations (45 CFR § 164.508) will have to be provided by "covered entities" that carry out the activities of health care payment, treatment, or operations (PTO). Clinical research–related uses and/or disclosures of PHI beyond PTO will require that a specifically defined authorization be obtained from a research subject. HIPAA-compliant authorizations will have to include the following core elements:

1. The authorization must be written in plain language.
2. It must contain meaningful description of the PHI, including whether the PHI is newly created, preexisting, or both.
3. It must identify the persons requesting the PHI and to whom the PHI will be disclosed.
4. It must give the date or event that will mark the end of the use of the disclosure.
5. It must acknowledge that the individual may revoke the authorization at any time.
6. It must state that used/disclosed PHI may no longer be HIPAA protected.
7. It must be signed and dated by the individual or by the authorized representative (and must state the relationship of the individual to the authorized representative).

The following additional elements may be required if the research is treatment based:

1. The statement that the subject may inspect or copy his or her information (with a stated, specific exception that postpones inspection or copying during a blinded period in a clinical trial until after the blind is broken).
2. A statement that the subject may refuse to sign the authorization without jeopardizing treatment (except research-related treatment in a clinical trial).
3. If applicable, a disclosure that the researcher will be remunerated, directly or indirectly.

Two logistical aspects of the Privacy Rule authorization should be noted. First, grandfather clauses will be implemented for research studies that began prior to the Privacy Rule's compliance date (April 14, 2003). Second, it should be noted that an IRB may approve a waiver of authorization if the use or disclosure of PHI would involve no more than minimal risk to subjects and if the IRB judges it impractical to conduct the research without the waiver and without access to the PHI.

XVI. ASSURING THAT REGULATORY OBLIGATIONS ARE ADEQUATELY IMPLEMENTED

The complexity of clinical research is evidenced by the associated regulatory and clinical documentation required before an IND is filed, throughout the clinical trial process, and, ultimately, during the preparation of an NDA filing. A sponsor must ensure that the studies supporting an NDA contain quality data that substantiates claims of safety and efficacy. This process is facilitated when a sponsor evaluates the acceptability of the regulatory obligations and responsibilities required by investigators and sponsors. Thus the penultimate concern regarding the safety and efficacy claims stated in a submission can be assessed. Although this chapter does not address the auditing and inspectional techniques used to identify potential deficiencies, it is important to understand why these regulations have been established, the type of deficiencies that are identified, and the impact of poorly implemented good clinical practices.

In 1986, the preamble to the IND rewrite stated that the detail of an inspection may be based on the knowledge that a sponsor has audited subject records. The preamble further reiterated that "FDA's policy to audit two or more critical studies will continue." These statements regarding the FDA's inspectional efforts, as well as the FDA Statement of Enforcement Policy (1990) and recent activities promulgated through the Office of Criminal Investigations, have encouraged sponsors of clinical trials to establish and implement quality assurance departments and programs. Internal clinical quality assurance departments have developed standardized procedures to provide objective, independent assessments of processes that will assure upper management that trials are being conducted according to good clinical practice procedures that include patient protection, safety, and welfare to produce accurate and reliable data. In addition, tools to identify and oversee corrective actions facilitate the speed and quality of submissions and provide opportunities for training in monitoring and the continuing improvement of standard operating procedures used in the oversight of clinical research. The ability to identify, correct, and prevent inadequacies that could result in disciplinary regulatory actions or, in the worst case, delay or prevent an approval, underscores the benefit of this proactive approach. Optimally, quality assurance personnel can facilitate the inspection process by helping to identify the appropriate staff in the functional area being inspected. Furthermore, a quality assurance presence can be helpful in advising functional personnel regarding study documents that are provided to the FDA, providing a scribe to generate minutes, facilitating daily debriefing meetings, and advising management of inspection findings and corrective actions. The importance of the IRB and IC regulations has also been highlighted by the FDA's recognition of the ICH Good Clinical Practice Guideline, which underscores these elements in the regulations.

XVII. AUDITS VS. INSPECTIONS

The focus of both audits and inspections is to review clinical research–related activities and associated documentation, to determine the adequacy of the conduct of the activities, and to determine the accuracy and reliability of the data reported. Historically, clinical research nomenclature commonly refers to audits as internally generated processes and inspections as official reviews by a government authority, e.g., the FDA. Both audits and/or inspections are actually assessments of the clinical research process and share the goal of identifying deficiencies for corrective action. The essential difference is that an audit initiated as an independent review by a company is often conducted proactively to identify and correct inadequate procedures and/or to verify the accuracy and reliability of data being collected for submission. Inspections are routinely conducted by regulatory authorities to protect the public safety and welfare, as well as to respond to potentially illegal or inappropriate research activities that have been exposed. Regulatory authorities can also impose punitive actions or pursue legal sanctions to promote the correction of inadequate or illegal clinical research activities.

Irrespective of whether audits are initiated by the IRB, a sponsor, or the FDA, a number of commonly identified deficiencies have been noted and are addressed below. It is important to note that investigational sites, sponsors, and IRBs are all subject to FDA-issued warning letters or repeat inspections to verify that deficiencies have been adequately corrected.

XVIII. COMMON AUDITING/INSPECTIONAL FINDINGS: IRBs

Clinical investigators routinely submit protocols and informed consent documents to IRBs to obtain an independent evaluation of the risk/benefit ratio of a study in order to meet their obligation to protect patients' safety and welfare. The Institutional Review Branch of the FDA's Division of Scientific Investigations conducts inspections of the IRBs that review and approve investigational studies for biologicals, drugs, medical devices, and food additives. Although the regulations specifically outline the IRB requirements and responsibilities in this review process, inspectional findings from routine surveillance, as well as directed inspections, have revealed seven commonly cited deficiencies that have resulted in regulatory or administrative actions:

1. A lack of sufficiently documented standard operating procedures describing an IRB's procedural responsibilities and activities.

2. Meeting minutes that do not fully detail actions taken or voting conducted at a meeting. Examples of insufficiently documented minutes may include inadequate reporting of voting on protocols or amendments to protocols, the basis for disapproving a protocol, or summaries of relevant discussions or issues.

3. Documentation that is not available to verify that a quorum was present at convened meetings to review proposed research and that a majority of those members present at the meeting approved the proposal.

4. Lack of documentation to verify that the IRB provided continuing review of research activities that it initially approved at intervals of no less than 1 year, but appropriate to the level of risk to the subject.

5. IRB membership lists or rosters that are not consistent with the elements required in 21 CFR 56 (see Sec. 4 of this chapter).

6. IRB records that do not adequately track or log research documents that have been submitted by the clinical investigator, including protocols, amendments, consent forms, Investigator Brochures, IND Safety Reports, advertisements, patient information sheets, and correspondence between the investigator and the IRB.

7. A lack of approval notifications, approval notifications that do not adequately identify the research document (or the version of the research document) that has been approved, and/or missing dates of approvals.

XIX. COMMON AUDITING/INSPECTIONAL FINDINGS: ICDs

Informed consent issues rank among the most commonly cited deficiencies reported by FDA inspectors. Findings can include deficiencies in the actual content of the informed consent as well as the actual informed consent administration process. Most frequently noted are the following inadequacies:

1. All the basic elements of the informed consent (according to 21 CFR 50.25) are not included.

2. The content of the informed consent is inadequate.
3. IRB approval of the consent or revised consent(s) has not been obtained.
4. The informed consent has not been properly administered to the subject of the clinical investigation or a legal guardian.

To limit inspectional findings related to informed consent deficiencies, auditor reviews of informed consents can be conducted proactively, i.e., before being submitted to IRBs for review and approval. Inadequacies regarding the lack of required content, the use of technical rather than lay language, readability above an eighth-grade level, and consents that are culturally and linguistically inappropriate for the anticipated population are examples of problem areas that are frequently overlooked. Also, it is important to ensure that subjects of clinical trials are provided with the most recent version of an IRB-approved informed consent. It is recommended that informed consents include the version number, date, and page number on the bottom of each page of the consent form that has been either signed or initialed and dated. In addition to a correctly signed and dated informed consent, it is often beneficial to provide patient information sheets or subject instruction sheets to clarify and/or reiterate the study procedures.

In conclusion, once the regulatory compliance issues regarding informed consent have been satisfied, it is essential to ascertain the subject's comprehension of the informed consent. Documentation of the administration and comprehension of the informed consent by the subject should be a routine component of the process.

REFERENCES

1. Advertising for Study Subjects, FDA Information Sheet, Rockville, MD: Public Health Service, Department of Health and Human Services, Food and Drug Administration, February 1989.
2. Clinical Investigator Information Sheets, Food and Drug Administration, 1989.
3. Code of Federal Regulations, Food and Drugs. Title 21, Part 50.
4. Code of Federal Regulations, Food and Drugs. Title 21, Part 56.
5. Code of Federal Regulations. Title 45, Part 46.
6. Declaration of Helsinki. Code of ethics on human experimentation. Helsinki, Finland, 1964; amended in 1975, 1983, 1989, 1996, 48th General Assembly.
7. IRB Information Sheets. Food and Drug Administration, 1989.
8. IRB and Clinical Investigator Information Sheets. Food and Drug Administration, 1995.
9. The National Commission for the Protection of Human Subjects of Biomedical

and Behavioral Research: The Belmont Report: Ethical Principles and Guidelines for the Protection of Human Subjects of Research. DHEW Publication No. (OS) 78-0012, Washington, 1978.

10. Institute of Medicine Committee on Assessing the System for Protecting Human Research Participants Report: Preserving Public Trust: Accreditation and Human Research Participant Protection Programs, 2001.

11. Standards for Privacy of Individually Identifiable Health Information. 45 CFR, Parts 160 and 164.

21
Quality Assurance

Earl W. Hulihan
META Solutions, Inc., Warren, New Jersey, U.S.A.

I. INTRODUCTION

The complexities involved in the new drug development (NDD) process have increased dramatically in the past 5 years. This has occurred mainly as the result of enhanced drug development techniques, significant regulatory initiatives (for example, the FDA's 21CFR§11, "Electronic Records, Electronic Signatures"), and efforts for global registration of products. Spurred also by the effort to maximize profits, this phenomenon has placed the quality process under increased and manifold stress. The quality assurance (QA) and quality control (QC) processes are placed in the forefront by any major drug development organization. The efforts of QA will be reviewed in this chapter.

Any review of the practices involved in defining and describing QA within the NDD process must begin by discussing the scope of QA activities.

For many large-scale pharmaceutical development organizations, QA exists throughout the complete life cycle of the drug development process. In the United States, the practice of QA is neither required nor defined by a regulatory standard within each of the drug development activities or stages for clinical research.

Although it is not required, the FDA acknowledges the QA department's importance and existence when it states "Identify all departments, functions, and key individuals responsible for areas sponsor activities such as protocol development, selection of investigators, statistical analysis, clinical supplies, monitoring, and quality assurance" and

> Clinical trial quality assurance units (QAUs) are not required by regulation. However, many sponsors have clinical QAUs that perform independent audits/data verifications to determine compliance with clinical trial SOPs and FDA regulations. QAUs should be independent of, and separate from, routine monitoring or quality control functions. Findings that are the product of a written program of QA will not be inspected without prior concurrence of the assigning DA headquarters unit. Refer to Compliance Policy Guide 7151.02 for additional guidane in this matter.*

The role of QA programs and their effect on influencing quality initiatives has also been acknowledged internatinally.[†] The assurance of quality is expected, however, by regulatory agencies for organizations that attempt to develop and market a new drug entity. In fact, drugs that use devices as the delivery system elevate the expectation for a regulatory base necessary for assurance activities, because in-process audits become a regulatory requirement.*

In the far broader scope of NDD and global submissions, global initiatives to introduce a more formal QA program to industry have been well received. As recently as 1996, the ICH[†] has included the activities of QA and QC as separate entities within its guideline for GCP.

Quality assurance associates will generally be using interviews, reviews, and audits[‡] as the mechanism to determine if the firm is compliant with regulations, current accepted practices (cGCP, cGLP, and cGMP activities), and internal procedures.

Internal written policies and procedures must be developed to define the scope of QA activities withinthe company. These policies and procedures should encompass those areas within the company that, after an assessment of risk, provide the most assurance that safety and integrity are designed into the drug development process.

Quality assurance should function in a reporting channel independent from the main operational development flow, yet a close working relationship with these same operations personnel should be a priority.

---

* Food and Drug Administration Compliance Program Guidance Manual, Program #7348.810, Part III.B.1.b(1) and Part III.B.4.d. February 21, 2001 Implementation date.
[†] "Optional Guideline for Good Clinical Practice Compliance and Quality Systems Auditing In Conformity with the Note for Guidance on GCP CPMP/ICH/135/95 (ICH GCP)" September 1998. ENGAGE: European Network of GCP Auditors and other GCP Experts.
[‡] Audit Definition (ANSI). To conduct an independent review and examination of system records and activities in order to test the adequacy and effectiveness of data security and data integrity procedures, to ensure compliance with established policy and operational procedures, and to recommend any necessary changes.

Internal QA procedures generally are sufficient in scope to utilize a thorough sampling process to determine internal operations' effectiveness in completing corporate objectives, policies, and procedures.

II. THE QUALITY ASSURANCE DEPARTMENT

The QA department will usually consist of a group of specialists, each having a high degree of knowledge and many years of experience in drug development. This background allows them to provide practical advice to the drug development departments with which they interact.

Auditors within the QA group usually possess very good cognitive skills, developed over many years within various aspects of the drug development process. They use their knowledgeand experience to provide assistance and practical applications and suggestions to departments and colleagues.

Other attributes typically observed with QA associates are refined communication skills, personal integrity, patience, and a penchant for detail.

The QA department may reside in a special pathway reporting directly to management. There may be a corporate oversight compliance group, as well as functional groups within each drug development pathway (Scenario 1). This pathway is the more common pathway experienced by drug development firms today.

Another scenario may exist in which there may be direct reporting within the research development pathway, yet with such a reporting relationship defined as outside of potential influence (Scenario 2).

In this scenario, key drug development operations are focused under one banner. Peer groups, with similar report structure and supervisors, administer responsibility for corrective and preventative actions. Indeed, in this age, a new corporate scenario (Scenario 3) has emerged. This scenario places the focus of responsibility within the team.

In this scenario, QA interacts with team members during the drug development process and reports observations to team members for their corrective and preventative action and documentation process.

The three scenarios are only a few of the designs utilized globally by drug development organizations. However QA may fit in the organization, the information supplied by the group can help to identify potential issue areas and compliance failures.

A. Operations Within the Quality Assurance Department

Most QA departments use a variety of methodologies to complete their objectives. These methods include discussions (group, individual), document and file reviews, direct examination of records, and indirect audits* (which correlate information from various sources to determine procedure compliance for a specific area).

Advance planning with development personnel can begin in many different ways. Typically, a project planning committee defines key stages in a new drug entity's life cycle. The committee will usually include the QA professional as a part of the team, which allows him or her to arrange a plan for monitoring the development life cycle from concept to submission.

A development strategy schedule will define those stages in the development of a new drug entity that require assurance of satisfactory completion. Two sources of information will fuel the decision for the new drug entity to advance satisfactorily to the point of NDA submission. One information pathway is focused on drug development typically called the clinical research department. Through the efforts of this department, case report information is transferred from the investigation site through the data management arm of the company and turned into cleaned, confirmed data for submission to the appropriate regulatory entity.

Traditionally, reviews and audits may be conducted in one of three ways:

Only by QA
Together with the operations department
With a third party

B. Effective Quality Assurance Can Influence Corporate Outcomes

Quality assurance activities can have a beneficial effect on corporate outcomes. Effective QA can save the firm money by discovering potential

---

* Direct and indirect audits. There are instances in which an indirect audit will prove of benefit within the organization. Examples of these may be the transition of information from another audit process or source such as drug accountability information from manufacturing's receipt of investigator returns with drug accountability logs and patient compliance information. Examples of direct audits include

Adverse event reporting
Operations area process
Management communications
Systems validation
Follow-up to an operations audit
Contractual responsibilities

problems early in the drug development process, allowing for early institution of corrective measures.

Quality assurance departments that demonstrate a history of effectiveness within the corporate culture and foster loyalty among their peers are usually known for fairness, constructive approach, cooperative attitude, and informative style.

In addition, QA can provide valuable assistance to associates by helping them understand their weaknesses in either knowledge or the implementation of regulations or corporate procedures. In some companies, a well-developed pathway from dissemination of information is present, to provide quick feedback to those audited.

Also, QA can assist management by assessing interdepartmental and intradepartmental inconsistencies. This can occur for example, by identifying associates who function inconsistently with other associates or those managers who expand procedures beyond corporate intent.

Periodically, colleagues will operate under different assumptions related to corporate policies and procedures. Quality assurance can provide valuable assistance to management, through immediate feedback, when differences occur in understanding and viewpoint.

Other QA activities that have proved effective in saving resources and costs include identifying protocol design and protocol implementation flaws; documentation deficiencies; deviations from procedures or regulations by the sponsor, monitor, investigator or contract firm; and providing gap analysis information to management on training deficiencies.

C. Quality Assurance Activities Within the Early Phase of Drug Development

Quality assurance activities actually begin early in the drug development process—in the analytical phase. United States requirements* are established as early as nonclinical laboratory studies. At this early phase, the audit program concentrates on in vivo and in vitro experiments, focusing on early

---

* Nonclinical Quality Assurance. Quality assurance unit means any person or organizational element, except the study director, designated by testing facility management to perform the duties relating to quality assurance of nonclinical laboratory studies. Nonclinical laboratory study means in vivo or in vitro experiments in which test articles are studied prospectively in test systems under laboratory conditions to determine their safety. The term does not include studies utilizing human subjects or clinical studies or field trials in animals. The term does not include basic exploratory studies carried out to determine whether a test article has any potential utility or to determine physical or chemical characteristics of a test article.

drug entities. These drug entities are tested under laboratory conditions to determine their potential safety risk. At this phase, human subjects (e.g., clinical studies) or field trials in animals are not involved.

Quality assurance efforts within this phase will focus on four types of studies conducted for safety evaluation: (1) safety studies on regulated products, (2) safety studies that encompass the full scope of laboratory operations, (3) studies that are significant to safety assessment, e.g., carcinogenicity, reproduction, chronic toxicity studies, and (4) studies that encompass operations for several species of animals.

At this phase of research development, QA efforts will consider adequacy of management reporting structures for delegation of responsibility (along with appropriate supervision and accountability) and assignment of qualified personnel. Additional areas reviewed by QA include study processes and conduct, documentation measures, QC mechanisms such as management oversight/monitoring and internal training requirements, adequacy of facilities, maintenance and calibration of equipment, and retention of regulatory-required sample procedures.

Additional efforts may be focused by QA for operations' compliance with cGLP regulations and monitoring for compliance with cGLP regulations where appropriate.

Non-GLP studies such as methods development, in vitro biochemical mechanisms, and other areas such as chemistry, pathology, microbiology, and food science studies for compliance with requirements may also be audited by QA. Further areas such as automated chemical data systems and analytical methods may also be audited.

D. Phase 1 Through Phase 3 Drug Development Activities and Quality Assurance

The QA programs focused during these phases contain many similar activities. These revolve around confirmation that appropriate regulatory requirements and corporate procedures are carried out by personnel associated with these activities.

Phase 1 through phase 3 areas in which QA reviews or provides audit activities may include the following (including categories generally reviewed):

1. Institutional Review Committee

Document review prior to study initiation
Investigator qualifications by a CV

Continuing review of investigation
Financial, coercion/undue influence
Membership
Written procedures

2. Investigator

Investigation products
Randomization procedures
Informed consent of trial subjects
Records and reports
Safety reporting
Trial termination or suspension
Qualifications
Agreements
Resources
Medical care of trial subjects
Communication with Institutional Review Committee (IRC)
Compliance with protocol

3. Sponsor

Quality controls
Medical expertise
Trial design
Trial management, data handling, records
Investigator selection
Allocation of responsibilities
Compensation to subjects
Notification to regulatory authorities
Confirmation of review by IRC
Information on investigation products
Manufacturing, packaging, labeling
Supply and handling of products
Record access
Safety information
Adverse drug reaction reporting
Monitoring
Noncompliance reporting
Clinical trial reports
Training and development

4. Data Management*

Procedures
Document design (e.g., CRF)
Document tracking
CRF correction
Data entry
Data coding
Quality control system
Computer system, software
Data reporting
Record keeping
Record retention
Training initiatives

5. Regulatory Submissions

Text consistency, grammar, spelling, headers, footers, pagination,
and spacing
Compare CRF data points with report
Protocol statements with report statements
Data validity and verification
Appropriate signatures

6. Compliance with Validation Requirements

System overview
Validation test environment including hardware, software
System security including passwords, network rights, functional
security, physical security, modem access, and virus
protection
Validation test environment including related documents, along
with standard operating procedures, user manuals, and system
development/maintenance and documentation
Validation assumptions, exclusions, and limitations
Responsibilities matrix
Validation data sets

---

* International Conference on Harmonization; Guideline on Data Elements for Transmission
of Individual Case Safety Reports. This document's efforts focus on quality control/quality
assurance endeavors to ensure accuracy and to promote validation in the handling of case safety
reports for both preapproval and postapproval periods. It covers both adverse drug reaction
and adverse event reports.

Acceptance criteria
Expected results
Execution of the validation plan
Resolution of errors
Documentation
Training records
Archives, storage, backup, and recovery procedures
Methodology and change control
Disaster, recovery, and contingency planing

7. Contract Vendors

Previous experience
Facilities
Affiliations
Qualifications of personnel
Services available
Offered procedures
Capability to complete project
Quality controls program
Quality assurance program
Review and approve contracts
Future compliance audits
Database management
Validation/verification needs
Contract laboratories
Procedures
Facilities/equipment
Personnel qualification
Training
Methodology

8. Contract Laboratories

QC program
QA program
Computer validation procedures
Results acceptance procedures
Documentation
Maintenance calibration
Record-keeping/retention
Computer system/software

Specimen handling/storage
Specimen analysis/reporting
Result reporting
Accreditation/licenses
Software system vendors/suppliers
Appropriate understanding of procedures

9. Contract Research Organizations

Organization
Staffing/resources
Experience
Controls/assurance
Standard operating procedures
Other items as identified above

III. SUMMARY

The QA function is responsible for assessing the localized accountability for performance by operations and assisting management in determining the impetus for training needs and measuring consistency among associates. By using audit results in trend analysis statistics, QA provides periodic management compliance review of observations from a procedural viewpoint, assists in determining the need to establish new SOP, the need to clarify existing SOPs, and the need for new or refresher training. Quality assurance also provides information to management on safety reporting compliance, ethical considerations, delegation of responsibilities, study medication compliance and procedural deficiencies, data problems, administrative documentation issues, and feedback on monitoring issues.

1.0   Definitions

1.46   Quality Assurance (QA). All those planned and systematic actions that are established to ensure that the trial is performed and the data are generated, documented (recorded), and reported in compliance with Good Clinical Practice (GCP) and the applicable regulatory requirement(s).

1.47   Quality Control (QC). The operational techniques and activities undertaken within the quality assurance system to verify that the requirements for quality of the trial-related activities have been fulfilled.

5.1   Quality Assurance and Quality Control

5.1.1   The sponsor is responsible for implementing and maintaining quality assurance and quality control systems with written SOPs to ensure that trials are conducted and data are generated, documented (recorded), and reported in compliance with the protocol, GCP, and the applicable regulatory requirement(s).

5.1.2   The sponsor is responsible for securing agreement from all involved parties to ensure direct access (see 1.21) to all trial related sites, source data/documents, and reports for the purpose of monitoring and auditing by the sponsor, and inspection by domestic and foreign regulatory authorities.

5.1.3   Quality control should be applied to each stage of data handling to ensure that all data are reliable and have been processed correctly.

5.1.4   Agreements, made by the sponsor with the investigator/institution and any other parties involved with the clinical trial, should be in writing, as part of the protocol or in a separate agreement.

5.19   Audit

If or when sponsors perform audits, as part of implementing quality assurance, they should consider:

5.19.1   *Purpose*

The purpose of a sponsor's audit, which is independent of and separate from routine monitoring or quality control functions, should be to evaluate trial conduct and compliance with the protocol, SOPs, GCP, and the applicable regulatory requirements.

5.19.2   *Selection and Qualification of Auditors*

(a)   The sponsor should appoint individuals, who are independent of the clinical trials/systems, to conduct audits.
(b)   The sponsor should ensure that the auditors are qualified by training and experience to conduct audits properly. An auditor's qualifications should be documented.

5.19.3 *Auditing Procedures*

(a)   The sponsor should ensure that the auditing of clinical trials/systems is conducted in accordance with the sponsor's written procedures on what to audit, how to audit, the frequency of audits, and the form and content of audit reports.

(b)   The sponsor's audit plan and procedures for a trial audit should be guided by the importance of the trial to submissions to regulatory authorities, the number of subjects in the trial, the type and complexity of the trial, the level of risks to the trial subjects, and any identified problem(s).

(c)   The observations and findings of the auditor(s) should be documented.

(d)   To preserve the independence and value of the audit function, the regulatory authority(ies) should not routinely request the audit reports. Regulatory authority(ies) may seek access to an audit report on a case by case basis when evidence of serious GCP noncompliance exists, or in the course of legal proceedings.

(e)   When required by applicable law or regulation, the sponsor should provide an audit certificate.

REFERENCES

1.   FDA Regulation 21 CFR Part 820—Quality system regulation. Source: 61 FR 52654, Oct. 7, 1996. Unless otherwise noted.
2.   The International Conference on Harmonization of Technical Requirements for Registration of Pharmaceuticals for Human Use.

22
Managing Clinical Trials

Andrea G. Procaccino
Johnson & Johnson Pharmaceutical Research & Development, LLC, Titusville, New Jersey, U.S.A.

I. OVERVIEW

What is a clinical trial? In its purest form, it is an activity designed to test a hypothesis and ultimately to reach a conclusion as to whether or not a drug/ biological or medical device product has any effect on the human body and the disease condition in which it is being tested. The goal is to demonstrate that the product will improve the subject's health or quality of life, have an advantage over the current treatment available for that disease or condition, and can be administered safely to the subject.

Clinical trials can be the most timely and costly part of new product development. They require thoughtful planning in trial design and careful consideration of the types of subjects to be enroled. Above all every evaluation must ensure the subjects' safety and well-being while participating in the trial. Therefore it is critical that all personnel involved in clinical trials understand the regulations and guidelines that govern the protection of human subjects while evaluating the efficacy of the products.

Timelines for product development are continually being shortened in an effort to get a compound on the market as quickly as possible. Current and future trends and industry paradigm shifts are changing the face of clinical trials so that the pharmaceutical industry can look forward to global approval of new and old pharmaceutical products.

At times, owing to insufficient preparation and management, the clinical trial falls by the wayside, creating delays in the timelines for market launches. This chapter will focus on the components of clinical trial management procedures from execution to closure.

II. REGULATIONS AND GUIDELINES

The conduct of clinical trials is regulated by the US government and regulatory authorities around the world. The US Code of Federal Regulations (CFRs) and the International Conference on Harmonization (ICH) Guidelines govern the conduct of clincal research using good clinical practices (GCPs) as the gold standards in the conduct of clinical trials. The US Food and Drug Administration (FDA) has the authority to ensure that the Code of Federal Regulations, containing GCPs, is adhered to by everyone involved in the conduct of clinical trials in the United States. Drug trials conducted outside of the US adhere to the ICH GCP Guidelines or the European Directives on Good Clinical Practices, depending in which country the clinical studies are conducted. Many countries also have their own local laws and regulations that govern clinical trials. A thorough understanding of these regulations and guidelines and how to apply them is vital in the process of conducting clinical trials. These regulations and guidelines detail the FDA's and the ICH's requirements that must be followed by the investigators, their staffs, sponsors, and monitors. Noncompliance to these regulations and guidelines can result in termination of clinical studies, penalties, and criminal prosecution. In the United States, the FDA imposes these regulations to protect consumers' safety from drugs, devices, foods, and cosmetics that are marketed in the US. The US Good Clinical Practice regulations can be found in 21 CFR Parts 11 (Electronic Records/Signatures), 50 (Protection of Human Subjects), 54 (Financial Disclosure), 56 (Institutional Review Boards), 312 (Investigational New Drug Process), 314 (Application for FDA Approval to Market a New Drug), 812 (Medical Devices). There are also additional regulations in the US that address federally funded studies, and they can be found in 45 CFR Part 46. Internationally, there are the ICH Guidelines on Good Clinical Practices, which are found in Section E6. These regulations and guidelines are readily available on both the FDA and the ICH websites.

III. CLINICAL TRIAL MANAGEMENT

There are key elements in managing clinical programs. Among them are investigator selection, preinvestigational site visits (PISV), study initiation visits (SIV), trial conduct and execution, legal aspects, periodic monitoring visits, product accountability, AE and ADR reporting, financial disclosure, study close-out visits (SCV), and final recommendations to the investigator on records retention and inspections. These important components of managing clinical investigations are detailed in this chapter with respect to their importance and practical application in completing clinical research trials successfully.

IV. INVESTIGATOR SELECTION

US GCP Federal Regulations and ICH GCP Guidelines mandate that a sponsor select only investigators qualified by training and experience as appropriate experts to evaluate an investigational product (21 CFR 312.53). A similar reference appears in the ICH GCP Guidelines as well (4.1).

As investigator selection is a critical step in conducting clinical trials, the following recommendations to identify potential investigators are the most frequently used:

Experience with investigators who conducted other studies for the sponsor's literature searches in the therapeutic area or disease state under study. These searches can be done in key medical publications (e.g., the Journal of American Medical Association, the New England Journal of Medicine) or via general searches on the world-wide web.

Medical or scientific meetings such as those of the American Psychiatric Association of the Gastrointestinal Society Annual Meetings, for example.

Clinical research professional organization directories such as those of the Association of Clinical Research Professionals (ACRP), the Drug Information Association (DIA), the Regulatory Affairs Professional Society (RAPS).

Referrals from other investigators with whom a sponsor company is already working on a particular product

Disease foundations (e.g., the American Cancer Society, the Lymphoma Research Foundation).

Site Management Organization—these are organizations that act as brokerages for investigators for certain therapeutic areas and often have a large geographic selection of investigators available.

It is important to remember, in the investigator selection process, that the sponsor company is entrusting this individual to research their investigational product that will result in quality, reproducible trial data. Most importantly, this individual will be managing the study subjects' safety and medical care during the trial and must have the proper credentials and specialty experience to do so. Other items to consider carefully during the selection process are:

Experience in clinical research and human clinical trials of the disease under study (for example, a gynecologist would not be appropriate for a study of a product for brain cancer).

Location of the site: is it in an area that is easily accessible to subjects? Is it in a center of excelence for the therapeutic indication under study?

Does this investigator have the appropriate subject population available to them to be able to recruit study subjects for the trial in a timely fashion? (A heterogeneous subject population is always more desired.)

Is the budget proposal from this investigator appropriate or is it cost-prohibitive? Does the institution require an overhead cost that is beyond budgetary restrictions?

Has the investigator been previously inspected by the US FDA or another regulatory authority and if so, what was the outcome of that inspection?

N.B. The FDA may disqualify an investigator from receiving investigational drugs, biologicals, or devices if the FDA determines that the investigator has repeatedly or deliberately failed to comply with regulatory requirements for conducting clinical studies or has submitted false information to the study sponsor. Investigators may also agree to certain restrictions on their conduct of future studies. The FDA publishes the list of those investigators that have at one time been disqualified, restricted, have made assurances in their use of investigational products, or have been prosecuted or had a criminal conviction. Where an investigator has been reinstated or restrictions have expired, this too is also noted on the list. The list can be found on the FDA website at: http://www.fda.gov/ora/compliance_ref/debar/debar.txt. The sponsor should check this list to make sure that the investigator is not on it, before they are selected to participate in a clinical program. Many sponsor companies have standard operating procedures (SOPs) that require that they not use any investigator who has ever appeared on this list. It is also prudent not to use investigators who have been reinstated from this list by the FDA. Industry often refers to this list as the FDA blacklist.

Can they complete the trial in the given time frame?

What methods will they have to employ to recruit subjects? Will they require extra assistance to recruit subjects?

Does the investigator have the appropriate staff available to assist with the conduct of the trial? Does the staff have the appropriate education and experience to conduct the trial?

Is there a study coordinator?

Have the investigators ever worked with the sponsor company in the past and if so, how was their conduct during the course of the trial?

Do the investigators have any other current research commitments that would compete with the trial you are trying to place at their site?

These questions are posed to potential investigators to examine the feasibility of their participation in the clinical program.

Once a potential investigator has been identified, the sponsor company will continue to be in contact with the investigator and the site to make additional assessments of their continued interest and capabilities to participate in the clinical program. This responsibility is assigned to personnel within sponsor companies that carry many different titles. Site managers (SMs), medical research associates (MRAs), clinical research associates (CRAs), and clinical research monitors (CRMs) are among the names used. For the purpose of this chapter, personnel with these responsibilities will be called monitors.

The monitor is an individual appointed by the sponsor who is familiar with the investigational product and the protocol developed for the clinical program and is responsible for coordinating, initiating, and overseeing the conduct of the clinical trial. Monitors ensure adherence to the protocol and regulatory requirements and act as liaisons between the investigators and their staffs and the sponsor company. It is important that monitors have the scientific and medical knowledge needed to oversee the clinical research program. They must understand the condition under evaluation and assure that all data recorded are entered correctly and reflected in the medical/hospital records. In addition, they should also have exceptional interpersonal skills.

> The sponsor may contract the monitoring or the entire execution of the trial out to a contract research organization (CRO). A CRO is defined as a person or an organization (commercial, academic, or other) contracted by the sponsor to perform one or more of the sponsor's trial-related duties and functions (ICH 1.20). Although the CRO assumes the sponsor's obligations, the sponsor is still ultimately responsible for the clinical trial (21 CFR 312.52 (b); ICH 5.2).

After an investigator and a site have been selected to participate in the clinical program, preliminary documentation is sent to the investigator. This includes:

A confidentiality statement or agreement
A copy of the protocol and case report form
A sample informed consent form
A contract with budget information

Once the investigator's site has had the opportunity to review these materials, the monitor will contact the site by phone to answer any questions and schedule a pre-investigational site visit.

V. PREINVESTIGATIONAL SITE VISIT (PISV)

After prescreening of potential investigators is established, it is vitally important that a PISV be conducted at the investigational site with the investigator and their staff to continue to assess their ability to conduct the trial.

The PISV is usually performed by the monitor or an authorized individual appointed by the sponsor company.

The sponsor representative(s) will have a face-to-face meeting with the principal investigator (PI) and their staff to ensure that they clearly and fully understand and accept their obligations in conducting clinical trials. Each person's qualifications will be reviewed and their curricula vitae (CVs) and medical licenses will be confirmed.

Among the staff members it is essential that an investigator appoint a study coordinator (sometimes referred to as the research nurse, clinical research coordinator, (CRC), or study nurse) who plays a key role in the execution of the clinical trial as a direct support to the principal investigator. Therefore careful consideration should be given to their qualifications and research experience.

If an investigator does not have a study coordinator, it is recommended that they should not be selected to participate in the clinical research program, or the monitor should suggest that they hire/train one immediately.

The study coordinator will have continuous interaction with the investigator and monitor during the trial. At the PISV the monitor will also assess the qualifications of any subinvestigators or other physicians who will be evaluating the subjects. It should be stressed that subinvestigators will have the same regulatory responsibilities as the PI; but the principal investigators must assure that they will oversee the entire clinical investigation including the involvement of the subinvestigators.

During the PISV the facility should be toured to ensure that all of the necessary equipment is available to fulfill the required study procedures and that the same examination rooms are available throughout the study to evaluate the study subjects. The equipment being used for the trial should be state of the art. The facilities should be clean and orderly, and storage for investigational product must be established. The storage area should be in a secure and locked area or cabinet with access granted only to that personnel assigned by the investigator. (The investigational products have not been approved by a regulatory authority for general market use. Therefore tight control over their availability and distribution must be adequately maintained.) Over-the-counter medications that may also be required for use in a clinical trial should also be stored under the same conditions. If the investigator does not have a storage facility to house investigational products one can be purchased by the sponsor company.

It is critical that the investigator understands their regulatory obligations and agrees to conduct the study accordingly. The FDA requires that each investigator sign a Statement of Investigator or FDA Form 1572 document. This lists the investigator's obligations during the trial. Any investigator conducting an investigational drug trial under a US Investigational New Drug Application (IND) must complete Form 1572. This form is not required by countries outside the US, but if the sponsor plans to submit the data from a foreign clinical trial in support of a product for US marketing, this document should be signed by the principal investigator from that country. Presently, this form is not required for medical device trials or for trials outside of the US that will not be filed in a US IND application. This federal regulatory document is a binding contract between the investigator and the FDA. Failure to comply with any of the obligations listed on this document could result in a citation on an FDA inspection report, a warning letter, or regulatory action by the FDA. Monitors should emphasize the seriousness of violating the requirements on a 1572 form to all who participate in a clinical program. By signing this document the investigator commits to the following obligations required by the US Code of Federal Regulations in 21 CFR Part 312:

Personally conducting or supervising the investigation
Obtaining informed consent
Reporting adverse experiences to the sponsor within the specified time
Reading and understanding the Investigator Brochure
Ensuring that the study staff is informed of their obligations in meeting these requirements
Maintaining adequate and accurate study records
Ensuring that the Institutional Review Board (IRB) complies with requirements
Agreeing to comply with all other requirements regarding the obligations of clinical investigators

The document also contains general information: the title of clinical trial, the names of the investigator and subinvestigators, the laboratory to be used for the trial, and the responsible IRB.

Since many trials are being conducted around the world and submitted to a US IND application, the FDA is working on a separate type of 1572 form to be used for these sites. The reason for this is that an ethical committee (EC), (the international version of our IRB), reviewing the research protocols and informed consents, is composed slightly differently from IRBs in the US. Independent ethical committees (IECs) follow ICH GCP guidelines, which differ slightly from CFR regulations.

The Investigator Brochure (IB) and the clinical protocol are reviewed at the PISV. The IB is a compilation of all of the nonclinical, preclinical, and clinical data collected to date on the investigational product. The investigator must review and understand this document in detail, because it provides information on pharmacology, toxicology, and other pertinent data confirming that the starting dosage to be administered to the subjects is reasonably safe. The protocol is reviewed and discussed in detail with the investigators and their staff during this visit. The protocol's objective, inclusion/exclusion criteria, study visit procedures, drug accountability requirements, adverse experience reporting procedures, and all logistical procedures are presented. Any questions that arise should be clarified.

At the completion of the PISV, the monitor will complete a written PISV report. This report will document any observations or findings from this visit as well as any agreements reached with the investigator and/or staff. All information gathered from this visit will be reviewed by the sponsor and based on the PISV, and a decision is made to include or exclude this investigator. A follow-up letter will be sent to the investigators informing them of this decision. When the investigator has been selected they will be required to submit the following documents to the sponsor:

> Signed Protocol page - it must be signed and dated by the principal investigator to document their agreement to conduct the trial as per the protocol.
>
> Signed and completed FDA Form 1572, Statement of Investigator (if the trial is to be filed in support of a US IND).
>
> Curricula vitae or CVs of the principal investigator and any subinvestigators listed on the FDA Form 1572. Some sponsors even request that a CV be submitted for the study coordinators, although this is not required by regulation.
>
> A signed and dated Clinical Trial Agreement or study contract between the investigator and the sponsor detailing any financial remuneration to be paid to the investigators for their participation in the trial; the study contract should include an indemnification clause that indemnifies the investigator and the institution against claims arising from the trial (not including claims that may arise from malpractice and/or negligence by the investigator or institution).
>
> IRB/IEC approval letter; this letter must clearly state that the protocol, informed consent, and any advertisement materials to be used for recruitment were reviewed and approved by the IRB/IEC. (This may take time, as these committees do not meet on a regular basis.)
>
> List of IRB/IEC members and their qualifications or, in the US, an IRB Assurance number to ensure that the IRB was properly constituted as per the requirements.
>
> Laboratory license or certification, laboratory normal values, and a CV for the laboratory director for each laboratory to be used in the trial. If a central laboratory is used, these documents will be obtained directly from the central laboratory by the sponsor, and copies will be sent to the investigator site for their files.

VI. INVESTIGATOR'S MEETINGS

When the sponsor company has selected all of the investigators and the investigative sites to participate in a clinical trial, they usually will hold an investigators' meeting. Representatives from each site (usually the principal investigator and study coordinator) will attend the meeting along with representatives from the sponsor's clinical team and from the regulatory affairs, data management, and quality assurance departments. If a central laboratory is being used for the trial, representatives from the laboratory will also participate. Investigators' meetings can be conducted in two ways. One type is a preparatory or peer group meeting, where the protocol is reviewed for comments by the investigators prior to being finalized. The second type is the more common and standard version, where the protocol has already been finalized; this meeting is a training session for the participants. A complete understanding of the protocol and how to conduct the clinical trial are usually the main objectives of this meeting. This is an excellent opportunity for the investigators and their staffs to ask questions about the trial and trial conduct. The following topics are typically addressed during an investigators' meeting:

Review of preclinical/clinical findings on the product
Protocol review
Case Report Form review and completion
Laboratory procedures for collecting specimens and how properly to ship them
Review of good clinical practices and investigator and staff obligations
Drug dispensation and accountability procedures
AE and ADR reporting
Recruitment techniques
Record retention

Attendance should be carefully monitored throughout the duration of the meeting to ensure that investigators and staff personnel are present. The CFR regulations and ICH GCP Guidelines require that the sponsor company train the investigator's staff on the protocol and protocol requirements. N.B. Investigators should pursue in-depth training on good clinical practices. Many clinical research professional organizations offer such training programs on GCPs for clinical investigators, CRAs, and clinical research coordinators. Some even offer certification programs. This is one of the new paradigm shifts in the clinical research arena. Sponsor companies are now being held responsible by regulatory authorities for investigator training in GCP obligations and the ethical conduct of clinical trials.

VII. STUDY INITIATION VISIT (SIV)

Once the PISV is complete, an SIV is the next step. (Some sponsor companies will combine the PISV and SIV into one visit to compress the time lines and to be more cost-effective. This occurs especially when the investigator has worked previously with the sponsor on past trials.) The monitor will schedule the SIV with the investigator and study coordinator via telephone or e-mail and send a follow-up letter confirming the date and time of the visit. All study staff personnel participating in the study should attend this important meeting. The investigator and their staff must be present for the entire meeting. Prior to this meeting, the monitor will also arrange for the initial shipment of the investigational product to be sent to the site along with any additional ancillary supplies that are required (e.g., syringes, alcohol swabs, Sharps containers for disposal). The site should await the monitor's review of the shipment at the SIV prior to logging the product in and storing it. The monitor will review the product and its storage at the initiation visit. The monitor will also send the Investigator Trial binder with copies of the documentation received to date in it. This binder will act as the central storage and filing of all required regulatory documents for the duration of the trial.

The initiation visit is also a training meeting. This is the last training on the protocol that the investigators and their staffs will have before beginning to recruit and enroll subjects into the trial. During this meeting, the monitor will review the following in detail:

Protocol—rationale, study design, inclusion/exclusion criteria, visit schedule and study procedures required at each visit, diagnostic tests and procedures, concomitant medications, publication requirements.

Adverse experience and serious adverse experience reporting–documentation, reports, whom to notify of serious adverse experiences and within what time frame and reporting requirements to the IRB/IEC.

The obligation of the investigator and the sponsor to report AEs and ADRs to the FDA or other applicable regulatory authorities in a required timely fashion is mandatory. (See Chap. on adverse experiences, adverse reactions, and interactions of drugs).

Product dispensation and accountability–The principal investigators are responsible for product accountability. They may delegate this responsibility to another qualified individual, e.g., pharmacist or study coordinator, but the investigator is accountable for prescribing the investigational product for the study subjects, and for assuring that dispensing and storage records account for all investigational products. The monitor is responsible for reviewing the documentation for product accountability prior, during, and at study closure.

Case Report Form (CRF) completion–The CRF is the data collection tool for the trial. The monitor will review in detail how to complete each evaluation on the case report form. Monitors should demonstrate proper correction procedures to ensure that data is not obliterated, that white-out is not used, and that the medical abbreviations are acceptable. For example, when an error occurs, the person completing the CRF will put a line through the incorrect information, record the correct information next to it, and initial and date the new entry. (It must be emphasized that the same person who entered the original data be the one to enter, sign, and date any corrections). The sponsor company may also create CRF Completion Guidelines to give to the site, which detail page by page how each data field should be completed. For a multi-center trial, this helps to ensure consistency in data collection and reporting.

Review of regulatory documents–The monitor will review what type of documentation should be collected during the trial and how and where to store it. These documents can be stored in a centrally located binder supplied by the sponsor or in a file drawer. Company-specific documents are also filed with the trial documents. Examples of company-specific documents are a monitoring or screening log. The monitoring log is used by the monitor to sign in at each monitoring visit, including the initiation and closeout visits. This tracks how and when the sponsor company monitored the trial. Upon an inspection by a regulatory authority, there is evidence that the sponsor met their obligations and that the sponsor monitored the progress of the clinical trial (21CFR Part 312.56 (a); ICH 5.18.2). The screening log keeps track of all the subjects that are screened for the trial, identifying them only by a screening number and their initials. Any other correspondence received by the investigator from the sponsor company, and all correspondence to/from the investigator and IRB/ IEC, should be maintained in this binder.

Source documentation–source data, as defined in the ICH Guidelines 1.51, is all the information in original office or hospital records, and certified copies of original records of clinical findings, observations, and other activities in a clinical trial necessary for the reconstruction and evaluation of the trial. Original data is contained in source documents. Source documents are composed of hospital records, office charts, laboratory data sheets, subject diaries, pharmacy dispensing records, recorded data from automated instruments, x-rays, etc. Source documents should be legible and should document that the subject is participating in a clinical trial. Some of the key areas to cross reference source documents to case report forms and regulatory criteria are the informed consent process, inclusion/exclusion criteria, adverse experiences, investigational product administration, concomitant medications administered to the subject during the trial, withdrawal from the study for any reason, and subjects lost to follow-up.

The investigator is responsible for the accuracy and completeness of then trial records and any discrepancies found in these records during an audit (ICH 4.9.1). The monitor will review the source documents for accuracy and completeness against the CRFs at each monitoring visit and will provide feedback on their acceptability to the investigators and their staff. Once the initiation visit has occurred, the study site is considered officially started and subject recruitment can begin.

VIII. PERIODIC MONITORING OF A CLINICAL TRIAL

Both the CFR and the ICH GCP guidelines require that the sponsor monitor the progress of the clinical trial at the site where the trial is being conducted. How frequently these monitoring visits should occur is not specified in the regulations and guidelines. It is up to the sponsor to make the determination of what that frequency should be. Most companies will have SOPs for monitoring that require periodic visits to occur every four to six weeks and will verify 100% of all data fields against the source documentation. This is not required under regulations or guidelines. The overall purpose of these periodic monitoring visits by the sponsor's monitor is to assure that the investigators and their staffs follow GCP regulations and guidelines and adhere to the protocol to assure that the rights of the subjects participating in the clinical trial are being protected and that the data reported is complete, accurate, and verifiable. Therefore it is extremely important to schedule monitoring visits based on the objective of the trial, the rate of enrollment, and the quality of data emanating from the investigational site. The first monitoring visit should occur upon the enrollment of the first few subjects into the trial, and subsequent monitoring visits are then scheduled on a regular basis according to the SOPs of the sponsor. During these visits the monitor must meet with the investigator to review any issues that need clarification or explanation and to entertain any questions that may arise on the general progress of the trial. The study coordinator must also readily be available during these visits to assist the monitors by retrieving source documents as needed, making any necessary corrections to the CRFs that come under their jurisdiction, and provide any needed regulatory documents. The site must ensure that it has a suitable area available to the monitor as a workspace during their visit and that the CRFs and their supporting source documents are readily available for review. After each monitoring visit, the monitor will complete a detailed monitoring visit report for internal use within the sponsor company. This report should contain information on whom the monitor met during the visit, any issues noted and the resolutions that were discussed, and any corrections made by the investigator or research coordinator or any other staff person.

The monitor is the main line of communication between the sponsor and the investigator. The following checklist can be used as a guide to underline the main responsibilities of the monitor at each site visit:

Ensure that the investigator is using their qualifications and resources to conduct the trial.

Ensure that the investigational product is stored, dispensed, returned, and disposed of properly.

Ensure that the investigator is adhering to the protocol and amendments.

Ensure that the appropriate CFR/ICH laws, regulations, and guidelines are being followed.

Confirm that all the subjects screened have signed an informed consent prior to undergoing any study related procedures.

Verify that only eligible subjects were enrolled in the clinical trial.

Ensure that the data on the CRFs are reflected in the source documents and is accurate and complete.

Review all adverse experiences and serious adverse reactions for each subject and ensure that the investigator reported them to the sponsor and the IRB/IEC appropriately.

Review the regulatory documents and check that they are being maintained at the site.

Perform product accountability, and ensure that the storage of the product is maintained, and that the amount of drug/device shipped to the sites, dispensed to the subjects, returned to the site, and disposed of are all accountable.

IX. TRIAL CONDUCT/EXECUTION

There are several other key components to trial execution that will require special attention: subject recruitment, the informed consent, IRBs/IEC review product accountability, adverse experience and adverse reaction reporting, financial disclosure, and record retention. Each is critical in the overall success of a clinical trial. If one of these is not handled or processed appropriately, the clinical trial will not be used in support of a new product application. Many of these components have been discussed previously in the context of monitoring. Adverse experience and adverse reaction reporting, informed consent, and IRB/IEC are detailed in Chaps. 11 and 20. The remaining key components relative to managing clinical trials will now be addressed.

X. SUBJECT RECRUITMENT

One of the surest ways to decrease the overall time to complete a clinical trial is to recruit subjects into the trial in the shortest amount of time. However, the demand for these subjects meeting protocol criteria can be very challenging, especially when there are competing trials at a given site. Regulatory agencies are also taking a closer look at how a site recruits and enrolls subjects. Questions arise such as Is the site coercing the subjects into entering a trial? Is the site influencing them inappropriately with money or gifts? The secret to effective subject recruitment is planning on how and where to recruit a subject population. The earlier in the trial process that a site or sponsor company does this, the more successful is the outcome. Sponsor companies and sites sometimes wait until a clinical trial is ready to begin before they address recruitment. In doing so, they find themselves in a "rescue mode." Rescue mode is a term used when one waits until the last minute to address a lagging recruitment rate with hopes to resolve it by allocating large budgets as an effort to rescue the recruitment.) In planning for recruitment, you must know and understand the subject population that will meet the protocol criteria. What motivates these subjects to participate in the clinical trial? What kind of medical treatment are they presently receiving, and who are they seeing to get this treatment? What is the present status of their medical condition?

Subjects' confidence with investigators and their staffs will greatly aid in recruiting them for the trial. For example, cancer subjects are highly motivated to receive promising therapies because of the seriousness of their condition and their enthusiasm for new therapies. They educate themselves very quickly about their disease via the internet and various disease foundations for information. On the other hand, migraine subjects act very differently and are more apt to have discussions with their physicians about other experimental treatments. These factors should be considered in the overall time for subject recruitment. Other considerations are the resources needed to complete the recruitment, i.e., money, time, people.

Once a strategy is created for subject recruitment and the trial has begun, the site must periodically review its success in recruiting subjects. If it is not working as planned, the reasons should be examined as to why the plan is not working, and alternative methods should be discussed and implemented. The old paradigm in clinical research was to plan lavish advertising campaigns that included newspaper, radio, and television ads. These methods are no longer very effective or efficient. The new paradigm is psychographics: the study of how subjects behave, where they shop, what they do, how they deal with their conditions emotionally, and so on. Sponsors now are testing the feasibility of subject recruitment before a clinical trial begins. Asking this question, in the protocol development stage, can save both the company and the site from expending precious time and resources in seeking subjects that will never meet protocol criteria. Future studies will experience even another paradigm shift as genomics will play an important role in how subjects are recruited.

XI. PRODUCT ACCOUNTABILITY

Clinical trials evaluate new investigational drug/devices which have not yet received marketing authorization from the appropriate health care authority. Therefore it is mandatory that strict control be maintained on any investigational product. The investigator is responsible for the accountability of the test product. Investigational products should only be prescribed by the investigator or authorized subinvestigators. The sponsor is responsible for retrieving/verifying the disposition of all used and unused product. Detailed records of product accountability must be maintained throughout a trial with information on the date dispensed, the quantity dispensed, the subject identifier (subject number), and the batch number of product prescribed.

When a health care authority inspects the site's product accountability records, every detail will be examined, i.e., dispensing, unused, and final disposition of product. Auditors will examine the product accountability procedure and evaluate its acceptability. At the end of the trial, the monitor will ensure the accountability of all investigational product. Any discrepancies will be investigated and documented accordingly in the source document data, the product accountability records, and/or in the monitoring visit report.

XII. FINANCIAL DISCLOSURE

One of the newest components of a clinical trial is financial disclosure. This regulation initiated in the United States on February 2, 1999, is required on all current or ongoing clinical trials filed in an IND. It is not retroactive to studies completed prior to this date. Financial disclosure is defined by the FDA as compensation related to the outcome of the study, proprietary interest in the product (e.g., patent), significant equity interest in the sponsor of the study, significant payments of other sorts to the investigator or institution (e.g., equipment, honorariums). The reason for this regulation is to assure the FDA that appropriate steps were taken to minimize bias in the design, conduct, reporting, and analysis of the studies even when the investigator has a financial interest in a new product. The investigator's responsibilities with respect to financial disclosure are to provide the sponsor company with sufficient and accurate information to allow for disclosure or certification to the FDA of no or any financial interest with the investigational product or with the sponsor. Therefore the sponsor company will collect the required financial disclosure information from the investigator. This information is required at the start of the study and one year after completion of the trials. Some sponsor companies may even request it at study completion. Anytime this information changes the investigator should send updated information to the sponsor company. The FDA will evaluate the financial disclosure information for each trial to determine its impact on the reliability of the trial data. Financial disclosure does not prohibit investigators from participating in clinical programs.

The FDA will consider both the size and the nature of the financial information disclosed, as well as what steps were taken during the conduct of the trial to minimize potential bias. The FDA will also look at the design of the trial as well as the number of centers that participated in the trial and at what percentage of the overall subject population was enrolled at that site where financial disclosure was revealed. If the FDA feels that there is a question about the integrity of the data or with the information disclosed, they can initiate agency audits for the investigator whose data is in question, request that the sponsor company submit further analyses of the data, request that the sponsor company conduct additional studies to confirm the study results, or refuse to treat that study as providing data that can be supportive for the agency's action to approve a compound and hence throw out that data. If the sponsor company refuses to reveal this information, the FDA can refuse to file its New Drug Application (NDA).

Closely related to financial disclosure is conflict of interest. Individuals involved in clinical research have the responsibility to maintain objectivity in research. Investigators and their staff must take precautions to prevent employees, consultants, or members of governing bodies from using their positions for purposes that are or give the appearance of being motivated by the prospect of financial gain. This is an area of growing concern and one the industry will most definitely be hearing more about in the future. Examples of conflict of interest would be a situation where a chairman of a department at a university acts as principal investigator on many studies and then appoints every faculty member on his staff to the IRB/IEC to review their studies. Another example would be if an FDA advisory panel had a consumer representative reviewing a product application and that same person happens to serve in an advisory capacity for a sponsor company submitting the new product application. As a result of the heightened concern with conflict of interest, there have been very controversial proposals discussed in editorials in industry publications, proposals such as blocking investigators from participating in clinical programs who have financial links to sponsors, having independent experts who have no financial investments in a product design protocols, execute the trials, and analyze the data. Another proposal stated that researchers should be required to inform potential study subjects of any financial conflicts of interest before they consider participating in a clinical trial. These debates are among many that have arisen in the past few years about conflicts of interest and are a growing concern in the new product development industry.

XIII. RECORD RETENTION

Record retention is critical to the ongoing viability of the study data. The FDA or other health care authorities may conduct an on-site inspection to verify the data from a given site at some time after submission of the New Drug Application (NDA). This information must be readily available at the site. Both the CFR and the ICH require that the records be retained for two years after the date of a marketing application is approved. If no application is filed or the file is rejected, the records must be retained for two years after the investigation is discontinued or withdrawn and the FDA or regulatory authority is notified. Records can be maintained as paper files, microfilm or microfiche, or as scanned documents in an electronic or web-based document management system. If the investigator should move during the retention period, records can be transferred and can be the responsibility of another person as long as the sponsor company is notified in writing and the new person is aware of their responsibilities in retaining these records.

XIV. STUDY CLOSURE VISITS (SCVs)

Once a trial is completed at an investigational site, the study must be appropriately closed. This cannot occur until all of the subjects have completed the course of the trial, or were dropped or withdrawn, and all data queries and issues have been addressed and resolved in the final evaluations. Only when this is done can the monitor proceed to a close-out visit. The following checklist will guide the monitor in completing the SCV:

All subjects entered in the trial have been accounted for.

All CRF pages have been completed and retrieved.

All data queries have been resolved.

All AEs and ADRs have been reported and followed up.

All investigational product has been accounted for and disposed of or returned to the sponsor.

All remaining supplies (CRFs, ancillary supplies) are returned or disposed of properly.

Regulatory records are complete and organized in the Trial Binder.

All outstanding issues are addressed. The monitor will meet with the investigator to conclude any outstanding issues and to review the IRB/IEC notification of study closure, i.e., filing of a study closure notification letter to the IRB/IEC (copy in regulatory file and copy sent to sponsor).

Review record retention requirements for investigator and staff (for all study-related records).

Review of the sponsor's publication policy.

XV. SUMMARY

Managing clinical trials requires a great deal of patience and integrity and tedious hours of attention. However, knowing that one has contributed in some small way to the improvement of a life or the treatment of a disease or condition can be very gratifying. With this comes an overwhelming responsibility to abide by and instill the rules and regulations and guidelines to assure the protection of subjects' safety. Everyone involved in clinical trials plays a key role in the product development process. They must take that role seriously and be educated on the regulations and guidelines designed to evaluate products safely and effectively for US and global submissions. New product development contributes not only to science and medicine but to the improvement of the overall health of the world population.

23

The European Union Directive on Good Clinical Practice in Clinical Trials: Implications for Future Research

Kent Hill
Biopharma Consulting Ltd., Colwyn Bay, United Kingdom

I. BACKGROUND

Since finalization in 1996, the International Committee on Harmonisation Tripartite Guideline for Good Clinical Practice (ICH GCP) underpinned by the ethical principles of the Declaration of Helsinki have been the cornerstones upon which most clinical research has been conducted outside the United States (1,2). However, in such a widely disparate and expanding territory as Europe (EU), the national differences in complying with local national requirements have presented a highly resource-hungry administrative workload for sponsors.

Multi-center clinical trials (CT) in EU countries known as 'Member States' (MS) currently present a formidable challenge to sponsors wishing to conduct a research study to the same protocol. The submission process to EU legally responsible governmental regulatory agencies known as 'competent authorities' (CA) and independent ethics committees (IEC) is varied. It may be conducted in parallel or in sequence, in some cases with IEC first and CA second or in other countries in reverse order, by a single national IEC with or without local IECs at all sites or by a single regional IEC followed by local IECs within a MS. Clearly, this creates varying timelines to approvals in each MS.

The need for drug import permits and additional IEC requirements vary with the national MS as do export licences if trials are not conducted under a US Investigational New Drug (IND). This variance in process translates into differing delays from initiation to receiving approvals to permit clinical start-up of between 2 and 26 weeks (3).

The initiation and management of multinational clinical trials in the EU therefore requires considerable coordination and effort. The centralized coordination of the national procedures is essential to make sense of the complexity, ensure consistency, and to avoid duplication of effort, thus saving time and money. Therefore, to transform the presently cumbersome disparate situation through the EU CT Directive into a single set of legally enforceable set of procedures is commendable in its purpose and desirable economically.

May 1, 2004, should herald the beginning of implementation as law by 28 Member States of the European Union (EU) Directive 2001/20/IEC on GCP in clinical trials (4). Thus, for the first time we can expect to witness a common legally binding and comprehensive set of laws supported by detailed guidance documents covering all aspects of clinical research on medicinal products covering the largest single pharmaceutical market of the world of over 450 million citizens (5).

The full title of the Directive is: "Directive of the European Parliament and of the Council on the approximation of the laws, regulations and administrative provisions of the Member States relating to implementation of good clinical practice in the conduct of clinical trials on medicinal products for human use". Other Directives previously implemented and in force in MS concerning medicinal products cover matters such as licensing requirements, manufacturing, distribution, and classification for supply, labelling, and advertising.

Agreement on this Directive was reached in February 2001 and the final version was published in the Official Journal of the European Communities on May 1, 2001, by the European Commission. After that point, Member States have had to transpose the requirements of the Directive into national legislation by May 1, 2003, and must implement them into domestic law by May 1, 2004.

II. PURPOSE

The overall purpose of the Directive is to unify the standards and procedures of ICH GCP as a common legally enforceable process for the protection of subjects participating in clinical trials within the EU through implementation into national European laws. In addition, it is envisaged that the Directive will allow the harmonization of regulatory requirements and country-specific nuances to be addressed, thus permitting a standardized approach to clinical trials to be adopted throughout the EU. The European Agency for the Evaluation of Medicinal Products (EMEA), referred to in the Directive as the "Agency", is the London-based decentralized regulatory agency assisted by the Committee for Proprietary Medicinal Products (CPMP) set up in 1995 to coordinate all clinical research applications leading to marketing authorizations subsequently granted by the Commission.

III. SCOPE

The Directive covers all current 15 EU Member States (MS) and European Economic Area (EEA) members (Norway, Iceland, and Liechtenstein) i.e., 18 countries populated by 382 million citizens and coincidentally by the deadline date of May 1, 2004, will be joined by a further 10 new members of close to 75 million persons bringing the total to about 457 million citizens (5). This is already by far the largest pharmaceutical market in the world by population and this position will by 2004 be further consolidated.

The scope of the Directive is very wide as the conduct of all CT in the European Union (EU) on human subjects involving medicinal products as defined in Article I of Directive 65/65/EEC will be covered. The term 'investigational medicinal product' applies to whether it is either medicinal by function, or is presented as treating or preventing disease in human beings. In effect, every CT involving medicinal products will be covered, irrespective of who sponsors it, whether industry, Government, research council, charity, or university.

In medical terms, the Directive will be all-encompassing for clinical research in citizens of the EU. It will cover trials from phase 1 in normal healthy subjects, via small phase 2 dose ranging efficacy trials in subjects expected to derive medicinal benefit, through large efficacy and safety phase 3 trials leading to Marketing Authorization application (MAA), the European equivalent to a US New Drug Application (NDA).

The Directive sets standards for protecting clinical trials subjects, including incapacitated adults and minors. Importantly, it will also establish ethics committees on a legal basis and provide legal status for certain procedures, such as times within which an opinion must be given. In addition, it covers certain competent authority (regulatory agency) procedures for commencing a clinical trial, lays down standards for the manufacture, import and labelling of investigational medicinal products (IMPs) and provides for quality assurance of clinical trials and IMPs. However, not all unlicensed chemical entities would be considered IMPs, as the Regulations (UK) would apply only to those that are medicinal products and are to be tested or used as a reference in a clinical trial. To ensure compliance with these standards Member States are required to set up inspection systems for GCP and good manufacturing practice (GMP). The Directive provides for safety monitoring of subjects in trials, and sets out procedures for reporting and recording adverse drug reactions and experiences. To help with the exchange of information between MS, secure networks will be established, linked to European databases for information about approved CT and for pharmacovigilance.

The provisions of the Directive do not distinguish between commercial and non-commercial clinical trials i.e., those conducted by academic researchers without the participation of the healthcare industry. Furthermore, 'non-interventional' trials where the medicinal product is prescribed in the usual manner in accordance with the terms of the marketing authorization are not within the scope of the Directive. In these cases the assignment of a subject to a particular therapeutic strategy is not decided in advance by a trial protocol, but falls within current practice and the prescription of the medicine is clearly separated from the decision to include the subject in the trial. Also, no additional diagnostic or monitoring procedure is applied to the subjects and epidemiological methods are to be used for the analysis of the collected data.

Notable changes in the UK as a result of the Directive will include abolition of the "Doctors and Dentists Exemption (DDX)" whereby practitioners have been allowed to prescribe novel agents which they believe on balance to have efficacious advantages that outweigh the risks to their subjects, not on behalf of a commercial organization or other non EU party (6). Furthermore, phase 1 trials in the UK will be subject to exactly the same regulatory agency scrutiny as other types of trials.

When fully implemented, the Directive will lay down significant new legislation that will affect clinical research and development of medicinal products in the MS and their national health services.

Theoretically, the currently notable heterogeneous central or regional IEC and regulatory agency hurdles will be reduced to more readily manageable levels under the Directive with the order and format of applications reduced to levels more acceptable to and welcomed by applicants.

IV. DEFINITIONS

The Directive provides detailed definitions for terms in common use within clinical research. The reader is urged to refer to the original document for details (4) with the multilingual glossary in European languages (7). These include 'non-interventional trial' as trials outside the scope of the Directive and 'investigational medicinal product' as a pharmaceutical form of an active substance or placebo being tested or used as a reference in a CT, including products already having a marketing authorization but used or assembled (formulated or packaged) in a way different from the authorized form, or for an unauthorized indication, or to gain further information about the authorized form.

V. PRINCIPAL ELEMENTS OF DIRECTIVE ARTICLES, DETAILED GUIDELINES AND GUIDANCE DOCUMENTS

In brief, the Directive sets standards for protecting CT subjects, establishes independent ethics committees on a legal basis and provides the legal status for certain procedures. It is largely structured as for ICH GCP but with some notable additions. The Directive will compel all IEC to operate within a detailed legal framework to provide a consolidated central approach to the ethical review of clinical trials. It also lays down standards for the manufacture, import and labelling of an investigational medicinal product (IMP) and provides for quality assurance of both CT and IMP. Notably, the provisions of the Directive do not distinguish between commercial and non-commercial clinical trials and the 1996 rather than the then-latest 2000 version of the Declaration of Helsinki is specifically referenced.

While the Directive as reasonably expected covers all aspects of the clinical research process, it is underpinned by the principles of ICH GCP and as such, only main definitions, modifications, and additions of note are described in the following sections.

A. Protection of Clinical Trial Subjects, Minors and Incapacitated Adults

Member States must legislate to protect from abuse individuals who are incapable of giving informed consent. Thus, a CT may be only undertaken if in particular the foreseeable risks and inconveniences have been weighed against anticipated benefit for individual trial subjects. The CT may only proceed if the IEC and/or the CA conclude that anticipated therapeutic and public health benefits justify the risks and continue only if compliance with this requirement is permanently monitored.

A clinical trial may only be undertaken if the informed consent of the minor's parents or incapacitated subject's legal representative has been obtained, representing the subject's presumed will and may be revoked at any time without detriment to the subject. The subject must receive information on the trial with risks and benefits in an understandable form from appropriately experienced staff. Investigators must heed the wishes of minors capable of forming an opinion or legal representatives to refuse or discontinue participation at any time. No incentives or financial inducements except compensation are to be given. Some direct benefit to this class of subject and relating to the clinical condition suffered by or uniquely in the subjects must be demonstrable. Particular attention is to be made to minimize pain, discomfort, and fear and to ensure potential benefits of the IMP outweigh any foreseeable risks or produce no risk in relation to the disease and developmental stage; the risk threshold and degree of distress must be specifically defined and constantly monitored. The IEC having specialized expertise or after taking specialist advice on clinical, ethical and psychosocial problems associated with these subjects must endorse the protocol in which the interests of the subject always prevail over those of science and society.

B. Independent Ethics Committee, Single Opinion and Detailed Guidance

Member States must take all necessary measures for establishing and operating independent ethics committees that must give its opinion on any issue before a trial commences. In preparing its opinion the IEC must particularly consider the relevance of the trial and its design, whether anticipated benefits and risks are satisfactory and justified in terms of the protocol, suitability of investigator and staff, quality of facilities, adequacy and completeness of the Information to Subjects and the Informed Consent form and procedures to be followed for obtaining informed consent, justification of research on persons incapable of giving consent.

Provision for indemnity or compensation in the event of injury or death of subjects attributable to the clinical trial, and for insurance or indemnity to cover liability of the investigator and sponsor must be described. The financial arrangements for rewarding or compensating investigators and trial subjects and relevant aspects between the sponsor and site and arrangements for recruiting subjects are to be documented.

Importantly, a MS may decide that the IEC is responsible for and giving an opinion on the indemnity, insurance and remuneration aspects; when this provision is applied, the MS must notify the Commission, other MS, and the EMEA.

The IEC will be limited to 60 days from date of receipt of a valid application to give its reasoned opinion to the applicant and to the CA. Within this period of examination, the IEC may send a single request for supplemental information to the applicant; the timeline is suspended until receipt of the information.

Extension to the 60-day period is only permissible for trials of gene therapy or somatic cell therapy or medicinal products containing genetically modified organisms. In such a case an extension of 30 days is permitted with a further extension of 90 days in the event of local MS consultation with a group or committee also allowed for, bringing the total to 180 days. There is *no* time limit for xenogenic cell therapy applications.

Member States are to establish procedures for managing multi-center trials limited to the territory of a single MS, irrespective of the number of IEC, in order to adopt a single opinion. Where the CT is to be conducted simultaneously in more than one MS, a single opinion is to be given by each MS.

The Commission in consultation with MS has published detailed guidance documents on the application format, documentation to be submitted in an application for an IEC's opinion paying particular attention to the information given to subjects and on appropriate safeguards for the protection of personal data. Some MS already have data protection legislation in place and the reader is encouraged to check this within each MS under consideration.

C. Commencement of a Clinical Trial

Member States must follow the following measures to ensure that the IEC and the CA have issued favorable opinions on the application before a clinical trial is allowed to start; the opinions can be sought in parallel. If the CA notifies the sponsor of grounds for non-acceptance, the sponsor may, on *one* occasion only, amend the content of the request to take due account of the grounds given. If the sponsor fails to amend the request accordingly, the request would be rejected and the CT not permitted to start.

Consideration of the request by the CA is expected as rapidly as possible and is limited to 60 days but the MS may lay down periods shorter than 60 days if in compliance with current practice; the CA may notify the sponsor of the approval at *any* time before the end of this specified period.

Written authorization is required before starting clinical trials on an IMP not having a marketing authorization and other IMPs with special characteristics such as those having as their active ingredient(s) or components or the manufacturing that is a biological product(s) of human or animal origin.

Specific reference is made to the application of 1990 Council Directives on the contained use of genetically modified microorganisms (8) and on the deliberate release into the environment of genetically modified organisms (9). Gene therapy trials, which could result in modifications to the germ line genetic identity of the subject, are *not* allowed.

D. Conduct of a Clinical Trial

These relate to amendments to conduct of a CT that is underway. Thus, the sponsor may make amendments to the protocol which, if substantial and likely to impact on safety of the trial subjects or change the interpretation of the scientific documents in support of the conduct of the trial, or are otherwise significant, the sponsor must advise the CA of all MS and all IEC.

In response, the IEC must give an opinion within a maximum of 35 days of receipt. If this opinion is unfavorable, the sponsor is disallowed from implementing the amendment to the protocol; under these circumstances the sponsor should either take account of the grounds for non-acceptance and adapt the proposed amendment accordingly or should withdraw the proposed amendment. But, if the IEC and CA approve the amendment, the sponsor is clear to proceed with its clinical application.

Should a new event arise likely to affect the safety of the subjects, the sponsor must take appropriate urgent safety measures to protect subjects from any immediate hazard and inform all CA and IEC accordingly of the new events and the measures taken.

Within 90 days of the end of a CT the sponsor must notify all CA and IEC; if the CT is terminated early, this period is reduced to 15 days and the reasons for termination clearly explained.

E. Exchange of Information, Suspension or Infringements, European Clinical Trials EUDRACT Database

The CA in whose territory the CT takes place enters the details into a new European Drug Regulatory Affairs Clinical Trial (EUDRACT) database. It allocates a unique EUDRACT number that cannot be reallocated to another trial if the original one does not proceed; if an International Standard Randomized Controlled Trial Number (ISRCTN) is available, this detail is also entered. These EUDRACT entry data are accessible only to the CA, the EMEA, and the Commission and details the request for authorization, the protocol, any proposed protocol amendments, approvals by the CA and IEC, any suspension, the declaration at the end, and reference to any GCP inspections.

Upon request by any MS, the EMEA or the Commission, the CA to which the request for authorization was submitted must supply all further information concerning the CT in question other than the data already in the European database.

In consultation with the MS, the Commission has published detailed guidance documents on the relevant data to be included in the database, which is operated with the assistance of the EMEA as well as methods for its secure and confidential electronic communication.

A MS having objective grounds for considering the conditions in the request for authorization at the outset are no longer met or has information raising doubts about the safety or scientific validity of the trial, may suspend or prohibit the trial and notify the sponsor. Except where there is imminent risk, the MS would ask the sponsor and/or the investigator for their opinion to be delivered within 1 week. In this case, the CA would advise other involved CA, the IEC concerned, the Agency, and the Commission of its decision with reasons to suspend or prohibit the trial.

F. Manufacture, Import and Labelling of Investigational Medical Products

All appropriate measures to ensure manufacture or importation of the IMP by MS are subject to applicants and subsequent "holder of the authorization" holding a valid authorization satisfying requirements in accordance with procedures referred to in a 2003 Council Decision (10).

The holder of the authorization must have at its disposal at least one "qualified person" (QP) who is authorized in the particular MS, to continue working permanently and continuously and providing expert services as laid down in the GMP Directive and detailed guidelines (see Table 1, p. 550). The QP is directly and independently responsible for satisfying him/herself of the purity and quality of production batches of the IMP manufactured locally or in a non-EU country. Where an IMP is a comparator product from a non-EU country having a marketing authorization, the QP is responsible for ensuring that the certification of *each* production batch has been manufactured under conditions at least equivalent to GMP standards. Investigational medicinal product(s) imported from another MS will not have to undergo further analytical checks if received together with batch release certification signed by the responsible QP.

The QP must certify in an up-to-date register available to CA or their agents for the period specified in the provisions of the MS concerned and not less than 5 years that each production batch satisfies the provisions of the Article.

Readers are also urged to refer to the "Commission Directive on the requirements to obtain an authorization to manufacture or import an investigational medicinal product and the requirements to be met by the holder of this authorization to implement the directive on Clinical Trials on medicinal products for human use" (10).

Labels must be in the official language(s) of the MS on the outer or immediate packaging of the IMP and published in accordance with existing regulations to ensure protection of the subjects, traceability and proper use.

G. Inspections, Verification of Compliance of Investigational Medical Products with Good Clinical Practice and Good Manufacturing Practice

Duly qualified Community inspectors appointed by the MS will inspect the CT sites, manufacturing facilities for the IMP, laboratories used for analysis

Table 1 EU Clinical Trials Directive: Principal Elements of Articles and Primary Applicable Draft Guidelines or Guidance Documents (December 2003) for Implementation

Principal Element	Article Title	Draft Detailed Guideline or Final Detailed Guideline/Guidance Document[a] Title Date and Document No.
	1. Scope	
	2. Definitions	
1. Protection of clinical trial subjects	3. Protection of clinical trial subjects 4. Clinical trials on minors 5. Clinical trials on incapacitated adults not able to give informed legal consent	Detailed guidance for request for authorization of clinical trial to competent authorities, notification of substantial amendments and declaration of the end of the trial. April 2003. ENTR 6416/01
2. Independent Ethics Committee	6. Independent Ethics Committee 7. Single opinion 8. Detailed guidance	Detailed guidance on application format and documentation to be submitted in an application for an Independent Ethics Committee opinion on the clinical trial on medicinal products for human use. April 2003. ENTR 6417/01
3. Commencement	9. Commencement of a clinical trial	As for Articles 3 and 6.
4. Conduct	10. Conduct of a clinical trial	*Detailed guidelines on the principles of good clinical practice in the conduct in the EU of clinical trials on medicinal products for human use. Draft 5.1, July 2002* *Detailed guidelines on the trial master file and archiving to implement the directive on Clinical Trials on medicinal products for human use. June 2002*
5. Exchange of information	11. Exchange of information	Detailed guidance on the European clinical trials database (EUDRACT Database). April 2003. ENTR 6101/02
	12. Suspension of the clinical trial or infringements	*Detailed guidelines on inspection procedures for the verification of GCP compliance to implement the directive on Clinical Trials on medicinal products for human use. June 2002*

Table 1 Continued

Principal Element	Article Title	*Draft Detailed Guideline* or Final Detailed Guideline/Guidance Document[a] Title Date and Document No.
6. Manufacture and import	13. Manufacture and import of investigational medical products	*Modifications to Commission Directive 91/356 of June 13, 1991 laying down the principles and guidelines of good manufacturing practice for Medicinal products for human use, as required by Directive 2001/20/IEC; June 2002.* Detailed guidelines on the Community basic format and the contents of the application for a manufacturing and/or import authorization of an investigational medicinal product for human use to implement the directive on Clinical Trials on medicinal products for human use. July 2002
	14. Labelling	*Revision of Good Manufacturing Practices Annex 13 to implement directive on Clinical Trials on medicinal products for human use. July 2002* Two-column informal working document. July 2002
7. Inspections	15. Verification of compliance of investigational medical products with good clinical and manufacturing practice	*Detailed guidelines on the qualifications of inspectors who should verify compliance in clinical trials with the provisions of good clinical practice for an investigational medicinal product to implement the directive on Clinical Trials on medicinal products for human use. June 2002* Detailed guidelines on inspection procedures for the verification of GCP compliance to implement the directive on Clinical Trials on medicinal products for human use. June 2002 Detailed guidelines on the qualifications of inspectors who should verify compliance in clinical trials with the provisions of good manufacturing practice for an investigational medicinal product to implement the directive on Clinical Trials on medicinal products for human use. June 2002

Table 1 Continued

Principal Element	Article Title	Draft Detailed Guideline or Final Detailed Guideline/Guidance Document[a] Title Date and Document No.
8. Adverse experiences	16. Notification of adverse experiences	Detailed guidance on the collection, verification and presentation of adverse reaction reports arising
	17. Notification of serious adverse reactions.	from clinical trials on medicinal products for human use. April 2003. ENTR 6101/02
	18. Guidance concerning reports	Detailed guidance on the European database of Suspected Unexpected Serious Adverse Reactions (Eudravigilance—Clinical Trial Module). April 2003. ENTR 6101/02
9. General provisions	19. General provisions	
	20. Adaptation to scientific and technical progress	
	21. Committee procedure	
	22. Application	
	23. Entry into force	
	24. Addressees	

Final Detailed Guidance for adaptation to suit national requirements.
Final Detailed Guideline meant to be legally binding i.e., a Commission Technical Directive.
[a] *Draft Guideline for consultation (in development).*

and/or the sponsor's premises in accordance with the Directive on behalf of the Community. Inspection findings are to be recognized by all other MS, coordinated by the Agency within the existing regulatory framework (Table 1) and reports given to the sponsor/inspectee and at their *reasoned* request to other MS, the IEC, and to the Agency. Should verification of compliance reveal differences between Member States, the Commission may request further inspections. Inspections are not limited to MS but may be conducted upon request at sponsor's premises, trial sites, and/or the manufacturer in non-EU countries.

Detailed guidelines are available for CT documentation constituting the trial master file (TMF) and archiving (11), qualifications of inspectors (12) and inspection procedures (13) to verify compliance are in accordance with published procedures laid down in Article 21.

H. Adverse Experiences and Serious Adverse Reactions Notification, Collection, Verification, Presentation and Reporting, SUSAR Database, Eudravigilance Clinical Trial Module Database

Serious AEs are to be reported immediately either verbally or in writing except where the protocol or IB identify as not required. Subsequent follow-up reports must be detailed and in writing; any further information on deaths of subjects must be provided by the investigator to the sponsor and IEC. Subject's anonymity will be preserved by a unique code numbering system.

Adverse experiences and/or laboratory abnormalities identified in the protocol as critical to safety evaluations shall be reported in accordance with requirements and timelines specified in the protocol. Sponsors must maintain detailed records of all AEs, which are to be submitted upon request by the MS in whose territory the trial was conducted.

All relevant information on suspected unexpected serious adverse reactions (SARs) considered *life threatening* or *fatal* must be reported to CA in all MS and to the IEC as soon as possible or within 7 days of the sponsor learning of them and all follow-up information within a further 8 days. All other reactions are to be advised within 15 days of *knowledge* by the sponsor. Member States are responsible for recording all SARs and sponsors for advising all investigators.

The sponsor must make an annual safety update to MS and the IEC of all SARs, outcomes, and safety aspects for all subjects. All MS will update the Eudravigilance database (see Article 11) and the Agency will disseminate this information to all CA.

The Commission in consultation with other parties has drawn up two detailed guidance documents on the collection, verification, and presentation of AEs/ARs with decoding procedures for SARs (Table 1, p. 552).

I. General Provisions, Adaptation to Scientific and Technical Progress, Committee Procedure, Application, Entry into Force and Addressees

The Directive came into force on its 2001 publication date, reaffirms that sponsors and investigators have "without prejudice" civil and criminal liabilities; the sponsor must be established in the Community and provide the IMP and any administration devices free of charge.

As intended, the Directive is being adapted by MS and CA in line with scientific and technical progress, the removal of technical barriers to trade. Should any amendments become necessary, this will be through the existing "Standing Committee on Medicinal Products for Human Use", which the Commission must consult; if the Commission disagrees with this Committee the matters would be referred to the Council.

The terms "Detailed Guideline" and "Detailed Guidance" are used for different purposes and use has been made of "Draft" and "Final" in describing versions for both in the normal manner. A total of 14 draft Guidelines were originally issued by the IEC shortly after publication of the Directive as consultation documents for all interested parties to comment upon and make suggested amendments until October 2, 2002, before finalization (Table 1). At the time of writing, four "Final Detailed Guidelines" are published on the European Drug Regulatory (EUDRA) website supporting the Directive; these *cannot* be altered by Member States (Table 1). The other five draft "Detailed Guidance" documents were designed to guide MS on the criteria for drafting their local legislative documentation for subsequent incorporation into their laws, heeding country-specific requirements.

VI. IMPLEMENTATION

The principles of the Directive should remove the complexity of clinical trial application, authorization and regulation in existing, new, and future Member States. Thus, substantial amendments to protocol that impact on safety of the subjects or where there is a change in the interpretation of data on the IMP must be notified under the legislation underpinning the Directive. This common process will obviate current disparate national procedures that range from a simple notification scheme to a complex authorization procedure. Implementation of the Directive cannot be expected to alter national requirements for provision to examiners of Information to Subjects and Informed Consent forms in local languages.

A common clinical trial application form will be used and will be accompanied by data on the Quality, Safety, and Efficacy of the IMP to the CA. The application process is an implicit approval within a maximum 60-day review period with one exception, for clinical trials with biotechnology IMPs, e.g., gene therapy, somatic cell therapy, and genetically modified organisms. In this case, written approval is mandatory and a 90-day review period will apply.

The immensity of the task of transposing guidelines into legislation is reflected in the timelines; its implementation has already been postponed for 12 months and in the UK, the July 16, 2003, edition of *Hansard* described a delay from July until October in completing the Statutory Instrument to be laid before Parliament.

The Spanish *Agencia Española del Medicamento* advised the Institute of Clinical Research in the summer of 2003 that it is currently working on the draft legislation; the first draft passed a public hearing before continuing along the approval procedure. The *División de Farmacología y Evaluación Clínica* expects the Royal Decree will be published before May 2004.

Whether individual MS succeed in this challenging quest to conduct clinical trials within their legal framework in accordance with the Directive from May 1, 2004, remains to be seen.

VII. IMPLICATIONS FOR FUTURE RESEARCH

Although the Directive is aimed at providing an environment for conducting clinical research that transparently protects participants without hampering the discovery of new medicines, several parties have expressed concern that this may not be the case and publication of their viewpoints is wide and unrelenting. The entire sector remains anxious about how well Member States put the new rules into local effect and some parties believe there are grounds for believing they will not make it easier to conduct international trials but could make them even harder.

Time is required after the May 1, 2004, deadline to assess the actual effects on clinical research within the EU and whether these anxieties for its global competitiveness in the marketplace were justified. Strategically, the attempt by the EU to boost local medicines research, and keep the industry afloat and actively able to supply the new products that subjects need, will be revealed in the near future.

Implementation of the Directive should lead to the better acceptability of EU clinical data by the FDA, a major factor given the global nature of the pharmaceutical research industry today and into the future.

Glossary

AE	adverse experience
CPMP	Committee for Proprietary Medicinal Products
CA	Competent authority
CT	clinical trial
EEA	European Economic Area
EMEA	European Agency for the Evaluation of Medicinal Products
EU	European Union
Eudra	European Drug Regulatory
EUDRACT	European Drug Regulatory Affairs Clinical Trial
FDA	Food and Drug Administration
GCP	good clinical practice
GMP	good manufacturing practice
HVT	healthy volunteer trials
IC	Informed consent
ICH	International Conference on Harmonisation of Technical Requirements for Registration of Pharmaceuticals for Human Use
IEC	Independent Ethics Committee
IMP	investigational medicinal product
IND	investigational new drug (USA)
MAA	Marketing Authorization application (EU)
MS	Member State
QP	Qualified Person
SAR	serious adverse reaction
SUSAR	suspected unexpected serious adverse reaction (Eudravigilance CT module)

REFERENCES

1. ICH E6 Guideline for Good Clinical Practice, CPMP/ICH/135/95/Step 5, July 1996.
2. World Medical Association, Declaration of Helsinki, Ethical Principles for Medical research Involving Human Subjects, 5th revision. 48th WMA General

Assembly, Somerset West, Republic of South Africa, October 1996 and the 52nd WMA General Assembly, Edinburgh, Scotland, October 2000.

3. Mermet-Bouvier P, de Crémiers F. Clinical Trial Initiation in Europe: Current Status. Regul Aff J July 2002; 571–578.

4. Directive 2001/20/IEC of the European Parliament and of the Council of 4 April 2001 on the approximation of the laws, regulations and administrative provisions of the Member States relating to the implementation of good clinical practice in the conduct of clinical trials on medicinal products for human use. OJ 2001; L121, 34–44.

5. EU Member States. Integration Office DFA/DEA http://www.europa.admin.ch/eu/expl/staaten/e/index.htm.

6. The Medicines (Exemption from Licences) (Special Cases and Miscellaneous Provisions) Order 1972. www.mca.gov.uk.

7. Vander Stichele R 2000. Multilingual Glossary of technical and popular medical terms in nine European Languages. http://allserv.rug.ac.be/~rvdstich/eugloss/welcome.html.

8. Council Directive OJ L 117, 8.5.1990; 1 Directive as last amended by Directive 98/81/IEC (OJ L 330, 5.12.1998; 13).

9. Council Directive OJ L 117, 8.5.1990, p. 15. Directive as last amended by Commission Directive 97/35/IEC. (OJ L 169, 27.6.1997; 72).

10. Commission Directive on the requirements to obtain an authorisation to manufacture or import an investigational medicinal product and the requirements to be met by the holder of this authorisation to implement the directive on Clinical Trials on medicinal products for human use. OJ L 262 14.10.2003; 22.

11. Detailed guidelines on the trial masterfile and archiving. http://pharmacos.eudra.org./F2/pharmacos/docs/Doc2002/june/tmf_06_2002.pdf.

12. Detailed guidelines on the qualifications of inspectors who should verify compliance in clinical trials with the provisions of good clinical practice for an investigational medicinal product to implement the directive on Clinical Trials on medicinal products for human use. June 2002. http://pharmacos.eudra.org./F2/pharmacos/docs/Doc2002/june/ins_gcp_06_2002.pdf.

13. Detailed guidelines on inspection procedures for the verification of GCP compliance to implement the directive on Clinical Trials on medicinal products for human use. June 2002. http://pharmacos.eudra.org./F2/pharmacos/docs/Doc2002/june/dtld_06_2002.pdf.

24
HIPAA: A New Requirement to the Clinical Study Process

Edith Lewis-Rogers
META Solutions, Inc., Warren, New Jersey, U.S.A.

Earl W. Hulihan
Regulatory Consulting Services, META Solutions, Inc., Warren, New Jersey, U.S.A.

Richard A. Guarino
Oxford Pharmaceutical Resources, Inc., Totowa, New Jersey, U.S.A.

I. INTRODUCTION

HIPAA is the acronym for the Health Insurance Portability and Account-ability Act of 1996. HIPAA evolved as a result of the rapid evolution of health information systems technology as well as the challenges for maintaining the confidentiality of health information. HIPAA was introduced initially as the Kennedy–Kassebaum bill, an outgrowth of the Clinton administration's attempt to revamp the health care system. The result in HIPAA was an effort to streamline and standardize the health care system and to establish the privacy of subject information. The result of this effort was the issuance of the final HIPAA rules in August, 2002, which establish the requirements that prevent the disclosure of individually identifiable health information (Privacy Rule) (1) without authorization from the subject. An accidental posting of individuals' health records and fraudulent use of medical records precipitated the passage of HIPAA.

Case 1. A Michigan-based health care system accidentally posted the medical records of thousands of subjects on the internet (references—The

Ann Arbor News, February 10, 1999). A speculator bid $4000 for the subject records of a family practice in South Carolina and then used them to sell them back to the former subjects (The New York Times, August 14, 1991).

Case 2. A Nevada woman who purchased a used computer discovered that the previous owner of the computer left a database with the names, addresses, social security numbers, and a list of all prescriptions received by the individual (The New York Times, April 4, 1997, and April 12, 1997).

HIPAA has some important provisions affecting research that are included in the Administration Simplification Provision under which the privacy rule evolved. In addition, it has another provision with respect to the fraud and abuse rule that made certain restrictions on inducement to subjects. With the implementation of HIPAA, subjects can now find out how their health information may be used. It also limits the release of information to a minimum time reasonably needed for the purpose of disclosure. In addition, it gives subjects the right to examine and obtain a copy of their health records, so they can request corrections. Most important, it allows individuals to control certain uses and disclosures of their health information. Subjects generally will have full access rights to their health care information under HIPAA. However, the rights may be waived if their authorization states that their health information will not be available during the clinical trial, or the authorization states whether the information will be available at the end of the trial and the subject has agreed to these waivers.

HIPAA and the Administration Simplification Provisions cover the electronic transactions and code sets, national identifiers for plans and providers, and employers and will include subjects, security, and privacy provisions that were intended to balance the simplification of the transaction and identifiers. The HIPAA privacy regulations are in Title 45 of the Code of Federal Regulations. Those who work in research and are familiar with the common rule, IRB, and informed consent regulations, also in Title 45, part 46. Administrative simplification and privacy rules can be found in Title 45, parts 160 and 164.

II. HIPAA'S IMPACT ON CLINICAL RESEARCH

HIPAA requirements for subject privacy is increasing the amount of documentation needed for the initiation of a trial. Besides the requirement for informed consent, which has evolved from the Declaration of Helsinki, there is now an additional need for authorization from the subject for release of the "individually identifiable health information" that the drug sponsor must enter into the data bank for statistical analysis to comply with requirements necessary for new product approvals. However, HIPAA does not include data needed for adverse experience reporting assessments for clinical trials.

III. COVERED AND NOT COVERED ENTITIES

A. Who Are the Covered Entities?

Directly covered entities of HIPAA are health care providers who engage in electronic transactions, and health care clearinghouses, which are billing agencies that some physicians' offices use to submit their claims and health plans. The covered entities are responsible for the privacy standards as well as for any other contracted individuals (called "business associates") to perform essential functions. Business associates do not include members of the covered entity's work force or volunteer medical staff. Among the business associates' functions or activities are legal, actuarial, accounting, consulting, clinical research, data analysis, processing or administration, quality assurance, and practice management. Contracts with business associates must be signed between the covered entity and the business associate, requiring the business associate to keep protected health information safeguarded. Components of a sample business associate agreement have been included in the HIPAA privacy rules as amended in August 2002.

HIPAA also allows for the creation of hybrid entities when certain parts of the entity are not engaged in the covered activities. However, research components of these hybrid entities that function as health care providers and engage in standard electronic transactions are subject to the privacy rule.

B. Who Are Not Covered Entities?

Anything that is not a covered entity e.g., pharmaceutical, biotech, or medical device companies or contract research organizations, typically are not covered entities. It is possible that a large organization may have a health clinic, or an infirmary on site, or there may be doctors there who may provide services, and those services may be billed to an insurer under those circumstances. It is possible that that part of a pharmaceutical or contract research organization is a covered entity. But for the most part, pharmaceutical companies, medical device companies, and contract research organizations are not health care providers, plans, or clearinghouses.

IV. APPLICABILITY

HIPAA applies to the use or disclosure of health information. The following are among the items considered to be part of the privacy rule:

Individual Identification—Identification includes name, birth date, admission date, treatment date, telephone number, Social Security number, photo, and vehicle identification numbers. Among the other items that are considered to make the subject identifiable are medical record numbers, health plan numbers, and device identifiers/serial numbers. Even zip codes with more than the first three numbers (except in some cases) will be considered subject identifiers.

Information relating to the individual's health, health care treatment, or health care payment.

Information maintained or disclosed in electronic format, or in hard copy. All information that is created or received by a provider, plan, clearinghouse, or employer relating to past, present, or future physical or mental health condition, provision of health care, or past, present, or future payment for the provision of health care that identifies the individual or reasonably could be used to identify the individual and it is transmitted in any form. Any information relating to the condition, care, or payment that could identify the individual.

V. PROTECTED HEALTH INFORMATION (PHI) AUTHORIZATION FOR CLINICAL TRIALS

A. Background

Investigators participating in clinical research must obtain from each subject authorization that accurately describes the uses and potential disclosure of PHI. The authorization (2) may be presented as part of the Informed Consent (see p. 565). In any event, authorization for access to PHI generated prior to research must be obtained from the subject (e.g., past medical history, previous treatments, hospitalizations). The authorization will state who will have access to the PHI and detail the specific duration of the use of the PHI; the expiration of use can be referred to a specific event, e.g., an FDA approval. If data will be used as a research database, then an expiration of "none" might be acceptable to the subjects. The authorization must disclose whether there is compensation to the researcher from a third party and the use or disclosure of the PHI, but the amount of compensation is not required. If the subject revokes the PHI authorization, information already obtained under the authorization may still be used to preserve the integrity of the clinical trial such as marketing application or ADR reporting. If this is the case, no new PHI on that subject may be collected or disclosed.

B. Enforcement of HIPAA

While enforcement authority for informed consents exists in the FDA and in other non-US national and regional health authorities, the enforcement agency responsible for HIPAA in the US is the Office of Civil Rights (OCR) within the Department of Health and Human Services (HHS). Monitoring of HIPAA will likely occur by the Office of the Inspector General.

There are civil and criminal penalties for violating the HIPAA. An individual who knowingly and wrongfully discloses or obtains individually identifiable health information faces fines of up to $50,000 and a year in prison. Individuals who disclose information with the intent to sell the data face a maximum $250,000 fine and 1 to 10 years imprisonment. It is important to understand that the Office of Civil Rights recognizes that this is a complex set of rules. They themselves are spending a fair amount of time trying to understand them. They have issued several guidances (5) to help comprehend the application of HIPAA. So one should not be in fear that we cannot do any more research because there now is a statute governing this and you might go to jail. Certainly, if one is in good faith trying to comply with these rules it is unlikely that there would be any serious challenge.

Individuals bound by the HIPAA privacy requirements (3,4) may be more reticent in releasing the needed information to the drug sponsors. Assurance of an adequate authorization statement from the clinical subject will be needed to overcome this concern. To insure that this information, on drug efficacy and safety, is made available for use and review by the product sponsors, the sponsors may need to include, in addition to the informed consent, a written authorization from the subject in a clinical trial that allows the sponsor to use the subject information in any future data analysis. A provision within the authorization should include that if the authorization is with drawn it may constitute grounds for the removal of subjects from specified clinical trials.

C. Authorization for Clinical Trials

How is the HIPAA framework applicable for clinical research? There are several different ways to disclose and use information for research including database research. There is nothing HIPAA and its application to research that is specific for databases. Each type of database research, whether it is in the creation of the database, the type of study using the database, the analysis, future analysis, etc., must be assessed with the same HIPAA privacy rules that apply to research, and the question must be asked, "How would this apply to this database and what is the best mechanism in order to be able to disclose the information for research purposes?"

The most effective way to gain authorization from the trial subjects is to obtain the consent/acknowledgment and written authorization from the subjects permitting the disclosure of and access to the clinical trial data.

A single consolidated authorization for the subject, which includes needed authorization for access to data for the clinical trial, can be included with the covered entities' authorizations for subject privacy, according to the HIPAA regulations. The drug sponsor's access to the needed data is best handled by a separate authorization from each subject for each clinical trial. In addition, a special authorization for subjects is needed for the release of records that involve psychotherapy notes. Drug sponsors should be sure that a special authorization is available for the drug sponsor's access to psychotherapy notes to complete the trial successfully.

The authorization needed to access the subject privacy must include the information that will be used for treatment, payment, or health care operations. Authorizations must be clearly written so that the subject can fully understand the document.

Authorization must include

Description of the subject information that will be reviewed.

Persons authorized to make the requested use or disclosure of this information. The drug sponsor should assure that this disclosure extends to all authorized parties involved in the clinical trial assessment, including Clinical Research Associates, Clinical Research Organizations, other consultants, etc.

Expiration date of the authorization—The best choice is for the use of "none" as the expiration date so that review of records can continue to be accessible for future reviews. Although one suggested expiration date was the end of research, the uncertain time frame may raise questions that will require additional resources.

Statement that the individual's access rights to inspect and obtain copies of their health records relative to the trial is suspended while the clinical trial is in progress and will be reinstated when the clinical trial is concluded.

In addition to the required elements, the authorization has to include a statement that the subject has the right to revoke the authorization. There are limitations about the right of the subject to revoke the use of the research information. For example if the data is already entered in the database and the subject then revokes the authorization, does that mean that all of their information has to be edited out of the results? The privacy rules make it clear that in so far as information has already been disclosed, and that the information has been relied upon, then there is no requirement that that information be removed. However, you would not be able to continue to put in further information on that particular subject into the database. If the removal of the information would have an impact on the results, you might have to do an analysis with and without the information to justify why it should stay in. In other words, if you can demonstrate how the analysis would be greatly affected by removing this data and therefore affect the integrity and impact of the final results, you can justify keeping that data. The privacy rules do allow for these exceptions.

D. Relationship to Informed Consent

The HIPAA authorization can be included with the informed consent document or it can be separate from the informed consent. See PHI authorization page. The information that must be included in the informed consent, along with the other data in the IC, as it pertains to the investigational product, must contain a specific and meaningful description of the information to be disclosed, including

Name of the person or class of persons authorized to make the disclosure, e.g., principal investigator, subinvestigators, research coordinators.

Name of the person or class of persons that will receive the disclosed information, e.g., sponsor, monitors, CROs, statisticians.

Statement that information received by the users may be used for future studies or statistics.

Expiration date or expiration event when authorities may disclose the information.

Statement containing a subject's right to revoke their authorization for disclosure.

Statement documenting the ability to condition enrollment on informed consent/authorization.

Statement documenting the possibility that the information may be redisclosed by the recipient (e.g., to the FDA).

Signature of subject and date of the signing of the HIPAA agreement.

The document should be written in a language understood by the subject, and a copy of the document must be given to the subject.

It should be noted that according to the HIPAA privacy rules, in the final form when research has obtained valid consent or waiver of consent from an IRB prior to the enforcement date of April 14, 2003, the research may continue without requiring a HIPAA authorization. Therefore if subjects in a clinical trial gave their informed valid consent prior to that date, the data can be continued to be collected and analyzed after the compliance enforcement date without an authorized waiver. On the other hand, if subjects were enrolled in a trial prior to April 14, 2003, and new subjects are then enrolled after that date, authorization or a waiver or creation of a limited data set must be obtained from these subjects.

E. Institutional Review Boards

Where HIPAA requirements are combined with the informed consent requirements, the entire document needs to be reviewed by the Institutional Review
Board (IRB). The Office of Civil Rights as well as the FDA's General Counsel,
as of April 7, 2003, had confirmed that IRB approval of subject authorization
for use or disclosure of protected health information required by the HIPAA
privacy rule is only required if the authorization language is to be part of the
IRB-approved informed consent document for human subjects review.

IRBs are also permitted to waive authorization requirements for a drug
sponsor using expedited review procedures permitted by the Common Rule.
Expedited review is permitted for each on-going research protocol when the
only addition is that of the subject authorization for the use or disclosure of
protected health information. This waiver may be permitted to a researcher
when the research is not possible without the waiver. The IRB must assure
that an adequate plan is available to protect identifiers and to be sure that the
identifiers are destroyed at the earliest possible date.

F. Privacy Boards

In cases where IRBs are not responsible for reviewing, the HIPAA Authorization Privacy Board may be formed to undertake this task. Members of
privacy boards should have varying backgrounds and appropriate professional competence. At least one member must not be affiliated with the covered entity or research sponsor. As with the IRB, there must be no conflicts of
interest on a case-by-case basis. A quorum consists of a majority of members.
Expedited review by the chairperson or designees is allowed for the waiver of
authorization.

G. IRB or Privacy Waivers of Authorization

Three criteria must be met for the IRB or Privacy Board to waive authorization for research:

> The use or disclosure of protected health information involves no more
> than a minimal risk to the privacy of the individual.
> The research could not practicably be done without the waiver.
> The research could not practicably be conducted without access to and
> use of the protected health information (PHI).
> The research will not adversely affect privacy rights or welfare.
> The privacy risks are reasonable in relation to anticipated benefits and
> the importance of the knowledge of the clinical results.

Before initiating the clinical trial, the drug sponsors need to have documentation of the waiver in their files. The identification of the IRB or Privacy Board should be included. The date of approval of the waiver, a statement that relevant waiver criteria have been met, a description of the information, and the statement of whether the action was taken under normal or expedited review procedures must be stated clearly.

H. Waiver of a Research Database

A research database using protected health information may be created by a noncovered entity without individuals' authorizations. Documentation must be obtained from the IRB or the Privacy Board that the specified waiver criteria were satisfied. This database could then be used or disclosed for future research studies as permitted by the Privacy Rule. Specifically, the database can be used as the basis for future research in which individual authorization has been obtained or where the IRB or Privacy Board grants a waiver.

Similarly, existing databases or repositories created prior to the April 14, 2003, compliance data can be disclosed for research either with individual authorizations or with a waiver from either the IRB or the Privacy Board. Approval from both the IRB and the Privacy Board is not required for the covered entity.

I. Study Recruitment

The covered entity's workforce can use protected health information to identify and contact prospective research subjects. The covered entity's health care provider can discuss the enrollment in a clinical trial with a potential subject before authorization is completed or there has been an Institutional Review Board or Privacy Board waiver of authorization. A clinician may use or disclose the PHI if such information is being used to treat the subject or using an experimental treatment that may benefit a subject. However, at no time can the research health care provider remove the protected data from the covered entity's site according to the HIPAA requirements.

If a researcher is not employed by the covered entity, the researcher can still have access to the protected information as a result of a partial waiver of individual authorization by an IRB or Privacy Board.

J. Limited Data Sets

HIPAA provides for the creation of limited data sets that can be provided to a researcher without obtaining the IRB or Privacy Board's waiver of authorization. All of the direct identifiers of the individual or of relatives, employers, or household members of the individual are required to be deidentified, with the following exceptions: admission, discharge, and service dates, date of death, age, and five-digit zip code.

Deidentification requires the covered entity to retain individual(s) who have experience using methods with generally accepted statistical and scientific principles and methods that mask identifying characteristics of information to assure that the information is not individually identifiable. For example, statisticians use scientific principles and methodology in statistical analysis.

Limited data sets must take into consideration the following direct identifiers of the individual, or of their relatives, employees, and household members, releasing which would be a violation of the HIPAA data use agreement.

Names
Postal addresses
Telephone/fax numbers
Electronic mail addresses
Social Security numbers
Medical record numbers
Health plan beneficiary numbers
Account numbers
Certificates/license numbers
Vehicle identifiers
Device identifiers/serial numbers
Web Universal Resource Locators (WURLS)
Internet Protocol (IP) address numbers
Biometric identifiers (including finger and voice prints)
Full face photographic images and any comparable images

The privacy to subject information that HIPAA commands is not totally unjustified, especially in the world of telecommunication we live in. However, it will put a great burden on investigators and sponsors who conduct clinical research in the process of new product development. This could delay the research progress that brings new products in the pharmaceutical field to market. One of the biggest obstacles in completing clinical research in a timely manner is the difficulty of adequate subject recruitment. HIPAA is another obstacle that could interfere with this essential step in conducting clinical research.

Possible solutions in overcoming this could be a two step authorization:

1. Giving initial authorization to permit investigators to use PHI to identify potential subjects that would meet the selection criteria as stated in a clinical protocol.

2. Giving authorization to allow study sponsors or others to disclose PHI. This information could be specifically directed in order to allow subjects to be enrolled in a clinical trial.

In summary, HIPAA is here to stay, and the most efficient way to act on it would be to create a HIPAA questionnaire that could be used on its own or incorporated into an informed consent. For now, sufficient assistance is available through the Internet to help guide and answer HIPAA questions (6,7).

REFERENCES

1. Privacy Rule guidance posted on the website for the NIH, which was approved by the Office of Civil Rights (http://www1.od.nih.gov/osp/ospp/hipaa/faq.asp and FDA April 7 response to the Internation Pharmaceutical Privacy Consortium).
2. HIPAA Informed Consent/Authorization Form (http://www.fda.gov).
3. Privacy Regulation. http://www.hhs.gov/ocr/hipaa/.
4. DHHS Fact Sheet. Protecting the Privacy of Subjects' Health Information. http://www.fda.gov.
5. Office of Civil Rights guidance. Standards for Privacy of Individually Identifiable Health Information. http://www.fda.gov.
6. Subscribe for updates on HIPAA documents and events. http://www.fda.gov.
7. www.urac.org.

25
Working with a CRO

Duane B. Lakings
Drug Safety Evaluation Consulting, Inc., Elgin, Texas, U.S.A.

PART I. CONTRACT RESEARCH ORGANIZATIONS (CROs)

I. INTRODUCTION

The use of CROs in discovery, nonclinical, clinical, and manufacturing drug development programs—or outsourcing, as the process is commonly referred to by the industry—is a common practice of many pharmaceutical and most biotechnology companies. At present, more than 450 CROs exist in the United States and Europe and the use of their services for all aspects of the drug discovery and development process is rising. The growth of outsourcing is expected to continue, with some CROs offering a complete drug development support system, from synthesis and characterization of the drug substance to conducting phase 3 safety and efficacy human trials and preparing NDA documents for submission to regulatory agencies. Other CROs specialize in selected aspects of the drug characterization process, offering services in such areas as pharmacology animal model development and implementation, formulation development and drug substance and drug product stability testing, bioanalytical method development and validation, or clinical trial protocol preparation and study support, such as site and investigator selection or data management.

This chapter discusses the processes commonly used to select a CRO for the nonclinical and clinical biological stages of drug development and the requirements for obtaining an appropriately completed study at a CRO. The processes and requirements for outsourcing the manufacturing program for a drug substance and the preparation and testing of a drug product are also areas of high growth and a number of CROs offer these services. However, the outsourcing of manufacturing processes, including the preparation of the chemistry, manufacturing, and control section for regulatory submissions, is not covered in this chapter.

II. NONCLINICAL CONTRACT RESEARCH
ORGANIZATIONS

A pharmaceutical or biotechnology company identifies a lead candidate that mediates a human disease and then conducts the required, GLP-driven preclinical research studies to obtain an IND, followed by the nonclinical and clinical studies necessary for an NDA submission. For several reasons, corporate management may decide to have some or all of these studies performed at a CRO. The drug development project team is informed of this management decision and is usually given the responsibility of coordinating the outsourcing program, as well as the internal research studies, and of ensuring that the development program stays on time and on track. For a small biotechnology company, this responsibility may fall on the shoulders of a single individual or a small group of two or three researchers, who need to have a good understanding of each of the scientific disciplines for which outsourced studies are being considered. A common practice for many biotechnology firms is to contract with a consultant or a consulting firm to assist in outsourcing, including the selection and management of the service providers and the review of generated results and study reports.

The first requirement for a successful program at a CRO is to identify which research studies or aspects of the nonclinical drug development program are to be conducted at a CRO. Then the projected time line for initiation and completion of the studies is needed so that results and technical or study reports are available at the appropriate time for decision making and regulatory agency submissions. As discussed in the chapter on project teams, a well-constructed drug development plan provides much of this information. The project team members whose scientific disciplines are part of the outsourcing program are typically assigned as scientific experts and the project team coordinator is given responsibility for contractual arrangements. These subproject teams need first to identify and then to select the appropriate CRO or CROs to conduct the desired research studies. These teams also need to monitor the CRO(s) to ensure that the studies are being conducted as designed and described in the study protocol and that the generated results are appropriately recorded in both the study records and the study report. The following sections provide more details on the CRO selection and monitoring processes for nonclinical drug development research studies.

A. CRO Identification and Selection

After a pharmaceutical or biotechnology company, commonly referred to as the sponsor, has decided to use CROs to support some or all of the nonclinical research effort in a drug development program, management or the project team responsible for the development of the drug candidate assigns individuals to identify and select the appropriate CROs. The steps in a selection process should include, but are not be limited to:

1. Preparing the study designs for each of the research studies to be outsourced. The more details provided in the study designs, the better. The CROs use the provided information to prepare a draft study protocol and a proposal with time and cost estimates. Examples of two study designs are shown in Table 1.

2. Determining which CROs should be considered as potential contractors. This aspect of the selection process is discussed in more detail below.

3. Soliciting cost and time proposals for each study design from each CRO. Generally three to five CROs that have the necessary expertise to complete the study successfully are requested to submit proposals for each study design.

4. Evaluating the proposals, which includes determining if the CRO understands the study design, and selecting those CROs to be considered further. At times, CROs will recommend additions to the study design, which may or may not improve the overall study and could provide additional information for the complete characterization of the drug candidate. When this occurs, the sponsor needs to evaluate critically the expanded study and determine if the increased costs, and possibly extended study duration, justify the additions to the study design.

5. Scheduling and conducting site visits to ensure that the CROs are qualified and have the facilities and personnel necessary to conduct the research studies. These site visits include assessments of GLP compliance, SOPs, and computer validation.

6. Negotiating time and cost for completion of the research studies. The original estimate in the proposal is usually not the final cost of conducting a research study at a CRO. Those CROs still on the short list should be asked to provide their "best and final" cost, the dates they can actually initiate the study, and the date they project the draft final report will be available for review. Some consulting firms specialize in this phase of interacting with CROs and will negotiate with the CROs for the sponsor, thus relieving the sponsor of the problems that can occur by pushing for the best price. As payment, these firms receive a percentage of the difference between the orig-

Table 1 Study Design Examples for Contract Research Organization Time and Cost Proposal Preparation

28–Day Toxicology in a Nonrodent Species

Purpose: To evaluate the toxicology of a protein test article in a nonrodent species after every-other-day subcutaneous dosing for 28 days

Test Species:	Beagle dog
Test article:	Protein therapeutic
Dose levels:	300, 100, 30, and 10 µg/kg plus vehicle control
Frequency:	Every other day (EOD), 14 doses total
Administration:	Subcutaneous, bolus injection; dosing solutions to be prepared daily; duplicate aliquots of each formulation level collected predose and postdose for the first, seventh, and thirteenth dose to be analyzed (using a validated analytical chemistry method to be transferred to the service provider) for test article concentration
Number:	Three animals per sex per dose group with four dose groups and a vehicle control group (30 animals total)
Evaluation:	Clinical signs of toxicity during in-life phase including general health, body weight, food consumption; clinical pathology (standard hematology, clinical chemistry, urinalysis parameters) predose, after fourth, seventh, and fourteenth doses; gross pathology including selected organ weights; histopathology at all dose levels
Toxicokinetics:	Blood specimens collected after the first, seventh, and thirteenth dose to be analyzed (using a validated bioanalytical chemistry method to be transferred to the service provider) for test article concentration to assess extent of exposure
Antibodies:	Blood specimens collected prior to the first, seventh, and fourteenth dose to be analyzed (using a developed assay to be transferred to the service provider) for antibodies to the test article
Timeline:	Projected start date and estimated completion date

Absolute Bioavailability, Pharmacokinetics, and Dose Proportionality in a Nonrodent Species

Purpose: To evaluate the absolute bioavailability and pharmacokinetics, including dose proportionality, of a small organic molecule drug candidate in a nonhuman primate

Test Species:	Rhesus monkey
Test article:	Small organic molecule, molecular weight less than 350
Route:	Intravenous, 100, 30, 10, and 3 µg/kg (or other dose range) Oral, 1,000, 300, 100, and 10 µg/kg (or other dose range)

Table 1 Continued

Frequency:	Multiple using balanced, crossover design with 7-day washout period between doses
Administration:	Intravenous, slow bolus injection at about 1 ml/min
	Oral, gavage
	Duplicate aliquots of each formulation collected predose and postdose to be analyzed (using a validated analytical chemistry method to be transferred to the service provider) for test article concentration
Number:	Equal to number of doses in crossover design
Specimens:	Blood for plasma; sufficient number to characterize the absorption, distribution, and disposition phases of the test article
	Possible series: 0, 5, 10, 20, 30, 45, 60, 90, 120, 180, 240, 360, 480, 720, and 1,440 minutes for intravenous doses and 0, 15, 30, 45, 60, 90, 120, 150, 180, 240, 300, 360, 480, 720, and 1,440 minutes for oral doses
	Urine; sufficient number of intervals to characterize the rate and extent of urinary elimination of the test article
	Possible series: 0–2, 2–4, 4–8, 8–12, and 12–24 hours for both routes
Bioanalytical:	Validated assay for plasma and urine specimens from rats to be cross-species validated by the service provider
Stability:	Test article stability in collected specimens to be determined from time of collection to projected time of analysis
Analyses:	Individual analytical runs to include all specimens of a given matrix for a test species or 30 plasma unknowns per run
Timeline:	Projected start date and estimated completion date

inal estimate and the final bid. The difference between original and final bids can be large, sometimes hundreds of thousands of dollars, for some studies such as carcinogenicity testing.

7. Selecting the CROs and awarding the contracts for each study to be outsourced.

The number of person-hours required for the identification and selection process depends on the size of the research program to be contracted. Normally, a minimum of 1 or 2 person-weeks is necessary to evaluate three or four CROs for each research study to be outsourced. This effort can be substantially reduced by the placement of more than one study at a CRO. Many biotechnology companies and some pharmaceutical firms use consultants or consulting firms to assist them in the CRO selection process. However, these firms need to ensure that the consultants have both expertise in scientific disciplines for the studies being outsourced and knowledge of how CROs operate. A common mistake is to hire a consultant with expertise in the disease area of the drug candidate but not in the nonclinical drug development process, or conversely, in regulatory compliance but not in the science necessary successfully to characterize a drug candidate. The sponsor should evaluate and select consultants who have the necessary knowledge of drug development and contract research to enhance the chance of a successful outsourcing program.

Pharmaceutical and biotechnology companies commonly use one of three strategies to identify CROs. These strategies can be designated virtual company, preselected, and special study.

1. Virtual Company Strategy

The virtual company strategy is used by companies, mostly biotechnology firms and many United States and European subsidiaries of Japanese pharmaceutical firms that do not have the infrastructure or resources to conduct GLP-regulated nonclinical research studies necessary to support regulatory agency submissions. The primary benefit of this outsourcing approach is that the various expertises, such as toxicologist, pathologist, and drug metabolism expert, and the infrastructure, such as facilities, quality assurance, and GLP compliance, needed to support regulated studies can be devoted to completing nonclinical development studies. This means the sponsoring company does not have to build the in-house groups and facilities necessary for ensuring GLP compliance and thus can avoid costly time delays. A primary limitation to this strategy is that the sponsoring company can be vulnerable to poor CRO selection or to mismanagement by the CRO. However, by using experts or consultants appropriately to assist in the identification and selection process and the monitoring aspects, discussed in the following section, a sponsor can usually avoid this limitation.

2. Preselected Strategy

In the preselected strategy, the first choice of many large and midsized pharmaceutical houses, a limited number—usually three to six—of CROs are prequalified to support a company's possible nonclinical drug development needs. The qualification process usually includes a detailed site visit to review the CRO's facilities, staff, and GLP compliance and to determine which types of nonclinical research studies, such as toxicology, drug metabolism, and formulation development, can be placed at the CRO. At times, long-term contracts are defined in which the CRO guarantees the sponsoring company a certain level of resources to be available to support projects and the company guarantees to provide a sufficient number of research studies to use effectively the committed resources. This strategy can provide a synergistic working relationship between the sponsoring company and the CRO, which in essence becomes an integral part of the development processes of the sponsor. The major drawback to the preselected CRO strategy is the unnecessary limitation of outsourcing. If a fairly large number of CROs, say 30, have the necessary expertise to conduct a nonclinical study or group of studies but the sponsoring company prequalified list contains only three CROs with the required expertise, the other 27 are not considered, even though some may be able complete the studies faster and cheaper or may have superior expertise and experience in the drug candidate's therapeutic area.

3. Special Study Strategy

The final strategy, the special study strategy, is used by some sponsoring companies to place single or a few nonclinical research studies with a CRO. If a company's internal resources are usually, but not always, sufficient to meet their nonclinical drug development needs, this strategy provides a means to have a critical study completed to meet the time line on a drug development plan. However, some companies use the special study strategy for all their nonclinical drug development needs and then attempt to integrate the results of the independent studies into a drug development story. For a company with substantial drug development expertise, this strategy may work but requires considerable effort in identifying and selecting CROs, in monitoring the various CROs, and in synthesizing the results from the various research studies. Contract research organizations are generally not in favor of this strategy because they become only "a pair of hands," have little understanding of the overall development program, and thus cannot provide the sponsoring company with their considerable expertise.

Whichever strategy is used, the sponsor should carefully select the CRO to conduct a nonclinical drug development study. One poorly conducted study can delay the drug development process until the study has been repeated and the results integrated into the overall story. If this delay is for a research study on the critical path, the projected time for regulatory agency submission has to be changed, thus delaying the date of approval for marketing and resulting in lost revenue for the sponsoring company.

B. CRO Monitoring

The identification and selection process is only the first step. The second aspect involves monitoring and managing the CROs to ensure that the outsourced research studies are conducted according to the study protocol, that

Table 2 Nonclinical Study Protocol Items Commonly Included in a CRO Conducted Research Study

Protocol title:	Descriptive title of the nonclinical research study
Objective:	Purpose of conducting the study
Study location:	Where and by whom the study is to be conducted
Sponsor:	Company that is sponsoring the study
Study monitor:	Sponsor's agent who is responsible for monitoring the study
Personnel:	CRO senior staff who will responsible for the various aspects of the study
Study dates:	Dates when the study is scheduled to be initiated, when the in-life phase is to be completed, and when the draft final report will be available for review
Compliance:	Statements on which regulatory guidelines, such as 21 CFR 58 for FDA GLP compliance, will be followed and on Animal Care Committee protocol review
Test article:	Information on the drug substance, which commonly includes the test article name or number, identification criteria, physical description, who is responsible for test article characterization, the concentration(s) to be used, recommended storage conditions, inventory maintenance, formulation procedures, reserve samples, retention samples, analyses for content and homogenity (if necessary), disposition, and safety precautions
Test species:	Information on the animal species to be studied, animal husbandry procedures such as housing, food, water, contaminants, environmental conditions, acclimation, and justification of selection
Study design:	Description of the number of test species groups, the dosage level to be administered to each group, the test article concentration or amount to be administered, the number of animals of each sex in each dose group
Assignment:	Statement on how animals will be assigned or randomized to each of the dose groups
Dose preparation:	Description of how the test article will be prepared for administration to the test species
Route of dosing:	Statements on how the test article will be administered, the frequency of dosing, and a justification for the selected route and dose levels

Table 2 Continued

Clinical observations:	Descriptions of how frequently the test species will be observed and what specific clinical signs are to be recorded in addition to unspecified signs
Body weights:	Information on how often the test species will be weighed during the in-life phase of the study
Food consumption:	Information on how food consumption will be determined
Physical exam:	Description of how often physical examinations will be conducted and by whom
Blood collection:	Information on when blood specimens will be collected for hematology, clinical chemistry, and toxicokinetics
Hematology:	Description of hematology tests to be conducted
Clinical chemistry:	Description of clinical chemistry parameters to be determined
Toxicokinetics:	Description of how blood specimens are to be processed and analyzed for test article concentration, including information on the testing laboratory, assay procedure, and storage and shipping procedures
Euthanasia:	Information on how the test species will be sacrificed at the end of the in-life phase of the study
Moribund or found dead animals:	Statements on how animals found moribund or dead during the in-life phase will be handled
Necropsy:	Information on the procedures to be used during necropsy
Organ weights:	Description of which organs are to be weighed and the procedures used to prepare organs for weighing and fixing for histopathological examination
Histopathology:	Statements on which dose levels, if not all dose levels, and which tissues will be examined and how the information will be recorded by the pathologist doing the reading
Statistical analysis:	Information on the statistical tests that will be performed on the results
Reports:	Description of what information will be included in the study report to be submitted to the sponsor
Raw data:	Information on how, where, and for how long raw data will be stored
Approvals:	Signatures of a sponsor representative, commonly the study monitor, the study director, and a corporate officer of the CRO

the results are obtained with appropriate techniques and procedures, and that the generated data are correctly recorded and documented in the study report. Monitoring studies at CROs should include, but are not limited to:

1. Reviewing and approving the study protocols prepared by the CROs and detailing the procedures to be followed to complete the study designs. The study protocol should provide information on all aspects of the study. Commonly included items in a nonclinical study protocol are listed in Table 2.

2. Monitoring various aspects during the research phase of each study. Each item listed in Table 2 is a possible point for potential study monitoring. Monitoring will ensure that the data collected are appropriately documented and do not contain "surprises" that can prevent the results from being used to support submissions to regulatory agencies.

3. When "surprises" do happen, and most outsourced studies will have at least one surprise, interacting with the CRO to characterize the problem or protocol deviation and to effectively correct the surprise or to amend the study protocol to document the problem and the solution.

4. Assisting in the evaluation and interpretation of results to ensure that the data are analytically acceptable and correctly correlated to tell the story of the experimental results.

5. Reviewing technical reports to ensure that the information provided accurately reflects the generated results, documents any deviation from the study protocols, and gives appropriate conclusions.

The number of person-hours required to monitor appropriately a research study conducted by a CRO again depends on the size of the outsourced research program. Normally, a minimum of 1 person-week for each in-life phase month of a research study is required and includes the time necessary to review and approve the study report. As noted above, some firms use consultants or consulting firms to assist with CRO monitoring and management and to ensure that the studies are conducted according to GLP guidelines. These consultants should be specialists in the scientific disciplines for the conducted studies. Having a toxicologist or pharmacologist consultant monitor the bioanalytical chemistry program to support a pharmacokinetic research study could result in an assay that is inappropriately validated or implemented and thus not capable of analyzing specimens for drug and drug metabolite concentrations.

III. CONCLUSION

This part of the chapter has provided information on the selection and monitoring aspects of conducting nonclinical research studies at CROs. By carefully evaluating and selecting CROs and then managing them during and after the study, the sponsoring firm can obtain the information needed to characterize their drug candidate and prepare the necessary submissions to regulatory agencies. A close partnering between the sponsor, or its designated agents, and the CRO is very important to ensure that the research studies are conducted as designed and within the planned time frame and budget.

PART II. CLINICAL CONTRACT RESEARCH ORGANIZATIONS

I. INTRODUCTION

The clinical portion of a drug development program constitutes the most labor-intensive and costly phase of drug development. Even large pharmaceutical companies sometimes find themselves understaffed and thus unable to embrace some aspects of a particular clinical development program. This situation is even more acute in most small biotechnology companies. If senior management in the sponsor company is not willing to support permanent increases in staff to accommodate the program's needs, or if sufficient numbers of qualified staff cannot be recruited and hired soon enough, the sponsor company will frequently turn to a CRO for the solution. The trend is increasingly in this direction and thus managers and directors of clinical programs need to adapt to this new way of conducting clinical research programs.

When properly managed, CRO services can provide a cost-effective solution and thereby enhance the ability of the sponsor team to achieve the corporate goals that are typically defined by time and budget constraints. However, if the relationship is mismanaged, valuable time and money will be wasted. A common reason for failure, probably the most common, is ineffective communication. Effective communication between the sponsor and the CRO has to occur at all stages of the relationship, including

1. At the onset, when the scope of the project is being defined and a CRO is being chosen.

2. During the conduct of the project, which includes collection and evaluation of the generated data for inclusion into the study report.

3. After completion of the study, when the study report is being drafted by the sponsor, the CRO, or a scientific writer.

Each of these phases of the relationship will be discussed in turn, with an emphasis on ways to achieve effective communication and a successful relationship.

II. DEFINING THE SCOPE AND CHOOSING A CRO

An entire clinical development program usually spans several years and includes many individual studies. Most sponsors will use CROs for some portion of the clinical development program but rarely for creating the overall development plan. Nevertheless, if a particular CRO has established experience in a particular therapeutic area, this service provider may be helpful in providing an independent assessment of draft plans prepared by the sponsor.

Contract research organizations can provide services for clinical trials whether they are the simplest phase 1 safety and tolerance studies or complex, multicenter phase 3 efficacy and safety studies. Table 3 identifies specific activities that may be considered for outsourcing. These activities are grouped according to four major categories: management of the study conduct at clinical sites, data management, data evaluation, and summarization.

The scope of the work to be outsourced is driven by the specific needs of the sponsor. In some instances all aspects of a particular study will need to be outsourced. In other instances, CROs are needed to provide only specific services to complement an almost complete team within the sponsor company.

Table 3 Scoping Out the Project

Prepare or review overall clinical development plan

Management of clinical study conduct
Protocol writing
   Site selection
   Investigator meetings
   Monitoring
      —site initiations and close-outs
      —primary and secondary monitoring
GCP audits
Data management
   Case report form design
   Database design
   Data entry
Data evaluation
   Programming for data listing and summary tables
   Statistical analyses and interpretation
Data summarization
   Medical interpretation
   Scientific writing

The bulk of the contracts awarded to CROs deal with one or more of the most labor-intensive portions of clinical research, namely, clinical monitoring of study sites, data entry, programming for data listings and summary tables, and writing clinical study reports.

Whatever the scope of the project, clear communication of the exact work plan is enhanced by providing a detailed description of the activities and the expectations. Merely listing activities, as presented in Table 3, is grossly inadequate and will result in numerous iterations in contract proposals as the CROs request more specific instructions and rework their proposals accordingly. Some questions to be considered when providing details of the work plan and deciding which CRO to select are as follows:

1. Does the CRO have experience in the particular therapeutic area under development? This is not always an absolute requirement but may be a strength when comparing CROs.

2. Does the CRO have access to the subject or patient population needed for the trial? For example, some CROs maintain specific patient pools, such as patients with hepatic impairment or renal impairment, which are often needed for clinical pharmacology studies.

3. If the study being outsourced is a pharmacokinetic or clinical pharmacology study, does the CRO have bioanalytical chemistry laboratory facilities and expertise appropriate for the analysis of plasma, serum, or other physiological fluid samples for the desired analyte(s)? Can your bioanalytical chemistry methods be transferred to their laboratories and validated or will samples be shipped to the sponsor or to another CRO that has the necessary method(s) up and running for analysis?

4. If the CRO is to prepare the detailed clinical protocol, are there other protocols from the same program that can be used as template?

5. Do you want the CRO to assist or participate in the investigator meeting?

6. If the CRO will be monitoring the study at the clincal site(s), will they be doing all of the monitoring for all sites or will some sponsor personnel also be monitoring?

7. If the trial is international, can the CRO provide monitoring services (or other services) in all jurisdictions? If a decision is made to work with separate CROs in each country, be sure to recognize the sponsor effort needed for coordination of all CROs.

8. Will the CRO be providing primary or secondary monitoring, or both?

9. When will the CRO get involved with sites—before site initiation or after selection and initiation are completed by the sponsor?

10. Who wil be negotiating the investigator grants for each clinical site, the CRO or the sponsor?

11. Will the CRO be asked to conduct GLP and GCP audits for selected clinical sites?

12. If the CRO is to design the case report forms, is there a set from a similar study that can be used as a template?

13. If the CRO will be asked to design the database, will the CRO need to standardize certain aspects with existing databases to allow them to be combined later? If so, provide some details on the required structure.

14. Have data conventions been established for other studies in the clinical program for a particular drug candidate that will need to be followed for this new study?

15. What are the standard procedures of the CRO for handling queries and corrections to the database?

16. What audit trail will be created to document data conventions and database corrections?

17. Has the CRO ever been audited by the FDA or other regulatory agency?

18. Will an independent GCP audit of the CRO's activities be undertaken?

19. If the CRO is asked to program data listings and summary tables, how many such listings and tables are expected? Do templates or examples exist from other clinical studies in the same program?

20. Are the final deliverables clear to all parties? For example, do you expect to receive the programs (for example, the SAS code) used to run the statistical analyses?

21. Does the CRO have experienced staff to provide statistical or medical interpretation of the data?

22. If the CRO is to write the clinical study report, does the sponsor have a standard template to be followed?

23. What word processing program is required? What are the expectations regarding in-text tables? Can they be imported directly from SAS, for example, or will significant word processing be required for new formats?

24. How many drafts are expected for a study report?

25. What are the time constraints for the activities being outsourced? Which dates are not negotiable? Which are subject to some flexibility?

26. Can the CRO offer assurance that personnel will be dedicated to your project?

27. What is the experience level of the specific individuals who will be assigned to your project?

28. Can the CRO provide names of previous customers with whom you can speak directly and privately?

29. What are the provisions in the proposed contract that deal with cost overruns and substantial increases in workload above what was originally anticipated?

30. What are the procedures for changing the scope of the project?

31. Does the CRO have the capacity to add more resources to the project if necessary?

32. How important is this project to the CRO? Is there a risk that your project will suffer because of competition for resources for higher status projects from other companies?

33. What are the provisions in the contract for dealing with poor performance?

34. Are the financial terms of the contract acceptable to the sponsor? How much is paid up front versus upon completion of major milestones?

35. Should the financial terms include penalties for significantly missed milestones or incentives for milestones completed ahead of schedule?

36. If the CRO is providing only selected activities to support a clincal study, how will the overall project be managed? Will a formal joint team be established with regular meetings?

37. How frequently will status reports be required from the CRO? Do these reports need to be written or verbal?

38. Will all contact be directed through one person in the sponsor company? How accessible to the CRO will other key personnel in the sponsor company be?

III. WORKING WITH THE CRO

The start-up of the relationship requires a considerable amount of time from sponsor personnel to ensure that the scope of the work is fully understood and that standards are clear. This highly interactive phase of the relationship may be ill-timed, unfortunately, because most companies decide to use CROs only after all possibilities of using internal resources have been exhausted, which often means that the sponsor personnel themselves are exhausted too! The sponsor staff may have a tremendous desire to hand off the project completely, and as quickly as possible, to the CRO but this will not be in the best interest of the project. Whereas working with a CRO can be an efficient way to expand the project's human resources rapidly, the sponsor needs to recognize that internal resources will still be needed. With such significant investments in clinical programs, it would be penny-wise and pound-foolish for sponsor management not to ensure that sufficient personnel exist in-house to oversee the performance of the CRO.

Usually one individual in the CRO and one in the sponsor company are given project management responsibilities for the contract activities. However, this should not be interpreted narrowly to mean that all communication has to go through these two individuals. Other individuals in each organization should have direct access to their counterparts in the other company for clarification of specific details. Joint working teams that discuss the details of the project at the level of implementation will enhance the quality of the communication between companies and increase the likelihood of the project's success.

The most effective working relationships are forged when the sponsor views the CRO staff as an extension of its own in-house team. If the CRO is providing supplemental services to complement an in-house study team (for example, providing additional clinical monitors or handling the data management and statistics for a trial that is monitored by the sponsor), then regularly scheduled joint team meetings will foster effective communication and standardization of efforts. Face-to-face meetings are ideal but not always possible, given the geographical distances existing between some parties. Teleconferences and videoconferences can be very effective. If the CRO is responsible for the entire conduct of a study, then regular update meetings are necessary to review progress and modify the activities as necessary to achieve the time and cost goals.

Even with the best intentions and careful review of the contract, either party may find, part of the way through the activities, that the scope, and perhaps the time line and cost estimates, need to be revised. Provisions for how to approach such discussions should be provided in the contract and these discussions may be best handled by senior management in both companies to preserve the working relationships of the members of any joint working teams.

Returning to the clinical activities listed in Table 3, some thoughts on the level of support that is realistic to obtain from CROs are as follows. A number of the labor-intensive activities, such as monitoring, auditing, database management, programming for listing and tables, and statistical interpretation, are relatively easy to outsource. Many CROs will have the necessary experience and capacity for these activities.

Protocol writing and case report form design go hand in hand and most CROs can handle these activities. But the sponsor should lead the strategic discussions on the study design and the statistical plan, taking into consideration the overall clinical development plan, which may include other indications, and the commercial objectives of the company. A high level of sponsor involvement in designing the study will increase the "ownership" of the project by the internal clinical team, even if 95% of the activities for running the trial are handled by contract services. This ownership is important to maintain throughout the trial, because in the end, the sponsor personnel will be defending the data to regulatory authorities such as the FDA.

Some CROs can be very helpful in identifying qualified clinical sites if they have previous experience in a particular therapeutic area. This can be of great use to small companies that are just starting new clinical development programs.

The process of data summarization, encompassing both medical interpretation and scientific writing, can be one of the more challenging aspects of a clinical program. The greater the level of sponsor involvement in these activities, the more internal ownership is reinforced and the sponsor is better able to defend the data. This is not to say that CROs cannot play an important role in these steps. Contract research organizations that have medically trained personnel with expertise in particular therapeutic areas can be an excellent resource for small companies that may have no internal medical staff.

Highly skilled medical writers are currently a limited commodity and difficult to recruit for most companies. Furthermore, the writing process itself is very time-consuming. For both of these reasons, companies are seeking these experts more and more through contract services, where the scientific writer is either an independent contractor or an employee of a CRO. If the sponsor has no medical writers, then having the CRO or an independent scientific writer complete the report might be best. However, the sponsor should seek medical interpretation from the sponsor clinical team, as necessary. If the sponsor does have experienced medical writers but the volume of work is too much, then a CRO or independent contractor could provide valuable assistance for the most labor-intensive parts of the writing, for example, by providing first and second drafts of the report. The sponsor team could then take over the report and provide the finishing "polish" on the interpretation of the data and standardization with reports for other trials in the same program.

IV. CONCLUSION

An effective relationship with a CRO is in some ways like a marriage. The key to success is open and honest communication, clear division of responsibilities, and patience while the relationship evolves into maturity. Once a match has been made, knowledge acquired in the first successful project can carry forward to subsequent contracts and efficiencies are then realized for both organizations. Many companies are finding it to their advantage to consider long-term relationships with desirable CROs, in which both parties provide some level of commitment to future projects, even before the exact details of those projects are known. Both parties benefit from such arrangements. The CRO can better manage personnel requirements when future contracts are guaranteed and the sponsor has the security of knowing that qualified resources will be available.

26

The Evolving SMO in the United States

Kenneth A. Getz
CenterWatch, Inc., Boston, Massachusetts, U.S.A.

I. INTRODUCTION

The past decade has not been smooth sailing for site management organizations (SMOs), by any stretch. Since 1997, the SMO market has been consolidating rapidly. Large numbers of SMO companies have exited the business owing to extremely slow adoption rates of their services, cash flow difficulties, and high operating costs. Yet, during the past 24 months, the SMO market has hit an inflection point, as growth is now accelerating.

Select SMOs have stayed the course and have carefully pursued business strategies designed to maintain financial stability and achieve higher levels of operating efficiency and performance effectiveness. Existing and new entrants are driving consolidation, international expansion, and diversification into a variety of service areas supporting study conduct. Approximately $250 million in sponsor grants was paid to SMOs in 2002.

Among a highly diverse collection of study conduct service providers—from academic medical centers to dedicated and part-time independent investigative sites—SMOs appear well positioned to meet growing demands for faster development cycle time, improved data quality, and controlled clinical trial costs. Conceptually, SMOs vie to support their positioning through the following mechanisms:

Centralized clinical research operations
Standardized contracts and operating procedures
Trained and accredited staff

New technologies to manage information and to track performance
Systematic management of patient recruitment and retention
Systematic management of clinical data
Streamlined regulatory and legal review and approval processes
Reduced fixed costs to offer more competitive pricing
Applied business and management principles

Industry insiders and observers now widely agree that the current operating environment for developing drugs and medical devices may drive biopharmaceutical companies and contract research organizations (CROs) to continue to expand their usage of site management organizations.

II. TODAY'S CLINICAL RESEARCH ENVIRONMENT

Most biopharmaceutical companies currently maintain a lean infrastructure, having faced several years of layoffs and attrition. Sponsors are now pursuing a complex array of strategies designed to drive sales growth and improve financial conditions. Promotional spending on marketed drugs is now growing at a much faster rate than is R&D spending. During the past five years, for example, R&D spending has grown 11% annually. In that same period, promotional spending, which reached nearly $26 billion in 2002, has grown 18% annually.

During the past several years, biopharmaceutical companies have modified their R&D strategies owing to a shortage of blockbuster NCE candidates and a strong desire to minimize large investments in risky, marginal development projects. Although the total number of new chemical entities in the R&D pipeline is growing by 12% annually, because of the impact of various discovery technologies, including high throughput screening, combinatorial chemistry, and genomics, the proportion of drug candidates entering clinical phases is actually declining.

Clinical research sponsors recognize the importance of maintaining a full pipeline of innovative medical therapies. Yet they are increasingly aware of their limited resources and financial pressures. Overall, $34 billion was spent on R&D in 2002. Spending as a percentage age of drug sales, however, has been declining steadily, as companies must reallocate their resources to improve their own financial performance. Whereas nearly 20% of every revenue dollar went into research and development each year between 1995 to 1998, between 1999 to 2002, 17% of sales went into R&D annually.

Development and approval cycle times continue to accelerate as sponsors push to achieve higher levels of performance. Drugs approved between 1994 and 1998 took 7.25 years to get there; this is compared with 5.92 years for drugs approved between 1999 and 2001. The FDA continues to improve its efficiency, and much of this is due to the impact of the User Fee Act. Between 1985 and 1988, the median approval time was 2.64 years, for example. Between 1999 and 2001, the agency took 1.15 years on average to approve an investigational drug. This represents a 56% improvement over 1985 levels.

This past year, major biopharmaceutical companies spent more than $9 billion on US clinical research activities. Within clinical research, phase I–III spending is growing at 12% annually, and phase IV spending is growing at nearly double that rate. Post-approval research programs—largely conducted among community-based clinical investigators—are designed to maximize a drug's performance in the market and to expand a drug's positioning after it has been introduced to prescribing physicians.

Sponsors have been actively improving and refining internal and contract service management operations. In 2002, nearly all of the top 20 pharmaceutical companies reported that they now manage their study monitors regionally. With regional structures in place, sponsor companies hope to interact more closely and responsively with their investigative sites in order to accelerate how studies are implemented and patients enrolled. Biopharmaceutical companies believe that effective partnerships with world-class investigative sites, including top SMOs, hold the key to continued drug development success. The study conduct arena offers many opportunities for incremental improvements in the clinical research process, from site selection through IRB approval, patient recruitment, retention, and enrollment, through data collection and management. In 2002, sponsor companies spent more than $4 billion on clinical research study grants to investigative sites, and a growing percentage of this total was allocated to SMOs.

Historically, sponsors and CROs have not completely understood, nor fully embraced, the SMO concept. The scope of most major clinical development projects often prevents sponsors and CROs from ever using SMOs as one-stop sources for study conduct services. As a result, sponsors typically apply a multivendor approach to working with SMOs. Biopharmaceutical companies appear reluctant to discard traditional site selection and site management practices. They now look to pick up a larger number of SMO sites, provided the sponsors continues to have direct relationships with each investigative site. This fragmented approach to working with SMOs' negates SMOs' ability to provide operating efficiencies across a large network of controlled research centers.

Whereas SMOs were used on 17% of clinical projects in 1999, sponsor and CRO companies report that they used SMOs on 23% of their projects in 2001. Other noteworthy findings on sponsor usage of SMOs include

> Sponsor and CRO companies report that SMOs are involved in more than two out of five clinical projects, 70% of them in phase III programs.

Almost two-thirds of sponsors and CROs report that their use of SMOs increased within the past two years.

The largest average number of SMO sites used in a single study is 15. For a given clinical study, about 20% of total investigative sites are from an SMO.

About 3 in 10 companies claim to now have a dedicated individual working with SMOs.

III. SMOs—CONSOLIDATION AND INTEGRATION PROVIDERS

Given the rich variety of study conduct business models in operation, industry has had a hard time reaching a consensus around a single definition of the SMO. The following are general characteristics of all SMOs:

1. They are business enterprises with multiple study conduct locations (regional and national).
2. They are managed centrally by a corporate structure.
3. They offer a full range of study conduct services, including, at times, both project management and study conduct services.
4. They focus on providing two primary assets: a large and diverse group of physicians and patients, and clean clinical study data.

Site management organizations have aggressive aims to reengineer and overhaul the clinical development process through consolidating the fragmented and unsophisticated market for site services. They hope to offer sponsors and CROs access to a consolidated base of investigators, quicker study start-up, faster time to study completion, and cleaner data. A major aspect of an SMO's strategy is to leverage various information technologies to improve the capture rate and management control of study data.

The corporate offices of SMOs typically handle a wide range of study conduct activities that are best provided through a systematic and centralized approach. These activities include regulatory and legal affairs, sales and marketing, business development, strategic planning and market research, contract and budget negotiations and approval, patient recruitment, and management operations (e.g., administrative, finance, IS, and human resources).

The traditional approach to monitoring has proved greatly inefficient. The typical study monitor travels as much as 75% of the time. This leads to "CRA burnout" and the challenge of replacing and training new CRA staff. Most importantly, it leads to costly delays related to poor data monitoring, interpretation, and follow-up. Site management organizations and site networks are looking at new approaches, through the use of technologies and internal staffing, to improve study-monitoring effectiveness. Regionally based in-house staff to provide monitoring services and advanced auditing and data capture technologies are approaches being used.

There are four broad approaches that SMOs have taken to structure and suppot their investigative site networks. Most SMOs in operation today favor one approach over another, but many of them have built site networks composed of multiple approaches (e.g., predominantly owned sites with a loose affiliation component).

A. Corporate-owned model
B. Physician-owned affiliation model
C. Loose affiliation model
D. Hybrid model

A. Corporate-Owned Model

The SMOs in this group own and operate the sites in their network. These providers primarily vary by whether each site in its network has a staff physician serving as the principal investigator, or whether the center primarily contracts with area physicians to fill the role of the principal investigators. Corporate-owned SMO providers that do not have staff medical directors will typically staff each of their centers with a site manager, study coordinator(s), and, lately, patient recruitment specialists. Physicians are paid on a fee-for-service or hourly basis. Depending on the trial, patients are seen either at the physician's office or at the SMO's own facilities.

Wholly owned SMOs recruit patients through the contract physician's database but must also rely on media advertising and their own patient data bases, particularly if physicians are on staff and not maintaining a clinical practice.

The perceived strength of owned SMOs is the ability to control all aspects of the study-conduct process. Because the sites are owned, the company can manage operating centrally to ensure that the sites in its network meet the performance standards. The investigative sites share a common mission: to treat clinical research as a business. Site personnel are company employees. In addition, this model may offer higher profit margins.

One major weakness of the corporate or wholly owned SMO, relative to other SMO models, is its access to patients. Sites must advertise for a high percentage of patients, which can be both time-consuming and costly. Patients identified through the use of broad-based media may be less attractive to sponsors, who often prefer to test their drugs among "real patients" being treated in the context of regular clinical care. This model may pose higher fixed costs.

Another weakness applies to the corporate-owned SMOs that contract with area physicians. Although these providers are able to tap into a larger community of physicians, the investigators do not become part of the company's core resources.

B. Physician-Owned Affiliation Model

In order to join a physician-owned SMO, physicians typically purchase stock in the company. These physicians then share in the profits of the business, and if these SMOs enter the public markets, physician-owners stand to gain a considerable return on their initial investment.

The strength of this model is that investigators are practicing physicians. In terms of patient recruitment, this type of SMO has access to a greater number of patients through its members' patient databases. The SMO may supplement this core resource with advertising and its own corporate database, but the majority of the patients are likely to come from the physicians' own patient community.

The SMO can draw on its members' scientific expertise to provide the sponsor with protocol design services. For this reason, most of the physician-owned SMOs have their origins in a specific therapeutic area. During the past several years, physician-owned SMOs have emerged in areas that include urology, neurology, psychiatry, rheumatology, and infectious diseases. By contrast, corporate or wholly owned SMOs have been largely multispecialty.

Physician-owned SMOs also offer sponsors an opportunity to hire physicians who are involved in providing direct patient care. Investigators from these networks can provide insights and feedback into how the investigational drug might be integrated into a patient's overall health program.

A major weakness of the physician-owned SMO is that the company does not have tight control of its study conduct operations carried out at each investigative site in the network. The common difficulties in managing physicians have been well documented in a variety of settings, including HMOs, PPOs, and PPM groups. Study coordinators are employed by the investigator and hence are more difficult for a central office to manage. Because investigators and their staffs receive revenue from their clinical practices, there is also some question about their commitment and motivation to be top performers in conducting clinical studies.

This lack of control can make it difficult for physician-owned SMOs to ensure quality performance across all sites. If a site is slow to enroll patients or is generating CRFs with a high incidence of errors, physician-owned SMOs are not necessarily empowered to improve an individual site's performance quickly. This is particularly troublesome because in a large multicenter trial, success hinges on the worst-performing site. Data cannot be locked and analyzed until all the sites are closed. Physician-owned SMOs may not have the same ability to conduct studies quickly and produce clean data as do the wholly owned SMOs.

C. Loose Affiliation Model

In loosely affiliated site network SMOs, the corporate office identifies, negotiates, and secures study grants, and typically it provides a variety of management services, including marketing and sales support, information systems support, and staff training. However, the investigators do not have an ownership stake, nor do they have exclusive arrangements with the corporate SMO. Investigative sites in these networks may secure most of their grants directly from their own contacts within sponsors and CRO companies.

The key strength of the loosely affiliated network SMO is its size. These SMOs have access to a large number of investigative sites. Because the relationship to its investigators is a nonexclusive one, the loosely affiliated networks can sign up many sites and therefore can grow quickly with minimal capital investment. In this way, as sponsors' development needs change, the loosely affiliated network SMO may respond faster than other SMO models. The weakness in the loosely affiliated network SMOs is an even greater lack of control over the performance of each site in its network.

D. Hybrid Model

The hybrid SMOs are establishing a position as providers of fully integrated contract clinical research services. Typically driven by CROs eager to enter the study conduct market, hybrid SMOs provide CRO services and own and operate study conduct centers. Traditional CRO activities like protocol design, project management, site monitoring, and data management are offered in conjunction with traditional site services like study initiation, patient recruitment, and data capture services. It is through this integration that hybrids hope to offer truly accelerated clinical development services.

Hybrid SMOs believe that inefficiencies exist within the study conduct arena and between project management and study conduct functions. The hybrid SMO promises to apply management controls across a broad range of clinical development activities—from project planning through implementation and NDA submission. It is this seamless integration that hybrid SMOs believe will be a competitive advantage in the long term.

Historically, only a few organizations have pursued the hybrid model. Many industry insiders hold that project management and study conduct services require unique and distinct skill sets that cannot be integrated. Others argue that the hybrid SMO has been slow to catch on, because a conflict of interest exists when investigative sites are monitored by the same company that owns them. Several industry observers believe the hybrid SMO will be unable to pursue a sizable portion of the overall clinical grants market because it competes with traditional CROs that are reluctant to place studies there. Interestingly, several major owned-site and affiliation model SMOs have recently announced their intentions to begin offering select CRO services.

IV. AN EVER-CHANGING SMO MARKET

The earliest entrants into the SMO market were VRG International and Future HealthCare. In the mid-1990s, both organizations offered centrally managed study conduct services across a network of investigative sites. Next came Affiliated Research Centers (ARC), Clinical Studies Limited (CSL), Collaborative Clinical, and Hill Top Research, followed closely by Health Advance Institute (HAI), InSite Clinical Trials, Integrated Neuroscience Consortium (INC) and Rheumatology Research International (RRI), as well as CRO-SMO integrated service providers Clinicor, MDS Harris, and Scirex.

By the end of 1997, SMOs had entered a new phase armed with venture capital and aggressive business development practices. Collaborative Clinical raised $42 million in a 1996 initial public offering. Phymatrix, a $200 million physicians practice management group acquired CSL for $85 million. ARC, INC, InSite, and HAI closed rounds of venture capital financing. The capital markets were putting their money behind the SMO concept, hoping to give the SMO a fair test in the marketplace. Many observers have drawn parallels with the emergence and success of CROs in the 1980s.

The year 1998 marked the beginning of a volatile period for SMOs. ARC appeared to be taking a more cautious and less aggressive stance. Other SMOs, such as InSite, Collaborative Clinical, and HAI, moved out of the spotlight to regroup and refocus. The largest national SMOs, CSL and Hill Top, along with two well-funded new entrants-ProtoCare and Radiant Research—drove a frantic pace of acquisition activity. In all, 22 investigative sites were acquired by SMO organizations in 1998. SMO market share held at approximately 7% of the total $3.4 billion clinical grants market.

During 1999 and 2000, SMOs faced unprecedented financial, operational, and marketing difficulties. While pharmaceutical and CRO companies were reluctant to embrace contracting with SMOs, site management organizations had to manage the burden of building networks of sites while supporting the rising costs of corporate overhead, business development, infrastructure, and the integration of acquisitions. With few exceptions, SMOs struggled to operate profitably at a time when the investment community began demanding results.

Despite having the ability to spread corporate expenses, infrastructure investment, and integration costs across a network of sites, most SMOs faced strained operating margins. CenterWatch estimates that the typical investigator generates a 10 to 12% operating margin each year. SMO corporate salaries, fixed costs, and investments in infrastructure and business development add as much as 20% in overhead for each site. Moreover, there are some indications that once an investigator's site is acquired, that investigator—now on a salary—becomes less productive. In these instance, despite an SMO's attempts to improve operating efficiency, individual site revenue and profits decline following acquisition.

Competitive intensity, market confusion, and financial volatility have become common characteristics of the SMO market environment. SMOs witnessed the departure of several notable affiliation models in 1999. These organizations included Collaborative Clinical, Valence, and Insite Clinical Trials. Despite this volatility, through 1999, SMOs were largely perceived as a cohesive group in terms of their overall business strategies.

The year 2000 marked a significant period of transition for the SMO study conduct segment. At this time, SMOs pursued very different strategic directions. One group—including Radiant Research, ICSL (formerly CSL), and nTouch (formerly Novum)—pursued acquiring higher numbers of investigative sites to fuel rapid growth and to spread operating costs across a larger base. The other group—including Protocare—anticipated steady growth through offering a focused network of efficient and productive sites.

Having raised more than $14 million in 1999, for example, Radiant Research surprised the clinical trials industry in May 2000 when it announced that it was purchasing peer SMO Hill Top Research. The acquisition of Hill Top's pharmaceutical research division added 20 investigative sites to Radiant's network, bringing the grand total to 38 sites. At the completion of the acquisition, Radiant employed more than 500 investigators and study staff with expertise across 16 therapeutic areas. This acquisition made Radiant the largest owned-site SMO.

In the spring of 2000, nTouch Research doubled the size of its investigative site network when it acquired peer SMO Health Advance Medical Research. Having raised $8 million in venture capital funding only four months earlier, nTouch wasted no time in executing an aggressive expansion strategy.

Other SMOs joined a growing list of enterprises that finally exited the clinical trials industry. InSync Research shut down its operations in 2000 after selling four of its seven sites to Radiant Research. Clincare, which had hoped to expand its regional network of eight owned sites, also went out of business in 2000.

In the fall of 2001, one market leader, ICSL, announced that it would be selling its SMO assets to Comprehensive Neuroscience. ICSL's problems stem from a long list of external and internal factors: a failed strategy to integrate clinical trials with a physician's practice management (PPM) network of prescribing doctors; an unwieldy cash flow due to a cumbersome $100 million debt burden left over following the divestiture of its PPM business; an inability to integrate disparate books of business; from health outcome services to medical billing management to a network of clinical trial sites; an inability to achieve profitability or to manage operating costs while expanding its investigative site network; and a top-heavy management team seeking high levels of compensation and incentives despite ICSL's growing financial woes.

Comprehensive Neuroscience, a relative new entrant and now a major player following the integration of ICSL sites into its network, has approximately 360 employees and revenues of $45 million to $50 million. Comprehensive Neuroscience's business includes a clinical trials division that consists of more than 34 managed investigative sites and a medical information technologies division.

During 2001 and 2002, an estimated 33 new SMOs entered the market, the vast majority, nearly 80%, being affiliated site networks. SMOs also acquired 67 sites, though only a few were individual sites. The majority of purchased sites were those offered by companies exiting the SMO business (e.g., Health Advance Institute, Hill Top Research, and Clinical Studies Limited). Radiant Research and nTouch Research added large numbers of new sites to their networks in 2000. In that same period, top SMOs have secured additional capital at a time when outside funding has been hard to come by. Radiant Research and nTouch Research raised more than $50 million.

Several SMOs have been diversifying their portfolio of services. Radiant Research acquired a call center when it purchased the assets of Hill Top Research. Radiant now offers patient recruitment services not only to support its own trials but also for investigative sites outside of its network. For several years, AmericasDoctor has been expanding its services to include patient recruitment. And in 2002, Rheumatology Research International (RRI) opened a patient recruitment division and announced its strategic intent to offer CRO services operating more as a hybrid SMO. Top SMO, nTouch Research, announced its plans to offer a biorepository and genetic sampling program in anticipation of a shifting clinical research enterprise toward personalized medicine.

In 2003, market leader Radiant Research is expected to complete the acquisition of Protocare, another top five SMO. This purchase further establishes Radiant as the largest global owned-site SMO. When completed, the acquisition will expand Radiant's network to nearly 60 sites with an estimated annual revenue of $90 million. With a network of this scale achieved, Radiant may at last be well positioned to achieve the study conduct efficiencies prematurely promised by many of the early entrant SMOs no longer in operation.

V. CONCLUSIONS

Economic turmoil now characterizes the clinical research enterprise. As the overall economy has tumbled, pharmaceutical companies have consolidated amid rapidly declining market valuations. Investigative sites are all facing project delays, slower grant payments, and revenue and profit shortfalls. Recently, an unprecedented number of investigative sites have exited the business, extended their credit lines, and sought alternative revenue sources. Ultimately, these changes contribute to capacity shortages at a time when sponsors and CROs need larger numbers of experienced investigative sites to support their development pipelines with strong performance.

Yet, in spite of the current operating environment, a resilient SMO market reports that it expects to see future revenues continue to grow at double-digit rates. Such growth makes the SMO market one of the fastest growing study conduct segments. Five to seven years ago, fledgling SMO companies were accused of overpromising and underperforming. Today, SMOs that have remained and expanded their operations are well positioned to play a larger role in providing study conduct services.

Following a shakeout in the late 1990s, the SMO market continues to grow and evolve steadily yet quietly. Biopharmaceutical and CRO companies are becoming more receptive and adept at working with SMO service providers. At the same time, many top SMOs are diversifying their portfolio of services in order to establish additional revenue streams. Looking ahead, top SMOs are more bullish that they will become a more dominant study conduct segment within the clinical research enterprise.

REFERENCES

1. SMOs: the race to consolidate. CenterWatch 1997; 4(4).
2. The difficulties of site integration. CenterWatch 1998; 5(11).
3. The ups and downs of SMO usage. CenterWatch 1999; 6(5).
4. Independent site alliances fight back. CenterWatch 1999; 6(12).
5. SMOs: is scale the answer. CenterWatch 2000; 7(8).
6. Modest gains in SMO usage. CenterWatch 2001; 8(5).
7. Large site networks quietly take the field. CenterWatch 2001; 8(8).
8. Characterizing the new SMO market. CenterWatch 2002; 9(12).

27
Accelerating New Product Approvals

Robert P. Delamontagne
EduNeering, Inc., Princeton, New Jersey, U.S.A.

I. INTRODUCTION

Few scientific or business processes carry greater costs and risks than do drug development and manufacture. Pharmaceutical product drug development is a costly endeavor, in terms of both time and money. Over the past three decades, especially in drug development, time has increased to an average of thirteen years, with a cost in excess of $800 million for each new product brought to market. Much of that time and cost are associated with meeting regulatory requirements for nonclinical and clinical research and manufacturing regulations. These are applicable not only in the country of origin but also in those countries targeted as potential markets for the new pharmaceutical products.

Companies in the pharmaceutical, biotechnology, cosmetic and food, veterinary, medical device, and nutraceutical industries may be subject to some of the 4,000 new regulations issued in a typical year, each one with the force and effect of law. Although these regulations may be imposed by US governmental agencies as diverse as the Federal Trade Commission and the Occupational Safety and Health Administration, the Food and Drug Administration (FDA) is the prime regulatory agency for drug, device, and biological product development.

The US government, however, is not the only national entity with which a US-based new product development team must be concerned. Regardless of where a new product is developed, the market for that drug—just like the condition it was developed to treat—is likely to cross all national borders. The global interchange of data has opened many new opportunities for the research community to collaborate, co-develop, and market new and old products. It also highlights the difficulties associated with meeting regulatory compliance under the laws of each country in which the drug may be offered.

II. THE GLOBALIZATION OF REGULATION

A. The International Committee of Harmonization (ICH)

In 1990, representatives from several governmental agencies met to address the need for harmonizing the supervision, regulation, and standards of medicinal products. The International Conference on Harmonization (ICH) was established by six founding members: the European Union; the European Federation of Pharmaceutical Industries and Organizations; the Ministry of Health, Labor and Welfare, Japan; the Japan Pharmaceutical Manufacturers Association; the US Food and Drug Administration; and the Pharmaceutical Research and Manufacturers of America. The goal of the ICH is to establish a common quality standard in the three market areas, eliminate duplicate research activities, and assist regulatory agencies in establishing a common standard for new drug development.

The ICH has received strong support not only from regulators but also from the pharmaceutical and biotechnology industries. Frank Douglas, Executive Vice President of Hoechst Marion Roussel noted, "Through ICH, the number of time-consuming, expensive Phase III trials required for an international launch will be reduced dramatically. This will not only save time and resources—it will save lives and improve the health of patients all over the world."[2] August Watanabe, President of Lilly Research Laboratories, was equally supportive, saying, "ICH has led to streamlined regulatory requirements across geographies while preserving focus on scientific quality in submissions."[3] Perhaps of most significance to US researchers, however, is the support provided by the FDA. Janet Woodcock, Director of the FDA's Center for Drug Evaluation and Research, offered a straightforward observation, noting, "Participation in ICH has focused FDA's attention on the organization, consistency, and scientific quality of our regulatory recommendations."[4]

Although much remains to be done in achieving true global harmonization of regulations and standards, the future of such harmonization seems inevitable. To date, ICH has released guidelines in four categories: quality topics, relating to chemical and pharmaceutical quality assurance; safety topics, relating to in vitro and in vivo preclinical studies; efficacy topics, relating to clinical studies in human subjects; and multidisciplinary topics, which include subjects such as medical terminology, electronic standards for the transmission of regulatory information, timing of preclinical studies in relation to clinical trials, and the common technical document (see Chap. 18). The ICH also had released a parallel set of guidelines relating to specific issues in biotechnological products.

The anticipated benefits to industry of this harmonized approach are straightforward. The need for duplicate studies in many clinical and biological areas is minimized. The common technical document will enable companies to prepare submissions more quickly, since a single technical dossier will be accepted by all authorities in the ICH areas. Overall, the drug development process will be streamlined, facilitating the process by which raw research is transformed into marketable drugs.

B. The Case for Training as a Core Business Process

Although efforts are under way to streamline the drug development process, it continues to suffer from excessive delays and inefficiencies, which result in undue costs. Much of the cost is associated with regulatory compliance and the delivery of workforce education. With increased globalization, employees are dispersed and are difficult to reach using the traditional instructional methods. In addition, the management and distribution of compliance-related information, including regulatory updates or changes to standard operating procedures, must be delivered promptly if compliance is to be achieved.

Just as the cost of compliance continues to rise, the risks associated with noncompliance show a corresponding increase. In 2001, the FDA conducted 18,649 inspections. Those inspections, in turn, led to 7,683 FDA 483s (Inspectional Observations) and 1,032 warning letters. That same year, 12 injunctions were filed, 27 seizures were approved, and more than 4,500 recalls were triggered.

Noncompliance can produce civil penalties or even criminal charges against a company and its employees. During the fiscal year 2001, the FDA's Office of Criminal Investigations made 422 arrests and obtained 360 convictions for violations of the Federal Food, Drug and Cosmetic Act and related statues. These investigations produced nearly $1 billion in fines and restitution. One of these cases involves the submission of false data in an attempt to obtain approval for a medical test kit. Two former corporate officers of the company were convicted and sentenced to serve 15 months in federal prison. The company was then sentenced to pay $150,000, and all three defendants were ordered jointly and severally to repay $297,000 lost by distributors in the scheme to sell the unapproved test kits. In another highly publicized case involving a multinational pharmaceutical company, a criminal fine of more than $23 million and a forfeiture of $10 million was levied against the company. The case centered on the intentional reporting of false manufacturing procedures in new drug applications and false records during the manufacture of bulk drugs.

Noncompliance creates a ripple effect far beyond the risks associated with civil or criminal prosecution. Insurance companies and potential investors may consider the company with a poor compliance history to be a poor business or investment risk. Employee recruitment and retention can be jeopardized. Public acceptance of the products that eventually are brought to market may be compromised by the bad publicity associated with noncompliance. Most important, drug development can be delayed or derailed as new products are prohibited from being brought to market.

The emphasis by regulatory agencies today is not merely on training, but on training as a core business process. Under the old paradigm, organizations could point to the number of hours of employee training they provided, implying the corollary that the more hours of training an employee received, the more knowledgeable the employee. This "more training, more knowledge" standard no longer can be substantiated. Today, the measure of training effectiveness is a basic business requirement. For training to be effective it must align the employees' work behavior with those stipulated by regulations and ensure conformity with standard operating procedures.

The regulatory focus on training under established regulations is far from the only reason to implement effective training programs. Regulations are not static. New laws are enacted, some to address new needs, such as the bioterrorism threats recognized by the US government since September 11, 2001. Existing regulations are modified, such as the 2002 modification of the FDA's new drug and biological product regulations, designed to ensure that certain human drugs and biologicals intended to reduce or prevent serious life-threatening conditions can be approved more quickly. New initiatives by regulatory agencies are inaugurated, such as the Division of Bioresearch Monitoring's expansion of inspection strategies, which is part of the division's reengineering effort.

Beyond the ever-changing network of regulations, science and technology demonstrate their own rapid evolution. Some experts believe that the time span between when knowledge is gained and when it becomes obsolete—the half-life of knowledge—is less than two years. In some cases, that half-life may be shorter than the time required to pass laws triggered by the new knowledge. Consider, for instance, the announcement on January 20, 2003, that scientists at the US Department of Energy's Pacific Northwest National Laboratory have extracted part of the human immune system and reconstituted it in brewer's yeast. According to the laboratory, the resulting technology might replace the need to produce antibodies within animals and could have major repercussions for fundamental biological science and for industries that use antibodies for senors, biodetectors, diagnostic tools, and therapeutic agents. As of January 21, 2003, the FDA regulated neither the technology nor its application, but that could change very quickly. Any regulation of the technology, its development, or its application inevitably would impose additional training requirements on laboratory and drug development staff.

Another factor fueling the need for training is the inevitable change in any organization's staff. As employees leave or join an organization, the existing level of knowledge about the specific research under way, the procedures required, and the standards maintained in that organization are vulnerable to mistakes, oversights, carelessness, and ignorance. An even greater impact may be imposed by the globalization of the drug development industry. Corporate acquisitions of companies from other countries typically require the integration of different approaches, cultures, and standards. Without effective training, the straightforward acquisition of a promising small company by a larger one could easily translate into unnecessary repetitions of research, inconsistent understanding of standard operating procedures, and potentially delayed compliance with applicable federal regulations.

III. THE ROLE OF THE INTERNET IN COMPLIANCE EDUCATION

The Internet has transformed the ways in which we share information. E-mail, in particular, routinely provides a method for communicating updated corporate policies, for scheduling meetings, and for linking colleagues. It is highly effective in that role, but e-mail is not the basis of an effective training program, even though some training courses now available are little more than expanded e-mail programs.

Information and instruction are distinguished by the ability of instruction to change behavior. Behavior change, in turn, is the one proven method that lowers the risk of noncompliance by aligning employee behavior with mandated work procedures. Instruction is an "engineered activity," specifically designed to meet identified learning objectives. Information, no matter how attractive or colorful, provides little stimulus to behavior change.

Traditional training relies on an instructor in a classroom setting. It offers a number of benefits, including the face-to-face exchange of information and concepts between instructor and learner. It also carries disadvantages, especially in today's fast-changing research climate. One particular disadvantage of instructor-led training is the timing of the courses and the typical need to coordinate the schedules of both instructors and learners. At one pharmaceutical manufacturing plant, for example, training of new employees was mandated by the company's standard operating procedure to occur within the first seven days of employment. Over a six-month period, the company was able to provide only 7 of 16 new employees with the required instruction within the designated time period. The main cause of delay was scheduling conflicts between the manufacturing department and the trainers.

Another substantial drawback to instructor-led training, especially in light of the industry's move toward globalization, is the lack of instructional consistency. The instructor at one facility may not be providing the same instruction as the instructor at another facility. The message inconsistency can be particularly problematical when the instructors and learners are located in different countries, allowing diverse cultural and language impacts to color the presentations.

For a training program to be successful in today's environment, it must be rapidly deployable; easily modified; accessible 24 hours a day, 7 days a week; and consistent in its instruction. The Internet is uniquely equipped to address those needs. E-learning—also known as on-line training or web-based training–provides a consistent message because the same instructional courses are available to any employee, regardless of location. It is capable of targeting instruction to each individual learner within an organization, and it is accessible 24/7. E-learning offers another advantage in its ability to document all training. In the event of regulatory audit, accident investigation, or legal action, the ability to produce documentation showing that the organization has taken measures to educate its workforce often is the company's first line of defense against penalties, civil litigation, or even criminal prosecution. Finally, when properly designed and implemented, on-line training is highly effective, with some studies showing learning gains of up to 56% for on-line learning when compared to traditional classroom training.

IV. E-LEARNING AND DRUG DEVELOPMENT

The inherent versatility of e-learning dovetails with the training needs of the drug development industry. Some of those needs are well illustrated by the guidelines that have been finalized by ICH in three categories: efficacy, quality, and safety.

ICH's finalized efficacy guidelines reflect the strict demands of regulators, both US and internationally. Efficacy guidelines have been issued in subjects ranging from clinical safety to dose response, ethnic factors, good clinical practice, and clinical trial design. ICH's quality category includes such subjects as stability testing of new drug substances and products, analytical validation, and biotechnological quality. The safety category focuses on issues of carcinogenicity, genotoxicity, kinetics, and toxicity.

It is worth noting how an e-learning curriculum might be developed to address these and related issues.

A core curriculum would likely begin with a basic understanding of the regulatory process. In the US, a review of the FDA's regulations might be followed by a series of basic courses on subjects such as good clinical practices (GCPs), good laboratory practices (GLPs); good manufacturing practices (GMPs); laboratory safety; an introduction to quality system regulations; personal protective equipment; principles of good documentation; the care and handling of drug product components, containers and closures; and understanding GMPs for facilities and equipment.

E-learning courses may be designed to prevent a learner from proceeding to the next level of learning until he or she has demonstrated competence in the basic course. Upon demonstrating that competence, learners could be focused on individual learning paths. One learner might focus on courses such as application of GMPs to analytical laboratories, change control, DEA compliance, environmental control and monitoring, and meeting process requirements for returned and salvaged drug products. Another individual might follow a course path that focuses on medical devices, with specific courses including compliance management for medical device manufacturers, design control regulations for medical device manufacturers, essentials of an effective calibration program, failure investigations for medical device manufacturers, handling a product recall, and understanding the principles and practices of process controls.

A third level of training might center on process validation with courses on subjects such as documenting validation activities; key concepts of process validation, Part 11: Electronic Records and Electronic Signatures; and writing validation protocols. Specialized courses might provide additional depth in targeted areas. For example, additional concentration on good clinical practices might include good clinical practices for new drug investigations, protection of human subjects in clinical studies, responsibilities of clinical research monitors, and the responsibility of the investigator in drug/biologicals clinical studies.

The US pharmaceutical and drug development industries have what some might consider an unlikely ally in the US Food and Drug Administration's Office of Regulatory Affairs (ORA), which launched a "virtual university" in 2001. The website, entitled ORA U, grew from a process initiated several years earlier to standardize training for the FDA's staff members and thousands of additional state and local regulatory staff who held responsibility for enforcing FDA regulations on food, drugs, and other commodities. That initiative occurred during the same period that the Federal Technology Transfer Act was promoting cooperative agreements between government agencies and the private sector to encourage collaborative research and development.

The FDA entered into its first learning technology Cooperative Research and Development Agreement (CRADA) in 1999 with EduNeering, Inc. The goal was to establish an e-learning training solution that would provide mandated training to the FDA's target audience more effectively and cost-efficiently than existing programs. Under the agreement, FDA provided the content for the web-based courses. EduNeering assumed responsibility for providing a comprehensive e-learning solution. This included highly interactive e-learning courses and a full-featured learning management system that enabled FDA administrators immediately to access information regarding the status of each learner in meeting statutory requirements.

ORA U has been highly successful for the FDA. Since its inception, training times for the FDA's new-hire investigators have dropped from between 6 and 12 months to just 3 months. Private companies can use the same training tools that are employed by the FDA to deliver over 100 courses either developed with or reviewed by the FDA. Those courses include basic and advanced GMP and GCPs and a specialty series entitled "Basics of Investigation for FDA Investigators." Among the individual courses are FDA 483s: Inspectional Observations, FDA Good Guidance Practices, Recall of FDA Regulated Products, Sample Collections, and Special Investigations.

With the curricula in ORA U, drug researchers and developers have been equipped with a solid foundation of training that covers the regulations, compliance requirements, and investigational procedures of the industry's premier regulatory agency. The courses of ORA U do not cover every aspect of drug development that might require training. For that, companies may develop custom courses or utilize existing classroom instruction.

V. DISTINGUISHING GOOD TRAINING SOLUTIONS

Effective e-learning solutions represent a blend of science and art. Employing a combination of technology, information, and instructional design, an effective course allows students to learn, retain the new knowledge, and apply the knowledge in their day-to-day work activities. To achieve that three-pronged goal, e-learning systems incorporate a number of key components, including the following:

Instructional design is the most important element of an effective web-based educational system. Effective design produces a more active and deeper engagement by the learner than more passive methods typically used to communicate information, such as memos or work procedures. Instructional design is, in fact, a science that—when implemented correctly—produces learning events that efficiently transfer knowledge and modify behavior. Some of the indicators of effective design are cueing of the learner, a statement of objectives, effective use of animations and graphics, a high level of inter-activity, and the variation of instructional treatment for varying levels of complexity in learning, such as facts, principles, concepts, and strategies.

Fail-safe documentation ensures that, in the event of regulatory audit, accident investigations, or legal actions resulting from employee injury, the company can demonstrate that it has taken measures to educate its employees in the correct and required work procedures. Often, that documentation is a company's first line of defense against penalties and expensive litigation. Certain regulatory agencies, including the FDA, require extensive documen-tation, information management, storage, and security measures as part of the regulatory requirements of a learning management system.

Technology infrastructure often determines the effectiveness of the learning experience. The effectiveness of the underlying code, the design and fundamental scalability of the database, the server configuration, and available bandwidth are all essential considerations. Because internal net-works often lack the speed and reliability required for compliance education purposes, many organizations are employing Application Service Providers for secure and specialized services outside the firewall of their internal networks.

Appropriate curriculum would seem to be self-evident as a key consid-eration. On-line courses must effectively address the regulatory requirements and offer the appropriate solutions for the individual organizations. Many organizations employ a blended approach comprising both classroom and on-line instruction. If on-line courses are used to complement instructor-led programs, the on-line courses should be matched against the appropriate job descriptions, work tasks, and regulations of the employees for whom the training is intended. For example, if 40 individual environmental health and safety courses are required to address the regulations adequately, they should be available to the designated workforce as part of the overall curriculum. In addition, these courses should represent "expert authority" and be supported and endorsed by industry experts and regulators.

Accessibility is one of the great advantages of web-based education. This 24/7 availability is compelling not only because it offers convenience but also because it provides for extensive cost reduction arising from lower travel costs, instruction time, administrative expenses, and consultants' fees. A study by Hambrecht & Co. concluded that corporations can save between 50 and 70 percent when replacing instructor-led training with electronic delivery. With the globalization of the workforce, it is common to have

US-based multinationals seek to extend a compliance training program to their offshore facilities. A web-based training strategy enables companies to reach out to an international workforce regardless of the boundaries of time and geography.

Usability is a core characteristic of any effective web-based training course. Courses must be intuitively logical, being effective for employees with a wide range of education and skill profiles.

Security has become a greater issue in recent years, and web-based educational systems must operate in a safe, secure environment so that data are protected and immediately retrievable when needed. Many highly regulated firms are turning to outside organizations that offer hosted services able to meet extremely high security standards.

The Internet has pervaded most aspects of corporate life, bringing greater efficiencies in its wake. It should be no surprise that it can bring equal benefits to the drug development process. The potential advantages of e-learning are significant; however, it will require organizations to think in new ways about compliance education.

Pharmaceutical and drug development companies have a strong financial interest in bringing the results of their research to market quickly and efficiently. With the globalization of both drug development efforts and the markets for new pharmaceuticals, companies are faced with a rapidly expanding need to accelerate their drug development process. Effective training stands as a fundamental requirement in meeting this core business objective.

Acronyms and Initialisms

AAAS	American Association for the Advancement of Science
AABB	American Association of Blood Banks
AACR	American Association for Cancer Research
AADA	Abbreviated Antibiotic Drug Application (FDA) (used primarily for generics)
AAFP	American Academy of Family Physicians
AAI	American Academy of Immunologists
AAP	American Association of Pathologists
AAPP	American Academy of Pharmaceutical Physicians
AAPS	American Association of Pharmaceutical Scientists
ABPI	Association of the British Pharmaceutical Industry
ACCP	American College of Clinical Pharmacology
ACE	Adverse Clinical Event
ACIL	American Council of Independent Laboratories
ACP	Associates of Clinical Pharmacology (USA), a group that certifies clinical research associates (CRAs) and clinical research coordinators (CRCs)
ACPU	Association of Clinical Pharmacology Units
ACRA	Associate Commissioner for Regulatory Affairs (FDA)
ACRPI	Association for Clinical Research in the Pharmaceutical Industry (UK)
ACS	American Chemical Society
ACT	*Applied Clinical Trials* magazine
ACTG	AIDS Clinical Trials Group (NIAID)

Adapted from CDER Acronym List, U.S. Food and Drug Administration. Compiled by Division of Biometrics III (www.Fda.gov/cder/handbook/acronym.htm).

ACTU	AIDS Clinical Trials Unit (NIH)
AD	Alzheimer's disease; antidepressant
ADAMHA	Alcohol, Drug Abuse, and Mental Health Administration (no longer exists)
ADAS	Alzheimer's Disease Assessment Scale
ADAS COG	Alzheimer's Disease Assessment Scale, Cognitive Subscale
ADE	Adverse Drug Experience/Effect/Event
ADI	Acceptable Daily Intake
ADME	Absorption, Distribution, Metabolism, Elimination
ADP	Automated Data Processing
ADR	Adverse Drug Reaction
ADRS	Adverse Drug Reporting System
AE	Approvable; Adverse Experience
AED	Antiepileptic drug
AEGIS	ADROIT Electronically Generated Information Service
AERS	Adverse Experience (Event) Reporting System (FDA)
AESGP	Association Européenne des Specialités Grand Public (European Proprietary Medicines Manufacturers Association)
AFCR	*See AFMR.*
AFDO	Association of Food and Drug Officials
AFMR	American Federation for Medical Research, formerly known as the American Federation for Clinical Research (AFCR)
AHA	Area Health Authority (UK)
AHCPR	Agency for Health Care Policy Research (NIH)
AICRC	Association of Independent Clinical Research Contractors (UK)
AIDS	Acquired immunodeficiency syndrome. *See also HIV and SIDA.*
AIM	Active Ingredient Manufacturer
AIP	Abbreviated Inspection Program
AMA	American Medical Association
AMA-DE	AMA Drug Evaluations
AMC	Academic medical centers
AMF	Administrative Management of the Files
AmFAR	American Foundation for AIDS Research
AMG	Arzneimittelgesetz (German Drug Law)
AMI	Acute myocardial infarction
ANADA	Abbreviated New Animal Drug Application
ANDA	Abbreviated New Drug Application (for a generic drug)
ANOVA	Analysis of variance
AOAC	Association of Official Analytical Chemists
AOAC	Association Pharmaceutique Belge (Belgium)
AP	Approved (COMIS term)
APhA	American Pharmaceutical Association
APHIS	Animal and Plant Health Inspection Service

AQL	Acceptable quality level
ARC	AIDS-related complex
ARDS	Adult respiratory distress syndrome
ARENA	Applied Research Ethics National Association
ASA	American Statistical Association
ASAP	Administrative Systems Automation Project (FDA)
ASCII	American Standards Code for Information Interchange (computer files)
ASCO	American Society for Clinical Oncology
ASCPT	American Society for Clinical Pharmacology and Therapeutics
ASM	American Society for Microbiology
ASQC	American Society for Quality Control
AT	Active (COMIS term)
ATF	Bureau of Alcohol, Tobacco, and Firearms
AUC	Area Under the Curve (an expression of exposure)
AZT	Zidovudine (HIV treatment)
BARQA	British Association of Research Quality Assurance
BB	Bureau of Biologics (now CBER)
BCE	Beneficial Clinical Event
BEUC	European Bureau of Consumer Unions
BfArM	Bundesinstitut für Arzneimittel und Medizinprodukte (Federal Institute for Drugs and Medical Devices, Germany)
BGA	Bundesinstitut für gesundheitlichen Verbraucherschutz und Veterinärmedizinn (Federal Institute for Health Protection of Consumers and Veterinary Medicine, Germany)
BGVV	Bundesgesundheitsamt (former German public health agency)
BID	Two Times per Day
BIND	Biological Investigational New Drug
BIO	Biotechnology Industry Organization
BIRA	British Institute of Regulatory Affairs
BLA	Biologic License Application
BMB	Bioresearch Monitoring Branch
BMI	Body Mass Index
BPAD	Bipolar Affective Disorder
BPI	Bundesverband der Pharmazeutischen Industrie EV (Germany)
BPM	Beats per Minute
BrAPP	British Association of Pharmaceutical Physicians
BRB	Biomedical Research Branch
BSA	Body surface area
BVC	British Veterinary Codex
C & S	Culture and sensitivity
CA	Chemical Abstracts; Competent Authority (regulatory body

	charged with monitoring compliance with European member state national statutes and regulations)
CAC	Carcinogenicity Assessment Committee
CACE	Committee for Advancement of Chemistry Education
CAD	Coronary Artery Disease
CANDA	Computer-Assisted New Drug Application. *See NDA.*
CAPLA	Computer-Assisted Product License Application. *See PLA.*
CAPLAR	Computer-Assisted Product License Agreement Review (FDA)
CAPRA	Canadian Association of Pharmaceutical Regulatory Affairs
CAS	Chemical Abstracts Service
CBC	Complete Blood Count
CBCTN	Community Based Clinical Trials Network
CBER	Center for Biologics Evaluation and Research (FDA)
CBF	Cerebral Blood Flow
CCASE	Coordinating Committee for Advancement of Scientific Education
CCC	Compliance Coordinating Committee (CDER)
CCD	Canadian Drugs Directorate
CCDS	Company Core Data Sheets
CCI	Committee on Clinical Investigations. *See also IRB.*
CCRA	Certified Clinical Research Associate. *See also ACP.*
CCRC	Certified Clinical Research Coordinator. *See also ACP.*
CDC	Centers for Disease Control and Prevention (Atlanta, GA)
CDER	Center for Drug Evaluation and Research (FDA)
CDRH	Center for Devices and Radiological Health (FDA)
CE	Continuing Education
CE	mark signifying compliance with EU harmonized standards and directives
CEN	Comité Européen de Normalisation (European Committee for Standardization)
CESS	CDER Executive Secretariat Staff
CFR	*Code of Federal Regulations* (usually cited by part and chapter, as 21 CFR 211)
CFSAN	Center of Food Safety and Applied Nutrition
CGMP	Current Good Manufacturing Practices
CH	Clinical Hold
CHD	Coronary Heart Disease
CIB	Clinical Investigator's Brochure
CID	CTFA Cosmetic Ingredient Dictionary
CIOMS	Council for International Organisations of Medical Sciences (postapproval international ADR reporting, UK)
CIR	Cosmetic Ingredient Review
CIS	Commonwealth of Independent States
CLIA	Clinical Laboratory Improvements Amendments
CMC	Chemistry, Manufacturing and Controls

CMCCC	Chemistry and Manufacturing Controls Coordinating Committee (CDER)
CME	Continuing Medical Education
CNS	Central Nervous System
COA	Commissioned Officers Association; Certificates of Analysis
COE	Code of Ethics
COIMS	Centerwide Oracle Management Information System (FDA)
COMIS	Center Office Management Information System
COSTART	Coding Symbols for a Thesaurus of Adverse Reaction Terms
CP	Compliance Program
CPMP	Committee for Proprietary Medicinal Products (EU)
CPSC	Consumer Product Safety Commission (USA)
CR	Cross Reference (COMIS term)
CRA	Clinical Research Associate
CRADA	Cooperative Research and Development Agreement (with NIH)
CRC	Clinical Research Coordinator. *See also CCRC.*
CRF	Case Report Form
CRO	Contract Research Organization. *See also IPRO.*
CS	Civil Service
CS	Clinically Significant
CSDD	Center for the Study of Drug Development
CSI	Consumer Safety Inspector
CSM	Commission for Safety of Medicines (UK Regulatory Agency) Committee on Safety of Medicines (UK)
CSO	Consumer Safety Officer (FDA)—Project Manager
CSR	Clinical Study Report
CSSI	Company Core Safety Information
CT	Computerized tomography
CT	Clinical trial
CTC	Clinical Trial Certificate
CTEP	Clinical Therapeutics Evaluation Program (NCI)
CTX	Clinical Trial Exemption Certification (MCA)
CV	Curriculum vitae
CVM	Center for Veterinary Medicine (FDA)
CXR	Chest X-ray
DAS	Drug abuse staff
DAWN	Drug Abuse Warning Network
DB	Double-Blind
DD	Department of Drugs (Swedish regulatory agency)
ddC	Dideoxycytidine, a cytidine nucleoside analogue
ddC	Didanosine, a purine nucleoside analogue
DDIR	Division of Drug Information Resources
DDMAC	Division of Drug Marketing, Advertising, and Communications

DEA	Drug Enforcement Administration (USA)
DEN	Drug Experience Network
DES	Division of Epidemiology and Surveillance
DESI	Drug Efficacy Study Implementation Notice (FDA, to evaluate drugs in use before 1962)
DGD	Now OGD (formerly CBER's Division of Genetic Drugs)
DHEW	Department of Health, Education, and Welfare (USA, now split into HHS and Department of Education)
DHHS	Department of Health and Human Services (USA)
DIA	Drug Information Association
DISD	Division of Information Systems Design
DMF	Drug Master File
DoD	Department of Defense (USA)
DPC-PTR Act	Drug Price Competition and Patent Term Restoration Act of 1984 (also known as Waxman-Hatch bill)
DRG	Diagnosis Related Groups
DRG	Division of Research Grants (NIH)
DSI	Division of Scientific Investigations (FDA)
DSM	*Diagnostic and Statistical Manual of Mental Disorders* (of the American Psychiatric Association)
DSMB	Data and Safety Monitoring Board
DSNP	Development of Standardized Nomenclature Project (FDA)
DUR	Drug Utilization Review
EA	Environmental Assessment
EAB	Ethical Advisory Board (term used in some nations for groups similar to IRBs and IECs)
EBSA	European Biosafety Association
EC	European Commission (in documents older than the mid-1980s, EC may mean European Community)
ECG	Electrocardiogram
ECJ	European Court of Justice
ECPHIN	European Community Pharmaceutical Products Information Network
ECU	European Currency Unit
ED	Effective Dose
EEC	European Economic Community (old term for EC, now EU)
EEG	Electroencephalogram
EEO	Equal Employment Opportunity
EER	Establishment Evaluation Request
EFGCP	European Forum on Good Clinical Practice (Evere, Belgium)
EFPIA	European Federation of Pharmaceutical Industries' Associations
EFTA	European Free Trade Association
EIA	Establishment Inspection Reports
EIR	Establishment Inspection Report (FDA)

ELA	Establishment License Application (biologics)
EMEA	European Medicines Evaluations Agency (UK)
EMS	Electronic Mail Service
EO	Executive Order
EOP1	End-of-phase 1
EOP2	End-of-phase 2
EORTC	European Organization for Research and Treatment of Cancer
EOS	End of Study
EP	European Parliament
EPA	Environmental Protection Agency
EPAR	European Public Assessment Report
EPL	Effective Patent Life
EPMS	Employee Performance Management System
EPO	European Patent Office
EPRG	European Pharmacovigilance Research Group
ER	Essential Requirements (EU)
ESRA	European Society of Regulatory Affairs
ESS	Executive Secretary and Staff
ETT	Exercise Tolerance Test
EU	European Union
EUDRACT	European Drug Regulatory Affairs Clinical Trial
EUP	Experimental Use Permit
FACA	Federal Advisory Committee Act 1972
FÄPI	Fachgesellschaft der Ärzte in der Pharmazeutischen Industrie e.V. (German Association of Physicians in the Pharmaceutical Industry)
Farmindustria	The Association of Italian Pharmaceutical Manufacturers
FAX	Facsimile
FCC	Federal Communications Commission
FCCSET	Federal Coordinating Council for Science, Engineering and Technology
FD & C Act	Federal Food, Drug and Cosmetic Act
FD 1571	Form Used to Submit IND
FD 1572	Statement of Investigator Form (accompanies IND)
FD 2252	Form Used to Submit NDA Annual Report
FD 2253	Form Used to Promotional Advertising or Labeling
FD 3500A	Form Used to Submit Drug Experience Report
FD 356H	Form Used to Submit NDA
FD 483	Form Issued by FDA upon Adverse Findings of Inspection
FDA	Food and Drug Administration (U.S.A.)
FDA-SRS	Spontaneous Reporting System of the Food and Drug Administration
FDLI	Food and Drug Law Institute
FFDCA	Federal Food, Drug & Cosmetic Act
FFPM	Fellow of the Faculty of Pharmaceutical Medicine (UK)

FMD	Field Management Directives
FOI	Freedom of Information
FOIA	Freedom of Information Act
FONSI	Finding of No Significant Impact
FPIF	The Finnish Pharmaceutical Industry Association
FPL	Final Printed Labeling
FR	Federal Register
FRC	Federal Records Center (Suitland)
FRCP	Fellow of the Royal College of Physicians, sometimes followed by a place name—for example, FRCP (Edin.)—that indicates a university medical school
FSIS	Food Safety and Inspection Service
FTC	Federal Trade Commission (USA)
FUR	Follow Up Request
GAO	General Accounting Office (US government)
GATT	General Agreement of Tariffs and Trade
GC	General Counsel (FDA)
GC	Gas Chromatography
GCP	Good Clinical Practice
GI	Gastrointestinal
GLP	Good Laboratory Practice
GMP	Good Manufacturing Practice
GP	General Practitioner
GPRA	Government Performance and Results Act
GRAS	Generally Recognized as Safe
GRASE	Generally Recognized as Safe and Effective
GRP	Good Review Practice
HAACP	Hazard Analysis and Critical Control Point (inspection technique)
HAI	Health Action International
HCFA	Health Care Financing Administration (HHS)
HF	Routing code for mail to the Office of the Commissioner of the FDA
HFD	Routing code for mail to CDER
HFM	Routing code for mail to CBER
HFS	Routing code for mail to CFSAN
HFT	Routing code for mail to NCTR
HFV	Routing code for mail to CVM
HFZ	Routing code for mail to CDRH
HHS	Department of Health and Human Services (USA, also called DHHS)
HIMA	Health Industry Manufacturer's Association (devices)
HIPAA	Health Insurance Portability and Accountability Act
HIS	Indian Health Service
HIV	Human immunodeficiency virus

HIV+	HIV-positive; HIV-infected
HIV-1	Human immunodeficiency virus type 1
HMO	Health Maintenance Organization
HPB	Health Protection Branch (Canada's equivalent of the FDA)
HPLC	High-pressure liquid chromatography
HRG	Health Research Group
HRRC	Human Research Review Committee
HRSA	Health Resources and Services Administration
HX	History
IACUC	Institutional Animal Care and Use Committee
IARC	International Agency for Research on Cancer
IC	Informed Consent
IC	Chemistry Information Amendment (COMIS term)
ICD	Informed Consent Document
ICH	International Conference on Harmonisation of Technical Requirements for Registration of Pharmaceuticals for Human Use
ICPEMC	International Commission for Protection Against Mutagens and Carcinogens
ICTH	International Committee on Thrombosis and Hemostases
IDB	Investigational Drug Brochure
IDE	Investigational Device Exemption (FDA)
IDR	Idiosyncratic Drug Reaction
IDSMB	Independent Data Safety Monitoring Board
IEC	Independent Ethics Committee. *See also EAB, IRB, NRB.*
IFPMA	International Federation of Pharmaceutical Manufacturers' Associations
IG	Office of the Inspector General (HHS)
IKS	Interkantonale Kontrollstelle für Heilmittel (Switzerland)
IM	Clinical Information Amendment (COMIS term)
IM	Intramuscular
INAD	Investigational New Animal Drug
IND	Investigational New Drug Application (FDA). *See also TIND.*
INDA	Investigational New Drug Application
INDC	Investigational New Drug Committee
INN	International Nonproprietary Name
IOM	Institute of Medicine (National Academy of Science, USA)
IPCS	International Program for Chemical Safety
IPRA	International Product Registration Document
IPRO	Independent pharmaceutical research organization. *See also CRO.*
IRB	Institutional Review Board, sometimes Independent Review Board. *See also IEC, EAB, NRB.*
IRC	Institutes Review Committee
IRD	International Registration Document

IRG	Initial Review Groups
IRS	Identical, Related, or Similar
IS	Information Systems
ISCB	International Society for Clinical Biostatistics
ISO	International Organisation for Standardisation
ISPE	International Society for Pharmacoepidemiology
IT	Toxicology Information Amendment (COMIS term)
IT	Information Technology
ITCC	Information Technology Coordinating Committee (CDER)
i.v.	Intravenous
IV	Interview
IVD	In Vitro Device; In Vitro Diagnostics
IVF	In Vitro Fertilization
IVF/ET	In Vitro Fertilization/Embryo Transfer
JCAH	Joint Commission for the Accreditation of Hospitals
JCAHO	Joint Commission of Accreditation of Health Care Organizations
JCPT	*Journal of Clinical Pharmacology and Therapeutics*
JCRDD	*Journal of Clinical Research and Drug Development*
JCRP	*Journal of Clinical Research and Pharmacoepidemiology*
JPMA	Japan Pharmaceutical Manufacturers' Association
KS	Kaposi's Sarcoma
L & D	Labor and Delivery
LAN	Local Area Network
LD	Lethal Dose
LD50	Lethal Dose (50%)
LEAA	Law Enforcement Assistance Administration
LERN	Library Electronic Reference Network
LIF	Swedish Pharmaceutical Industry Association
LKP	Leiter der klinischen Prüfung, under the German Drug Law, the physician who is head of clinical testing
LNC	Labeling and Nomenclature Committee
LOA	Letter of Agreement
LOC	Level of Concern
LOCF	Last Observation Carried Forward
LOD	Loss on Drying
LRC	Lipid Research Clinic
LRI	Lower Respiratory Infection
LTE	Less Than Effective
LVP	Large Volume Parenterals
MA	Marketing Authorization
MAA	Marketing Authorization Application (EC)
MAH	Marketing Authorization Holders
MAPP	Manual of Policy and Procedures
MBC	Minimum Bactericidal Concentration

MCA	Medicines Control Agency (UK)
MDA	Medical Devices Agency (UK)
MDD	Medical Device Directives (EU)
MDI	Metered-Dose Inhaler; Manic-Depressive Illness
MDR	Medical Device Reporting
MDV	Medical Device Vigilance
MECU	Million ECU
MEDDRA	Medical Dictionary for Drug Regulatory Affairs
MEDLARS	Medical Literature Analysis and Retrieval System
MEDWATCH	MedWatch Adverse Experience (Event) Reporting System (3500A)
MEFA	Association of the Danish Pharmaceutical Industry
MEMO	Medicines Evaluation and Monitoring Organisation
MEP	Member of the European Parliament
MHW	Ministry of Health and Welfare (Koseisho, Japan's drug regulatory agency)
MI	Myocardial Infarction
MIC	Minimum Inhibitory Concentration
MOU	Memorandum of Understanding (between FDA and a regulatory agency in another country) that allows mutual recognition of inspections
MPCC	Medical Policy Coordinating Committee (CDER)
MRA	Medical Research Associate
MRI	Magnetic Resonance Imaging
MTD	Maximum Tolerated Dose
NA	Not Approvable
NABR	National Association for Biomedical Research
NADA	New Animal Drug Application
NAF	Notice of Adverse Findings (FDA postaudit letter)
NAFTA	North American Free Trade Agreement
NAHC	National Advisory Health Council
NAI	No Action Indicated (most favorable FDA postinspection classification)
NAS	National Academy of Sciences
NAS	New Active Substance
NAS-NRC	National Academy of Sciences–National Research Council
NATRIK	National Reporting and Investigation Centre (UK)
NCCLS	National Committee for Clinical Laboratory Standards
NCE	New Chemical Entity
NCHGR	National Center for Human Genome Research (NIH)
NCHS	National Center for Health Statistics (in CDC)
NCI	National Cancer Institute (NIH)
NCPIE	National Council on Patient Information and Education (Washington, DC)
NCRP	Northwest Clinical Research Professionals (Portland, OR)

NCRR	National Center for Research Resources (NIH)
NCS	Not clinically significant
NCTR	National Center for Toxicological Research
NCVIA	National Childhood Vaccine Injury Act (1986)
NDA	New Drug Application (FDA)
NDE	New Drug Evaluation
NDS	New Drug Study (Canada's new drug application)
NEFARMA	Dutch Association of the Innovative Pharmaceutical Industry
NEI	National Eye Institute (NIH)
NEJM	*New England Journal of Medicine*
NF	National Formulary
NHLBI	National Heart, Lung, and Blood Institute (NIH)
NHS	National Health Service (UK)
NHW	National Health and Welfare Department (Canada's equivalent of DHHS)
NIA	National Institute on Aging (NIH)
NIAAA	National Institute on Alcohol Abuse and Alcoholism (NIH)
NIAID	National Institute of Allergies and Infectious Diseases (NIH)
NIAMS	National Institute of Arthritis and Musculoskeletal and Skin Diseases (NIH)
NICHD	National Institute of Child Health and Human Development (NIH)
NIDA	National Institute on Drug Abuse (NIH)
NIDCD	National Institute on Deafness and Other Communication Disorders (NIH)
NIDDKD	National Institute of Diabetes and Digestive and Kidney Diseases
NIDR	National Institute of Dental Research (NIH)
NIEHS	National Institute of Environmental Health Sciences (NIH)
NIGMS	National Institute of General Medical Sciences (NIH)
NIH	National Institutes of Health (DHHS)
NIMH	National Institute of Mental Health (NIH)
NINDS	National Institute of Neurological Disorders and Stroke (NIH)
NINR	National Institute of Nursing Research (NIH)
NLEA	Nutrition Labeling and Education Act (1990)
NLM	National Library of Medicine (NIH)
NME	New Molecular Entity
NMR	Nuclear Magnetic Resonance
NOEL	No Observed Effect Level
Non-Mem	Non-linear Nixed Effect Model
NR	No Reply Necessary (COMIS term)
NRB	Noninstitutional Review Board, also known as an Independent Review Board. *See also* EAB, IEC, IRB.
NRC	National Research Council
NRC	Nuclear Regulatory Commission

NSAID	Nonsteroidal Anti-Inflammatory Drug
NSF	National Science Foundation
NSR	Nonsignificant Risk
NTP	National Toxicology Program
OAI	Official Action Indicated (serious FDA postinspection classification)
OAM	Office of Alternative Medicine (NIH)
OASH	Office of the Assistant Secretary for Health
OB-GYN	Obstetrics-Gynecology
OC	Office of the Commissioner; Office of Compliance (CDER)
OCD	Office of the Center Director (CDER)
OCPB	Office of Clinical Pharmacology and Biopharmaceutics (CDER)
OCR	Office of Civil Rights
OCR	Optical Character Recognition
OD	Right Eye
ODB	Observational Database
ODE	Office of Drug Evaluation (CDER now has five such offices: ODE I, II, III, IV, and V)
OEA	Office of External Affairs
OEB	Office of Epidemiology and Biostatistics (CDER)
OECD	Organization for Economic Cooperation and Development
OGC	Office of the General Counsel
OGD	Office of Generic Drugs (CDER, formerly DGB)
OGE	Office of Government Ethics (formerly part of Office of Personnel Management, separate executive branch in 1989)
OHA	Office of Health Affairs
OHRM	Office of Human Resource Management
OJC	Office Journal of the EU-C Series (Information)
OJL	Office Journal of the EU-L Series (Legislation)
OLA	Office of Legislative Affairs
OM	Office of Management (CDER)
OMB	Office of Management and Budget (USA)
ONDC	Office of New Drug Chemistry (CDER)
OP	Open (COMIS term); Office of Policy
OPA	Office of Public Affairs
OPD	Orphan Products Division Directorate
OPM	Office of Personnel Management
OPRR	Office of Protection from Research Risks (NIH)
OPS	Office of Pharmaceutical Science (CDER)
ORA	Office of Regulatory Affairs
ORM	Office of Review Management (CDER)
ORO	Office of Regional Operations
OS	Left Eye
OSHA	Occupational Safety Health Administration (USA)

OTA	Office of Technology Assessment (USA; abolished by Congress, Fall 1995)
OTC	Over-the-Counter (refers to nonprescription drugs)
OTCOM	Office of Training and Communications (CDER)
OTR	Office of Testing and Research (CDER)
OU	Both Eyes
P	Priority
PAHO	Pan American Health Organization
PAI	Preapproval Inspection
PAITS	Pre-Approval Inspection Tracking System
PAR	Postapproval Research
PB	Privacy Boards
PC	Personal Computer; Protocol Amendment–Change (COMIS term)
PCC	Parklawn Computer Center; Poison Control Center
PCP	*Pneumocystis carinii* pneumonia
PD	Position Description; Pharmacodynamics
PDA	Parenteral Drug Association
PDQ	Physicians' Data Query (NCI-sponsored cancer trial registry)
PDR	*Physicians' Desk Reference*
PDUFA	Prescription Drug User Fee Act (of 1992, USA)
PEM	Prescription Event Monitoring
PEP	Performance Evaluation Plan
PERI	Pharmaceutical Education & Research Institute, division of PhRMA
PET	Positron Emission Tomography
PFT	Pulmonary Function Tests
PHI	Protected Health Information
PhRMA	Pharmaceutical Research and Manufacturers of America (previously PMA)
PHS	Public Health Service (USA)
PI	Package Insert (approved product labeling)
PI	Principal Investigator
PI	Protocol Amendment–New Investigator (COMIS term)
PK	Pharmacokinetics
PLA	Product License Application (biologics) (UK)
PLA/ELA	Product License Application/Establishment License Application
PM	Project Manager
PMA	Pre-Market Approval Application (FDA); Pharmaceutical Manufacturers Association (now PhRMA) (equivalent to NDA for Class III Devices)
PMCC	Project Management Coordinating Committee (CDER)
PMDIT	Project Management
PMS	Postmarketing Surveillance

PN	Protocol Amendment–New Protocol (or Pending Review) (COMIS term)
PO	Per Os (by mouth)
PPA	Poison Prevention Act
PPI	Patient Package Insert
PPM	Physician Practice Management Organizations
PPO	Preferred Provider Organization; Policy and Procedure Order
PR	Pulse Rate
PR	Public Relations
PRIM&R	Public Responsibility in Medicine and Research (Boston, MA)
PRN	As Needed
PROG	Peer-Review Oversight Group (NIH)
PSUR	Periodic Safety Update Reports
PTCC	Pharmacology/Toxicology Coordinating Committee (CDER)
PUD	Peptic ulcer disease
QA	Quality assurance
QAU	Quality Assurance Unit
QC	Quality control
QD	Once daily
QID	Four times a day
QL	Quality of life
QNS	Quantity not sufficient
QOD	Every other day
QOL	Quality of Life
QSAR	Quantitative SAR
R&D	Research and Development
R&TD	Research and Technological Development
RAC	Reviewer Affairs Committee (CDER)
RADAR	Risk Assessment of Drugs–Analysis and Response
RAPS	Regulatory Affairs Professionals Society
RCC	Research Coordinating Committee (CDER)
RCH	Remove Clinical Hold
RCT	Randomized Clinical Trials
RD	Response to Request for Information (COMIS term)
RDE	Remote Data Entry
RDRC	Radioactive Drug Research Committee
RDT	Rising-Dose Tolerance
RFA	Request for Approval
RIF	Reduction In Force
RKI	Robert-Koch-Institut, Bundesinstitut für Infektionskrankheiten und nich-über tragbare Krankheiten (Federal Institute for Infectious and Non-communicable Diseases, Germany)
RL	Regulatory Letter (FDA postaudit letter)
RMO	Regulatory Management Officer

RTF	Refuse to File, the decision by the FDA to refuse to file an application
RUG	Resource Utilization Group
Rx	Prescription
S	Standard
SAE	Serious Adverse Experience (Event)
SAL	Sterility Assurance Level
SAR	Structure Activity Relationship
SBA	Summary Basis of Approval
SBIR	Small Business Innovative Research Program (USA)
SC	Subcutaneous
SC	Study coordinator. *See also* CCRC, CRC.
SCSO	Supervisory Consumer Safety Officer
SCT	Society for Clinical Trials
SD	Standard deviation
SDAT	Senile dementia of the Alzheimer's type
SE	Standard Error
SEA	Single European Act of 1987
SEER	Surveillance, Epidemiology, and End Results (Registry of NCI)
SES	Senior Executive Service
SIDA	The Spanish (síndrome inmunodeficiencia adquirida), Italian, and French abbreviation for AIDS. *See also AIDS.*
SMART	Submission Management and Review Tracking (FDA)
SMDA	Safe Medical Devices Act (1990)
SME	Significant Medical Event
SMO	Site Management Organization
SmPC	Summary of Product Characteristics
SNDA	Supplemental New Drug Application
SNIP	Syndicat National de l'Industrie Pharmaceutique (France)
SoCRA	Society of Clinical Research Associates
SOMD	Safety of Medicines Department (UK)
SOP	Standard Operating Procedure
SPM	Society of Pharmaceutical Medicine
SQ	Subcutaneous
SRS	Spontaneous Reporting System
SSCT	Swedish Society for Clinical Trials
SSFA	Società di Scienze Farmacologiche Applicate (Italy)
SSM	Skin Surface Microscopy
STD	Sexually Transmitted Disease
STT	Short-Term tests
SUD	Sudden unexpected death
SUPAC	Scale-Up and Postapproval Changes
SVP	Small-Volume Parenterals
SX	Symptoms

TB	Tuberculosis
TGA	Thermographic analysis
TID	Three times a day
TIND	Treatment IND. *See also* IND.
TK	Toxicokinetics
TMO	Trial Management Organization
TOP	Topical
TSH	Thyroid-stimulating hormone
UA	Urinalysis
UKCCR	UK Coordinating Committee on Cancer Research
UNESCO	United Nations Educational Science and Cultural Organization
USAN	US Adopted Names Council
USC	*United States Code* (book of laws)
USCA	U.S. Code Annotated
USDA	United States Department of Agriculture
USP	United States Pharmacopeia
USPC	U.S. Pharmacopeial Convention
USP-DI	United States Pharmacopeia–Drug Information
USP-NF	United States Pharmacopeia–National Formulary
USUHS	Uniformed Services University of the Health Sciences
VA	Veterans Administration (officially, United States Department of Veterans Affairs)
VAERS	Vaccine Adverse Experience (Event) Reporting System
VAI	Voluntary Action Indicated (FDA postaudit inspection classification)
WD	Withdrawn (COMIS term)
WHO	World Health Organization (also used to refer to WHO glossary for coding AEs)
WHOART	World Health Organization Adverse Reaction Terminology
WI	Inactive (COMIS term)
WL	Warning Letter (most serious FDA postaudit letter, demands immediate action within 15 days)
WNL	Within Normal Limits
WRAIR	Walter Reed Army Institute of Research (DoD)
WTO	World Trade Organization

Index